Nutrition Basics

FOR BETTER HEALTH AND PERFORMANCE

THIRD EDITION

LIZ APPLEGATE, PH.D.

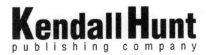

Kendall Hunt
publishing company

Kendall Hunt
publishing company
www.kendallhunt.com
Send all inquiries to:
4050 Westmark Drive
Dubuque, IA 52004-1840

Contents

To students; thank you for your dedication to learning.

Acknowledgments

This third edition of *Nutrition Basics for Better Health and Performance* reflects the new U.S. Dietary Guidelines for Americans published in early 2011 and other new research and updates on the previous edition's text.

Creation of this book took numerous dedicated and supportive individuals who had the vision for its completion and were willing to see to every last detail.

As you look through this text, please note the wonderful illustrations/graphics, much of which was created by Steve Oerding of UC Davis' Mediaworks Information and Education Technology Group. His expert work has given me the opportunity to put concepts and ideas in nutrition to life. What once were mind-boggling concepts have now become enjoyable and understandable for students. Thank you Steve. Thank you too to the Regents of the University of California for giving permission to utilize these illustrations.

I also wish to thank teaching assistants past and present for their help with this text. Marlia Braun and Sandra Samarron gave much time and insight to earlier editions of this book. This year, I looked to teaching assistants Rachel Scherr and Mary Nicole Henderson for guidance on how to clarify this text given their expertise in the Nutrition 10 course. Thank you for your help.

Thanks to the amazing team at Kendall Hunt Publishing who made everything run so smoothly. Editor Beth Klipping and project manager Amanda Smith's organization, guidance and creativity are without parallel.

My family provides a tremendous source of support to me—I'd like to thank my husband Jeff and my children Grant and Natalie.

Lastly, I'd like to thank the thousands of inquisitive and energetic students whom I have had the honor to instruct. With some quick math, I realized that I have taught over 60,000 students during my 30+ year career and these students helped to shape the delivery and course content. They also continue to inspire me to reach for my best as a teacher.

—Liz Applegate, Ph.D., UC Davis, 2016

SPEAKING OF NUTRITION... SOME BASICS

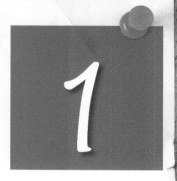

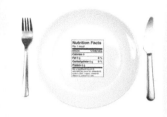

Welcome to the world of nutrition, the study of food and health. Taking this class means you have an interest in your health and fitness. I applaud you for wanting to take charge of your body—learning about what your body needs for optimal health for today and a lifetime. Your food choices impact your performance today as well as set the stage for health and disease prevention later in life.

In this course, you will learn that while many people tend to categorize foods as "good" or "bad," such as carrots and oranges versus burgers and fries, that all foods fit in your diet. Some do provide you with an array of substances better for your health than others, but eating and living well is about making balanced choices. During this course, you will have the opportunity to assess your food choices by completing the Diet Project. As you learn about the roles of protein, fiber, fat, vitamins, and more in your body, you can compare how your diet rates with recommendations for optimal health, and then learn how to best meet your needs through foods and understand where supplements may be an option.

Before we can explore specifics about what's best for you to eat, a few basics must be introduced. So let's get started!

WHAT ARE NUTRIENTS, THEIR BASIC FUNCTIONS, AND HOW MUCH DO YOU NEED (THE RDA)?

How much food do you eat in a year's time? Or, what about the amount of food you may eat over the next four decades? Like many college students, you most likely average about 1 million calories a year or in 45 years almost 70,000 pounds of food. So where is all this food going? What could your body possibly be doing with such a tremendous amount of food energy and material? This food and energy goes into making the "parts" that make you up and help to maintain your "appearance." Every day your body renews itself—making new cells, tissue, hair, and more. In fact, take a look in the mirror. Even though you look the same as you did a year ago (perhaps you may have a new hair color or style, or an ear piercing), you are not the

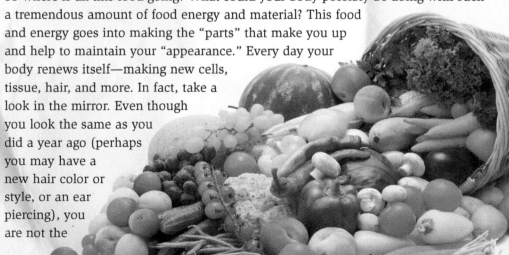

same person. You actually have an entirely new skin surface, newly remodeled bones, and fresh lining to your intestinal tract. In fact:

*   About 1% of your blood cells are new every day.
*   The cells in your intestine renew themselves every three to five days.
*   Your skin is sloughed daily (which is some of the dust in your dorm room or apartment!).
*   You're busy growing new body hair daily.

The food that you eat supplies you with the parts and fuel—nutrients—needed to keep up this type of rebuilding and renewing schedule. Food supplies nutrients that:

*   provide energy
*   serve as building materials
*   help to maintain or repair body parts

There are six categories of nutrients (all totaled there are 50 nutrients):

1. Proteins (made of 20 different subunits)
2. Carbohydrates (simple and complex)
3. Fats (two categories with several types)
4. Minerals (15 plus minerals)
5. Vitamins (13 different ones)
6. Water (a single nutrient in a class by itself)

Foods, such as fruits, vegetables and whole grains, contain other substances that may have biological activity in disease prevention and health promotion. These substances, called **phytochemicals**, of which there are thousands in whole foods, help protect the plants we eat from UV light, insects, and other pests. Once we eat these colorful phytochemicals in carrots, peppers, oranges and the like, these substances promote better health and help protect us from chronic diseases, such as cancer. Scientific studies show that phytochemicals in soybeans called isoflavones help lower risks for certain cancers.

All six categories of nutrients are present in the body but in differing amounts or percent of your body weight as follows:

1. **50–60% water**—males generally have about 60%, and females have 50% due to differences in body fat and muscle content.
2. **15–25% fat**
    *   Desirable levels: 15% for males and 22–25% for females
    *   Body fat levels influence body water content because fat tissue is very low in water content (about 23%) compared to muscle or brain tissue (70%).
    *   As body fat increases, body water decreases; as body fat decreases, body water increases. This explains why most males have a higher percentage of body water than females.
3. **18–20% protein**—males have more than females due to higher lean or muscle mass.
4. **4–5% minerals**—the body's mineral content is primarily in bones and teeth. This varies by gender (males have higher levels than females) and race (blacks have more than whites, who have more than Asians).

Nutrition Bite

Fun fact about your hair—you grow over 350 miles of hair in a lifetime!

Nutrition Bite

Is there a best body fat level for athletes?

Here are some numbers for body fat in collegiate athletes (see Figure 1.1). And as you'll see in Chapter 7, there is not a perfect or ideal body fat level that depicts optimal health but rather there are ranges.

PERCENT BODY FAT VALUES IN ATHLETES		
	MALES	**FEMALES**
Basketball	7–12	18–27
Distance Running	3–8	8–18
Gymnastics	7–12	16–22
Soccer	4–10	14–25
Swimming	5–12	10–20
Tennis	12–16	15–22
Nonathlete, avg.	15–16.9	20–26.9

Figure 1.1

5. **Less than 1% carbohydrates**—storage of carbohydrates in the muscles and liver is vital for fuel during exercise and rest (especially for the brain).
6. **Less than 1% vitamins**—very trace amounts exist in each cell.

Foods, as well as the body, contain all six categories of nutrients in varying amounts. Must you eat all 50 nutrients or only some?

Essential nutrients are those nutrients that the body cannot make or cannot make at a rate sufficient to meet your needs. Therefore, the diet requires them. For example, calcium is a mineral that originates in soil (rocks), gets into plants that cows eat, and then gets into milk, and eventually gets into our bodies. We are incapable of making calcium, so we must get it from the food we eat.

On the other hand, water is made every day in our bodies as we metabolize food for energy. However, we only make about a cup each day, which falls short of the several cups we need. Therefore, water is essential in the diet.

How Do Nutrients Function in the Body?

1. **Energy**—Only proteins, carbohydrates, and fats (the macronutrients) contain potential energy. Elements, primarily carbon, are connected to each other via chemical bonds that are much like tiny stretched rubber bands. When let go, the energy is released. The energy released from chemical bonds is measured as calories. (We'll learn more about this in Chapter 3.)
2. **Structure**—Nutrients, such as protein and calcium, are the building material and structure for bone and teeth.
3. **Regulation**—As regulators, nutrients help manage and oversee many processes in the body such as building new hormones, regulating fluid balance, or catalyzing a reaction such as enzymes, which are made of protein. Regulatory nutrients are much like traffic lights that help regulate the flow of vehicles on busy streets.

How Do We Express Our Nutrient Needs or Requirements?

The amount of protein, Vitamin C or other nutrients a person needs depends on a host of factors including:

- Gender
- Age
- Physiological state (e.g., pregnant or breastfeeding)
- Illness
- Genetics traits

While we all need the same nutrients, the amounts vary depending on these and other factors. Setting nutrient standards is the task of an arm of the government—the Food and Nutrition Board. Health professionals and others call these standards **Dietary Reference Intakes (DRI)** (see Figure 1.2) and use them in establishing nutrient intakes for planning and assessing the diets of healthy individuals.

These nutrient requirements are designed to prevent deficiency diseases, such as scurvy from too little Vitamin C or rickets (a bone deformity) due to too little calcium and Vitamin D. The DRIs are also designed to promote optimal health and the reduction of chronic disease risks, such as cancer, potentially from a marginal intake of Vitamins C, D, and calcium.

Under the umbrella term of DRI, there are four separate nutrient standard values of which the Recommended Dietary Allowance (RDA) is one.

In addition, the DRIs are designed to set an upper limit of intake to avoid the risk of adverse reaction due to overdose.

You are probably familiar with or at least heard of this term before. In this course, we will make reference to the RDA, what it means, how the RDA for a given nutrient is determined, and how best to meet your needs. While the other nutrient standard values are important in the world of nutrition, in this course we will not utilize these except for making reference to the Tolerable Upper Intake Level or UL. This standard represents the highest level of daily nutrient intake that is likely to be safe and not pose any adverse health effects to most people in the population. But

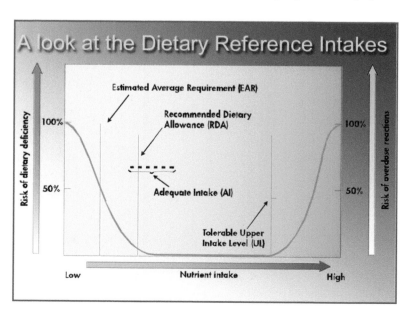

Figure 1.2

dietary or supplement intake exceeding the UL for a certain nutrient, such as iron, may present some health problems. As we will cover in the topic of supplements in Chapter 9, not only can we get too little of a nutrient, but excessive intake through foods that are fortified with nutrients, such as vitamins as well as supplements, pose health risks.

A Closer Look at the RDA

The RDA is the daily amount of nutrient considered adequate to meet the needs of nearly all healthy people in the population (about 98% of us), while decreasing risk of chronic diseases. The RDA is NOT a minimum amount nor is it an average need but instead a generous value. And the RDA is set based on scientific information.

- The RDA has been determined for protein and other nutrients (vitamins, minerals, etc.).
- The RDA is established for several age groups, gender, and physiological states (pregnancy and lactation).
- The RDA is designed to be an average over several days. (In other words, you don't have to meet the RDA each day, but instead averaged it over several.)
- Adjustments are made when setting the RDA based upon several factors that we will highlight as each nutrient is covered, such as the quality of the diet (as in protein covered in Chapter 2), bioavailability (as with minerals covered in Chapter 8), and losses due to food preparation (as with vitamins covered in Chapter 9).

You will not need to memorize each RDA (except for protein) but instead know what goes into setting the RDA and what it means to you.

HOW DOES YOUR BODY COPE?

Ever wonder why you still function even though you haven't eaten all day, or why your body's internal temperature hovers around 37 degrees Celsius or 98.6 degrees Fahrenheit despite freezing or scorching temperatures outside?

The reason is actually more of a concept or process called **homeostasis**. This is the maintenance of relatively constant internal conditions (such as body temperature and blood sugar levels) through the efforts and control of many systems in the body.

The concept of homeostasis will be emphasized throughout this course to help us predict as well as understand why our bodies respond and perform the way they do. For example, once you grasp the concept of homeostasis, you will soon understand why taking large amounts of a particular supplement such as vitamins or amino acids (components of protein) will not drastically change or alter the way your body or cells work so as not to upset other systems in your body.

Let's use the example of body water content to help understand homeostasis as well as learn more about the nutrient water. Recall that about 50% to 60% of your body weight is water. Figure 1.3 depicts the fluid inside and outside the body cells; the distribution of body water is determined and controlled by several factors such as hormones, the action of the kidneys, and the mineral and protein levels in body fluids.

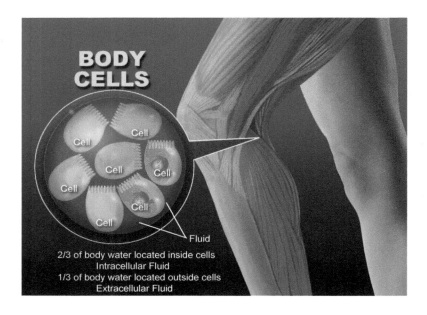

Figure 1.3

Your body water content as fluid homeostasis is regulated well. On average a typical person takes in about 2 ½ liters of fluid daily and loses the same (see Figure 1.4).

On your final, you will be asked to define homeostasis and give an example of a nutrient under homeostatic control. By the end of the course, you'll surely have many ideas for your answer.

INSIDE WORK—THE PROCESS OF DIGESTION AND ABSORPTION

How do we process food and prepare it to enter our bodies? Our bodies accomplish this task through the process of digestion and absorption. **Digestion** is the process by which food is broken down into a form that can be absorbed by the intestines. **Absorption** is the process of moving nutrients into the body or bloodstream. Digestion occurs in the digestive tract, which begins at the mouth and is 26 feet long. Visualize the digestive tract as "outside" your body; that is, the digestive tract is a

Nutrition Bite

The surface area of your intestinal tract would cover about a third of a football field.

FLUID BALANCE			
INTAKE:		**OUTPUT:**	
Fluid	1.2 liters	Urine	1.5 liters
Food	1.0 liters	Stool	0.1 liters
Metabolic	0.3 liters	Sweat and breath vapor	0.9 liters
	2.5 liters		2.5 liters

Figure 1.4

tube that runs through your body, but the contents (if you swallow a golf ball, for example) are not really inside of you. Absorption only occurs when the food (its components) is transported from the small intestine into the circulation.

Figure 1.5 illustrates the digestive tract (with each part identified) along with some of the accessory organs, collectively called the digestive system.

There are two phases of digestion.

1. **Physical digestion:** the moving and grinding of food. This starts in the mouth with chewing, though you do not have to chew your food (despite that mom told you to chew your food well before swallowing) to completely digest your food. Once you have chewed (or just swallowed) your food, the bolus (swallowed food) moves down your esophagus into the stomach where it is "blenderized." The stomach, which has a 4-cup capacity, is much like a blender (strong muscles) that makes a smoothie out of your swallowed food.

2. **Chemical digestion:** the chemical breakdown of food through the use of digestive enzymes (actual breaking of chemical bonds in foods and stomach acid). This process starts in the stomach with a majority occurring in the small intestine. The digestive enzymes needed to break these bonds are secreted by the pancreas into the small intestine. Once the process of chemical digestion is complete, the food has been digested and the process of absorption occurs.

Absorption is the process of taking these small food fragments from the small intestine and transporting them into the blood. The surface of the small intestine is where absorption occurs. The surface of the small intestine, as shown in Figure 1.6, is designed for maximum surface area. The folds, the folds on these folds called villi, and then hair-like structures on villi called microvilli all contribute to a tremendously large surface area that allows the nutrients an opportunity to be taken up into the body and eventually into the circulation. Figure 1.7 illustrates villi and microvilli structures and the placement of capillaries that allow for transport of absorbed small food units into the body via the circulation.

Urban Myth

Myth: "We should eat food, such as fruit, separately because our digestive tracts can't handle different foods at once."

The design of our digestive enzymes and intestinal tract allows for the processing of different food types, such as fruits, meats and vegetables, all at once. In fact, nutrient absorption improves when a variety of foods are present. There is no need to separate foods when eating.

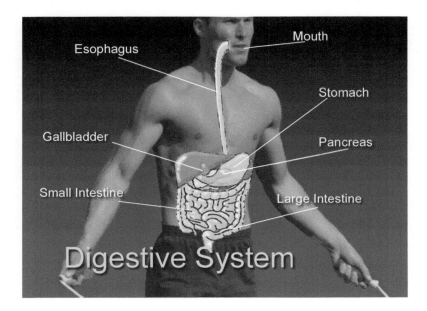

Figure 1.5

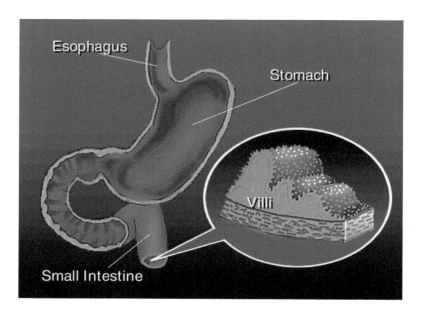

Figure 1.6

However, some food is not digested and absorbed. These items, such as fiber (or if you happened to swallow a food wrapper), move into the large intestine where the body extracts water and minerals, and prepares the remnants as stool. The stool then represents material that never got into the body in the first place, but only passed through the digestive tract. You might have wondered what urine represents. This metabolic waste represents substances, such as excess sodium that the body (kidneys) have filtered from the cells, blood, and elsewhere, and sends out in the urine.

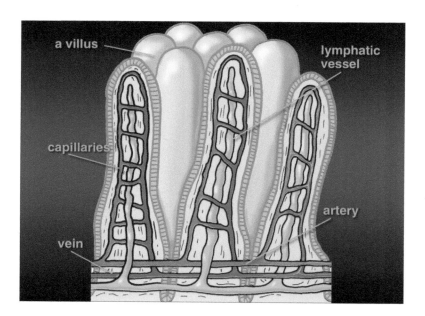

Figure 1.7

Quiz Yourself

1. Most of the enzymes responsible for the digestion of the energy nutrients come from the:

    a. mouth

    b. stomach

    c. liver

    d. pancreas

2. What is the approximate average body water content of a young adult human expressed as a percent of body weight?

    a. 10–20%

    b. 30–40%

    c. 50–60%

    d. 70–80%

    e. 90%

3. List the six classes of nutrients, give a food source example and note which ones provide energy.

    1. _____

    2. _____

    3. _____

    4. _____

    5. _____

    6. _____

4. What are the three basic functions of nutrients?

    1. _____

    2. _____

    3. _____

5. Most of the body's water occurs in extracellular fluid compartments (outside of the body cells.

    a. true

    b. false

6. Define an essential nutrient.

_____

_____

_____

_____

Give an example of an essential nutrient:

_____

7. Define the Recommended Dietary Allowance (RDA) and list three factors that are taken into consideration when establishing the RDA.

_____

_____

_____

_____

1. _____

2. _____

3. _____

8. Define digestion and describe the two types of digestion.

_____

_____

_____

_____

9. What is absorption and where does it occur?

_____

_____

_____

_____

PROTEIN—THE VERSATILE NUTRIENT

No doubt you have good feelings about protein—usually thoughts of muscle strength and good health come to mind with protein. For millions of dieters, high-protein diets have become a way of life in an effort to shed unwanted pounds. In this chapter on protein, you will discover how vital this nutrient is for an array of duties in the body including immune health, muscle strength, and recovery along with the truth about high-protein diets as a means to lose weight.

UNDERSTANDING PROTEIN STRUCTURE AND FUNCTION

The word *protein* means "primary." Early scientists of the 1700s and 1800s knew that a source of protein was vital for life. In those early days of nutrition, scientists believed that there was one single substance "protein" and that this substance contained the element nitrogen. These early researchers also knew that the element nitrogen was in the air that both humans and animals breathe but that a dietary source of nitrogen (thus protein) was vital for life. During this time, scientists also knew that nitrogen was unique to protein.

By the 1900s, scientists discovered that rather than one single substance, there were many, even thousands of different proteins, all of which contained the element nitrogen. Different proteins were discovered in the human body, such as proteins in the blood and protein in hair, while other unique proteins were discovered in foods such as in eggs and beef. How did all of these proteins differ from each other? A look at protein structure will explain these differences along with

Chapter Objectives

In this chapter, we will cover four major areas regarding protein:

- How protein structure makes each protein different from the other and affects their function.
- How the body processes protein and its building blocks—the amino acids.

- The consequence of protein deficiency—how much protein you need and the impact of exercise and other factors on protein requirements (along with whether protein supplements are needed).
- How to meet protein needs and make healthful food choices (meat vs. vegetarian diets).

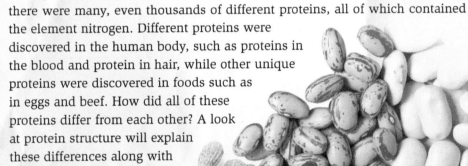

getting us on our way to understanding why we need protein, how much we need, and how best to meet that need.

Chemical Structure of Protein

We will use two examples in discussing the chemical structure of protein: a protein in food that you might eat, such as beef, and a protein found in your body, such as a blood protein. Figure 2.1 shows these two proteins.

- Notice that each protein exists as a three-dimensional shape, much like a rope folded up in a specific way. This 3-D shape is different for each protein, whether in food or in the body, and as we will learn, the shape of each different protein is designed to suit that protein's function (such as carrying a vitamin in the blood, which is why this protein has an opening or dish-like shape).
- If we snipped a piece from each of these 3-D structures, upon close inspection, we would find that rather than a rope, the protein is made up of a chain of linked subunits—hundreds of them.
- These subunits are called amino acids, as shown in Figure 2.2. There are 20 different amino acids reflected in Figure 2.2 as different colors and numbers. Amino acids are linked together by peptide bonds.

Amino Acid Structure

Now let's take a look at what makes up an amino acid, and very importantly, how amino acids differ from one another.

Elements that make up amino acids (and other nutrients) follow certain rules when it comes to making chemical bonds. The four elements that make up amino acids are: carbon (C) with four bonds, oxygen (O) with two bonds, hydrogen (H) with one bond, and nitrogen (N) with three bonds. In Figure 2.3 illustrating a generic amino acid, the amino group (N) and the acid group (i.e., COOH group) are identified. Every amino acid has both of these chemical groups.

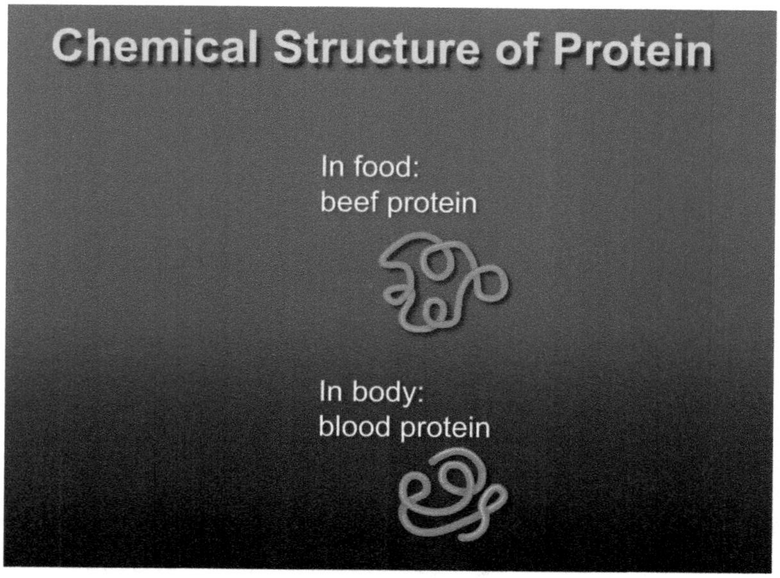

Nutrition Bite

You may come across the term *peptides* when looking at protein supplements available on the Internet or in a store. This term is used to describe a few amino acids joined together. Peptides are essentially small fragments of a protein, and offer nothing special over eating proteins whole from foods.

Chemical Structure of Protein

In food:
beef protein

In body:
blood protein

Figure 2.1

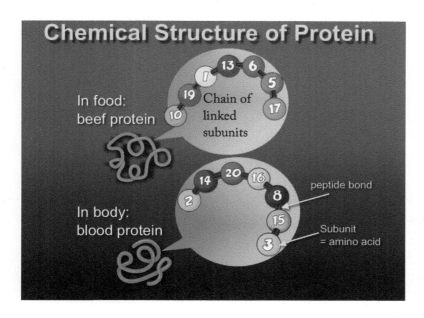

Figure 2.2

The R group pictured over the middle carbon represents a chemical group (rather than an element with the abbreviation "R"). There are 20 different R groups—20 different chemical groups. This means there are 20 different amino acids, each with their own name. A few examples are shown in Figure 2.4.

- Many of the amino acid names sound the same and often end in "ine." In this course, we won't worry about their names, but instead will differentiate between amino acids by referring to them with the numbers 1 through 20 as shown in Figures 2.2 and 2.5.
- Each R group has specific chemical properties. Some R groups may like to interact with a watery environment, while others might be attracted to other R groups. This is very important when it comes to a protein's 3-D structure and function.

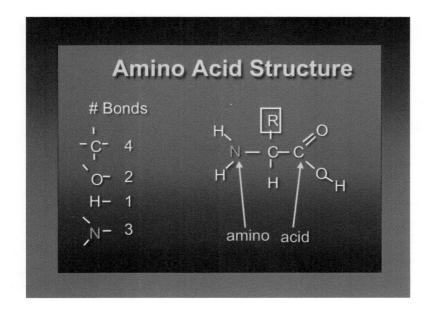

Figure 2.3

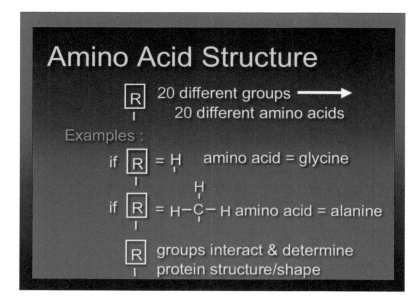

Figure 2.4

- Upon inspection of one protein (beef) compared to another (blood), we notice that the sequence or order of amino acids differ, as shown in Figure 2.5. This in turn determines how a protein is shaped. R groups interact with other R groups down the chain and fold up depending upon the sequence of amino acids in the protein chain.
- In the beef protein example, note the sequence of amino acids. Amino acid #10 interacts with amino acid #17. This interaction causes the chain to fold, creating the loop on the right. This R group interaction dictates how the protein folds. Because each protein has a unique sequence of amino acids, this makes the shape or structure of the protein unique.
- How was the amino acid sequence determined for a specific protein? We will discuss this more in another section, but each cell in animals and in plants comes equipped with a set of instructions (genetic material) that determines

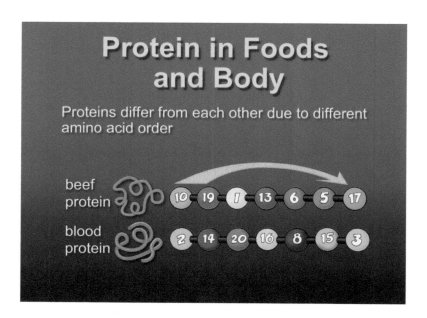

Figure 2.5

what proteins each cell type will make. So in a cow's muscle cells, the genetic material instructs a contractile protein to be made with a unique amino acid sequence that differs from that of a blood protein made by the liver. We in turn eat this protein when we eat beef (among many other types of proteins found in beef).

Amino Acid–Protein Analogy

Let's use an analogy—letters of our alphabet spelling words to help clarify how amino acids' sequence determines shape and shape determines function of a protein.

- Amino acid order is like spelling a word (the order of letters).
- Folding of the amino acid chain into a 3-D shape (structure) is like the pronunciation of that word (since the letters in that order follow phonetic rules).
- The protein function is like the meaning of the word.

Use this example of seven letters shown in Figure 2.6 and you can see how letter sequence is vital to the word meaning just like amino acid order is vital to protein shape and structure.

- Just as words can have more than one of the same letter, such as the words "pepper" or "school," proteins also can have duplicate (or more) of a given amino acid. Also, proteins vary from one another in the profile or amounts of each of the 20 amino acids.

Amino Acids—Are They All Essential or Just Certain Ones?

- Of the 20 different amino acids, nine are essential. This means these specific amino acids can't be made in the body and must come from foods that contain those nine essential amino acids in the food's protein. These amino acids are referred to as the essential amino acids or EAA for short. The reason is primarily because the R group on these nine essential amino acids can't be made by our metabolic machinery.

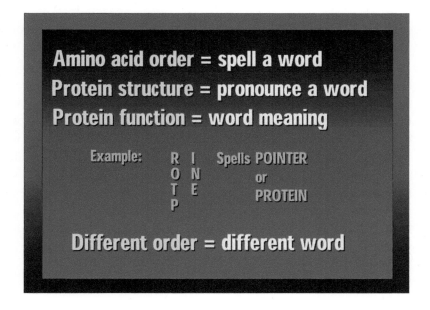

Figure 2.6

- The other 11 amino acids are called nonessential amino acids or NEAA for short. These do not need to be in your diet since you have the ability to make the NEAA from other components in your diet (carbon from fat or carbohydrate, for example). But you do need a source of nitrogen in your diet to build a NEAA. Remember those early scientists proved that protein supplied this element.

This brings us to two important reasons why protein is needed in our diet:

- A source of EAA
- A source of nitrogen (needed to make NEAA)

Function of Protein

Recall the three basic functions of nutrients: structure, energy, and regulation. Protein is a versatile nutrient and performs all three.

1. **Structure**
   - Bone: minerals, calcium, and phosphorous intertwine with a protein, honeycomb-like structure that forms bone.
   - Connective tissue: a structural protein called collagen acts much like glue that holds us together—literally keeping teeth in the gums, blood vessels intact and joints held together. Collagen makes up about 25% of the protein in the body making this structural protein of great significance. (Collagen will be discussed in Chapter 11 when vitamin C is covered, because this vitamin is needed for the formation of healthy collagen.)
2. **Energy**
   - Protein (specifically food protein) possesses potential energy in its chemical bonds. This energy is released in the form of heat or calories (more in Chapter 3) and this energy can be used by the body.
   - There is no storage of protein or amino acids. This means that all protein in the body is actively working. So using functional tissue for a source of energy means that protein from tissue loses its ability to do its job as that protein. This contrasts with fat and carbohydrate, which are stored as fuel reserves.
3. **Regulation** Thousands of proteins perform regulatory roles in your body from building a new strand of hair to helping your cells regulate water level. Here are a few examples of protein in a regulatory role:
   - **Hormones:** Some hormones are made of protein, but not all. Insulin, a hormone made by the pancreas, is involved in carbohydrate homeostasis.
   - **Enzymes:** All enzymes are made of protein and these are chemical catalysts that facilitate or allow a reaction in the body to occur. For example, to build a new muscle protein, an enzyme is needed to bring together the amino acid building blocks and form the muscle protein.
   - **Immune system:** Specialized cells that fight off infection are built with protein.
   - **Fluid balance:** Special proteins in the blood and inside cells keep the fluid balance at the delicate one third outside of cells and two thirds inside of cells.

Think about these important regulatory roles for our discussion of protein deficiency. Would fluid balance be maintained or would an infection be a risk for a person not getting enough protein?

PROCESSING PROTEIN IN THE BODY

Now let's take a look at how your body processes protein from its digestion to its use inside cells for protein synthesis. Follow what happens to a sample meal, consisting of a glass of soy milk and a turkey sandwich, as these food proteins are digested.

Protein Digestion

The proteins pictured at the top of Figure 2.7 (representing the mouth and throat) are from the soy milk and from the turkey sandwich (though there are other proteins in these foods). These proteins have different 3-D shapes (different proteins) and thus different amounts of each of the 20 amino acids.

- The physical digestion of protein begins in the mouth with chewing the food and mixing it with saliva. But, there's actually no need to chew your food at all or for a certain number of times (maybe your mom told you to chew your food seven times before swallowing). The rest of your digestive track can handle unchewed food although swallowing slightly chewed food is more comfortable.
- Once swallowed, the soy milk and turkey sandwich travel down your esophagus and land in your stomach for the remainder of physical digestion. Here in the stomach, the food is "blenderized" much like a smoothie. Also, special cells in the stomach secrete acid, and this mixes with your soymilk-turkey smoothie (see Figure 2.8).

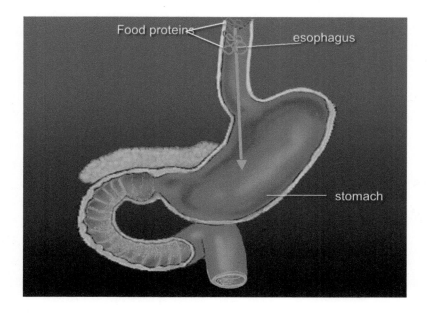

Figure 2.7

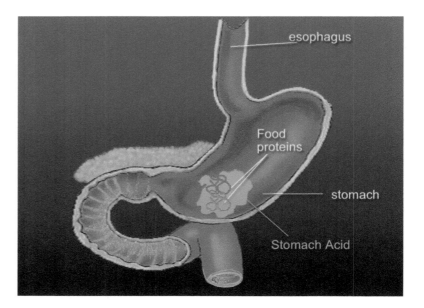

Figure 2.8

- The acid disrupts the R groups of the amino acids in the strand of protein. This causes the protein structure to denature, or unfold, as shown in Figure 2.9. This is the beginning of chemical digestion for protein.
- These unfolded strands of protein then move into the small intestine where a digestive enzyme from the pancreas is secreted to complete chemical digestion (Figure 2.10). This enzyme, protease (hint: "prot" = protein; "-ase" = enzyme), chemically breaks the peptide bonds releasing individual amino acids into the small intestinal space, as shown in Figure 2.11.
- Both EAA and NEAA are present, thousands and thousands of each. The intestinal tract cannot tell which amino acid came from which food.

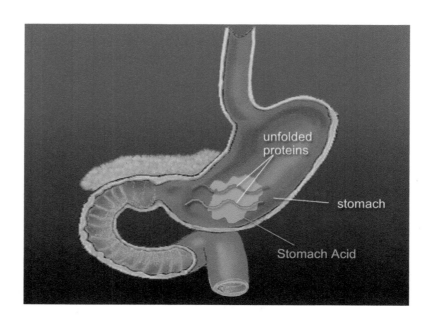

Figure 2.9

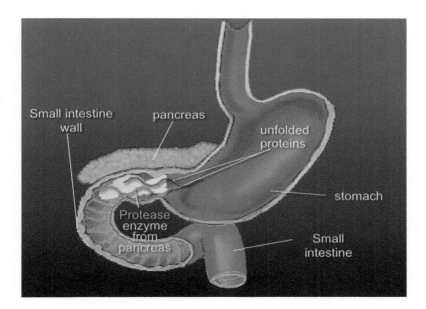

Figure 2.10

- Additionally, intestinal tract cells are sloughing off and being digested along with the food. The proteins from these cells are also digested in the same way (see Figure 2.11).
- **The end product of protein digestion is individual amino acids from food and from digested intestinal tract cell protein.** These individual amino acids are absorbed through the wall of the small intestine (see Figure 2.12).

Now let's take a look at how your body uses these absorbed amino acids.

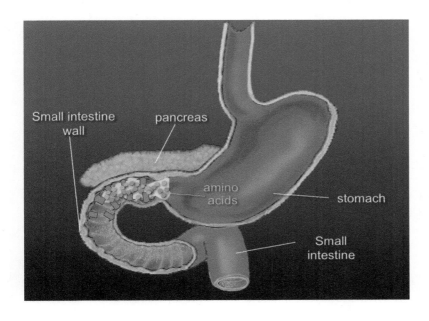

Figure 2.11

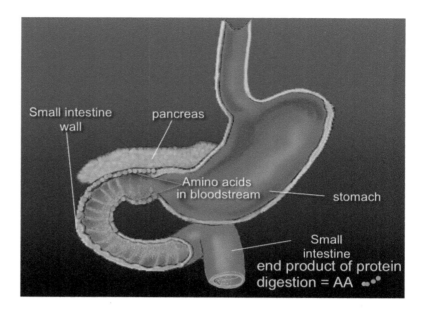

Figure 2.12

How the Body Uses Protein

After the meal of soy milk and a turkey sandwich is digested in amino acids and assimilated (absorbed), these new amino acids are now surging through your blood vessels heading off to muscle cells, liver cells, and even eye ball cells for use.

Figure 2.13 shows a generic body cell along with a few crucial parts of the cell. The DNA is the set of instructions that are "read," dictating what proteins are made. The process of the protein synthesis from amino acids occurs in the endoplasmic reticulum (E.R.). Use figures 2.14 to 2.17 to follow how each cell uses amino acids.

- Inside a body cell (such as liver or muscle cell), consider the mix of EAA and NEAA as a "bucket" of amino acids. Based upon the set of instructions that a specific cell has (for example, a muscle cell has instructions to make contractile protein and a liver cell may have instructions to build a fluid–balance protein),

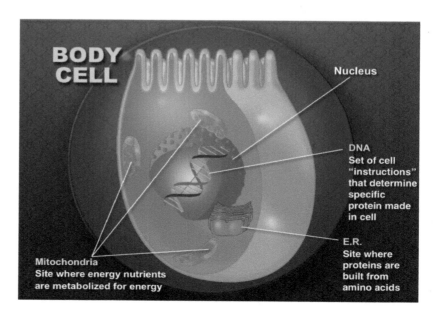

Figure 2.13

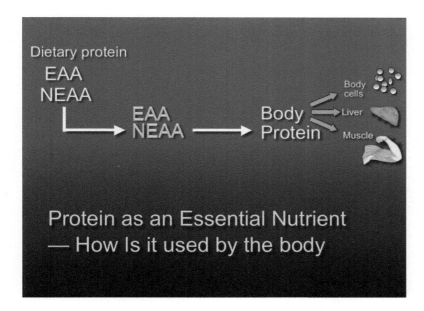

Figure 2.14

the cell pulls the amino acids needed to build the proteins it is instructed to make out of the "bucket." The cell will make only what it is instructed to make (i.e., type of protein) and only in the amount needed. This means that even if the bucket is "overflowing" (loads of amino acids because of extra protein in the diet), only the amount of protein needed will be made. (Remember homeostasis?)

- Also, the right profile or proportion of amino acids must be present in the "bucket" to make the protein. If a particular NEAA is missing from the bucket, the cell has the ability to make that amino acid if given a source of nitrogen, which would come from other amino acids. If a particular EAA is missing, the protein will not be made. A substitution with another amino acid in the chain would mean that the strand of amino acids would fold up differently due to the R groups and thus the structure and function would be different. Back to the alphabet–amino acid analogy—putting the wrong amino acid in would be like creating a typo instead of a word.

- Take another look at Figure 2.14. The amino acids are made into a protein, and then they break down again. Amino acids ⇆ protein implies that proteins are being made, and then broken down again to their building block components, and then made into other proteins again, and so on. Why would the cell do this? It seems like a waste of energy.

The process of **protein turnover** (see Figure 2.15) is a very good thing because it allows us (our bodies) to make more of a protein that we might need immediately and less of another protein that is not quite crucial at the time. Here are some examples.

- If you were to swallow a rock or sharp object with your food and damaged your intestinal tract, it's nice to know the damage would be repaired in about three to five days since this area does turnover quickly. If you didn't repair yourself in a timely fashion, then your intestinal tract damage may impair your ability to digest and absorb food and subsequently get the nutrients you need to stay healthy.

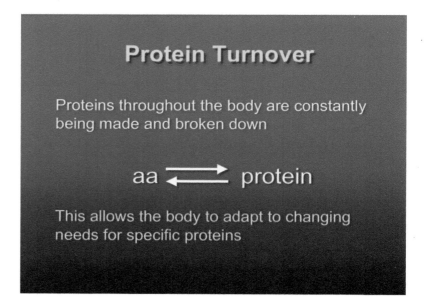

Figure 2.15

- If you get sick with a serious illness, such as chicken pox, you would want your body's immune system to rise to the occasion and kick the virus, rather than just produce a set number of immune fighters that may not be designed to fight this specific infection. In the meantime, your body can make less of other proteins such as the enzymes that break down alcohol. You probably won't be drinking much when you are sick!

The rates at which some proteins turnover are shown in Figure 2.16. Make note of the high turnover proteins which are affected more dramatically than slow turnover proteins during protein deficiency. Which condition—intestinal trouble versus brain damage—would a person more likely recover from once adequate protein was consumed?

- Not all proteins turn over; some are lost to the body. These are known as the "dead-end" proteins because the body doesn't get them back after they are

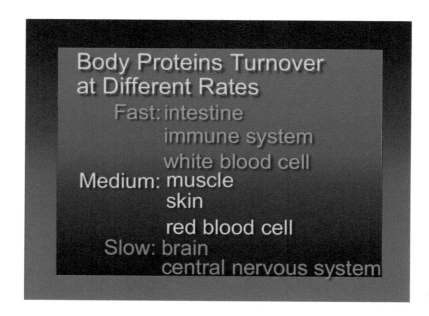

Figure 2.16

made. These include the proteins in hair, skin, nails, and stool (from unab-sorbed dietary protein and sloughed-off intestinal cells). Think of these dead-end protein losses as a hole in the bottom of a water tank, where water leaks out steadily. The water must be replaced to keep the fill line constant. In your body, dietary protein must be consumed to replace these dead-end protein losses.

- Let's now complete the diagram by adding Figure 2.16 and look at what happens with amino acids when we have an excess amount—in other words, our "bucket" is overflowing. We've already established that with excess amino acids, more proteins are NOT made. So what happens to the excess?

As shown in Figure 2.17, the nitrogen is stripped off the amino acid, leaving what is called a "carbon skeleton." So now we have two items to track: **nitrogen** and **carbon skeleton**.

Nitrogen: The option is there, as the arrow indicates, that the nitrogen could be used to make a nonessential amino acid. But since amino acids are in abundance, the need to do this is unlikely. Instead, the nitrogen must be removed because it is a toxic substance that the body wants to get rid of soon. In the kidneys, the nitrogen is transformed into a substance called urea, which is then excreted in the urine. It costs calories to perform this process, but the body is willing to put in the extra cost since nitrogen is a toxic substance. So, if you have consumed more protein than what you need, you will excrete the excess nitrogen in your urine.

It's important to point out that you always have some nitrogen (urea) in your urine at all times, not just if you are consuming extra protein. This is because at any given moment in time, a cell is pulling the nitrogen off to use the carbon skeleton to make another amino acid or some other substance.

Carbon skeleton: This "skeleton" of an amino acid contains potential energy in the chemical bonds. This energy can be utilized immediately, that is, broken down with the chemical bonds being broken and heat released—your body can extract about 4 calories for every gram of amino acids/protein (more on this in Chapter 3). But what if you weren't in need of immediate energy? This potential energy in the carbon skeleton does not go to waste. Instead, with a bit of chemical magic, the carbons are rearranged into fat. This means that **amino acids or protein**

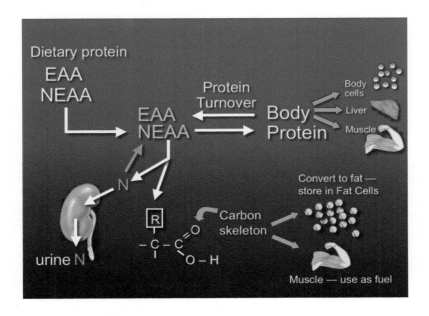

Figure 2.17

eaten in excess of need can be converted to and stored as fat. Since most Americans exceed their protein needs (our "bucket" is overflowing) and many don't exercise or expend enough calories, the carbon skeletons often end up being converted to fat (remember, the nitrogen goes to the urine).

Does Taking an Amino Acid Supplement Make a Difference?

With what you've just learned about amino acids, their use by the body and how your cells treat excess amino acids, let's take a look at adding more to the mix. Many people take an amino acid supplement in hopes of improved muscle weight gain, or perhaps another benefit touted on the supplement label. Now that you know how amino acid metabolism works, you can decide whether an extra amount of one or more amino acids will make a difference in protein synthesis.

Refer to Figure 2.18. If a person takes an amino acid supplement, eaa_3 for example, this ends up in the "bucket." The amount in supplements is quite small, and the extra will go virtually unnoticed. But more importantly, will extra of an amino acid increase the amount of protein being made? No extra protein will be made for two reasons. First, extra of one amino acid does not mean more of an entire protein will be made (similar to saying you could spell more words if you have more of the letter "e"). And second, the body is programmed to make a certain amount of each protein (remember homeostasis?) so no extra will be made. Now what do you think—is taking this supplement of amino acids helpful?

Key Concepts about Protein

It's time to pull a few items together to make sure we have a good understanding about key protein concepts.

- Each protein has a unique order or sequence of amino acids.

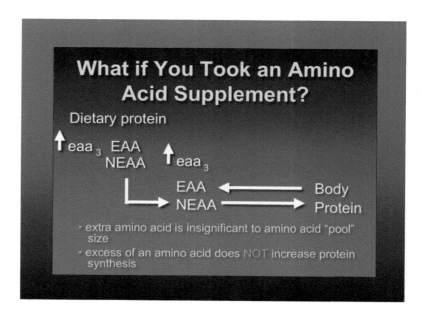

Figure 2.18

- There are 20 amino acids. Nine amino acids are essential, and all 20 are found in your body proteins and food proteins. Each protein has different proportions and sequences of each of the 20 different amino acids.
- Proteins in the body turn over.
- There is no storage of protein or amino acids in the body.

PROTEIN DEFICIENCY AND REQUIREMENT

In this section, we'll take a look at what happens when too little protein (or insufficient EAA) is consumed as well as how much protein is required and what factors, such as exercise or severe illness, impact protein needs.

Protein Deficiency

Before we can discuss protein deficiency, we need to review a few things about growth stages. Intuitively, you might agree that protein deficiency in a young child would have a different impact, more severe, compared to an older child or an adult. This has to do with the impact of growth on protein needs.

Stages of Growth

The first stage of growth occurs during fetal development up to the first 18 to 24 months of life. Growth during this stage is accomplished by an increase in the number of cells in an organ and tissue. For example, the brain increases in size due to an increase in cell number, as shown in Figure 2.19, therefore, nutritional status is very important at this stage in life. Inadequate intake of protein or other nutrients such as vitamins can lead to permanent damage or stunted growth (permanently reduced height and stature).

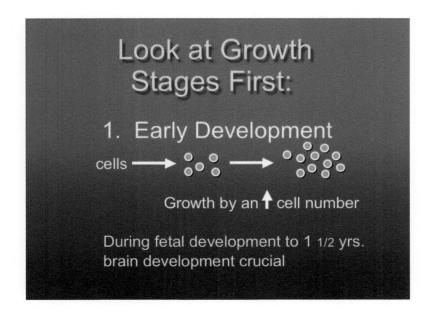

Figure 2.19

During this later stage of development pictured in Figure 2.20, growth occurs mostly by an increase in cell size. This stage occurs in children and teens, while there is still some increase in cell number during these years. The results of a nutritional deficiency at this stage is not as devastating if proper nutrition is provided soon.

Consequence of Protein Deficiency

High turnover proteins (recall those with a high turnover rate) will be affected most dramatically with protein deficiency. These high turnover proteins rely on a constant supply of amino acids.

Protein deficiency during early development results in:

- developmental delays
- reduced growth or stunting (permanent)

In young children, teens, and adults protein deficiency results in:

- **Edema**—retention of fluid, giving a puffy swollen appearance. Proteins involved in fluid balance are not being made, so that fluid leaves the inside of cells and moves to the extracellular space giving a swollen appearance.
- **Intestinal problems**—diarrhea and poor absorption of nutrients. Without sufficient protein, the individual cannot keep up with the rapid turnover of intestinal cells (every three to five days). The intestinal tract surface becomes smooth, and with the reduced surface area, nutrients are not absorbed so diarrhea results as water is drawn into the intestinal tract.
- **Distended abdomen**—fatty liver and fluid retention cause the belly to protrude. Fluid buildup in the abdominal cavity causes a distended abdomen. Also, the liver is unable to make proteins necessary to package up fats and send them out into the bloodstream. The liver then builds up with fat and enlarges. This is seen in alcoholics because of a poor diet and alcohol interferes with liver function (more on this in Chapter 10).

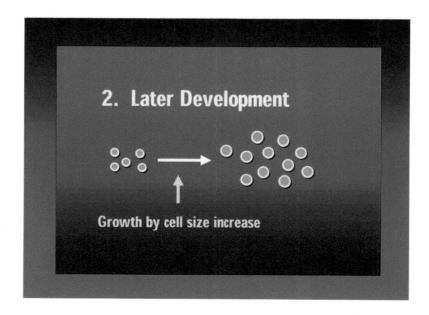

Figure 2.20

- **Infections**—eye, lung, and skin infections develop due to reduced immune response. Without adequate protein, the immune system becomes weak and invading bacteria and viruses take hold. Often, people with protein deficiency succumb to these infections.

  Conditions seen with protein deficiency:

- **Kwashiorkor**—this means "the evil spirit that infects the first child after the second child is born." This condition occurs in young children (usually in underdeveloped countries) that are weaned from breast milk at about 6 to 9 months of age when the mom becomes pregnant with a second child. The weaning food given to this first child is generally low in protein and the child becomes very sick by the time the second child is born. Often this first child has edema, which then progresses to an emaciated look.
- **Protein-calorie malnutrition**—severe wasting of muscle and fat as the person is starved for total food or energy. The body breaks itself down and muscle wasting appears.

Protein Requirement

The time has come to figure out your protein requirement. This method is going to involve just a bit of math in a three-step process. In the end, you will know your RDA for protein.

  Why do you need protein?

- source of essential amino acids
- source of nitrogen (to make NEAA)

  Three-step process to compute the RDA for protein:

1. Compute the minimum amount of protein needed for an average person.
2. Adjust this figure to account for population variability.
3. Adjust this figure for quality of protein in the diet.

STEP 1

Start with an average adult, male or a female (who is not pregnant or lactating because these factors would alter protein needs), weighing 70 kg (about 155 pounds). How much protein does this person need every day?

  Recall that the body is like a tank with a leak of water—how much water do we need to put in to cover water losses? Now think of our body and the protein we lose every day—hair, skin, nails, urine, and stool. These losses could be collected (very tedious) and used to calculate how much minimum protein is needed to cover daily losses. The amount of nitrogen in these items is measured since nitrogen is unique to protein—nitrogen is our marker for protein.

Nitrogen Losses Reflect Protein Needs

This average male or female loses nitrogen daily that we can measure—let's say that it is 5 grams daily. This value must be converted to grams of protein per day (and this would represent the "leak" in the tank). To do this, we are going to make a conversion of grams of nitrogen to grams of protein. We will use a factor of 6.25 grams of protein for every gram of nitrogen. (This factor comes from the fact that 16% of the weight for all proteins is nitrogen. So 100 grams of protein has 16 grams of nitrogen or divide 100 by 16 and you get 6.25 grams protein/gram nitrogen. *Note:* This is only a conversion factor and has nothing to do with your RDA for protein!)

For Our Average Male and Female

$$5 \text{ grams nitrogen} \times \frac{6.25 \text{ grams protein}}{\text{gram nitrogen}} \approx 31 \text{ grams protein}$$

This means that 31 grams represents the minimum amount of protein these two people weighing 70 kg would need each day ("leak" in their tank). There's a catch though. The protein needed must be perfect protein, protein that supplies all nine EAA in the amounts needed to make body proteins. Only two proteins meet this description: human breast milk protein and egg white protein. Thus, this 70 kg man and woman must eat 31 grams of egg white protein daily to cover their protein losses/needs.

STEP 2

In this step, we take into account variation in the population. Let's take into consideration that not everyone is average, that is, not everyone loses 5 grams of nitrogen daily.

As shown in Figure 2.21, the need for protein falls on a distribution curve. So to meet the needs of *nearly all* people in the population, let's add to 31 grams and push it up to 40 grams of perfect protein daily. This amount of perfect protein should meet virtually everyone in the population who weighs 70 kg. (By the way, we got the number 40 by adding two standard deviations to the average value.)

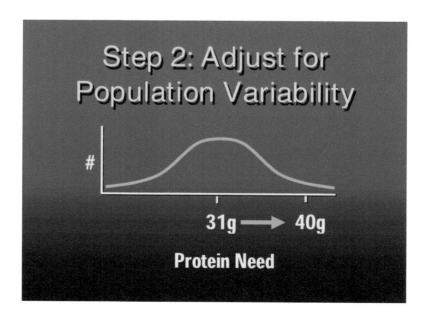

Figure 2.21

STEP 3

This final step takes into account that we eat a mix of proteins each day rather than just eating egg white protein. Food proteins contain all of the 20 amino acids and the nine essential amino acids. But various food proteins have these nine EAA in different amounts.

We'll be discussing protein quality in the next section. For now, let's say that if we gave egg white a quality score of 100, the protein in most people's diets would score about 70 considering a person may eat peanut butter, milk, fish, soy, beans, and grains. Each of these food protein sources vary in their essential amino acid composition. The ratio of 100 to 70 is used to adjust the 40 grams to 56 grams per day for a 70-kg adult male or female. This means that a 70-kg male or female could meet their protein needs on 56 grams of proteins from a variety of sources.

But since not everyone weighs 70 kg, we need to express this as a requirement based on 1 kg of body weight, in a way that all of us can use (56 grams/70 kg =):

> The RDA for protein for adult men and women is 0.8 grams protein/kg body weight per day

This value represents the amount of protein from a mix of food sources that should meet the needs of nearly all healthy people in the population. Also, this amount is averaged over several days and does not represent a minimum value.

Let's use the RDA for protein in a calculation. How much protein does a 50-kg woman require?

$$50 \text{ kg} \times 0.8 \text{ g/kg per day} = 40 \text{ g protein/day}$$

This value represents the amount of protein that should be more than adequate for her from a variety of food sources.

Factors That Change Protein Needs

The RDA for protein above is for an adult man or woman. As you might expect, the protein needs for a child, teenager, and pregnant or lactating woman are different. How does injury, illness, and exercise impact protein needs?

1. **Growth**

   The RDA for infants is about 2 grams of protein/kg body weight per day. This is much greater than the RDA for adults due to the infant's rate of growth compared to that of an adult. Consider that each day a growing baby is ending the day with more cells than it started with (so, of course, the need for more protein). Look at the numbers in Figure 2.22 to see how the protein requirement changes with age as growth rate slows down. *Note:* The only time there is a gender difference is during the late teen years, due to differences in growth rate. Girls are finished growing by approximately age 15 or so, while boys continue to grow and therefore need more protein.

   The table in Figure 2.22 expresses protein needs based on body weight or what's referred to as relative protein needs. Don't confuse this with the overall protein need of a given individual expressed in grams per day. With this in mind, who requires more protein: an infant who weighs 10 pounds or

A Question for You...

Her 50-kg male friend requires more protein. True? False?

False!
Protein requirement is not a function of gender, so he would require the same amount.

RDA FOR PROTEIN BASED ON AGE	
AGE (YR) RDA	**PROTEIN G/KG BODY WT**
0–0.5	2.2
0.5–1	1.6
1–3	1.2
4–6	1.1
7–14	1.0
15–18	0.9 male
15–18	0.8 female

Figure 2.22

an adult weighing 150 pounds? The adult would need more simply because he or she is so much larger than the baby. But if you were asked who needs more on a relative basis, the infant would (2g/kg versus 0.8 g/kg).

2. **Pregnancy and Lactation**

   Over the course of a pregnancy, a woman typically puts on about 22 to 27 pounds of body weight. Much of this weight gain is due to an increase in blood volume, and an increase in her fat stores, uterine size, and breasts along with the weight of the baby. If this is all taken into consideration, a woman needs 25 grams of extra protein daily above her RDA.

   Lactation or breast-feeding requires additional dietary protein as the mother produces milk (protein source) for the newborn. An extra 25 grams per day is needed for a lactating woman.

3. **Injury and Illness**

   Remember that the RDA meets the needs of nearly all *healthy* people in the population. What about people who are sick with a severe illness, such as pneumonia—do they need more protein? Or if a person is injured such as with burns or extensive surgery, how are protein needs impacted? These are individual situations that alter protein needs and must be considered. A health professional, such as a physician or dietitian, could assess the protein needs for an individual who is seriously ill or injured. When you get sick with a cold or flu, your protein needs are not dramatically altered, so there's no need to worry about eating more protein during those times of illness.

4. **Exercise**

   The RDA for protein is computed for a person who is NOT engaged in regular, vigorous exercise, such as weight lifting or running. Studies show that people who engage in regular exercise for about an hour daily need more than the RDA for protein. The amount over the RDA depends upon many factors, such as the type of exercise—its duration, frequency, and intensity.

   For weight-training athletes or those involved in contact sports, such as football, muscle mass increases. There is also some muscle damage that occurs during impact exercise. Research studies show that an extra 0.4 g/kg body weight or 50% above the RDA is needed.

For endurance athletes (runners, triathletes, and cyclists), another situation occurs. Protein contributes a small amount to total energy use—about 10% overall. For the average person not participating in these types of sports, protein needs would not be altered. But consider that some of these athletes train for hours every day. This translates to an increase in protein needs of about 0.4 g/kg body weight or 50% above the RDA.

Since many athletes take in more calories than a non-athlete, they typically get enough protein and there is no need to supplement to get this amount. However, for some athletes who have difficulty making good food choices, a protein powder mixed with juice or made into a smoothie is a good way to meet protein needs.

The milk protein whey (often a staple in protein powders) offers a quickly digested and usable form of protein that may further augment protein rebuilding after a workout. Milk proteins and lean proteins from meats and egg provide a dose of essential amino acids that according to research leads to greater rebuilding of muscle protein following a workout compared to lower quality protein types.

Protein on Food Labels— The Daily Value for Protein

Now that you know your personal protein requirement based on your weight, how can you use that information to make food choices based on the Nutrition Facts food label? As you might guess, food manufacturers couldn't list everyone's protein requirements on the label—it just wouldn't fit! Instead, the Daily Value for protein is used as a point of comparison for consumers. We'll be learning more about the Daily Value, or DV for short, in future chapters. The DV is set for a variety of nutrients, such as protein, fat, saturated fat, fiber, and more and is based on an average consumer (age four and older) taking in about 2,000 calories daily. The DV represents a suggested intake for good health and the prevention of chronic disease. (More on this in Chapter 6 when we cover fat and heart disease.)

The Daily Value for protein is 50 grams. This means that the average consumer eating approximately 2,000 calories daily needs about 50 grams of protein. Food labels list the amount of protein in a serving of the food, as shown in Figure 2.23. (The Food and Drug Administration recently updated the Nutrition Facts panel layout and details, which food manufacturers must adopt by mid-2018.) Food labels are NOT required to list the percentage this product provides of the DV for protein unless a specific claim is made on the label in regards to protein, such as "excellent source of protein," as might be stated on a box of protein-enhanced breakfast cereal.

However, you can calculate what percent of the DV a serving of food provides with some simple math. Here's how it's done for a serving of cheese casserole (see Figure 2.24).

Using food labels or the chart on page 33, which lists the protein content of several types of food, practice calculating the percent of DV. Many foods such as canned tuna, chili, and others provide a substantial proportion of the DV for protein.

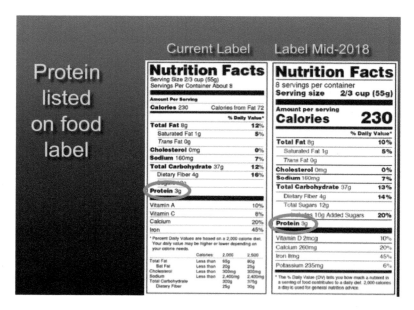

Figure 2.23

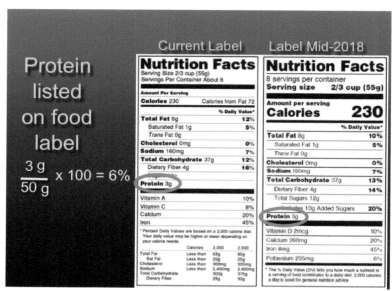

Figure 2.24

MAKING PROTEIN FOOD CHOICES

Now that you know how much protein you need, and that food proteins (like body proteins) differ in their amino acid content, let's consider making protein choices. Since food proteins differ in their amino acid profile, do you think that the protein in peanut butter would meet your need for protein as well as egg protein? Intuitively you might say no, and you're right. This is what protein quality is all about, and understanding this can aid us in making choices from including meat in the diet to adopting a vegetarian plan.

Protein Quality

Food sources differ in the quality of protein present. All proteins contain the EAAs and provide a source of nitrogen. But, as mentioned before, proteins differ in the amount (or proportion) of each of the essential amino acids they provide. It's the EAA content of a food protein in relationship to our need that determines the quality of a food protein.

FOOD, SERVING SIZE	GRAMS OF PROTEIN
milk, low-fat, 8 ounces	8
soy milk, 8 ounces	7
refried beans, 1 cup	12
yogurt, low-fat, cup	13
lentils, 1 cup cooked	18
Thai-style fish curry	17
soy burger, a 2-ounce patty	18
skinless chicken breast, grilled, 4 ounces	28
canned tuna, 3 ounces	22
beef chili, 1 cup	24
Clif Builder Bar	20
smoothie (Jamba, w/protein), 24 ounces	20
fast-food items • Pizza Hut Veggie Lover's, pan, medium 12", 1 slice • Taco Bell Burrito Supreme • McDonald's Grilled Chicken Classic Sandwich • Burger King Whopper	 10 17 32 29

The quality of a food protein can be assessed directly (measuring the EAA content of the food protein) or indirectly (assessing the growth of a laboratory animal eating a diet that contains the test protein). We will cover two protein quality tests—one indirect and the other direct. First, we need to provide some definitions used in discussing food protein sources.

Complete Protein

- Complete protein contains all nine essential amino acids.
- The essential amino acids are present in proportion to need.
- The food protein is digestible.

Examples of complete proteins:

- beef
- poultry
- fish
- dairy
- egg
- soybean (soy products)

Egg protein and human breast milk protein are complete proteins and are perfect; that is, they're the best complete proteins you can get. In general, animal sources of protein are complete and when you think about it, many animal proteins are similar to our own proteins (muscle or flesh, for example), which would mean that essential amino acid profiles would match our needs fairly well. Many protein powders containing whey or casein, which are both cow's milk proteins, are complete sources of protein. Soy protein is the only plant protein source that is complete. So tofu, soy burgers, soy milk, and other soy foods are good-quality protein sources.

Incomplete Protein

Incomplete proteins do not contain all nine essential amino acids in amounts proportional to need. Examples of incomplete proteins are shown in Figure 2.25.

GRAINS	BEANS (LEGUMES)	NUTS	SEEDS
oats	kidney	peanuts	sesame
wheat	garbanzo	cashews	sunflower
barley	navy	almonds	pumpkin
rice	pinto	walnuts	

Figure 2.25

What if you only eat incomplete protein sources? Many vegetarians do this. It is certainly possible to meet your needs for EAA but you must use some care. More on this later.

What type of protein are shown here in Figures 2.26 and 2.27?

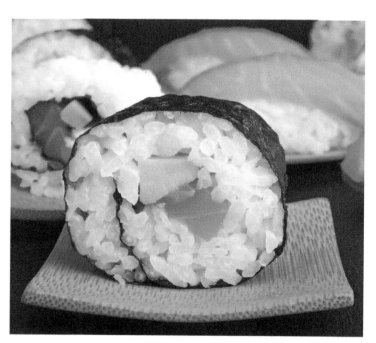

Figure 2.26

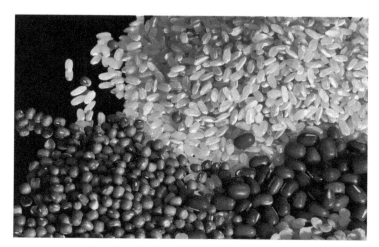

Figure 2.27

Protein Quality Tests

Protein quality tests measure either indirectly or directly EAA content. Let's take a look at two protein quality tests: Protein Efficiency Ratio and Chemical Score.

1. **Protein Efficiency Ratio or PER**

   This is an indirect measurement of EAA content. In this test, growing laboratory animals, such as rats, are fed a diet containing the protein in question, corn protein for example. Each day, weight gain is measured and the amount of food (protein) eaten is determined. The PER is a ratio of weight gained to protein eaten.

$$PER = \frac{weight\ gained}{protein\ eaten}$$

   A high PER would mean that the protein was utilized (meaning, good EAA content) and the animal grew well. A low PER would mean the EAA content was poor because the animal's growth was not good. Some PER values are shown in Figure 2.28.

   As you may notice, complete proteins have a high PER and incomplete proteins have a low PER. Does this fit with our definition of complete and incomplete proteins? There are a few limitations using the PER quality test.

   - The PER does not reveal which EAA might be in low amount in the protein.
   - Also, how well a laboratory rat grows on a specific protein may not reflect how well a person might utilize the same test protein.

   With these two things in mind, measuring protein quality may be better assessed using a direct measure of EAA content.

2. **Chemical Score**

   This protein quality test is a direct measure of essential amino acid content. The protein to be tested is put into a machine that can tell you how much of each amino acid is present and what the relative percentages are, that is, percent by weight. These percentages are then compared to the percentages found in our

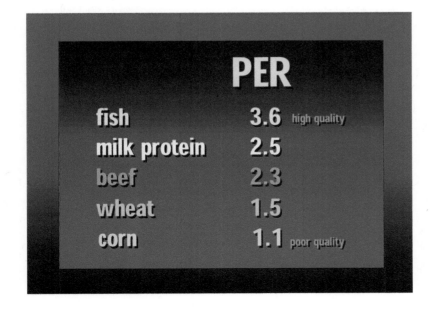

PER		
fish	3.6	high quality
milk protein	2.5	
beef	2.3	
wheat	1.5	
corn	1.1	poor quality

Figure 2.28

"gold" standard egg white protein. This is chosen because egg white's essential amino acid content best reflects our need for the nine essential amino acids.

For simplicity, only five of the nine essential amino acids are listed in Figure 2.29 for egg white and our test protein from white flour. This is done to save space, but in a true chemical score test, values of all nine essential amino acids would be listed.

In Figure 2.29, the amount of each of the EAA as a percent by weight is listed for egg white and the test protein. Also, thrown in to test your understanding of protein quality is the value for glycine, a nonessential amino acid. Don't be fooled by this because if you follow on with the calculation for chemical score and don't omit the glycine, you will obtain the wrong number. Ask yourself, do we care how much of a NEAA is in a food protein? Does this impact the quality? No to both of these questions! So be sure to cross out this value for the NEAA, glycine.

The next step is to compute what percentage of each EAA of our test protein white flour compared to egg white protein (see Figure 2.30).

CHEMICAL SCORE

AMINO ACID	EGG WHITE	WHITE FLOUR PROTEIN
lysine (EAA)	7.0	2.1
methionine (EAA)	5.6	4.0
leucine (EAA)	8.6	7.0
tryptophan (EAA)	1.7	1.1
valine (EAA)	6.6	4.1
glycine (NEAA)	2.2	0.5

Figure 2.29

CHEMICAL SCORE

AMINO ACID	EGG WHITE	WHITE FLOUR PROTEIN	%
lysine (EAA)	7.0	2.1	$2.1/7.0 \times 100 = 30$
methionine (EAA)	5.6	4.0	$4.0/5.6 \times 100 = 71$
leucine (EAA)	8.6	7.0	$7.0/8.6 \times 100 = 81$
tryptophan (EAA)	1.7	1.1	$1.1/1.7 \times 100 = 64$
valine (EAA)	6.6	4.1	$4.1/6.6 \times 100 = 62$
~~glycine (NEAA)~~	~~2.2~~	~~0.5~~	
Chemical Score = **30**			

Figure 2.30

The **chemical score** of a protein is the lowest percentage computed—in the case of white flour protein lysine has a value of 30 (30 percent of the lysine content of egg white). If glycine had not been canceled out, then the score would have been computed as 23, which is incorrect since this NEAA does not impact the quality of the protein.

The score also tells us which EAA is in the lowest amount relative to our need. This is called the **limiting amino acid—the essential amino acid in a food protein in the lowest amount relative to need**. All incomplete proteins have one or more limiting amino acids.

Most grains (flour, barley, rice) are limiting in lysine and most beans (legumes, such as kidney and black beans) are limiting in methionine. This actually is great when combining these sources of protein in vegetarian meals and diets because grains and beans compliment each other and form a complete protein. (More on this in the next section.)

Is Protein Quality an Issue for Children and Adults?

How big of an issue is protein quality when you make your daily food choices? To answer this, we need to look at how much of your daily protein needs must be as the essential amino acids. (Recall that you need protein as a source of EAA and a source of nitrogen.) As you might imagine, the EAA needs for an adult would be different than that for an infant or child because of growth.

- **An adult needs only 0.09 g of EAA/kg of body weight or 11% of the RDA for protein as EAAs.** This means that the other 89% can be any amino acid since they all supply nitrogen. If you wanted to meet your need for EAA by eating an incomplete protein source exclusively, this could be done. You would need to eat, for example, one loaf of bread (grain protein) to meet your need for EAA—a doable but boring diet. Nonetheless, you could eat a loaf of bread in one day, but this is not the case for a young child.
- **Infants require 0.7 g of EAA/kg of body weight or 40% of their RDA for protein as EAAs.** Why the big difference? Infants are making new proteins every day above those that are just turning over as an adult would. (We are in maintenance.) Could an infant meet their need for EAA by eating one incomplete protein source exclusively? If it takes four loaves of bread to meet the EAA need of a one-year-old child, it would be impossible to get such a small child to eat so much! So feeding an incomplete protein source as the exclusive protein source would not meet the child's needs. Instead, a complete protein source would be better. Any suggestions? How about breast milk, or if the child is old enough, fish, soy, beef, or dairy products would all be good choices.

Vegetarian Diets

Now with a good understanding of protein quality, let's take a look at vegetarian diets. Perhaps you are a vegetarian, or considering adopting a vegetarian meal plan. This section will help you put together plant sources of protein that will meet your need for protein, particularly EAA.

Humans have long been meat eaters. In fact, we have teeth designed for tearing flesh (canine teeth) and others (molars) for grinding nuts, berries, and seeds. Vegetarian diets arose in biblical times for religious reasons. Today people choose vegetarian diets for a variety of reasons—religious, ethical (in objection to slaughtering of animals for meat), economical (animal sources of protein are typically more expensive than plant sources), or for better health and environmental (animal protein requires use of greater resources, such as fuel and land compared to an equal amount of vegetable protein).

The health benefits of vegetarian diets have been known for some time and research studies show that vegetarians tend to have lower risk for a variety of diseases related to diet, such as heart disease, certain cancers, and obesity. But vegetarians also tend to lead more healthful lives overall—exercising more regularly, not smoking or using drugs or engaging in other safe lifestyle habits, such as wearing seatbelts more often. So some of the health attributes of a vegetarian diet may be due to other healthy practices other than diet.

As you go through this course, you may opt for more vegetarian meals or even choose to be a vegetarian as a way to eat more fiber and key nutrients that promote good health and to help prevent chronic disease. Strict vegetarian or "vegan" diets include no animal products in their diets. Other forms of vegetarianism include "ovo-vegetarian" (eggs are eaten) and lacto-vegetarian (dairy is consumed). People may also consider themselves vegetarian if they include chicken or fish but no red meat, but these are not forms of vegetarianism.

The issue for vegetarians is paying attention to combining protein sources in order to complement incomplete proteins. For example, if you combine grains and legumes, you will get enough of the limiting amino acids (lysine and methionine, respectively) as shown in Figure 2.31. Eating soy on a regular basis also ensures that you will get ample EAA since this is a complete protein. If you're planning on including more vegetarian meals in your daily fare, check out the vegetarian menu provided on page 39 to give you some ideas.

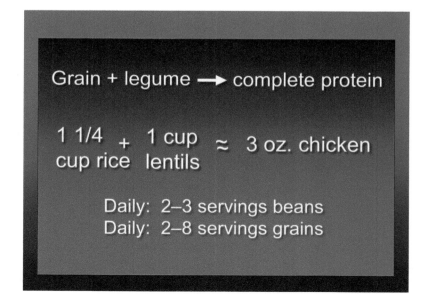

Figure 2.31

VEGETARIANS

To get all of the nutrients you need from non-meat sources, just follow this food plan.

Breakfast

- ½ cups nine-grain cooked cereal topped with 1 ounce chopped almonds
- ¾ cup blueberries
- 2 tablespoons honey
- 8 ounces soy milk

Morning Snack

- 2 ounces trail mix (raisins, dried papaya, pumpkin seeds)

Lunch

- One bean burrito (1 cup black beans, ½ cup rice, 1 ounce soy cheese)
- ¼ cup salsa
- 1 cup fruit salad (kiwi, apple, and melon)

Afternoon Snack

- One banana spread with 2 tablespoons peanut butter
- 8 ounces cranberry juice

Dinner

- Spinach pasta with "meat" sauce (1 cup spinach pasta, ¾ cup red sauce, two (soy) veggie burgers crumbled into sauce)
- 1 cup steamed broccoli
- 1 ½ cup dark greens tossed with 1 tablespoon olive oil vinaigrette
- 1 ounce dark chocolate

Calories:	2,500
Protein:	92 grams
Carbohydrate:	413 grams
Fat:	26% calories

Plant-based Protein Powders

Many plant-based protein powders use a single or a combination of different plant proteins. Here's a rundown on the most commonly used varieties:

Soy: A vegetarian source of protein, soy supplies just as many key building blocks called essential amino acids (EAA) as milk proteins. Soy also contains health-boosting isoflavones shown to lower risk of certain cancers and heart disease.

Hemp: Extracted from cannabis seeds, hemp protein supplies less overall protein compared to milk and eggs, but hemp comes with some key essential fats and fiber, which helps you feel full and aids digestion.

Pea: A vegan protein source that digests well but does not have an EAA profile equal to milk or egg, but pea protein is better than most grains such as brown rice. When combined with brown rice and hemp proteins, pea protein makes for a great addition for your morning smoothie.

Brown Rice: A common ingredient in vegan protein powders, brown rice protein is incomplete so in combination with pea or soy protein help round out the essential amino acid profile.

Quinoa: This seed, more closely related to beets than an actual grain such as wheat, supplies protein that is of slightly better quality than rice and wheat, which means the amount of the EAA is a greater.

Quiz Yourself

CHAPTER 2

List a good food source for each:

- a complete protein _____

- a protein with a low chemical score _____

- a protein with a high PER _____

- an incomplete protein _____

1. Which of the following has the highest relative protein requirement expressed in grams of good protein per kg body weight per day?

    a. 2-year old child

    b. an adult man

    c. a teenager

    d. all have the same protein requirement

2. A 60 kg female eats 1 cup of vegetarian chili that provides 15 grams of protein.

    a. What is the percent of DV for protein from the 1 cup of the chili?

    b. What is the percent of RDA for protein from the 1 cup of the chili for the 60 kg female?

3. Would you expect the amino acid profile (the amount of amino acid) to be the same from protein in beef, almonds, refried beans, and a human blood cell? Why or why not.

    _____

    _____

    _____

4. Protein quality is primarily determined by the amount of each of the 20 amino acids.

    a. true

    b. false

5. Which of the following food proteins have a limiting amino acid?

   a. Peanut butter

   b. Refried beans

   c. Wheat bread

   d. Tofu

   e. a through c above

6. The Recommended Dietary Allowance (RDA) for protein represents the average amount of "perfect" protein needed by most of the healthy population.

   a. true

   b. false

CALORIES—THE ENERGY BASIS OF NUTRITION

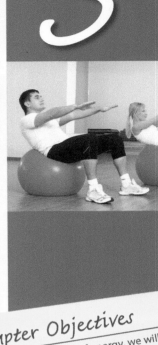

With our first nutrient under out belt, we must divert a bit and discuss the topic of energy. You undoubtedly have tossed around the term *energy* before, often in conjunction with feeling low "energy" or describing a person's demeanor as high "energy." In this course, **energy** means the ability to do work: either metabolic work (building a protein in a liver cell for example) or physical work (moving furniture or running).

ENERGY VALUE OF FOODS

Several scientists took up exploring the energy value of food centuries ago. One in particular, Lavoisier, made the comparison between how much energy is released when a carbon-containing food (such as bread, vegetables, butter, or meat—these all contain the macronutrients carbohydrate, protein, and fat) is burned and how much energy is released when an animal eats this same food. (See Figure 3.1.)

The carbon in the food, in the presence of oxygen, is burned and gives off carbon dioxide (CO_2) and heat. Our body's metabolism, or that of an animal, can be thought of as similar to the burning of food. The carbon in the food is combined with oxygen and the chemical bonds are oxidized (or burned), releasing their potential energy as heat.

When we eat food, we (1) break chemical bonds in the macronutrients protein, carbohydrate, and fat; (2) release the energy in the form of heat, and (3) release the carbon as the gas CO_2, which we exhale. (See Figure 3.2.)

Rather than just referring to energy released as "heat," let's give it a unit of measure: the **Calorie**.

A **Calorie** is the heat needed to raise 1 liter (about 4 cups) of water 1 degree Celsius.

Chapter Objectives

During our discussion of energy, we will cover two areas:

- The energy value of foods—how it's measured and how to calculate what amount of energy is in the food you eat.
- Your energy requirement—how much energy you need to support your metabolism and other activities.

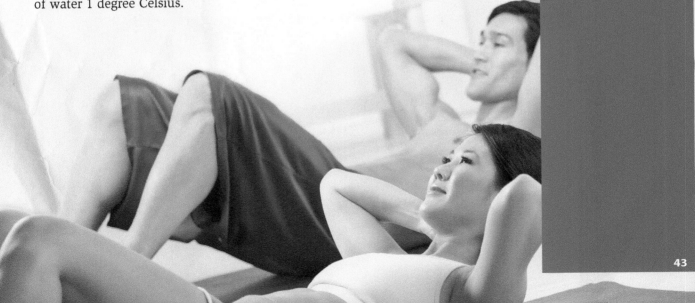

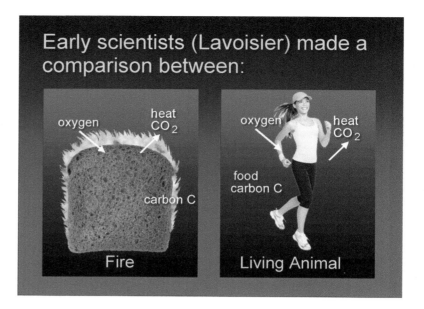

Figure 3.1

You may have taken a chemistry course and learned about a calorie being the amount of energy needed to raise *one gram* of water 1 degree Celsius. Chemists use this much smaller unit of heat energy. But in nutrition, a calorie is 1,000 times the size of a chemistry calorie. You needn't worry about making any conversion because at all times when the term calorie is used in this course, on food labels and on calorie expenditure charts, we are referring to the nutrition calorie. Sometimes I use the abbreviation kcal or kilocalorie to signify calorie. (This simply means 1,000 chemistry calories and is scientific lingo but you should still read kcal as "calorie.")

Calorie: a measure of heat energy

1 calorie = heat to raise 1 liter of H_2O by 1 degree Celsius
1 calorie = 1 kilocalorie = 1 kcal → "nutrition" calorie

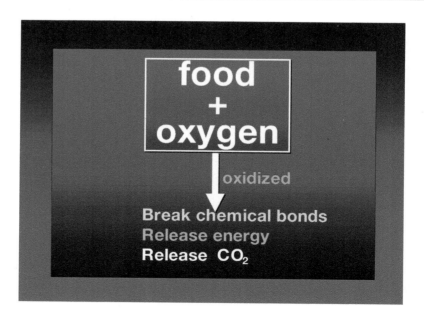

Figure 3.2

Now let's figure out how much potential energy or calories are in carbohydrate, fat, and protein. A specially designed machine, a more sophisticated version of Lavoisier's device as pictured in Figure 3.3, called a bomb calorimeter, is used to determine the potential energy or calorie value of foods. This clever machine consists of a small container where the food in question rests ready to be burned with an ignition wire. A larger chamber of water maintained at a set temperature surrounds the smaller container. Once the food is ignited and burns, heat is given off and the water heats up. From the change in temperature in the water chamber, the number of calories in the food can be calculated. This value represents the **total potential energy released from the food** and is displayed in calories (or kcal) /gram.

Here is the potential energy in the macronutrients. (You needn't memorize these numbers.)

Carbohydrate	4.2 kcal/gram
Fat	9.4 kcal/gram
Protein	5.7 kcal/gram

Do you think our bodies are as efficient as a bomb calorimeter machine when we eat? Lavoisier thought so, but his device was crude, and he wasn't able to measure the fact that living creatures cannot extract all the potential energy in foods. We lose some energy due to indigestible losses (after all, the machine doesn't have to chew and digest the food) and metabolic energy losses in the urine (with protein energy metabolism only).

The amount of energy that is physiologically available to us from the macronutrients is slightly lower than the total potential energy.

Refer to Figure 3.4. Some portion of the carbohydrate we eat, about 5%, is not digested and absorbed and will be lost in the stool. (Thus, your stool has some potential energy due in part to undigested carbohydrate.) You are left with 4 kcal/gram of carbohydrate, which is the **Physiological Fuel Value** for carbohydrates. This is the amount of energy your body gets when you eat 1 gram of carbs.

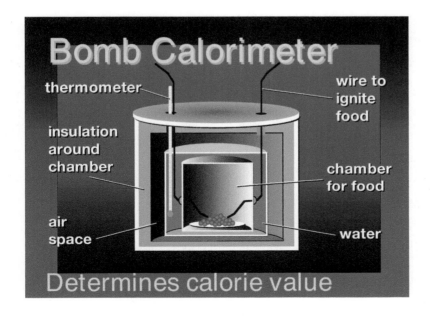

Figure 3.3

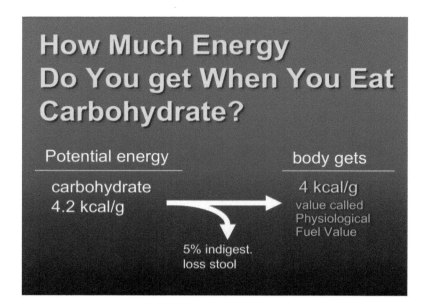

Figure 3.4

Refer to Figure 3.5. As with carbohydrates, a small portion (5%) of fats are not digested and absorbed and go into the stool, which represents a loss of potential energy. Thus, fat has a Physiological Fuel Value of 9 kcal/gram.

Matters get a bit more complicated with protein because the element nitrogen is part of the amino acid structure. This nitrogen must be disposed of through a means that costs the body calories. Refer to Figure 3.6. We start with 5.7 kcal/gram and we lose in the first step about 10% of the energy due to indigestible losses. Some vegetable sources of protein—remember the incomplete proteins, which are not well digested.

If an amino acid is used for energy or converted to fat for storage, the nitrogen must be taken off. Can we just let the nitrogen hang around and use it later? No, nitrogen is toxic, and we need to get rid of it right away. Our bodies must make

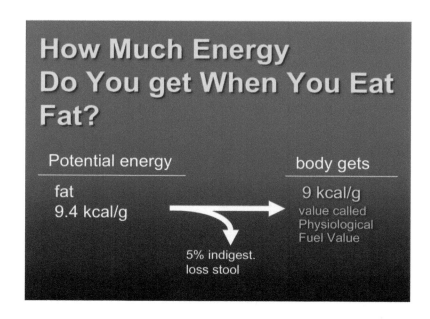

Figure 3.5

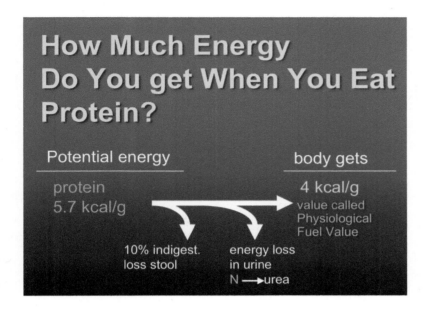

Figure 3.6

urea at a caloric cost, which serves as a vehicle for nitrogen to leave the body via the urine. This means that your urine has metabolic energy waste from the breakdown of protein, a loss of approximately 20%. In addition, don't forget that 10% of the protein consumed is not digested or absorbed, which also represents a loss of energy in the stool. So while we started out with a potential energy of 5.7 kcal/gram and a loss of energy occurs, we end up with 4 kcal/gram as the Physiological Fuel Value for protein.

Figure 3.7 shows the Physiological Fuel Values for the three macronutrients. (These are the same values that appear on food labels.) These values are very important for you to learn. You will use them in calculating the calorie value of foods as well as what percent of the calories in a food or meal come from either carbohydrate, fat, or protein.

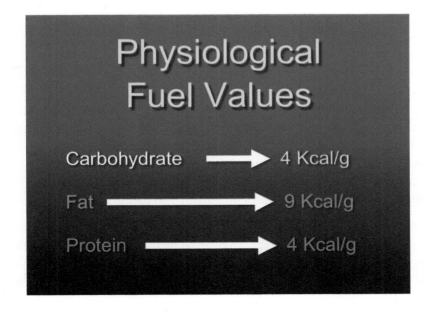

Figure 3.7

Let's put these numbers to work and calculate the number of calories in a food like a hot dog with a simple three-step process.

1. Note the number of grams of carbohydrate, fat, and protein there are in each turkey hot dog.
2. Multiply each by its respective Physiological Fuel Value. (Make sure you also write down the units of kcal/gram.)
3. Add up the resulting products to get the total available energy (kcal/g).

One turkey hot dog (wiener only!) contains:

Carbohydrate	1 gram	$\times$	4 kcal/g	=	4 kcal
Fat	16 grams	$\times$	9 kcal/g	=	144 kcal
Protein	7 grams	$\times$	4 kcal/g	=	28 kcal
TOTAL				=	176 kcal

What if you wanted to know the percentage of calories from fat in a turkey "dog?" Simply divide the number of fat calories by total calories and multiply by 100 to get a percentage.

$$\frac{144 \text{ fat calories}}{176 \text{ total calories}} \times 100 = 82\% \text{ fat calories}$$

Wow!! Looks more like a "fat" dog. There are other types of hot dogs available, reduced-fat, soy, and other versions that are lower in fat. As you'll learn in later chapters, keeping total fat intake to less than 30% of the total calories helps reduce risk for chronic diseases, such as cancer and heart disease.

You can also calculate the percent of calories from carbohydrate and protein. On your diet project, you'll be doing exactly that as well as doing these types of calculations on the exam.

Here are a few final notes on calorie value of foods:

1. Calories in a meal are additive.
   - This means the calories in your hot dog get added with calories in the bun, condiments you may use, along with a soda and chips you may also eat with your hot dog.
   - This also means that there is no such thing as a "negative calorie" food (regardless of what your friends may tell you). For example, chewing celery does not provide you with negative calories.
2. Water, cholesterol (a fat-like substance present in foods in a very small amount), vitamins, and minerals all have NO calories. Remember, only the macronutrients, protein, carbohydrate and fat, can be burned for energy. Alcohol in beer, wine and distilled spirits also contains physiologically available energy, but alcohol is not a nutrient (more covered in Chapter 10).
3. Fiber, which is an indigestible carbohydrate, cannot be broken down in the intestinal tract and therefore is excreted in the stool. Thus, fiber has no available energy to us; however, fiber is very important as we will learn in the next chapter.

On food labels, total calories are listed per serving. Calories contributed by fat are also listed prominently but will no longer be featured in the new label format. Both total calories and fat calories are expressed as physiologically available energy, not total potential energy (see Figure 3.8). The new label also features calories per serving in a larger font.

Urban Myth

Myth: "Some foods like celery have negative calories because it takes more energy to digest the food than are actually in the food."

While foods, such as celery and lettuce, contain few calories, digestion burns still fewer.

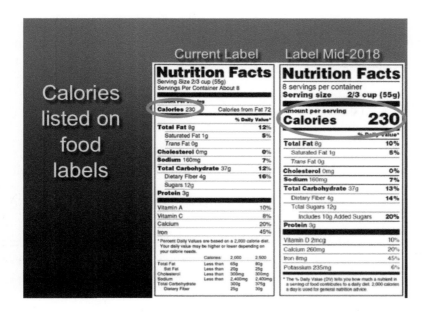

Figure 3.8

DETERMINING ENERGY NEEDS

Now that we know the definition of energy and how much energy is in food, let's figure out how many calories (or how much energy) you need to support normal body functioning.

Your daily energy needs reflect the sum of three components:

1. **Basal Metabolic Rate (BMR)**
   - This is the amount of heat/energy/calories needed to keep basic body functions going such as your heart beating, lungs breathing in and out, as well as your liver doing its maintenance duties. The **BMR** is measured in a person at rest, no food (fasted for about 12 hours), without exercise or strenuous physical activity for 24 hours (hard workouts cause your metabolism to rise), and in an environment (room) where the temperature is neutral.
   - The BMR is typically the largest component of daily energy needs and values usually fall between 1,000 to 2,000 calories daily.

2. **Activity**
   - This is energy needed to perform any activity above the basal metabolic rate—sitting, standing, jogging, taking notes in class.
   - The activity component is usually equal to or less than your BMR, depending upon your movement during the day.

3. **Thermic Effect of Food (TEF)**
   - This is the amount of energy needed to digest and assimilate food.
   - The TEF represents the smallest component of your energy need and values usually fall between 50 to 200 calories.

4. **Growth**
   This energy need component supports the cost of building new tissue as well as the actual cost of the material that makes up tissue, such as muscle or bone. We will not be computing this in class, but you need to know that growth must be taken into consideration when determining a child's energy requirement.

Summary:
- Component 1 + 2 + 3 = the total energy requirement for adult men and women who are NOT pregnant or lactating.
- For children, you must also compute a fourth component, the amount of energy needed for growth.

Fat Gain or Loss

Before we move on to computing energy requirements, let's consider what happens if a person is over or under eating. That is, what happens if you consume in excess of your energy needs or less than your energy needs? This would mean that you are not in energy balance (calories in = calories out) (see Figure 3.9) and that the excess calories (calories in > calories out) would be stored as fat, and weight would be gained (more on this in Chapter 7). And if you were in a calorie deficit (calories in < calories out), the deficit would be met by taking calories out of storage (fat), thus weight loss.

The number to compute weight gained or weight loss is **3,500 calories per 1 pound of body fat** gained or lost (in excess or deficit). We will use this number later in a calculation so you can see how works. (See calculation on page 55.)

Now let's compute the three components of your energy requirement.

Computing the Calorie Cost of BMR

The amount of energy you need to maintain basic bodily functions depends upon several factors: body weight, age, gender, and body surface area. A University of California Davis professor some years ago determined the relationship of body surface area to BMR. Computing BMR based upon body surface area would take some doing and a bit too complicated for us. There are other ways to approximate, so in this class, we will use a very simple method based upon body weight and gender.

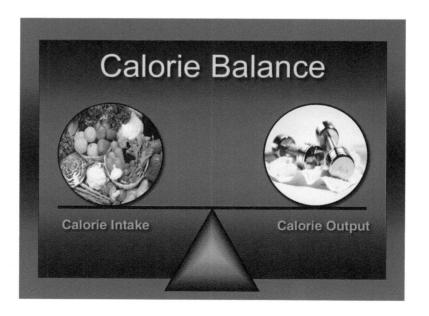

Figure 3.9

The following equations yield an estimate for a person's BMR:

Males: 1 kcal/kg body weight per hour
Females: 0.9 kcal/kg body weight per hour

Men have a greater BMR per unit of body weight because of body composition differences (more lean or muscle tissue, which costs more to maintain than women who have proportionately more body fat, which is a less "expensive" tissue to maintain). Here's a sample calculation:

What is the BMR for a 55 kg woman?

$$0.9 \text{ kcal/kg} \cdot \text{hour} \times 55 \text{ kg} \times 24 \text{ hours/day} = 1{,}188 \text{ kcal/day}$$

Her BMR falls right into the range of 1,000 to 2,000 calories/day given earlier. (It's important for you to double-check your number to make sure you did the calculation properly and always include the units.)

Factors That Alter the BMR

There are several factors that can change how many calories you burn just to maintain your basic bodily functions.

1. **Age.** You guessed it; getting older puts a damper on your BMR. After about age 20, your BMR drops about 2% to 3% for every decade. So a 60-year-old would have a BMR that was about 12% lower than in her twenties. This drop in BMR with age is mostly due to a decline in activity that in turn leads to a loss of muscle mass with age, since muscle requires more energy to maintain than fat tissue. But you can hedge off this slump in BMR by maintaining muscle through resistance exercises such as calisthenics or weight lifting. And it's never too late to boost your muscle mass—even a 90-year-old can get buff!

2. **Fasting.** When you skip eating altogether, your BMR drops about 10% to 20% within 24 hours. This is a smart response by your body as it tries to conserve energy. Think back to prehistoric days when cave people went without food for days because it was scarce. Those people who could survive by slowing their BMR passed on their genetic material. (Low and behold, we are their descendants!)

3. **Exercise.** Participating in physical activity boosts your BMR. The effect is variable and may last only 30 minutes to as much as 24 hours; it depends upon the type of exercise—its intensity and duration. The more vigorous, the greater the BMR boost. After exercise your body recovers by rebuilding proteins and storing up carbohydrate fuel that was spent. This all costs calories, which shows up as a greater BMR. The amount may be a mere 25 calories or over 250 calories daily. No matter what the boost in BMR, exercise is great to do and good for you!

Computing Calorie Costs of Activity

Estimating calorie costs of activity can be done several ways.

1. **Time and activity method:** Activity costs are based on total time spent in each activity multiplied by the caloric cost of that activity. (Check Figure 3.10 for some values.)

$$\text{time (min)} \times (\text{kcal/min} \times \text{kg}) \times \frac{\text{kg body weight}}{} = \frac{\text{kcal spent}}{\text{on activity}}$$

Nutrition Bite

Many supplements sold on the Internet and in stores claim to "rev up your metabolism" (or BMR). One supplement sold as a skin patch delivers the mineral iodine, which is a component of the thyroid hormone responsible for setting the BMR. But remember homeostasis? Extra iodine doesn't mean the body will start wasting calories. Truth be told, these supplements fall short on their claims.

ENERGY EXPENDITURE DURING VARIOUS ACTIVITIES

	MALE 70 (KG) KCAL/MIN	FEMALE 55 (KG) KCAL/MIN
Basketball	8.6	6.8
Cycling (10 mph)	7.5	5.9
Running (7.5)	14.0	11.0
Sitting	1.7	1.3
Sleeping	1.2	0.9
Walking (3.5 mph)	5.0	3.9
Weight lifting	8.2	6.4

Figure 3.10

This method is tedious. You have to keep very good records or carry a recording device for documentation of every single activity you perform during the day. While this method is used in research, we won't be doing this in class because it's so time-consuming!

2. **Activity profile expressed as a percentage of BMR:** This method categorizes a person into one of four activity profiles. Each profile represents a percentage of the BMR that would then be added along with BMR and TEF to estimate the daily energy requirement. The four activity levels:

CATEGORY	% BMR
Sedentary	+ 30%
Light	+ 50%
Moderate	+ 70%
Strenuous	+ 100%

Which category best fits you?

Sedentary: typical student, lots of sitting (studying), watching TV, computer time, maybe exercise two to three times per week, ride bus to campus. Any job held is not very physical—a desk job, for example.

Light: more daily movement, not much sitting, bike or walk to school, exercise three to four times weekly. Any job held has some walking, stair climbing, and other movement involved.

Moderate: very active days, workout four to five times weekly. Active job that involves being on feet hours a day—childcare, for example.

Strenuous: implies males exercise vigorously most days of the week, little sitting. Physically demanding job, such as landscaping.

Let's compute how many calories a 55 kg woman would burn on activity with a moderate activity level.

1. **Calculate BMR**

$$55 \text{ kg} \times \left(\frac{0.9 \text{ kcal/kg}}{\text{body weight}} \times \text{hour} \right) \times 24 \text{ hours/day} = 1{,}188 \text{ kcal/day}$$

2. **Activity = 70% of BMR**

$$0.7 \times 1{,}188 \text{ kcal/day} = 831.6 \text{ kcal/day needed to support activity}$$

Once you compute your calorie cost of activity, the number should either be equal to or less than your BMR. (If the number you get is greater than the BMR, go back and check your work.)

Computing Calorie Cost of Thermic Effect of Food (TEF)

The energy needed to digest and assimilate food is generally between 5% and 10% of the daily calorie intake. Fat and carbs take around 5% for processing while protein costs 10%. In our calculation, we'll use 5% of calorie intake needed for TEF. The best estimate of total calorie intake is the sum of BMR and activity.

Let's compute how many calories are needed for TEF for a person with a BMR of 1,000 kcal and activity level of light or 500 kcal daily.

$$BMR = 1{,}000 \text{ kcal/day} \qquad \text{Activity} = 500 \text{ kcal/day}$$

$$TEF = 0.05 \,(1{,}000 + 500) \text{ kcal/day}$$

$$= 0.05 \,(1{,}500 \text{ kcal/day})$$

$$= 75 \text{ kcal/day to digest and assimilate food}$$

Double-check your math. TEF should fall between 50 and 200 kcal/day.

Computing Total Energy Requirement

Now let's put everything together and calculate the energy requirement for the following person. Let's go through the example in Figure 3.11 step by step: BMR, then Activity, then TEF, and finally add these three components together to determine the energy requirement.

1. **BMR**

$$0.9 \text{ kcal/kg} \times \text{hour} \times 52 \text{ kg} \times 24 \text{ hours/day} = 1{,}123 \text{ kcal/day}$$

2. **Activity**

$$\text{Strenuous activity level} = 100\% \text{ BMR} = 1{,}123 \text{ kcal/day}$$

3. **TEF**

$$0.05 \,(BMR + \text{Activity}) = 0.05 \,(1{,}123 \text{ kcal} + 1{,}123 \text{ kcal}) = 112 \text{ kcal/day}$$

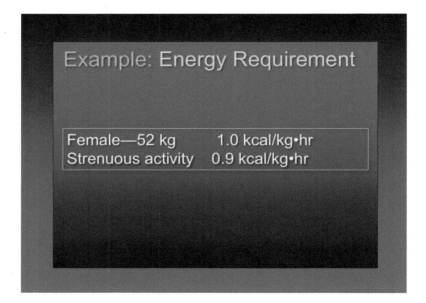

Figure 3.11

4. **Total Energy Requirement**

BMR + Activity + TEF or (1,123 kcal + 1,123 kcal + 112 kcal)

= 2,358 kcal/day

At each step, double-check your numbers. Is the BMR within (or near) the range of 1,000 to 2,000 kcal/day? Is the Activity value in keeping with the BMR? Is the TEF between 50 and 200 kcal/day?

Now ask yourself, do all women who weigh 52 kg have the same energy requirement? The answer is NO. Not all 52 kg women have this activity level. Energy needs must be computed based on activity level as well as body weight and gender.

Computing Total Energy Intake

Now let's add a twist: gaining or losing weight and how this impacts computing energy intake for a person (note: not an energy requirement).

Let's compute the energy intake for the example in Figure 3.12. In this example, we now must account for the fact that this man is overeating or gaining weight at the rate of 500 kcal/day. This will impact the TEF (more food, therefore, a greater cost of digesting and assimilating the food). Follow the same sequence as the first example, but now account for the gain.

1. **BMR**

1.0 kcal/kg × hour × 70 kg × 24 hours/day = 1,680 kcal/day

2. **Activity**

Activity = 50% BMR

= 0.5 (1,680 kcal/day) = 840 kcal/day

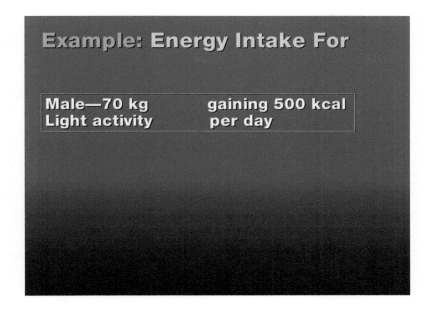

Example: Energy Intake For

| Male—70 kg | gaining 500 kcal |
| Light activity | per day |

Figure 3.12

3. **Gain**

   (We now add in the gain—which is equivalent to the amount he is overeating—the number of calories in a double-decker fast-food burger each day!)

   $$= 500 \text{ kcal/day}$$

   (*Note:* Even though he is overeating and technically gaining weight, do not adjust his body weight in computing the BMR.)

   (*Note also:* If he were losing at the rate of 500 kcal/day, you would simply subtract the 500 kcal = –500 kcal/day.)

4. **TEF**

   $$5\% \,(\text{BMR} + \text{Activity} + \text{Gain})$$

   $$0.05 \,(1{,}680 \text{ kcal} + 840 \text{ kcal} + 500 \text{ kcal}) = 151 \text{ kcal/day}$$

   (*Note:* If he were losing weight, the loss would be subtracted, thereby lowering the TEF.)

   Remember to double-check all your numbers to see if they are reasonable.

5. **Total Energy Intake**

   $$\text{BMR} + \text{Activity} + \text{Gain} + \text{TEF}$$

   $$(1{,}680 \text{ kcal} + 840 \text{ kcal} + 500 \text{ kcal} + 151 \text{ kcal}) = 3{,}171 \text{ kcal/day}$$

   This is his energy intake, NOT his energy requirement. Why not? Because he is overeating exceeding his energy requirements.

   How much fat would this man gain in one week?

   $$500 \text{ kcal/day} \times 7 \text{ days/week} = 3{,}500 \text{ kcal/week}$$

   This translates to 1 pound of fat gained in one week. (Recall that 3,500 kcal = 1 pound fat.)

You now have mastered two important concepts surrounding energy:

1. Energy value of foods
2. Computing our energy requirements

Go practice your new skills on the diet project or these sample problems.

Quiz Yourself

3

CHAPTER

1. When looking at a Nutrition Facts food label, the energy value of a food is expressed in _____ and represents the _____ present in food.

   a. milligrams / total potential energy

   b. calories / total potential energy

   c. calories / physiologically available energy

   d. milligrams / physiologically available energy

2. Males always have a greater basal metabolic rate than females (expressed in kcal/day).

   a. true

   b. false

3. Determine the calorie content of 2 tablespoons of peanut butter (SHOW YOUR WORK).

Fat	16 g
Carbohydrate	16 g
Protein	18 g
Fiber	2 g

   Calculate the percent of calories coming from fat, protein and carbohydrates.

4. Calculate the total energy intake for the following person (SHOW YOUR WORK).

   • Female; 68 kg; light activity; losing 1 lb every 2 weeks

5. List and define the three components of your energy requirements. List approximate values for each component.

    1. _____

    2. _____

    3. _____

6. Describe three factors that affect your BMR.

    1. _____

    2. _____

    3. _____

7. What is a calorie?

    _____

CARBOHYDRATES—THE ENERGY NUTRIENT

4

Following our discussion of the energy value of foods and energy requirements, the second major nutrient, carbohydrate, follows logically. Known primarily as the "energy nutrient," carbohydrate-rich food provides the majority of calories in your diet.

CARBOHYDRATE STRUCTURE AND FOOD SOURCES

The word *carbohydrate* means just what it says: "hydrated carbon," or simply carbon with water attached. Most carbohydrates come from plants—apples, potatoes, wheat, and sugar (from sugar cane plant or sugar beets). (The exception to the plant carbohydrate rule is the sugar found in dairy products.) Plants are able to make carbohydrates by trapping the sun's energy by means of photosynthesis.

As shown in Figure 4.1, plants take up water from their roots, CO_2 (carbon dioxide gas) from the air along with the sun's energy (solar energy) and combine this to form carbohydrate, which the plant then stores (potato, apple, wheat kernel, etc.). Ask yourself where the CO_2 came from? (Recall from Chapter 3 that CO_2 is exhaled in your breath when foods are oxidized during energy metabolism.)

The sun's energy is now trapped as potential energy in a carbohydrate unit. We will cover how this energy is released in more detail later in this chapter. For now, know that this energy represents carbohydrate's major function in the body—energy source. About half of your calories come from carbohydrates. Carbohydrate energy is specifically necessary for brain function and during high-intensity exercise.

Now let's take a closer look at carbohydrate, specifically its structure.

Carbohydrate Structure

The three levels of carbohydrate structure, which are all present in foods and in your body, are: monosaccharides, disaccharides, and polysaccharides.

Chapter Objectives

In this chapter, we'll cover four major areas for carbohydrate:

- Carbohydrate structure and food sources
- Carbohydrate digestion
- Understanding the power of fiber
- Carbohydrate energy metabolism, including the impact of diabetes, exercise and a no-carbohydrate diet

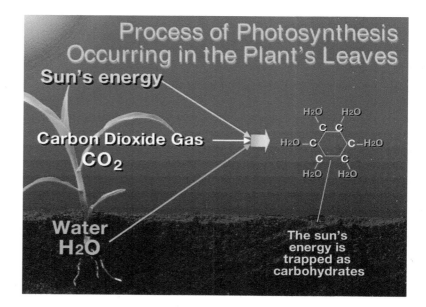

Figure 4.1

1. Monosaccharides

The most basic structure of carbohydrate is a six-carbon ring with water attached to each carbon. "Mono" means "one" and "saccharide" means "sugar."

There are three different monosaccharides, all with six carbons, but with slight variations on the arrangements of the attached water and chemical bonds. Monosaccharide food sources are referred to as **simple sugars** or **simple carbohydrates**.

Rather than looking at the detailed chemical structure, each monosaccharide is represented with a symbol. (See Figure 4.2.)

Be familiar with food sources of monosaccharides.

As noted above, the monosaccharides are part of the next levels of structure—disaccharides and polysaccharides.

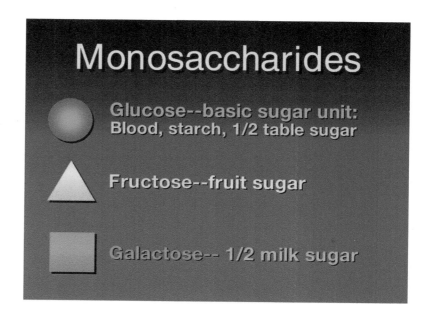

Figure 4.2

2. Disaccharides

With disaccharides, the sugar rings are joined together—"di," which means two. Like monosaccharides, food sources of disaccharides are referred to as **simple sugars** or **simple carbohydrates**. There are three disaccharides of significance in your diet: sucrose, maltose, and lactose.

- Sucrose is one glucose and one fructose molecule joined together. (See Figure 4.3.) Food sources include cookies, candy, soda, or anything made with table sugar, corn sweetener, and other forms of sucrose such as brown sugar (white sugar with a small amount of molasses), powdered sugar, and crystallized sugar or "sugar in the raw."

- Maltose is two glucose molecules linked together. (See Figure 4.4.) There are very few food sources of maltose. It is a breakdown product of starch (a polysaccharide found in potatoes, pasta, etc.) during digestion. In fact, if you chew a piece of bread for several minutes, the maltose will begin to

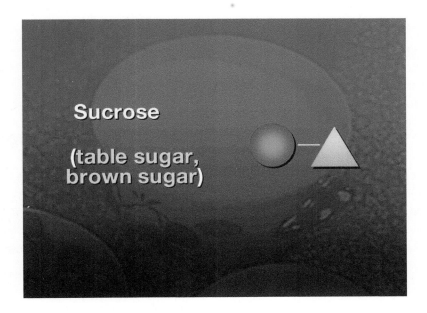

Figure 4.3

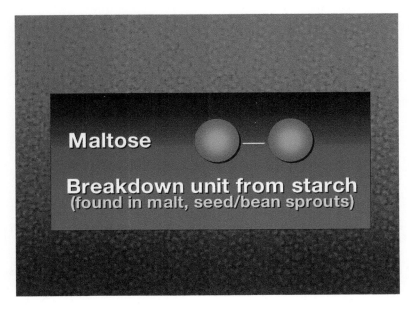

Figure 4.4

be released in your mouth (more on carbohydrate digestion later) and this tastes slightly sweet, almost nut-like. Bean and other seed sprouts contain maltose. Maltose is also added in the making of beer (malt) and is used as a flavoring agent in some foods.

- Lactose is one glucose and one galactose molecule linked together. (See Figure 4.5.) Known as milk sugar, lactose is found in dairy products, such as milk (including human breast milk), yogurt, ice cream, and cheeses. Lactose is one of the few sugars made by animals and hence, found in some animal products.

High Fructose Corn Syrup

As shown in Figure 4.6, high fructose corn syrup (often called corn syrup) is similar in composition to sucrose or regular table sugar. Corn syrup is made from corn treated with enzymes that essentially converts the starchy carbohydrate to the monosaccharides glucose and fructose.

What's Honey?

- Honey is a supersaturated solution of sugars and water made by bees from their collection of nectar from flowers. As shown in Figure 4.7, honey is a mixture of fructose, glucose and some sucrose.
- Honey versus table sugar: Gram for gram, honey is sweeter tasting because of the fructose content. Per teaspoon, honey has more calories than table sugar (23 vs. 16 calories per teaspoon). However, honey is a solution of sugars and more carbohydrate is present per teaspoon than table sugar.
- Since honey is collected from plants, it contains very small amounts of substances called antioxidants that may have health benefits. (We'll cover more on this in Chapter 9.) Research is ongoing to determine if any extra nutritional benefits result from honey. Most likely, the amounts of antioxidants are so small that a teaspoon of honey here and there in your diet provides no nutritional

Nutrition Bite

How much honey does a bee make in its lifetime? About an eighth of a teaspoon, that's all! So next time you enjoy some honey on a slice of bread, think about the effort that goes into that delicious bite.

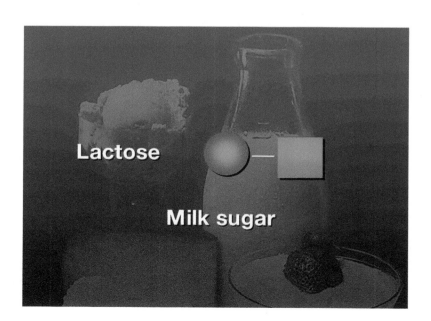

Figure 4.5

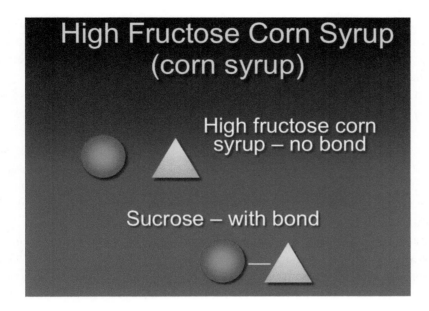

Figure 4.6

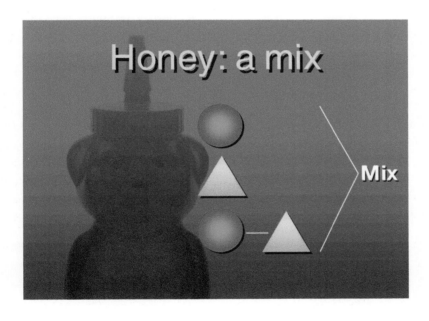

Figure 4.7

advantage over table sugar. For centuries, however, honey has been known to have healing properties that fight bacterial infection in skin wounds, such as burns and ulcers. Special compounds are present in honey from the small amounts of bee saliva that act in combating infection.

Sour on Added Sugars

We love sweets. Sugar is added to literally everything from beverages to pasta sauces. And according to new research, some people enjoy the taste of sugary treats more than others thanks to evidence that penchant for sugar may be wired in our genes. But bitter news about the impact of added sugar has been mounting. Studies show an association of sugary food and beverage intake with a host of ailments including higher rates of heart disease and Type 2 diabetes. Whether added sugar actually "causes" these conditions is hotly debated among scientists. Consuming too many calories, regardless of their source (sugar, fat, other carbs etc.), leads to obesity, which greatly ups the rates diabetes along with heart disease, certain cancers and more (more on this in chapters 6, 7, and 12.)

The Food and Drug Administration and U.S. Department of Agriculture put a cap on sugar intake—no more than 10% of total calories or about 50 grams (12½ teaspoons) of added sugar for the typical consumer eating a 2000 calories diet, well below our current consumption levels of almost 75 grams. Studies show that eating much over the recommended limit of 50 grams of added sugar daily, makes it hard to get the 50 + essential nutrients like fiber, iron, zinc and vitamin E we need for good health. Curbing empty calories from added sugar, which FDA hopes will happen with the new cap, may help obesity and diabetes rates fall.

Currently, food labels do NOT list "added sugars." Unfortunately, it's a bit of a guessing game as to how much added sugar in a serving a packaged food. "Sugar" listed on label represents both naturally occurring sugars such as lactose in milk or fructose in raisins (fruit) as well as added sugar such as sucrose or high-fructose corn syrup. The new label (fully implemented by the FDA by mid-2018) will list "Added sugar" in grams. If a food has little fruit or milk (dairy), the grams listed on the label are predominantly added sugar (see Chapter 12).

For those foods with both naturally occurring sugars and added sugars, you have to make a comparison between products to estimate. [for example: 8 oz. low-fat milk 13 grams sugar (lactose) 8 oz. chocolate low-fat milk 24 g (13 g lactose + 11 g added sugar)

Sugar and its aliases: Check the ingredient list for names of added sugars that all count toward your added sugar budget. If an added sugar is listed in top five ingredients best to look for a lower-sugar alternative as a way to improve the nutrient quality of your diet byavoiding empty calories from added sugars: *Sucrose, brown sugar, corn syrup, dextrose, fructose, high fructose corn syrup, honey, maple syrup, maple syrup, raw cane syrup/sugar.*

FOOD	GRAMS ADDED SUGAR (TEASPOONS) [1 TSP. = 4 GRAMS SUGAR]
Instant oatmeal, cinnamon, 1 packet	13 g (3)
Breakfast cereal, Frosted Mini-Wheats®, 1 oz.	12 g (3)
Jarred pasta sauce, 1.2 cup	12 g (3)
BBQ sauce, 2 T	12 g (3)
Bottled sweetened iced tea, 16 oz.	48 g (12)
Sports drink, 16 oz.	28 g (7)
Yogurt, fruit flavored	28 g (7)
Chocolate milk, 8 oz.	11 g (2.5)
Starbuck caramel macchiato, 16 oz.	16 g (4)

Intense Sweeteners

Manufacturers make diet sodas, sugar-free desserts, and sugarless candies, along with a wide array of other sugar-free products, with intense sweeteners that give the sweetness of sugar without the calories. But what are these substances and are there any health concerns about their uses?

People have used intense sweeteners, often referred to as artificial sweeteners (though some are natural compounds extracted from plants), for almost 100 years. There are several different ones currently in use today sweetening beverages, processed foods, candy, chewing gums and more. Most of these compounds are synthetically made and, due to their chemical structure, they taste 200 to over 1,000 times sweeter than regular table sugar. As a result, it requires very, very small amounts to sweeten foods and beverages. Sucralose (Splenda®), for example, is 600 times sweeter than sugar and requires only 6 milligrams (a speck!) to replace the sweetening power of a teaspoon of sugar (4,000 milligrams). Some sweeteners can be used in baking (heat stable) while others cannot and thus are only used in carbonated diet drinks. Stevia, extracted from an herb leaf, is 200 times sweeter than sugar and is used in many beverages and as a table sweetener. Even though Stevia comes from a plant leaf, the body breaks this compound down and excretes byproducts.

Once consumed in a food or beverage, some intense sweeteners pass through the body unabsorbed (ending up in stool), such as sucralose and acesulfame-K. Products that the body can further process absorb and metabolize others, such as aspartame (Nutrasweet®). Even though some intense sweeteners break down in the body, such small amounts are added to foods and beverages that there is no addition of calories.

Before a company can add an intense sweetener to foods or beverages, a detailed review by the Food and Drug Administration must take place regarding any safety concerns and health implications. The intense sweeteners in use today are some of the most heavily tested food additives, and the FDA has deemed them safe; that is, researchers have not shown that aspartame, Sucralose and others cause cancer, birth defects or other potential health problems. While the FDA has set an Acceptable Daily Limit that it advises consumers not to exceed, this amount corresponds to a large amount of sweetened beverage or food (such as 20 diet sodas in the case of aspartame.)

A question that many consumers have about using intense sweeteners is, will a person crave more sweet foods and perhaps even gain weight if she drinks and eats products with artificial sweeteners. A majority of the scientific research examining the use of intense sweeteners does not support an increased craving for sweet foods. And, in fact, researchers have shown that using intense sweeteners is an effective way for people to cut out sugar calories from their diet and even lose weight. Additionally, intense sweeteners do not bring on a rise in blood sugar levels, thus they do not aggravate the onset of Type 2 diabetes (next sections.)

3. Polysaccharides

As you might guess, polysaccharides are many simple sugars (six-carbon rings) linked together. Polysaccharides containing foods are also called **complex carbohydrates**. We will cover three polysaccharides: starch, fiber, and glycogen.

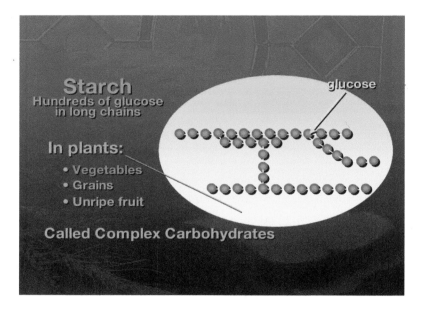

Figure 4.8

Starch

- As shown in Figure 4.8, starch is made up of hundreds of glucose units linked together in a straight chain, or a branched chain as shown.
- Starch is the most common polysaccharide in food. It comes from plant foods such as grains (wheat, rice, barley, oats), foods made with these grains (pasta, bread, muffins), and vegetables (corn, potatoes). Starch is also in unripe fruit (which you probably don't eat); during the ripening process, this starch converts to fructose, explaining the sweet flavor of fruit.

Fiber

- Shown alongside starch from a potato for comparison in Figure 4.9, fiber is also made up of hundreds of glucose units. But the linkage between glucose units is different (at a different angle than the chemical linkage in starch); this

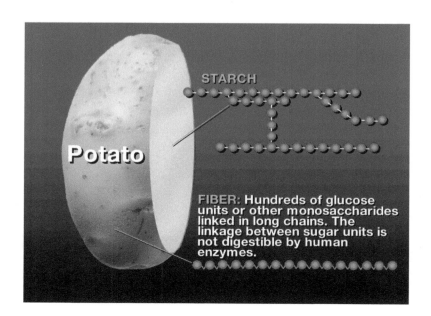

Figure 4.9

simple difference makes fiber indigestible for humans because we lack the enzyme to break this chemical bond. Since this fiber is not digested, and it is too big to be absorbed, the fiber passes through our intestines into the stool. Thus, we end up losing a source of potential energy. (This means fiber would yield calories only in the bomb calorimeter, but fiber has no physiologically available energy for you.) Despite this loss, fiber has a number of health benefits that will be discussed in another section of this chapter.

- A group of animals called ruminants can break this bond in fiber. Cows, sheep, and other ruminants can digest fiber (with the help of bacteria in their stomach, which actually makes the enzyme to do the job). These animals can get much of their nourishment from grasses and hay that contain potential energy in the sugar units because their digestive systems can break down the fiber for usable energy.
- Fiber is only found in plant products and represents the structural material in plants that makes up the cell wall. Food sources of fiber include whole grains, vegetables, and seeds in their unprocessed states. There will be more about food sources in another section.

Glycogen

- This polysaccharide **differs** from starch and fiber because it is found in living humans and mammals in their muscles and liver. Like starch, glycogen is made of hundreds of glucose units. But glycogen's glucose is arranged in a highly branched chain (Figure 4.10).
- The unique design of glycogen allows for many exposed ends that can be clipped off, yielding many glucose units in times when energy is needed such as during exercise (muscle glycogen) or in maintaining blood sugar levels (liver glycogen). Compare glycogen to starch's structure. Plants do little running (none, actually) so the structure of starch is adequate for their need of glucose for fuel to support growth. However, for humans and other mammals, the design of glycogen allows for rapid release of glucose for fuel, which enables you to run or do another intense activity (more on this later).

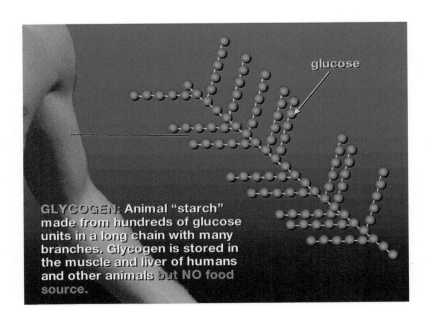

GLYCOGEN: Animal "starch" made from hundreds of glucose units in a long chain with many branches. Glycogen is stored in the muscle and liver of humans and other animals but NO food source.

glucose

Figure 4.10

- There are NO FOOD SOURCES of glycogen. Despite the fact that beef or other animal flesh may seem like a source, by the time we get it in the store, the glycogen has broken down and there is none present in the meat.
- Humans store about 1,600 calories worth of glycogen in the muscles (primarily) and the liver. This supply of carbohydrates as we will discuss in another section lasts about 24 to 36 hours in a person who is resting but not eating. This lasts only 2 to 3 hours if the person is rigorously exercising, such as running a marathon.

CARBOHYDRATE DIGESTION

In this section, we'll detail carbohydrate digestion by using a sample meal that you might consume—a glass of milk and a whole wheat bagel topped with jam (Figure 4.11).

This meal contains different carbohydrates:

- The milk contains lactose.
- The bagel contains starch and fiber.
- The jam contains sucrose. (Even though there is some fructose from the fruit, you will see this sugar requires no digestion.)

The two disaccharides (lactose and sucrose) are in fairly simple form, so for now we can ignore their digestion until they are farther down in the small intestine. At first, we'll track starch and fiber, the two polysaccharides, during digestion.

In the mouth: Saliva contains an enzyme called "salivary amylase," made by the salivary glands, that starts the process of chemical digestion of starch. (See Figure 4.12.) (The bonds that connect the glucose units in fiber, however, are left untouched.) Amylase works to break off smaller chains of starch. This chemical digestion of starch was most likely important in prehistoric times when some of the plant foods consumed took time to digest. But now, we could skip this step all together—you could swallow your bite of bagel without chewing (though a bit

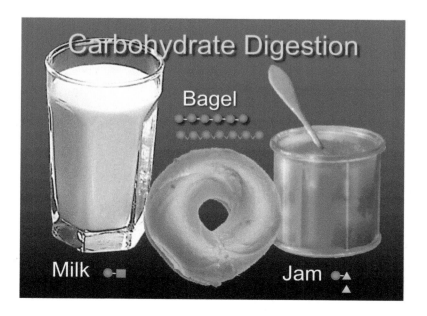

Figure 4.11

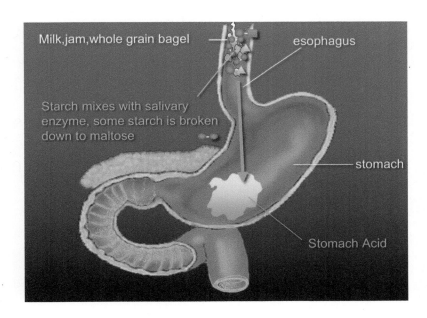

Figure 4.12

uncomfortable) and digestion would not be compromised. However, if you were to chew the bite of bagel long enough, it would start to taste mildly sweet as the maltose is released into your mouth.

In the stomach: Here, the chemical phase of digestion for starch stops because the acid in the stomach "kills" the enzyme. (Remember that enzymes are protein and proteins denature and become inactive in the stomach.) Although chemical digestion comes to a halt, physical digestion goes into full swing when the stomach makes a "smoothie" of the bagel-milk-jam meal. (See Figure 4.13.)

In the small intestine: The "smoothie" moves into the small intestine where the pancreas squirts in an enzyme called "pancreatic amylase" (the same enzyme as before, just from a different source). Chemical digestion restarts and the starch is broken down completely to maltose. As in the mouth, the bonds in fiber are not digestible so the fiber passes through untouched. (See Figure 4.14.)

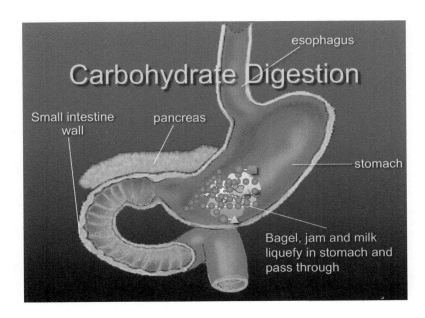

Figure 4.13

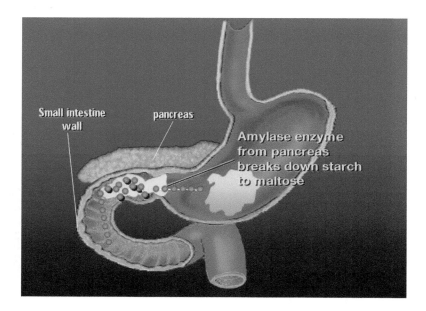

Figure 4.14

At this point, our meal has been processed into three disaccharides: maltose (from the bagel), lactose (from the milk), and sucrose (from the jam). These disaccharides, however, are still too big to be absorbed through the wall of the small intestine, therefore, more chemical digestion must occur.

On the surface of the small intestine specific enzymes are made that break apart the specific disaccharide. As shown in Figure 4.15, each disaccharide is broken down into two monosaccharides.

Maltase is the enzyme that breaks apart maltose, **sucrase** breaks apart sucrose, and lactase splits **lactose**. In the next section we'll cover issues with lactose digestion.

As noted below, the end product of carbohydrate digestion is monosaccharides. Notice that the fiber is passing through undigested and unabsorbed. (See Figure 4.16.)

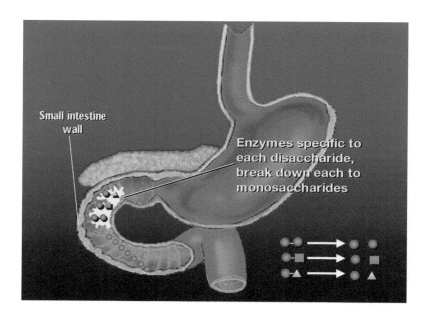

Figure 4.15

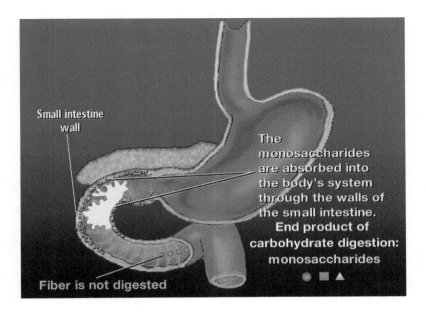

Figure 4.16

Lactose Intolerance

Some people, an estimated 10% of young adults, have limited ability to digest the milk sugar lactose. Most of these people either lack the enzyme lactase or have very little, so when a cup of milk is consumed, there is not enough lactase available to digest the milk sugar.

Trouble develops when lactose is not digested as shown in Figure 4.17. Since lactose is too big for absorption, it moves on down "the line" into the large intestine (colon). There the bacteria go to work and start digesting it and their digestion products draw water into the area. This causes bloating. Also, gas forms. Get the picture? Lots of discomfort, even diarrhea may occur.

Note that lactose intolerance is NOT an allergy to milk but rather an inability to digest milk sugar.

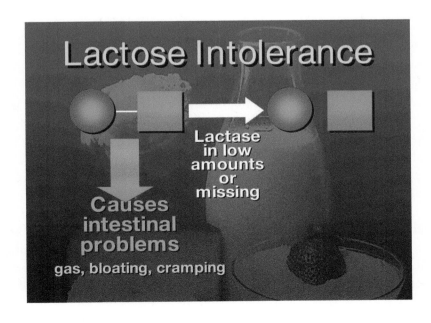

Figure 4.17

Lactose intolerance is not uncommon and appears to be more prevalent in certain cultures. The ability to digest lactose decreases with age in most mammals. For example, dogs can drink milk when they are puppies, but as adults a bowl of milk can create discomfort. Since most mammals get their nutrition as babies from mother's milk, it makes sense to have lactase. And when weaning occurs, the amount of lactase declines. This doesn't appear to happen in humans as we retain some lactase activity. People of specific ethnic backgrounds seem to have retained the lactase enzyme. Those people who have maintained dairy herds as part of their culture, such as peoples from Northern Europe, tend to have more lactase activity as adults than those who traditionally did not, such as most Asian, African, and Native American peoples.

UNDERSTANDING THE POWER OF FIBER

No doubt you have heard before to get more fiber in your diet because it is good for your health. Studies show that people who eat ample fiber in their diet have lower risk for certain cancers and heart disease, and can assist weight loss compared to people who eat a low-fiber diet. But you have also learned that fiber is not digestible. So technically, fiber does not get into your circulation. How could it be that an indigestible substance can have such powerful health benefits?

Let's take a look at fiber: what it is, fiber types, and its health benefits.

What Is Fiber?

- Fiber is only in plants.
- Fiber is the structural material in plants such as the cell wall.
- Fiber is not digestible by human enzymes.
- Fiber does contain potential energy, but this energy is NOT available to us.

There are two fiber types with distinct properties in the intestinal tract that relate directly to their health benefits.

1. Water-Insoluble Fiber

- In technical terms this fiber type is called cellulose and hemi-cellulose. (Both are much like wood sawdust or the stringy material from celery and other vegetables.)
- Food sources of water-insoluble fiber include the outer husk or shell of wheat grain kernels (bran layers) and vegetables (especially the skins and peels).
- When water-insoluble fiber comes in contact with water (such as in your intestinal tract that is a very watery environment), it swells up. Think about a bowl of bran cereal—pour milk on it and the cereal swells as the little pieces of cereal absorb and hold water rather than dissolving.
- This "water holding" characteristic of water-insoluble fiber is key in your intestinal tract. As it moves through your intestines, it holds water and bulks up. This larger bulk swells, pushing against the intestinal wall, causing the muscle of the colon to "push back." (Just think of yourself in a line for a concert and someone pushes on you as the crowd swells; you push back and hold your ground, right? Well, so does your intestinal tract.)

- This pushing helps speed the passage of waste through the intestinal tract, which, in effect, tones or "works out" the muscles of the intestinal tract. As the waste moves through, it does so with ease and exits the body easily as soft, bulky stool. Ultimately, this process avoids constipation, or the straining of a bowel movement.
- From this action comes several health benefits. Let's take a look at what happens if you eat a low-fiber diet and its consequences to understand the benefits of an ample fiber intake.

Figure 4.18 shows a comparison of a large intestine while on a low-fiber diet and a large intestine on an ample fiber intake.

Low-Fiber Diet

- With a low-fiber intake, there is not much mass of waste material to move through. This smaller amount of waste moves through the intestinal tract slowly, allowing more time for the body to pull water out, making it even smaller, harder, and drier.
- This hard, compact dry stool is difficult to move or evacuate. Thus, it will take some "effort" to expel this waste. If you have to strain or apply effort to have a bowel movement, you are constipated. Constipation is NOT about the number of times you have a bowel movement—once a day, or once every other day. Constipation is about having to "work" at it.
- If constipation is a regular occurrence, this frequent straining can put pressure on the blood vessels that are at the anus (the opening) and ultimately leads to the formation of **hemorrhoids**—varicose veins (bulging, swollen vessels) that become very painful.
- In addition, when this hard, dry, and slow-moving material sits in the intestines, it can lead to other health problems, such as **diverticulitis**—when the lining of the colon wall becomes inflamed and forms small pouches as shown in Figure 4.19. It is possible that these small out-pockets may burst and infiltrate the intestinal cavity with waste material, which can lead to acute medical problems. (See Figure 4.20.)

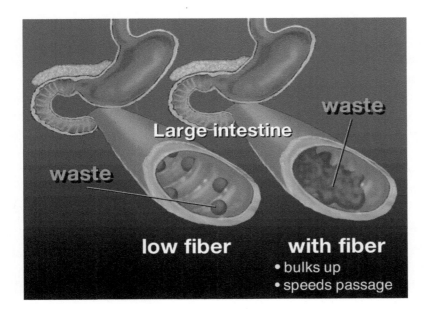

Figure 4.18

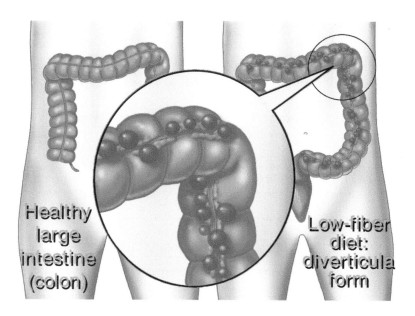

Figure 4.19

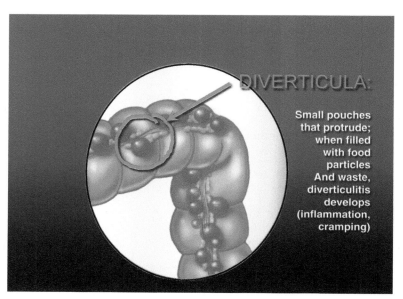

Figure 4.20

- Another problem with a low-fiber diet is that this waste material most likely contains cancer-causing agents (often referred to as carcinogens). Slow movement of waste through the colon increases exposure time of the large intestinal wall to these harmful substances may lead to cancer of the large intestine (cancer of the colon) years down the road—a serious form of cancer that is linked to a low-fiber diet.

High-Fiber Diet

Take a look at the low-fiber versus high-fiber diagram in Figure 4.19 again, and let's see what health benefits stem from getting ample fiber in your diet.

- The mass of waste material is larger and softer in the higher fiber situation. As a result, this mass moves through faster, and you don't have to strain to have a bowel movement.

HERE'S THE DIETARY FIBER CONTENT OF VARIOUS FOODS

FOOD, SERVING SIZE	GRAMS FIBER / SERVING
Rice Krispies	0
White bread, 1 slice	1
100% wheat bread, 1 slice	3
Broccoli, 1 cup	2
Carrot, 7″	2
Prunes, 5 each	3
Steel cut oats, cooked, 1 cup	5
Banana, 1 large, 9″ long	4
Raisin bran cereal, 1 cup	4
Apple, 1 large, 4″ diameter	4
Bagel, whole grain	6
Artichoke	7
Lentil soup, 1 cup	7
Kidney beans, 1 cup	8
Soy burger on whole wheat bun, 1 each	8
Vegetable chili, 1 cup	13
Fiber One Cereal—½ cup	14
Fast-Food • McDonald's Quarter Pounder • Taco Bell bean burrito, 1	 2 13

- Bottom line, you have a reduced chance of becoming constipated.
- This in turn means lower risk of developing hemorrhoids and diverticulitis.
- Since material doesn't sit for long, any potential carcinogens have little time for contact with the intestinal wall, and the potentially harmful substances become effectively diluted with the larger mass of waste material. Additionally, the fiber can bind carcinogens, preventing their entry into the body. Studies also show that bacteria ferment fibers in the large intestine and thereby products of fermentation may inhibit cancer growth. All this results in a lower risk of colon cancer in a diet that provides ample fiber from fruits, vegetables, beans, and whole grains rather than from fiber supplements.

2. Water-Soluble Fiber

- This fiber type is called gums and pectins in technical terms. (You may notice gums and pectins on the ingredient list for some foods, such as jams.)

- Food sources of water-soluble fiber include fruits, beans (kidney, black, pinto, and other beans), and oats.
- When water-soluble fiber comes in contact with water or other liquids, such as milk (or your intestinal juices), it forms a gel. (Think of a bowl of oatmeal that has sat for awhile; it becomes gel-like and holds a shape.)
- In your intestinal tract, this gel property helps to slow the emptying of your stomach content into the small intestines. This slowing may help you feel full longer (reduce your hunger levels) and studies show this fiber type may help with weight loss.
- Water-soluble fiber's gel-like quality also works to lower circulating cholesterol (a fatty, waxy substance covered in the next chapter) absorption in the body. This fiber "traps" cholesterol from your food or cholesterol by-products that are recycled in the intestinal tract. More on this will be covered in Chapter 6 when heart disease is covered.
- Once bound to the fiber, cholesterol is no longer available for absorption and it leaves the body in the stool with the fiber. This action effectively lowers your circulating level of cholesterol. As covered in Chapter 6, high blood cholesterol is a risk factor for heart disease.

Soluble fibers also slow the rate at which the stomach empties its contents into the small intestine, which slows glucose absorption as well as helping you feel full longer. This means a more gradual release of glucose into the bloodstream and subsequently more steady blood sugar control. Soluble fibers may assist with Type 1 diabetes control (see next section).

The health benefits of water-soluble fiber are:

- Helps to reduce appetite and control the feeling of hunger after a meal
- Lowers blood cholesterol level
- Lowers heart disease risk
- Lowers Type 2 diabetes risk

How Much Fiber Do You Need?

For starters, you need both types of fiber in your diet. Although some food sources of fiber may have more of one fiber type than another, wheat bran (water insoluble) and oat bran (water soluble) for example, most unrefined fruits, vegetables, beans, and grains supply both fiber types.

The Dietary Reference Intake (DRI) for fiber has been established for men and women and is based on 14 grams for every 1,000 calories eaten:

38 grams / day for men
25 grams / day for women

This amount of fiber should be averaged over several days and include a mix of fibers from a variety fruits, vegetables, beans, and whole grains. The less processed or refined the food, the greater the fiber content as milling grains along with various cooking techniques can reduce the fiber content.

How much fiber do you take in daily? Your Diet Project assignment will reveal how you stand compared to your needs. The average American gets only 15 grams of fiber daily. This low intake may help explain why many suffer from chronic ailments, such as heart disease and obesity-related health problems.

Note that some foods contain what's called **functional fiber**, which represents fibers that, added to foods, have health benefits. Functional fiber may represent insoluble or soluble fibers extracted from plants or manufactured.

Fiber on Food Labels

The Food and Drug Administration has established a Daily Value for fiber based on the typical consumer of age 4 or older eating 2,000 calories per day.

Daily Value = 25 grams fiber/day from a mix of fibers

Listed on the food label, as shown in Figure 4.21, is the amount of fiber in a serving of the specific food and the percent Daily Value (DV) that this represents.

You calculate the percent DV for a breakfast cereal. Is your calculated value listed the same as the label?

$$\frac{4 \text{ grams fiber}}{25 \text{ grams fiber}} \times 100 = 16\% \text{ DV}$$

CARBOHYDRATE ENERGY METABOLISM

Time to go back now to our meal of milk, a whole wheat bagel, and jam and let's see what happens to the carbohydrate in these foods. After digestion, the end products were the individual monosaccharides—glucose, galactose, and fructose. We'll now track how these monosaccharides, once absorbed into the body, are used for energy.

As shown in Figure 4.22, the three monosaccharides make a brief stop at the liver. There fructose and galactose are converted into glucose. Glucose is the basic "currency" of energy in the body. When someone says "my blood sugar" is low, glucose is the "sugar" they are talking about. As glucose travels through the circulation for uptake into cells, such as muscle cells, it will then use this glucose for fuel or store it for later use.

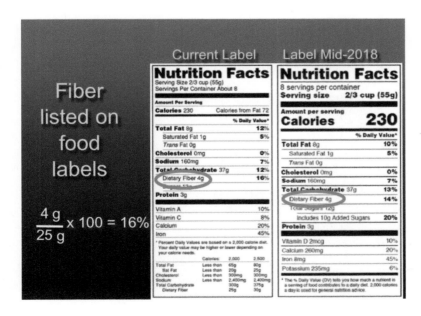

Figure 4.21

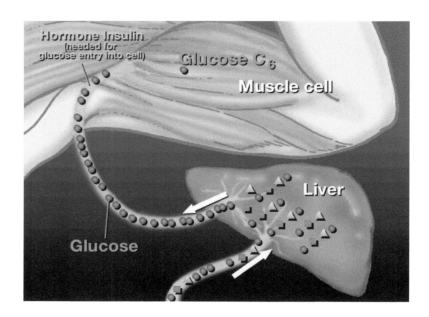

Figure 4.22

However, the glucose must "get permission" to enter the cell. Glucose entry into most cells requires the hormone **insulin** made by the pancreas. Insulin is much like a monitor in a school that "knocks" on the "door" (cell receptor) of a cell for the door to open up and let glucose in as shown in Figure 4.23.

Once the cell recognizes that glucose is seeking entry, the "door" opens up and glucose marches inside for the cell for use. (See Figure 4.24.)

This process of glucose entry into cells does not occur that smoothly for some individuals. Unfortunately, some people do not make insulin; they are people with Type 1 diabetes and must take a replacement of insulin via an injection (or use of a pump) that puts insulin directly into the circulation. If insulin is lacking, the glucose accumulates in the bloodstream as shown in Figure 4.25. This pileup of glucose wreaks havoc on the body by damaging blood vessel walls, which leads to poor circulation, heart disease, and loss of eyesight (see Figure 4.26).

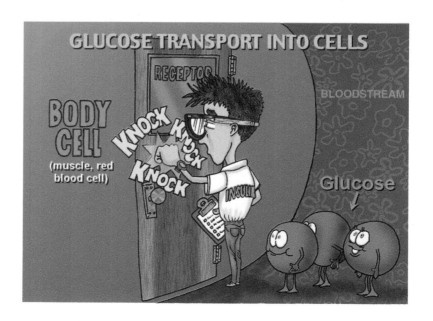

Figure 4.23

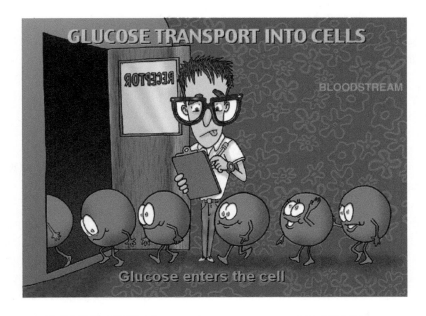

Figure 4.24

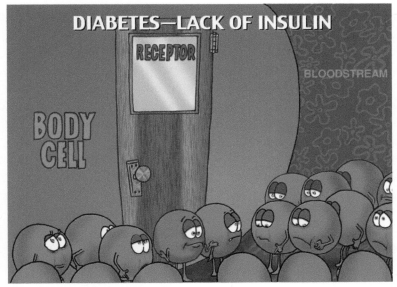

Figure 4.25

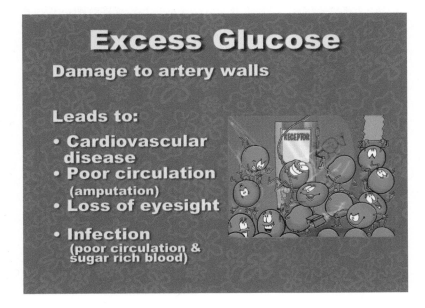

Figure 4.26

There is another form of diabetes, which actually represents about 90% of the diabetes in the United States. Called Type 2 diabetes, this condition is hallmarked by insulin that does not work very effectively; that is, the cell does not "hear" the insulin "knocking," as shown in Figure 4.27. Since glucose is not getting access into the cells, the pancreas secretes more insulin so that glucose may enter the cell. But in the meantime, glucose accumulates and causes the same devastation on the body as Type 1 diabetes. Millions of Americans suffer from Type 2 diabetes, primarily due to a lack of exercise and obesity, which directly impacts the cell receptors to be less sensitive to insulin. The American Diabetes Association estimates 17 million Americans have been diagnosed with diabetes. Unfortunately, another 7 million people are unaware that they have the disease.

Once glucose does enter the cell, it has an opportunity (depending upon the body's need for immediate energy) to be used as fuel or to be stored as glycogen.

Let's take a look at carbohydrate storage first. As shown in Figure 4.28, glucose enters a muscle cell. (Recall that glucose has six carbons—C_6—which becomes an important detail for later when we look at glucose's use as an energy source.) Hundreds of glucose units can be strung in branched chains called **glycogen**, which is **the body's storage form of carbohydrate**. We learned about glycogen in our discussion of carbohydrate structure.

Most of the body's glycogen is stored in the muscles. Some glycogen is also stored in the liver (about ¼ to ⅓ of the total carbohydrate stored in the body). Liver glycogen is a vital source of glucose for the bloodstream when you haven't eaten for a while. Also, recall that your brain relies on glucose for fuel. If blood sugar levels start to fall below normal, the pancreas sends a hormone signal to the liver to release glucose units from its stored glycogen.

The glycogen in the muscle serves that specific muscle as glucose storage. All told, the body can store about 1,600 calories of glycogen in the muscles. You can tuck away even more if you are physically fit and have been doing some endurance training such as running. As we'll see, storing more glucose energy makes sense because it is used during exercise. A fit person can store a few hundred extra calories worth of glucose as glycogen (a loaf of bread's worth of carbohydrate all together).

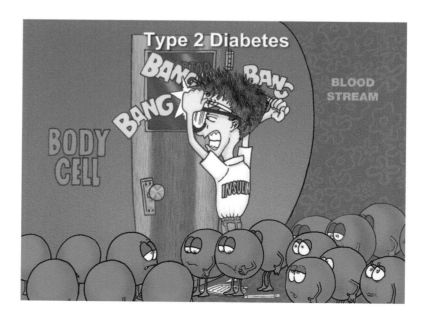

Figure 4.27

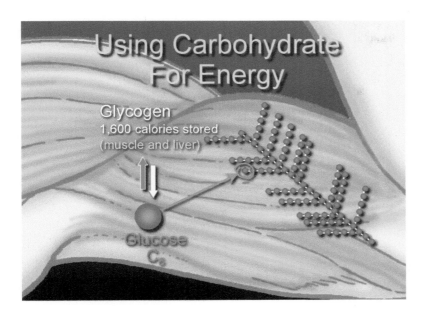

Figure 4.28

Now let's take a look at glucose being used as fuel by the muscle. (See Figure 4.29.) Glycogen can be broken back down into glucose or, the glucose enters the cell and is immediately used as a fuel source.

Glucose is a six-carbon molecule and in this first step, glucose is broken in half to release the potential energy out of these chemical bonds and give two three carbon units—C_3. (While it is shown in Figure 4.30 as one step, it actually takes a series of reactions to yield these three carbon units.)

There is something very special about this breakdown of glucose (C_6) to C_3 units for energy. Unlike the breakdown of fat and protein for fuel, glucose can be broken down for fuel WITHOUT oxygen (you'll learn about this in the next chapter). This type of energy metabolism for carbohydrate is called **anaerobic**, which means "without oxygen."

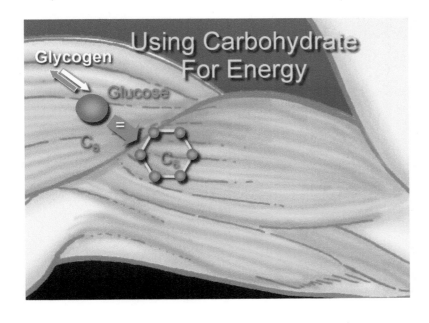

Figure 4.29

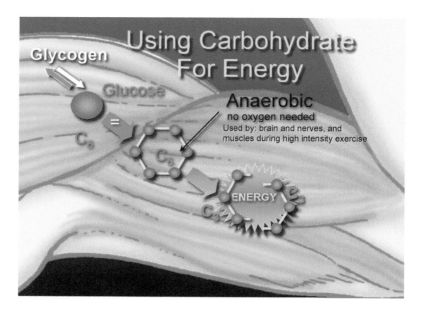

Figure 4.30

- The brain and central nervous system use glucose for fuel anaerobically.
- There are also times when your body needs energy but little if any oxygen is present. During intense exercise for example, this breakdown of glucose for fuel provides immediate energy for hardworking muscles. The muscles, however, can only sustain this anaerobic energy metabolism for a short period of time—less than a few minutes—due to the accumulation of substances that hamper muscle contraction. The body must then slow down and take in oxygen for the further breakdown of glucose.

There is still more potential energy in the three carbon—C_3—units that can be released. These next steps however require the presence of oxygen. This process is called **aerobic** energy metabolism. As shown in Figure 4.31, oxygen is used when C_3 units are broken down to C_2 units and their carbon (C) is released as carbon dioxide—CO_2 and exhaled from the lungs. Since chemical bonds are broken, energy

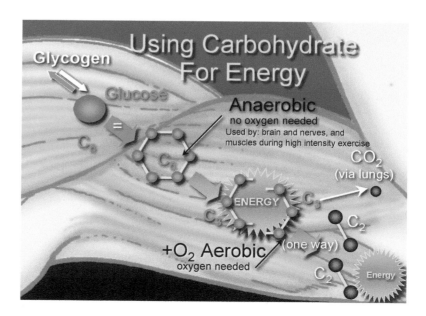

Figure 4.31

is released, which is used by the cells such as the muscle to drive contraction or carry out another metabolic processes, such as building new protein.

- An important side note: The step of $C_3 \rightarrow C_2$ is a one-way process (as noted by the one-way bold arrow). This means that once C_2 is made, the reverse process cannot occur. This fact becomes important when we discuss how the body resorts to making glucose when stores have run out.

There is still potential energy left in the C_2 units—right? (This means a chemical bond at least connecting the two carbons.) The body recognizes this and would not let this potential energy go to waste. Aerobic energy metabolism continues as shown in Figure 4.32 and the C_2 units are completely broken down for fuel and the carbon is released as CO_2. This, as in the previous step, is blown off via the lungs. In addition to CO_2, water is made during the aerobic energy metabolism when the C_2 units completely break apart and energy is released. This process of breaking down C_2 units for energy, while shown here as "one" step is actually several biochemical reactions and is collectively called the Tri-Carboxylic Acid (TCA) cycle. (You may learn about this energy metabolism cycle in another class.) As you will see in the next chapter, this cycle is the same cycle for the energy metabolism of fats and protein.

Now carbohydrate energy metabolism is complete.

- The end products of carbohydrate energy metabolism are:

$$\text{Energy (4 calories/gram of carbohydrate)} + CO_2 + H_2O$$

Carbohydrate Excess

During anaerobic and aerobic carbohydrate energy metabolism, energy is released for the cells to use. But what if you ate more carbohydrate than what your body needed for fuel at the time? Let's say you overate at your bagel meal and had a few bagels with lots of jam or a couple glasses of milk. If the body didn't need the fuel and glycogen stores are filled, what would happen to this potential energy?

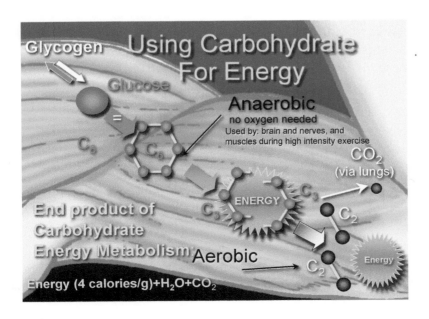

Figure 4.32

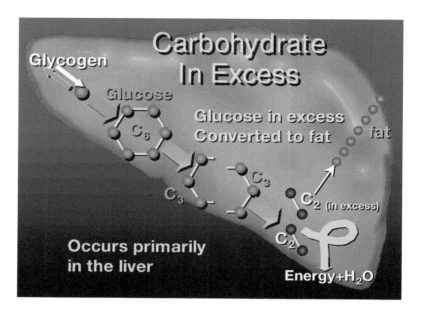

Figure 4.33

Various metabolic signals go into place to tell the liver that excess carbohydrate energy is present. The liver takes the C_2 units and strings them together to build a fat (technically called a fatty acid) as shown in Figure 4.33.

The potential energy that was in the C_2 units has now been transformed into another molecule that contains potential energy—fat. This fat is packaged up into a carrier and then sent off into the circulation for eventual storage into fat cells. (This will be covered in detail in the next chapter.)

- So in the end, **carbohydrate eaten in excess of energy needs is converted to and stored as fat**.

Carbohydrate "Deficiency"

Up to this point, we have discussed the use of carbohydrate for fuel. What if carbohydrate is lacking in the diet, or at least inside the cell? What does the body do in this case since carbohydrate fuel is specifically necessary for the brain and central nervous system to function? Also, muscles rely on glucose during high-intensity exercise. Additionally, other cells in the body use only glucose for fuel, such as red blood cells, so there is a specific reliance on carbohydrate in the body.

The following are situations when a "deficiency" of carbohydrate may occur:

- During a fast, when a person has not been eating anything for 24–36 hours or more
- During a very low carbohydrate diet such as popular weight-loss diets (Atkin's diet) that emphasize protein consumption
- When insulin is lacking so that glucose does not get into cells (the cell is essentially "starving" for glucose fuel despite the fact there is plenty in the bloodstream), which may occur in a diabetic who is not taking replacement insulin.

The first action taken by the body is to break down any stored glycogen for glucose fuel. The glycogen in the muscle serves that specific muscle. The glycogen

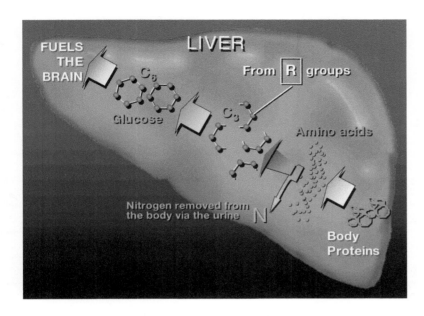

Figure 4.34

in the liver supplies the blood with glucose, which is in turn where the brain gets this sugar.

But stores of glycogen run out in about 24 to 36 hours. Usually liver glycogen runs out in less than 24 hours. If you are exercising, the use of glucose is greater so the glycogen stores may run out in two to four hours.

With stores of glucose depleted, the body must resort to making its own glucose because the brain MUST have glucose for fuel. As shown in Figure 4.34, the process of making glucose occurs in the liver and involves breaking down protein for conversion into glucose.

Hormonal signals that alert the body to this "no glucose" situation stimulate body proteins, such as those in muscle and elsewhere, to break down into individual amino acids and then get shuttled to the liver. As you may recall from Chapter 2, each of the 20 amino acids has a unique R group, and it's this R group that comes to the rescue. The nitrogen is pulled off each of the amino acids and excreted in the urine as urea. The remaining carbon skeletons, which contains the R groups, have the option of being converted into glucose.

Here's How It Works

- If the R group chemically "looks" enough like C_3 it gets converted into a C_3 unit.
- This C_3 unit combines with another C_3 unit to make a glucose.
- This glucose then gets shuttled out into the bloodstream and can fuel the "hungry" brain.
- This process, called gluconeogenesis, is very costly to the body because vital proteins are used at the expense of making glucose. But this must happen since the brain needs carbohydrates for fuel.
- Also, this process of making glucose can only supply enough glucose fuel for the brain's central nervous systems and red blood cell's energy use, but not enough to restock glycogen stores so that a person can go run a marathon or do an extended session of exercise.

HERE IS THE CARBOHYDRATE CONTENT OF COMMON FOODS

FOOD, SERVING SIZE	GRAMS OF CARBOHYDRATE / SERVING
Low-fat milk, 1 cup	13
Sports drink, 1 cup	15
Peach, 1 medium	17
Crackers, Triscuit (7 ea)	21
Cereal, cornflakes, 1 cup	24
Apple, 1 large	32
Banana, 1 large	36
Quinoa, 1 cup	40
Energy bar (Clif)	42
Rice, white long grain, 1 cup	45
Baked potato, 1 medium	51
Beans, barbeque, 1 cup	50
Fast-Food • McDonald's french fries • Pizza Hut, pepperoni, medium 12″, 1 slice	 46 21

- If the R group is not chemically similar to C_3, it is converted to C_2 units and used for fuel in the TCA cycle (not pictured). This means that not all the amino acids get converted to glucose, which is another reason why this process of converting protein to glucose is so costly—you lose 2 grams of amino acids for every gram of glucose you make.

Need for Carbohydrate

So during a fast, high-protein/low-carb diet, or without insulin if you are diabetic, your body loses functional protein tissue (muscle, enzymes, and other body proteins).

- To prevent this protein breakdown, some carbohydrate is needed in the diet—about 130 grams of carbohydrate is necessary each day.
- For optimal health, the Food and Nutrition Board suggests between 45 to 65 percent of calories come from a variety of carbohydrates (whole grains, vegetables and fruit). The Food and Drug Administration (the government agency in charge of food labels) has set the **Daily Value for carbohydrate at 300 grams**. This amounts to 55% of the calories for a typical consumer eating 2,000 calories per day.

Key Points about Carbohydrate Energy Metabolism

Let's review carbohydrate energy metabolism because grasping this will assist you in the next chapter when energy metabolism of carbohydrates, protein, and fats is integrated.

- Glucose (from a meal) can be stored as glycogen in the muscles and liver. (See Figure 4.35.) Glycogen stores lasts about 24 to 36 hours if you are at rest, or about 2 to 3 hours if you are exercising.

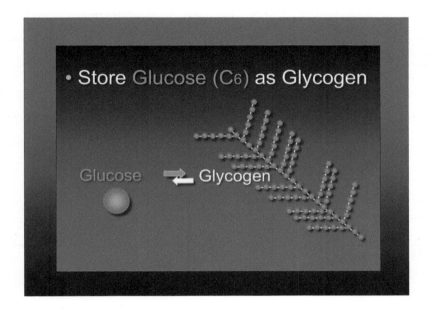

Figure 4.35

- Glucose can be broken down as an energy source in the absence of oxygen (anaerobically). (See Figure 4.36.) This process is especially important for the brain and central nervous system. Also, during intense exercise, anaerobic carbohydrate energy metabolism is vital. Fat and protein cannot be utilized this way.

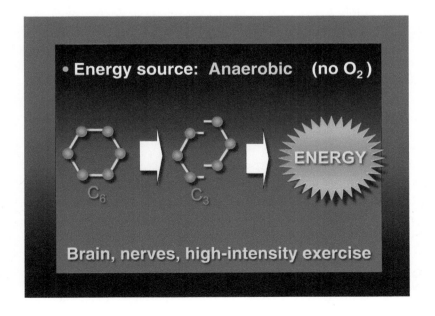

Figure 4.36

Figure 4.37

- In the presence of oxygen, glucose can be broken down completely to release 4 calories per gram of energy, water is made and CO_2 is released. (See Figure 4.37.) If carbohydrates are eaten in excess, glucose is broken down to C_2 units and converted to and stored as fat.

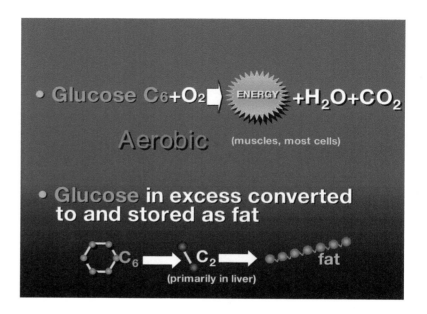

- In the absence of dietary carbohydrate (or when insulin is lacking as in Type 1 diabetes), glycogen stores are depleted; thus, glucose must be made so that the brain can function. Glucose is made from protein, which is broken down into amino acids, which in turn are converted to glucose. (The nitrogen is excreted in the urine.) Making glucose from protein means a loss of functional tissue. (See Figure 4.38.)

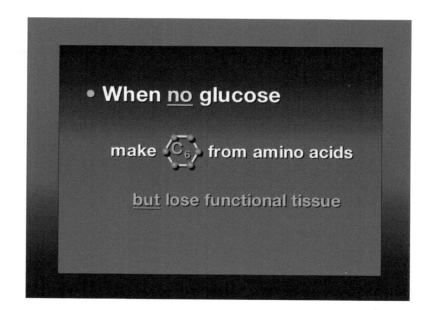

Figure 4.38

Quiz Yourself

4

CHAPTER

List good food sources of

- Insoluble fiber _____
- Glycogen _____
- Lactose _____
- Polysaccharide _____
- Disaccharide _____
- Simple sugar _____
- Water-soluble fiber _____

1. The major monosaccharide found in the body is:

   a. glucose
   b. fructose
   c. galactose
   d. sucrose
   e. maltose

2. The *storage* form of carbohydrate in the body is:

   a. glucose
   b. cholesterol
   c. glycogen
   d. fat
   e. glycoprotein

3. What is the percent Daily Value for fiber in 1 bean burrito with 8 grams of fiber?

4. Describe the two types of fiber, give their actions in the intestine, health enefits, and list a food source for each.

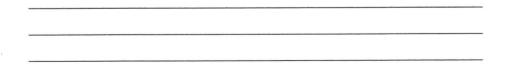

   _____

   _____

   _____

   _____

5. What is lactose intolerance?

_____

_____

_____

6. Describe what happens when carbohydrate is eaten in excess of energy needs.

_____

_____

_____

7. How many calories are released during the aerobic energy metabolism of carbohydrate?

a. 2 calories/g

b. 4 calories/g

c. 6 calories/g

d. 9 calories/g

8. What is diabetes?

_____

_____

_____

9. How long do glycogen stores last for a person who is inactive but not eating?

a. 1 hour

b. 12 hours

c. 24–36 hours

FAT—THE MISUNDERSTOOD NUTRIENT

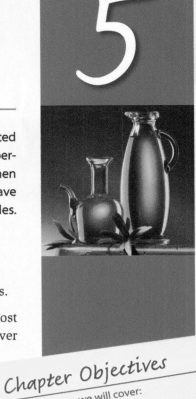

5

No doubt you have thoughts about "fat" already. Most likely you have contemplated cutting back on fat in your diet, or perhaps you view fats as "bad" in general. Your perspective on fats may change after reading this chapter. Fats are not created equal when it comes to your health. While this nutrient *is* vital in your diet, certain types of fats have a negative impact on your health, while other fat types are essential for a variety of roles.

THE FUNCTION OF FAT

Like protein and carbohydrate, fat performs all three basic functions of nutrients.

1. **Energy:** Fat supplies 9 calories/gram and is an excellent energy source. Most Americans eat about a third of their calories from fat—this translates to over 270,000 calories in fat per year or 6,000 teaspoons of fat! As we will discuss in future chapters, high-fat diets are linked with chronic diseases, such as heart disease and cancer.

2. **Regulation:** Fat performs numerous regulatory roles in the body mediating a number of processes. An example is hormones. Some hormones, notably the sex hormones testosterone and estrogen, are made from fat and cholesterol.

3. **Structure:** Fat serves the body a number of ways as a structural nutrient. Fat surrounding organs, such as the kidneys, help protect and cushion them from shock. Fat is also a very important component in the structure of cell membranes. As we will discuss in a later section, certain fats make up cell membranes and give the membrane its fluid characteristic and ability to serve as a selective barrier. This presence of fat in every single cell of your body means that you could never get rid of all your body fat even if you tried extreme dieting and exercising—about 3 to 4 percent of your body weight is fat in this capacity.

Chapter Objectives

In this chapter, we will cover:

- The function of fat
- Fat types and food sources
- Essential fats and their role in health
- Fat in foods: processing and fat replacements (fat-free foods)

- Fat digestion and transport
- Fat energy metabolism
- Bringing it all together—energy metabolism (protein, carbohydrate, and fat)
- Cholesterol—its vital roles and transport in the body

FAT TYPES AND FOOD SOURCES

Let's examine fat's chemical structure in food fat, such as butter or a vegetable oil, as well as fat from a person (let's say fat has been "sucked" out and is in a bowl). The chemical structure is the same in all three examples. All three of these fat examples consist of **triglycerides**—the basic unit of fats.

The triglyceride shown in Figure 5.1 consists of **fatty acids** on a three-carbon backbone (called glycerol). For now, we are going to "pluck" off the fatty acids from the glycerol and take a look at these to understand their structure and characteristics.

Fatty Acids

There are two categories of fatty acids—saturated and unsaturated. It is the difference between these two categories that explains why butter is solid, olive oil is liquid at room temperature, and fish oil stays liquid even in icy cold temperatures. Fatty acids are long chains of carbon that are typically even in number and range from about 4 carbons to 26 carbons long (with 16 and 18 carbons in length being the most common fatty acid length in foods).

1. **Saturated Fatty Acids**
    *   "Saturated" means that each carbon is fully saturated with hydrogen atoms (recall that each carbon must bond four times to a neighboring element). The particular fatty acid in Figure 5.2 has 16 carbons and is called palmitic acid. Palm oil, a type of tropical fat from palm kernels and used in snack foods and cookies, consists of triglycerides with many of their fatty acids as palmitic acid.
    *   Notice below the C–H structure of palmitic acid in Figure 5.2 is a simplified drawing of this fatty acid that reflects the characteristic of this fatty acid—straight and stiff like a piece of wood. Thus, on the triglycerides, the saturated fatty acids tend to align themselves and stack up to form a solid fat at

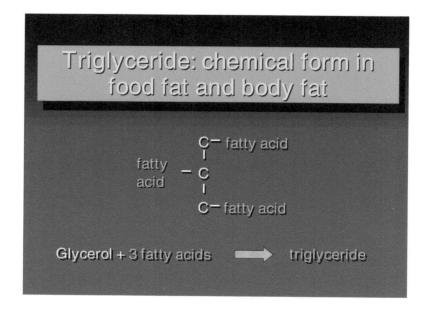

Figure 5.1

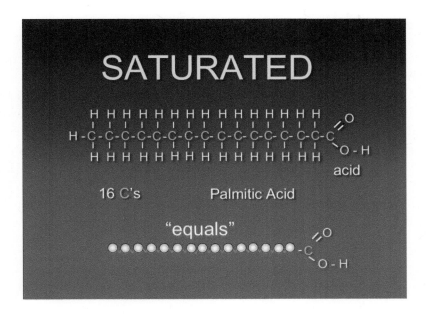

Figure 5.2

room temperature. If a food fat (triglycerides) has predominately saturated fatty acids, then it is **SOLID** at room temperature.

- Saturated fatty acids have an even number of carbons, such as 6, 12, and up to 26 carbons.
- The most common saturated fatty acids are palmitic acid (16C), and stearic acid (18C). (*Note:* The number indicates the number of carbon atoms.)

2. **Unsaturated Fatty Acids**
   - Notice in Figure 5.3 that compared to the saturated fatty acid, two hydrogens are missing. Thus, the fatty acid is not fully "saturated" with hydrogen, or **unsaturated**. These carbons still must maintain the four-bond rule, so they end up bonding twice with each other. The chemical bond between the two carbons is called a **carbon-carbon double bond (C = C)**, which characterizes the unsaturated fatty acid. The fatty acid in Figure 5.3 is called oleic acid and is the predominate fatty acid found on the triglyceride from olive oil.

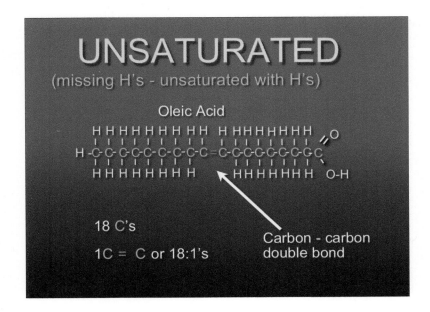

Figure 5.3

- Another way to represent this fatty acid is "18:1," which reflects the number of C atoms: number of C=C bonds. "18:1 fatty acid has 18 carbon atoms and one C=C bond and is called a monounsaturated fatty acid ("mono" means one).

- Let's take a look at how this double bond changes the property of the fatty acid. As shown in Figure 5.4 in the simplified drawing of the fatty acid, the double bond puts a bend or crimp in the strand of carbons. This changes everything. Now the triglycerides with these unsaturated fatty acids do not stack up neatly and increases movement which causes the fatty acids to be **LIQUID** at room temperature.

- Unsaturated fatty acids with more than one C=C bond are called polyunsaturated fatty acids. (Generally, fatty acids have no more than six C=C bonds.) (See Figure 5.5.)

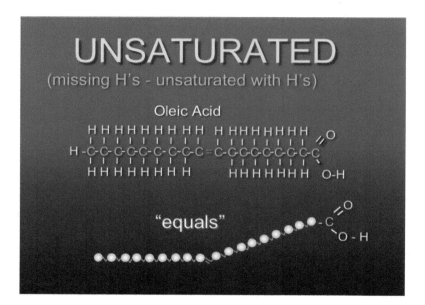

Figure 5.4

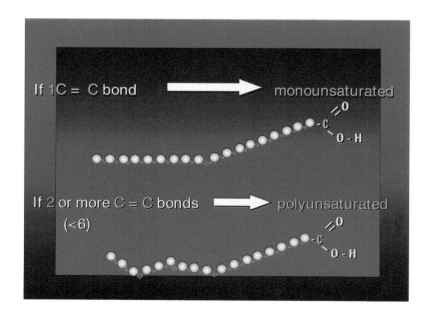

Figure 5.5

- The placement of the C=C bond is very important. In oleic acid, the C=C bond is in the "9" position; that is, it is 9 carbons in from the left. Your body, primarily in the liver, makes fatty acids and can make oleic acid if it wants. The body cannot make C=C bonds in the "3" and "6" positions. However, these resulting fatty acids have vital roles in the body, which makes them **essential fatty acids**. You must eat a dietary source of these fats that have essential fatty acids as components of their triglycerides.

  Figure 5.6 illustrates the common unsaturated fats and lists their food sources.

Notice that the two essential fats—18:2 linoleic (18 C's and 2 C=C bonds) and 18:3 linolenic (18 C's and 3 C=C bonds)—have an even more crimped structure. This imparts an even more "liquid" nature to these fats. Linolenic (18:3) is an essential fat found in flaxseed meal and oil, and a slightly longer version is found in fish, especially cold-water fish. This fatty acid is also called omega-3 fat. With the extra C=C bond, this fatty acid is very liquid at room temperature, and in cold seawater it doesn't solidify. (Just think, if fish did have monounsaturated or saturated fatty acids as part of their bodies, the fish would be "stiff as a board" and find it impossible to swim!)

ESSENTIAL FATS AND THEIR ROLE IN HEALTH

These vital fats are needed for important roles in the body—cell membrane structure and prostaglandin formation.

1. **Cell membrane structure**

   As shown in Figure 5.7, the cell membrane is made up of two layers of fatty acids (referred to as a "lipid bilayer"). Essential fats are components of this layer and allow the cell membrane to have a very fluid character while at the same time serving as a barrier.

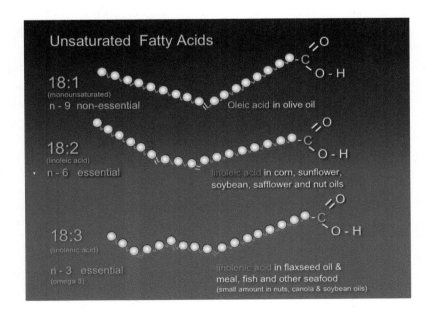

Figure 5.6

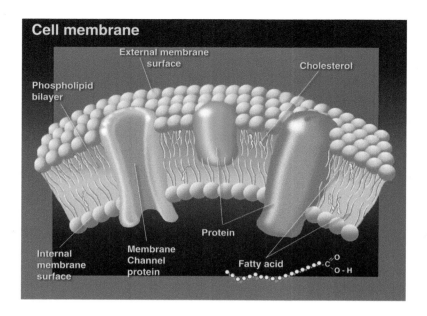

Figure 5.7

2. **Prostaglandin formation**

Essential fats are converted to a series of substances called prostaglandins, which act much like hormones in specific locations in the body such as in blood vessels and in the uterus, mediating blood clot formation and uterine contractions (during menstrual bleeding). Prostaglandins also mediate the inflammatory response such as with swelling from an injury. The aspirin that you might take to ease the pain actually works against certain prostaglandins to lessen the inflammation.

How Much Essential Fatty Acid Do You Need?

- **Linoleic 18:2**—We need 12 to 17 grams or 5 to 10 percent of our total calories from this fat or about three teaspoons of corn oil daily. Most Americans easily get this amount from a variety of foods that contain vegetable oils.
- **Linolenic 18:3**—We need 1.1 to 1.6 grams or about 1 percent of our total calories as omega-3 fat daily. This would mean eating fish (a 3–4 ounce serving) a few times per week; something most Americans don't do. Researchers feel that we fall short on our intake of this essential fatty acid. In fact, we have an imbalance of 18:2 to 18:3 fats, which may contribute to the development of age-related diseases such as heart disease and certain cancers. The theory is that the imbalance of essential fats creates changes in the cell membrane and prostaglandin profile in the body that promotes these chronic diseases. (See Chapter 12 for specific dietary recommendations for fish intake.)

What Happens If You Have a Deficiency of Essential Fatty Acids?

Essential fat deficiency is quite rare. Since our need is very little (about a teaspoon of oil daily) and we get plenty of vegetable oils in our diet, falling short on 18:2 (or linoleic acid) is not a risk. However, we tend not to get enough of 18:3 (or omega-3 fats). Even though this does not present an immediate problem, long-term imbalance, as mentioned above, may lead to age-related ailments. In rare situations, an essential fat deficiency may develop; for example, in a person with stomach or bowel disease typically on tube feeding (getting all their nutrients through liquid fed via a tube) in which too little or none of the essential fats were added to the mixture. In this case, growth failure results and dry flaky skin.

FAT IN FOOD—PROCESSING

Let's go back to our original look at fat's chemical structure—the triglyceride. Fatty acids are attached as part of the triglyceride structure and don't exist in foods "unattached." (See Figure 5.8.)

As alluded to earlier, not all the fatty acids on a triglyceride are identical. As you'll note, fats in foods (triglycerides) are a mix of saturated, unsaturated, and polyunsaturated fatty acids (See Figure 5.9).

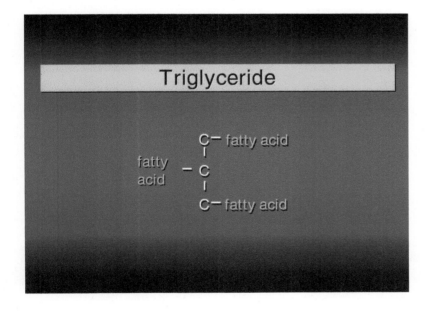

Figure 5.8

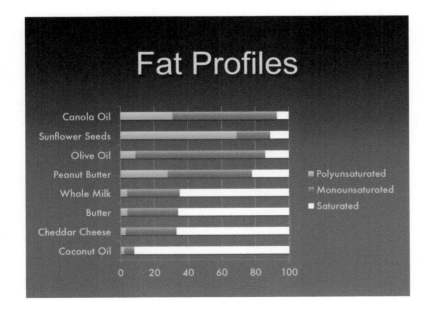

Figure 5.9

- A food fat is called a "saturated fat" if a majority (not all) of its fatty acids are saturated.
- Similarly, a food fat is called "unsaturated fat" if most (not all) of its fatty acids are unsaturated.

Let's look at a general comparison of food fat from animal and vegetable sources. (*Note:* By "vegetable" what is meant are plant sources typically from a plant seed such as a sunflower seed, which is rich in fat, not a "vegetable" such as a carrot or lettuce.) (See Figure 5.10.)

Know your food sources of saturated and unsaturated fats. Figures 5.11, 5.12, and 5.13 show some examples.

FOOD FAT	
ANIMAL	**VEGETABLE**
• Saturated fat	• Unsaturated fat
• Low 18:2 (linoleic) 18:3 (linolenic)	• High 18:2 • (very small amount of 18:3)
• Solid	• Liquid
Exceptions: Fish (18:3), chicken, egg	*Exceptions:* Coconut, palm oil

Figure 5.10

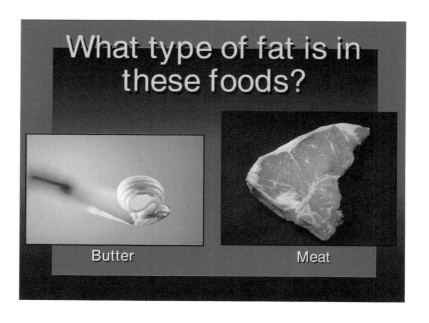

Figure 5.11

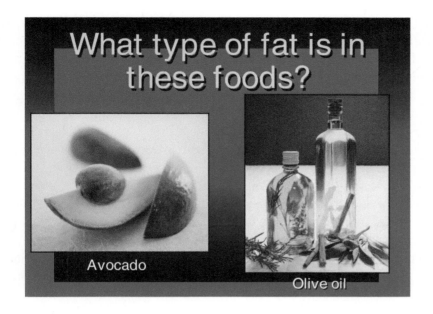

Figure 5.12

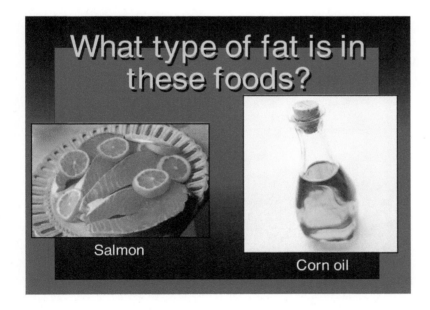

Figure 5.13

Fats and Food Processing

You may have been wondering up to this point why certain food fats, such as margarine and vegetable shortening, have not been mentioned. These fats are "manufactured" by processing natural food fats to change their properties, and hence, texture in foods. Margarine and vegetable shortening were developed decades ago (around the time of World War II) because butter was in short supply and inexpensive vegetable oils were plentiful. But the $C = C$ bond in unsaturated fats presented a challenge. This bond is very fragile. Exposing an unsaturated fat to oxygen in the air will cause the bond to "come undone" or, in scientific terms, oxidize and form free radicals as shown in Figure 5.14.

When a food fat is allowed to sit, let's say in a bowl or open bottle, exposed to the air, the free radicals that form can change the taste and appearance of the food. This off-taste is called **rancidity**. Obviously, food manufacturers don't want their food to become rancid, but they still want the ability to use these inexpensive vegetable oils. So the process of **hydrogenation** was "invented" as a way to stabilize the unsaturated fats by changing their chemical configuration about the C = C bond making the fat saturated, as shown in Figure 5.15.

Hydrogenation converts an unsaturated fatty acid to a saturated one. Hydrogen gas is bubbled into a vat of vegetable oil, such as corn oil or cottonseed oil, in the presence of a catalyst to start the reaction of "undoing" the C = C bond. Hydrogen is added to the C = C bond making the oil a saturated fat, thus changing a liquid fat

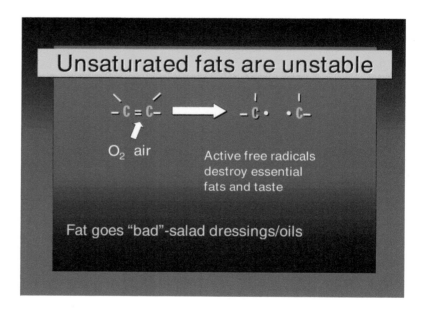

Figure 5.14

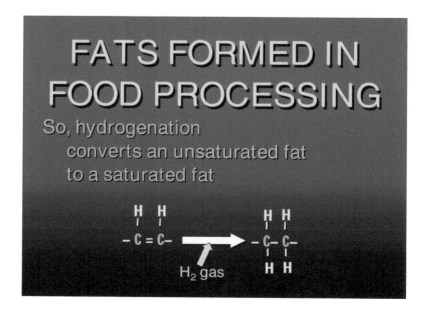

Figure 5.15

to a solid fat. You may see the term "partially hydrogenated" on an ingredient list of a food. This simply means that the vegetable was "partially" hydrogenated; thus, most of its fatty acids were converted to saturated fats.

Hydrogenation results in several important changes to the original vegetable oil:

- The fat is now more stable having a longer shelf-life, and it now can be stored at room temperature.
- The fat has changed from a liquid to a solid at room temperature.
- Unsaturated fatty acids become saturated.
- By removing the $C = C$ bonds, the fatty acids that were once 18:2 linoleic or 18:3 linolenic (small amount in vegetable oils) NO longer possess double bonds. That is, hydrogenated vegetable oils are NOT a good source of the essential fats.
- The process of hydrogenation also forms a new type of fatty acid called "*trans*" fatty acids.

Let's take a closer look at *trans* fatty acids because scientific research shows that foods with these types of fatty acids on the triglycerides have health implications, specifically increasing the risk for heart disease.

Trans Fatty Acids

To compare how trans fat may impact health, let's remind ourselves how saturated and unsaturated fatty acids look. In these next few illustrations, we'll look at the simplified drawings of saturated and unsaturated fatty acids that reflect their straight and bent nature, respectively.

In Figure 5.16, the chain of carbon atoms in a saturated fatty acid is straight and stiff, allowing them to stack easily (as part of the triglyceride structure). This characteristic makes saturated fats solid at room temperature.

Now let's look at an unsaturated fatty acid and compare this to a saturated fatty acid. See Figure 5.17. The double bond causes a "kink" in the carbon chain that doesn't allow the fatty acids (while part of the triglyceride structure) to stack nicely. This is what keeps unsaturated fat liquid at room temperature. This particular type

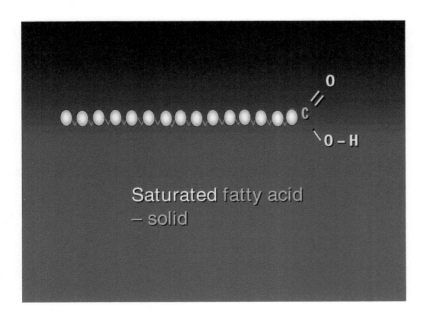

Figure 5.16

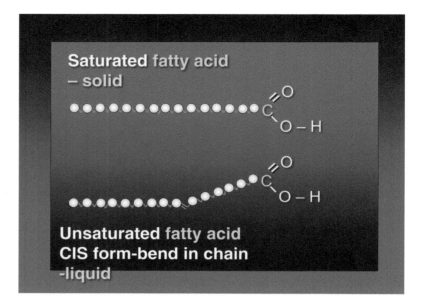

Figure 5.17

of "kink" caused by the arrangement of the C = C bond is called a "*cis*" configuration. (In the world of chemistry, this has to do with how the chain of carbons is oriented about the C = C bond.) The *cis* configuration is the way unsaturated fatty acids exist in nature.

Now let's take a look at what happens to some of the fatty acids during hydrogenation or partial hydrogenation. See Figure 5.18. During the hydrogenation process, many, but not all of the fatty acids are converted into saturated fatty acids. Some of the unsaturated (*cis*) fatty acids are tweaked a bit—the double bond comes "undone," but does not get filled with hydrogen atoms, but rather goes back to a double bond with a different configuration. This new arrangement about the C = C bond is called "***trans***" and as pictured, the chain of carbons is straight just like a saturated fatty acid despite its C = C bond. Thus, a trans fat is straight and stiff, solid at room temperature. This helps give margarine and other foods made with hydrogenated vegetable oil their texture.

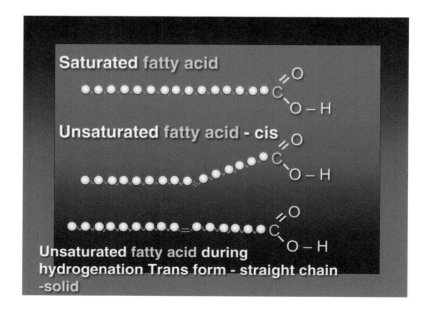

Figure 5.18

Health Concerns about Trans Fats

Perhaps you've heard about the dangers of *trans* fat in the news, or seen products such as margarines that state "*trans* fat-free" on the label. All the fuss about *trans* fats has to do with how they behave like saturated fats, not only in food, but also in your body. As we'll discuss in our next chapter on heart disease, saturated fats increase your risk for this ailment by indirectly boosting your blood cholesterol levels. Unfortunately, *trans* fats do the same thing. Research shows that diets that supply several grams of *trans* fat from margarine, snack foods, and cookies all made with hydrogenated or partially hydrogenated vegetable oils increase risk for heart disease. Therefore, the Food and Drug Administration requires that amounts of *trans* fat in food be listed on the Nutrition Facts food label. This will allow consumers to see how much *trans* fat is in a food. A Daily Value (or suggested limit) for *trans* fat intake is not set, but instead the U.S. Department of Agriculture suggests to avoid foods with *trans* fat from hydrogenated and partially hydrogenated oils (see Figure 5.19).

FAT DIGESTION, ABSORPTION, AND TRANSPORT

Fat is tricky stuff when it comes to its digestion, absorption, and transport in the body. Think about trying to dissolve a stick of butter in a pitcher of water versus dissolving a cup of sugar. There is no problem stirring the sugar into the water and watching it dissolve, but try as you may, the butter is not going to dissolve in the water. Fat and water don't mix, and this is the challenge the body is faced with since the body is over one-half water. The blood, for example, is mostly water. Fat must be made soluble every step of the way—during digestion, absorption, and transport. Emulsification is the process of making fat soluble in water. During fat digestion, absorption, and transport, emulsification on some level takes place for the fat to be "accepted" by the body.

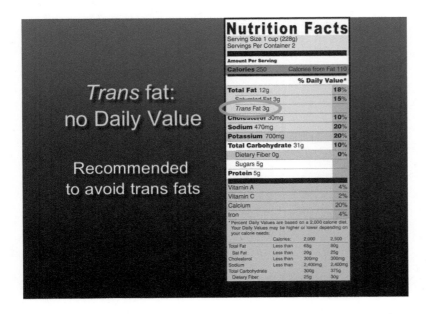

Figure 5.19

Fat Digestion

Unlike protein and carbohydrate, there is no digestion of fat in the mouth or stomach. Digestion takes place in the small intestine as fat is made soluble in the watery environment and then fat can be chemically digested.

In the small intestine, as shown in Figure 5.20, triglyceride from a meal such as a bagel with cream cheese (which is about 90 percent fat, by the way) mixes with a substance called **bile**. Much like soap that you would put on a shirt or other fabric to wash away grease, bile acts to emulsify triglycerides and "wash" them into the digestive juices. Bile is made in the liver from cholesterol (more on this in another section) and is stored in the gallbladder. When you eat a meal, the gallbladder dispenses bile much like a pump dispenser of soap alongside a sink.

Once the triglyceride has been emulsified into solution, the enzyme **lipase** ("lip" = lipid or fat; "ase" = enzyme) secreted from the pancreas starts to chemically digest triglycerides. Lipase breaks off fatty acids from the triglycerides leaving monoglycerides (single fatty acid attached to the glycerol) and free fatty acids. As shown in Figure 5.21, fat droplets form a droplet called **micelles**, which contain a combination of fatty acids and monoglycerides. These small micelles are much like the tiny droplets of oil you see when you shake a bottle of oil and vinegar salad dressing.

Fat Absorption

Once the micelles have formed, they migrate to the surface of the small intestine where they are absorbed. In the interior of the small intestine wall (before passing into the circulation), the triglycerides reform (fatty acids and monoglycerides rejoin). But before the triglyceride can move into the blood, as shown in Figure 5.21, the fat must be made soluble again.

A protein "coating" is put on the outside of the triglycerides to make the fat "acceptable" to travel in the blood since protein is soluble in water (and the blood is mostly water). This new fat + protein combination is called a **chylomicron**. (See Figure 5.22.) As we are about to see, chylomicrons venture out into the circulation as

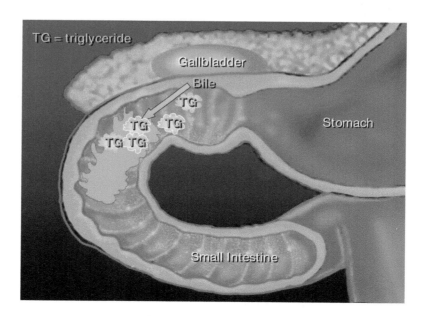

Figure 5.20

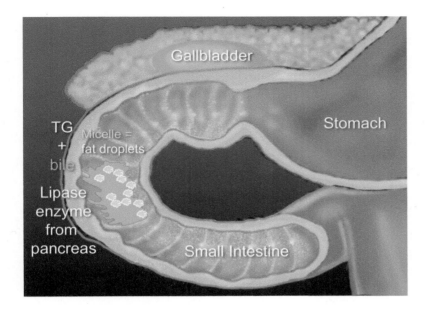

Figure 5.21

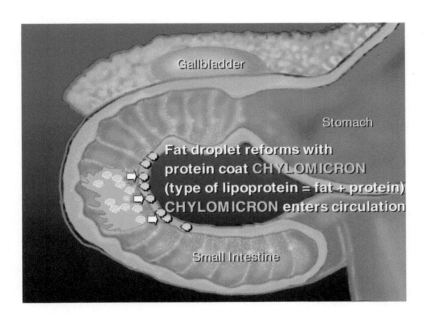

Figure 5.22

a transport vehicle for triglyceride to cells. Chylomicrons are one of several types of **lipoproteins**, which are **the transport form of fat in the circulation**, as described in the next section.

Fat Transport

Chylomicrons migrate from the small intestine wall into the circulation to deliver triglyceride to the cells of the body. As mentioned, chylomicrons are a type of lipoprotein—fat + protein coating—that transports fat through the circulation.

To help visualize a chylomicron (as well as other lipoproteins that we will be introduced to), think of them as a special kind of bus. The outer shell of the bus is made of proteins (the outside advertisement signs represent different proteins), and the passengers inside (that we have met so far) are triglycerides.

This bus (chylomicron) travels around the body; stops at muscle and fat cells, as pictured in Figure 5.23, opens its doors; and drops off its passenger—triglyceride. Most of the triglyceride "passengers" get off the bus and enter these cells, but not all. Which cell type—muscle or fat cell—depends upon your energy balance. If you're exercising and fit, the chylomicron likes to stop off at muscle cells so the triglyceride can be used immediately as fuel; but if you're sedentary, most likely this lipoprotein will stop at fat cells to put triglyceride away in storage for a rainy day when you do need the fat as fuel.

After a while, the chylomicron "fatigues" with delivering triglyceride to cells and heads to the liver. (See Figure 5.24.) Much like a bus depot or headquarters, the liver repackages the remaining triglyceride along with any new fat that has been made from excess protein or carbohydrate. This regrouped triglyceride now gets on a new "bus" and is shipped out of the liver. This new lipoprotein is called **VLDL** (short for **V**ery **L**ow **D**ensity **L**ipoprotein). The term *density* relates to the amount of

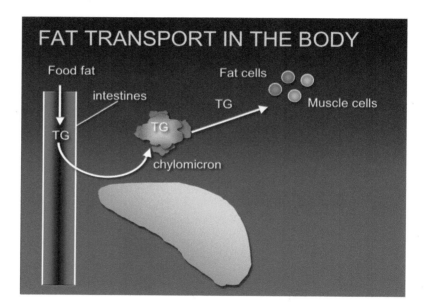

Figure 5.23

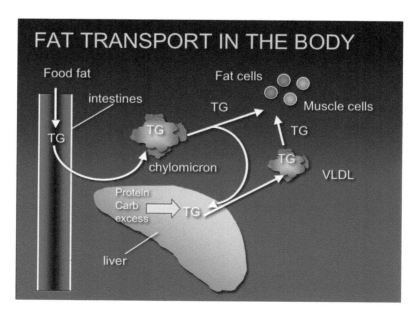

Figure 5.24

triglyceride in the lipoprotein and its density in water—the more fat, the less dense or the more it floats in water.

VLDL is another lipoprotein—fat with a protein coat—and it also transports triglyceride to cells. Just like the chylomicron, VLDL "opens" its doors and drops off triglyceride to fat and muscle cells depending upon the need for energy. VLDL is a more compact or smaller version of a chylomicron with different proteins (different outside advertisements on the outside of the "bus").

This complex scheme of fat transport via the lipoproteins (chylomicrons, and VLDL) results from fat's insolubility in water (the blood). There's more to the fat transportation story—other lipoproteins and one more passenger in the lipoproteins, namely cholesterol, will be discussed in the last section of this chapter.

FAT ENERGY METABOLISM

Once the chylomicrons and/or the VLDLs have delivered triglyceride to cells, what happens to this fat? If put away in fat cells, the triglyceride waits until it is called upon to come out of storage for use as fuel by other cells. This would occur when a person has not eaten for several hours or when calorie intake falls below calorie expenditure for the day. More on this will be covered in Chapter 7 when we discuss obesity and weight loss.

If delivered to muscle cells, the triglyceride is used as fuel. Recall from Chapter 3 that fat contains 9 calories per gram, so it has potential energy in its carbon bonds.

Inside of a muscle cell, triglyceride is broken apart to release the fatty acids. (For sake of simplicity, we'll ignore the glycerol backbone and what happens to it.) These fatty acids contain potential energy and are broken down into C_2 units. (See Figure 5.25.) Energy is released and oxygen is used. This process is aerobic—with the presence of oxygen.

These C_2 units are just like the C_2 units from when carbohydrate was broken down aerobically. There is more potential energy in these two-carbon units, and they are sent through the TCA cycle to release more energy—all told, 9 calories per gram. At the same time CO_2 is released and water is made.

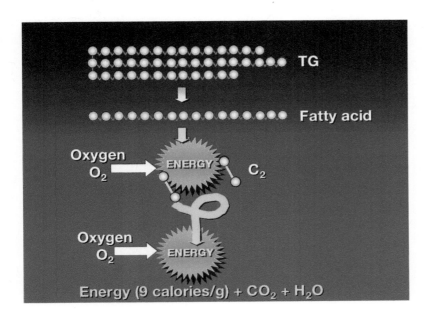

Figure 5.25

The end products of fat energy metabolism are energy (9 calories/gram) + CO_2 + H_2O.

Now that we know the end products of fat and carbohydrate aerobic energy metabolism are the same, when does the cell decide to burn fat or carbohydrate as a fuel source? Well, BOTH are used simultaneously. In fact, both carbohydrate and fat must be burned together for operations in the C_2-burning (TCA) cycle to work best. When you are sedentary or not very active (such as walking), the body burns about 60 to 70 percent fat and 30 to 40 percent carbohydrate. However, as you step up the intensity of your activity, the muscle cell shifts to using more carbohydrate and less fat. So during a run (good effort) you are burning about 70 percent carbohydrate and 30 percent fat for fuel.

BRINGING IT ALL TOGETHER—ENERGY METABOLISM (PROTEIN, CARBOHYDRATE, AND FAT)

Let's integrate now what we know about how protein, carbohydrate, and fat are used for energy in the body. Energy metabolism is the collective term used to describe the body's use of fuel depending upon its status or state of energy balance. What the body uses for fuel, or what the body may decide to store for later use as fuel, depends upon different situations.

Let's take a look at three different energy metabolism "conditions" that your body may be routinely faced with and how energy metabolism works in each of these three situations.

1. After you eat a meal.
2. Several hours without eating, such as when you first wake up in the morning.
3. Without food for at least 24 hours—you are fasting.

For each of these three situations, we will look at Figure 5.26, which tracks each of the energy nutrients—carbohydrate, fat, and protein. Then we'll summarize energy metabolism for each situation in a table.

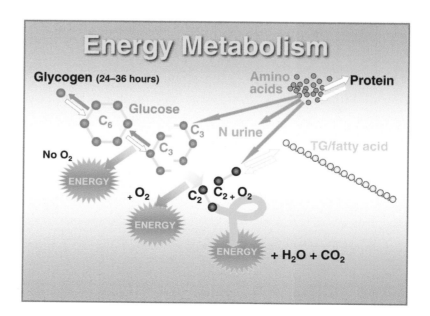

Figure 5.26

Figure 5.26 shows the possibilities for each of the energy nutrients. Carbohydrate (glucose), which can be stored as glycogen, used anaerobically and aerobically for energy, and in excess, can be stored and converted to fat. Which the body chooses to do depends upon the current energy metabolism situation (situation 1, 2, or 3 listed previously).

1. After Eating a Meal

When you eat a meal, it is similar to taking a trip to the grocery store and coming back to your apartment. What do you typically do with the bags of groceries? You put them away—in the refrigerator, freezer, and pantry. Your body does the same thing with energy nutrients. **Following a meal, energy nutrients are put away into storage.** Follow along with each of the energy nutrients as they are put away in storage by following Figure 5.26. Figure 5.27 is a simplified diagram that shows the storage of energy nutrients following a meal.

Carbohydrate (Glucose)

After you eat a meal containing carbohydrate, it is digested, absorbed and transported to body cells as glucose. Glucose then enters the cell and can be used if needed for energy ($C_6 \rightarrow C_3 \rightarrow C_2 \rightarrow CO_2 + H_2O + energy$).

Chances are, you've eaten a bit more than you need at the time for fuel so that you restock glycogen stores. Once these are filled in the muscles and liver, the excess glucose is converted to fat (in the liver), shipped out into the circulation via a VLDL and sent to fat cells.

Fat

Fat from your meal is already fat, and if you don't need it immediately for a fuel source in the muscle (that is, you're lounging around after your big meal), food fat is readily stored as body fat. Via a trip in a chylomicron, this excess fat from a meal makes a journey to fat cells for storage.

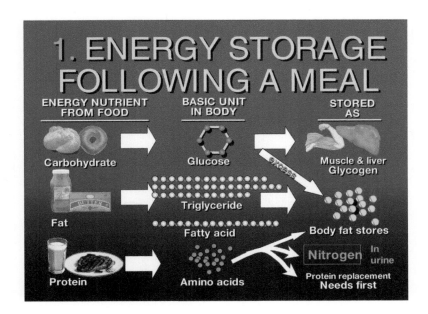

Figure 5.27

Protein

Protein from your meal is broken down to amino acids and used for protein replacement needs (replenish or make any new proteins). If you've consumed more protein than what your body needs, the excess amino acids are stripped of their nitrogen (goes into the urine) and the leftover carbon skeleton is converted to fat (via conversion of C_2 units). Like carbohydrates, this is done in the liver and the fat is shipped out (via the VLDL) and sent to fat cells for storage.

2. Several Hours after Eating

When you first wake in the morning, it's been several hours since you have last eaten—dinner the evening before or perhaps a late night snack (overnight "fast"). This energy metabolism situation is much like you going into your kitchen when you are hungry and looking for something to eat but there's nothing out on the counter for munching. So what do you do? You open the cupboards or refrigerator and bring food "out of storage." This is exactly what your body does when you haven't eaten for a while. **Energy nutrients are brought out of storage when you haven't eaten for several hours.** Follow along using the integrated energy metabolism diagram in Figure 5.26 on page 108. Also, Figure 5.28 represents a simplified diagram that illustrates energy nutrients being brought out of storage after several hours without eating.

Carbohydrate (Glycogen)

Your brain and other parts of your body still need carbohydrate as fuel and even though you haven't eaten anything in the past few hours, there are readily available stores of carbohydrate for use—glycogen. This storage form of carbohydrate in the muscles and liver provides the body with carbohydrate fuel. Glycogen in a muscle is used by that specific muscle for fuel. (The right biceps muscle glycogen store, for example, is for that muscle, not some other part of the body.) Liver glycogen on the other hand, is used primarily for the brain and nervous system. (Glycogen breaks down to glucose and this moves out into the circulation to fuel the brain.)

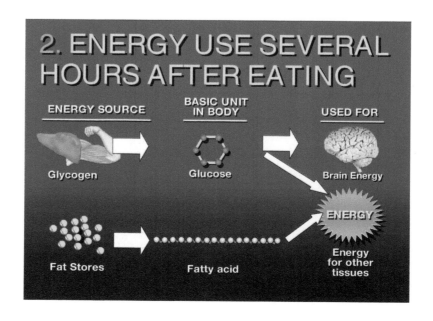

Figure 5.28

Fat

Body fat stores are signaled that fuel is needed and triglycerides are brought out of storage. These are first broken down to C_2 units (aerobically) and then all the way to energy—9 calories/gram + CO_2 + H_2O.

Protein

At this point, the protein in your body (which is all functional tissue—no "storage") is not touched since you have plenty of carbohydrate fuel. In other words, there's no reason to break protein down to make glucose since you have a supply of glycogen to last you about a day.

3. Fasting—without Food for at Least 24 to 36 Hours

This final energy metabolism situation is much like when you walk into your kitchen to get something to eat because you are famished, but unlike the previous situation, there's not much left in the cupboard or refrigerator. In fact, you're out of ready-to-eat food like breakfast cereal so you have to scrounge to find something edible. In your body, when you have gone without eating for 24 hours or more, and your store of carbohydrate—glycogen—is out, so you have to make your own source of glucose.

So the primary difference with the previous situation is that **with fasting, glycogen stores in both the liver and muscle have run out**. Follow along using the energy metabolism diagram in Figure 5.26 (page 108) to track how the body converts protein to glucose as well as using fat as fuel during a fast.

Glucose (Carbohydrate)

The stores of glycogen in muscle last approximately one day with fasting. These stores of glucose can run out sooner if you exercise, lasting about 2 to 4 hours of continuous exercise. Liver glycogen stores also run out in about a day's time.

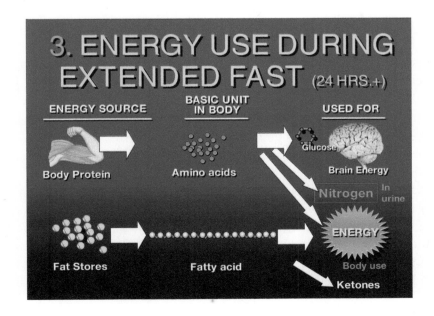

Figure 5.29

Dangers of Fasting

If you ever fast for an extended period of time, you need to know the dangers associated with reintroducing food. When fasting (or in starvation mode) for several weeks, such as hunger strike participants or victims of concentrations camps from World War II, the body is geared up for breaking down proteins. That is, the enzymes responsible for breaking down proteins to amino acids and then taking the nitrogen off are going full throttle. Thus, if a big steak meal—lots of protein—is given to a fasted person, this may present a life-threatening situation. With a big dose of protein, these enzymes go to work and break apart the protein and release the nitrogen, which then spikes in the blood. High blood nitrogen can be toxic; in fact, it may lead to instant death. Unfortunately, victims from concentration camps were given hearty meals upon their release and some died from this nitrogen poisoning. In addition, the intestinal tract becomes weakened with fasting, so food must be introduced slowly as the intestinal tract surface rebuilds to handle digestion and absorption of nutrients.

Protein

With glycogen stores gone, and the brain and other cells in the body, such as nervous tissue and red blood cells needing glucose, the body sends a signal to make carbohydrate from protein. Functional protein tissue, such as muscle proteins, enzymes, and organ proteins are broken down into the amino acid building blocks. Recall from Chapter 4 that this occurs in the liver where the amino acids are stripped of their nitrogen, which gets excreted by the kidneys into the urine. The remaining carbon skeletons are converted to C_3 or C_2 units (depending upon the R groups). The C_3 units are "glued" together to form glucose (in the liver), which is then sent out into the circulation to fuel the brain and other needy tissues. This process is limited in that you can't make enough glucose to load up muscles with glycogen. In fact, you'll feel pretty weak during a fast, or even light-headed as glucose needs are barely met. The remaining C_2 units are used as fuel by the body.

Fat

At the same time, protein is being broken down, hormones signal fat stores to initiate triglyceride break down to fatty acids, which are in turn broken down to C_2 units, and finally CO_2 + H_2O + energy. *Note:* Fatty acids are NOT converted to C_3 units; thus, they *cannot* be used to make glucose. This is why protein is lost—functional tissue—during a fast, in addition to body fat.

Another consequence occurs during a fast—the formation of **ketones**, which are a by-product of fat metabolism, are formed from C_2 units. Ketones form as C_2 units build up in part because carbohydrates are lacking to turn the cycle efficiently (you'll recall that CHO and fats work together in the TCA cycle to generate energy). This formation of ketones gives a person who is fasting a characteristic breath odor of acetone (a type of ketone). This metabolic state is called **ketosis**. It occurs in people who have fasted for a few days or more or following for several days a high-protein/low-carbohydrate diet, or untreated diabetes. During the first few days, a "quick" five pounds of weight is lost. This occurs due to water loss as the glycogen stores run out. Water that is normally "packed" around glycogen is also lost. This rapid weight loss gives people the impression that fasting is a great way to lose weight or that a high-protein diet is a very effective way to lose weight quickly. Actually, the rate of weight loss slows down as the body adapts by slowing energy expenditure and lowering the Basal Metabolic Rate. In addition, the state of ketosis can be dangerous for people with kidney trouble because this puts a strain on kidneys to excrete these extra products.

This shift in energy metabolism during a fast can be simplified using the diagram in Figure 5.29. The key thing to remember is that glycogen stores have run out and the body must make its own glucose from body or food protein.

CHOLESTEROL—ITS VITAL ROLES AND TRANSPORT IN THE BODY

Let's finish our discussion about fat and its transport through the circulation. We need to meet one more member of the fat family—cholesterol.

Cholesterol is a fatty, waxy-like substance in the body and is handled like fat. Its chemical structure—shown in Figure 5.30—looks a bit like cyclone fence wire and belongs to the chemical family called sterols. Cholesterol performs several essential regulatory functions in the body, but cholesterol is NOT broken down to C_3 or C_2 and therefore provides no energy.

Cholesterol's functions include the following:

1. **Precursor to bile:** Recall that bile is just like a "soap" that the liver makes to emulsify fats in our small intestines so that fat can be digested and absorbed.
2. **Precursor to sex hormones:** The sex hormones testosterone and estrogen are also made from cholesterol. (In fact, their chemical structures look very similar to cholesterol and are considered in the "sterol" family based upon their carbon-ring structure.)

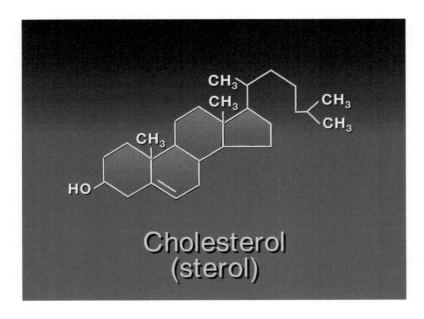

Figure 5.30

3. **Precursor to vitamin D:** Cholesterol goes through a series of modifications in our body for eventual conversion to vitamin D. One of the first steps is the "activation" of cholesterol in the skin by ultraviolet light from the sun. We'll cover this in greater detail when we discuss vitamin D in Chapter 9.

4. **Component of cell membrane structure:** As shown in Figure 5.31, cholesterol sits in the cell membrane as the vital component giving the membrane its ability, in part, to control what goes in and gets out of the cell. Thus, cholesterol is a normal part of every cell in our body, and all mammals. (Remember this when we think about food sources of cholesterol.)

Even though cholesterol has all these vital roles in the body, it is not an essential nutrient. This must mean that the body can make cholesterol and make enough to meet its needs. Cholesterol is made in the liver of all mammals—you included. As shown in Figure 5.32, cholesterol is made from C_2 units that result from the breakdown of fats, protein, or carbohydrate.

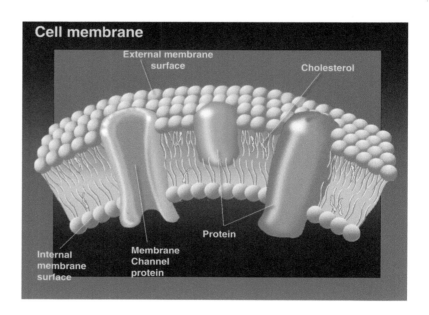

Figure 5.31

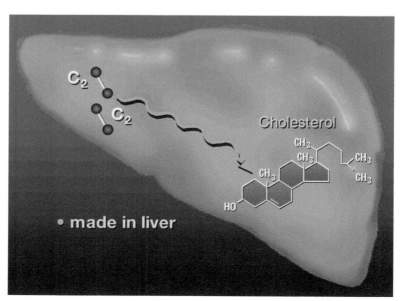

Figure 5.32

Sources of Cholesterol in the Body

- Each day the body manufactures about 1,000 to 1,500 milligrams of cholesterol.
- Each day you take in about 200 to 400 milligrams—this depends upon your diet (specifically how much you eat in the way of animal products—meats, milk, eggs, fish).

Food Sources of Cholesterol

Think about where cholesterol is made and then translate this to possible food sources. Any food that comes from something with a liver—in other words, any animal product—contains cholesterol.

Examples of foods that contain cholesterol: beef, chicken, seafood, eggs, milk (even skim milk), and, of course, liver and other organ meats.

How about avocado? Or what about olives or margarine? Even though these foods are high in fat, they are plant products and therefore contain NO cholesterol. Cholesterol is a type of fat, but that does not mean that only high-fat foods contain cholesterol. In Chapter 6, we'll discuss how high intakes of saturated fat and trans fats can indirectly elevate circulating levels of cholesterol and ultimately increase the risk for heart disease.

This brings up how cholesterol moves through the body via the circulation.

Cholesterol Transport

Let's go back to our discussion about lipoproteins and the transport of fat. We now have a new "passenger"—cholesterol. Since cholesterol is a type of fat, it is not soluble in water (hence, the blood), thus, it needs a ride in a lipoprotein as a means of transport through the body so cholesterol ultimately gets to cells and carries out its duties.

When you eat a food that contains cholesterol, it is absorbed along with fat in the micelle in the small intestinal wall, and then moves through the circulation as a "passenger" in chylomicrons, as shown in Figure 5.33. **Chylomicron, a type of lipoprotein, is made up of three items—triglyceride, cholesterol as "passengers," and a protein coat.** As we'll see, **all lipoproteins are made of the same items,** just in different proportions.

As the chylomicron delivers triglyceride to fat and muscle cells, the cholesterol stays on board the "bus" and after several hours ends up at the liver. Here the cholesterol is repackaged with triglyceride (both cholesterol left over from the chylomicron along with new triglyceride made from excess carbohydrate and protein) and sent out in the **VLDL—Very Low Density Lipoprotein.** VLDL is also made of triglyceride, cholesterol (both "passengers"), and a protein coat.

Recall that the VLDL's job was to drop off triglyceride at fat and muscle cells, and while it does this, cholesterol stays on board. As this happens, the VLDL transforms—it becomes smaller and becomes proportionately richer in cholesterol (although it still has triglyceride on board). This is now a new lipoprotein—**LDL** or **Low Density Lipoprotein.**

LDL, which is made of the three same items (triglyceride, cholesterol, and a protein coat—just different proportions compared to chylomicrons and VLDLs),

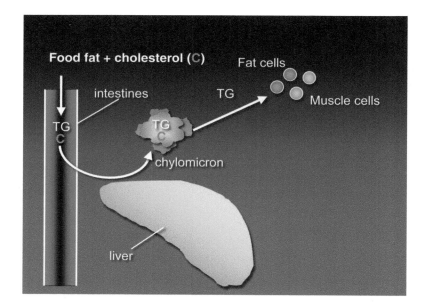

Figure 5.33

now travels through the circulation with a job to do that is different from the chylomicron and VLDL. LDL delivers cholesterol to cells, as shown in Figure 5.34. LDL looks for cell receptors (similar to a bus stop sign) on the surface of cells to know if the LDL should make a stop there and deliver cholesterol. Every cell needs cholesterol for normal functioning. You may have heard about LDL as the "bad" cholesterol. In Chapter 6, we'll see how LDL cholesterol transport can go awry and lead to heart disease.

There's one more lipoprotein to this fat and cholesterol transport story. **HDL** or **High Density Lipoprotein** is also made up of triglyceride, cholesterol, and protein coat. But this lipoprotein is proportionately richer in protein so it's "heavier." HDL originates from the liver and has a very specific job—it acts like a scavenger. HDL picks up loose cholesterol that has fallen from lipoproteins or from dying

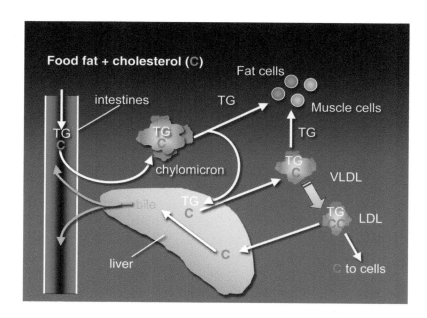

Figure 5.34

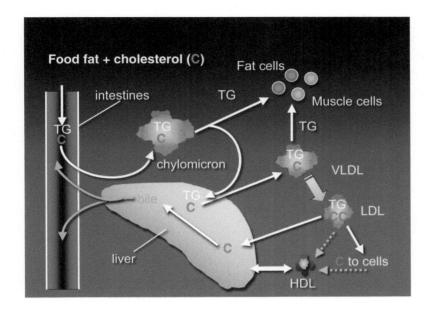

Figure 5.35

cells. Once on board, the HDL travels to the liver where the cholesterol can get off and have the opportunity to become bile and leave the body or be recycled back on board a VLDL (as shown in the completed cholesterol and fat diagram in Figure 5.35).

HDL is frequently referred to as the "good" cholesterol since high levels of HDL is associated with a reduced risk for heart disease—more on this in Chapter 6. But we'll leave this discussion by noting that HDL levels can be boosted with exercise. It seems that with regular exercise, such as running, levels of HDL are increased due to a shift in lipoprotein transport, helping to explain why exercise lowers risk for heart disease. Also women tend to have higher levels of HDL compared to men. This is related to their greater estrogen levels. However, once women go through menopause in their late 40s to early 50s (estrogen levels fall), levels of HDL decline as this hormone plays a role in the formation of HDL. This helps explain why heart disease risk subsequently goes up for women during these years.

The lipoproteins, chylomicrons, VLDL, LDL, and HDL are made in the body and transport fat and cholesterol. **There are NO food sources of these lipoproteins.**

Quiz Yourself

5

CHAPTER

1. List a good food source for each of the following.

   - Monounsaturated fat _____

   - Polyunsaturated fat _____

   - Saturated fat _____

   - Cholesterol _____

   - Trans fat _____

   - LDL _____

   - 18:2 (linoleic) _____

   - 18:3 (linolenic) _____

Multiple Choice

2. Fat is transported through the circulation system to various to tissues, such as muscle and adipose, as:

   a. small droplets made exclusively of triglyceride

   b. lipoproteins, composed primarily of triglyceride, cholesterol, and protein

   c. cholesterol droplets, which can accumulate on arterial walls to form fatty deposits

   d. separate droplets containing either cholesterol, triglyceride, or phospholipids and coated with protein

   e. c and d above

3. Hydrogenation is a process that makes unsaturated fats:

   a. more solid

   b. have a higher cholesterol content

   c. more resistant to oxidation

   d. a and b

   e. a and c

4. Bile is made from and functions in:

   a. calcium / fat digestion

   b. cholesterol / fat digestion

   c. prostaglandins / carbohydrate digestion

   d. cholesterol / carbohydrate digestion

   e. prostaglandins / fat digestion

5. If you eat more protein than you need at any given time, in an otherwise adequate diet, the excess amino acids are largely converted to:

    a. cholesterol

    b. fatty acids

    c. fructose

    d. muscle protein

    e. hormones

6. The end products of fat energy metabolism are:

    a. fatty acids plus glycerol

    b. monosaccharides

    c. CO_2, H_2O plus energy

    d. same as carbohydrate energy metabolism (aerobic)

    e. c and d above

7. You've just finished stuffing yourself at an all-you-can-eat buffet. Describe energy metabolism following this large meal (use Figure 5.27).

    _____

    _____

    _____

8. Describe energy metabolism during a 24- to 36-hour fast (use Figure 5.29).

    _____

    _____

    _____

KEEP YOUR HEART HEALTHY WITH THE RIGHT FOODS

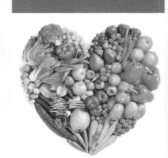

Congratulations! You just increased your knowledge about fats and cholesterol and their transport through the body as part of lipoproteins. Now, we can move into unraveling the origins of heart disease, the leading cause of death in the United States for both men and women. The chance that, years from now, you may suffer from this age-related disease, or at least have a family member or close friend who suffers may not quite move you today. But perhaps knowing that the process of vascular damage—the buildup of cholesterol in your arteries—has most likely already started in your body may prompt you to sit up and take notice.

THE LIPOPROTEIN STORY AND HEART DISEASE

Let's take a look at what vascular disease is and how it gets started.

Figure 6.1 shows a cross section of a normal artery that supplies blood flow (oxygen) to a muscle such as your heart (which pumps blood and, like other muscles in your body, it needs oxygen). The cross section shows a clear and unobstructed path for blood flow. Your arteries looked like this when you were a newborn and perhaps the first few years of life. Probably by age 10 or even sooner, LDL particles start "crashing" into your artery walls. White blood cells, platelets and immune cells, then attack the area to fight off what they see as invaders. Cholesterol, which spills out of the LDLs, is deposited and hardens, making "plaque" (a different plaque than plaque on teeth). We refer to this condition of plaque build-up and its hardening as **atherosclerosis**. Over time, this process continues with "crashing" LDLs' cholesterol and its oxidation progressively builds up. (See Figure 6.2.)

As the opening for blood flow narrows, danger of a heart attack or stroke lurks. When you exercise or climb a flight of stairs, your heart demands more oxygen. With limited blood flow, or even

Chapter Objectives

In this chapter, we will cover:

- Lipoproteins and their implications for heart disease
- Heart disease risk factors
- Diet and heart disease connection
- Dietary recommendations to reduce your risk for heart disease

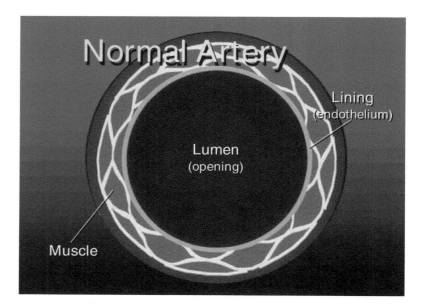

Figure 6.1

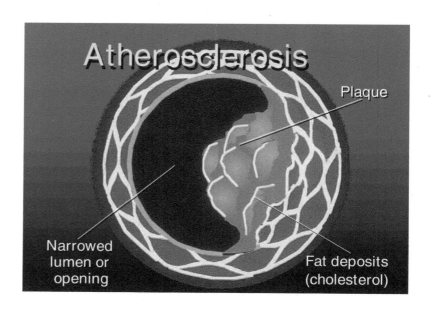

Figure 6.2

blockage when plaque breaks off and lodges in a narrowed artery, you feel chest pain and radiating discomfort down your left arm (or even flu-like symptoms). Your heart muscle is starved for oxygen, and you suffer a heart attack. Atherosclerosis in the arteries that feed the heart is called **coronary heart disease**. If atherosclerosis occurs in your brain, you suffer from a stroke when a portion of the brain is also starved for oxygen. This is usually the first sign of vascular disease. Unfortunately, the disease is quite progressed at this point because it has been developing for decades.

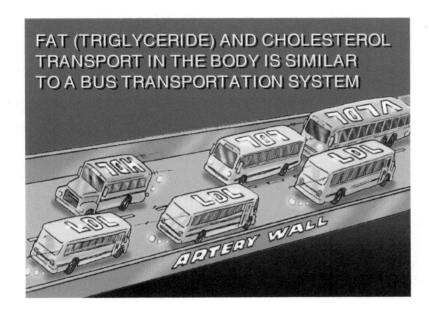

Figure 6.3

In Chapter 5, we referred to lipoproteins and their transport much like buses traveling through freeways and roads transporting the passengers, triglycerides, and cholesterol. Using a cartoon analogy can help you understand this process of vascular disease, which in turn may assist you in making dietary and other lifestyle changes that may decrease your risk for heart disease. (See Figure 6.3.)

Remember that lipoproteins are made up of the same three components—triglyceride, cholesterol, and a protein coat—each lipoprotein with a different job to do "delivering" its passengers. (See Figure 6.4.)

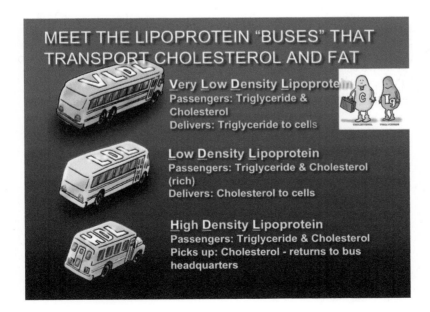

Figure 6.4

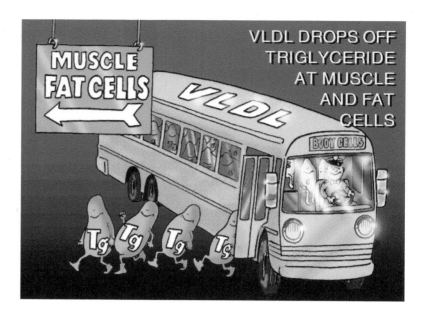

Figure 6.5

Figures 6.5, 6.6, and 6.7 show Very Low Density Lipoprotein's (VLDL), Low Density Lipoprotein's (LDL) and High Density Lipoprotein's (HDL) transportation roles.

As the LDL travels through your roadways (arteries), the transportation of cholesterol can go awry. Picture an LDL "bus" driving around for a long time with

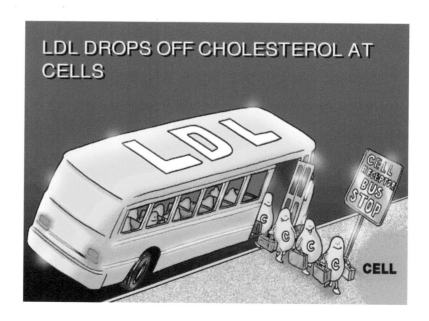

Figure 6.6

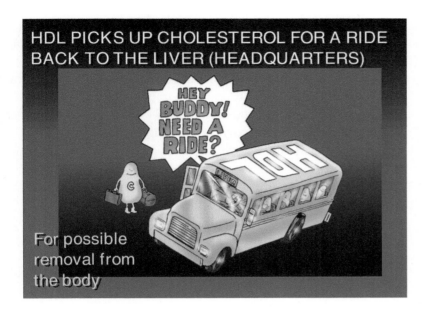

Figure 6.7

no place to go and becoming very tired. As time drags on, the LDL can become damaged (referred to as oxidation) and drive out of control, "crashing" into the side of the road. This process of LDL infiltrating or "crashing" into artery walls is more likely to occur in smokers or in those with a poor diet low in fruits, vegetables, and whole grains. (See Figure 6.8.)

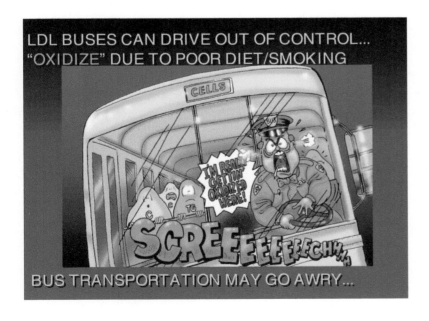

Figure 6.8

Much like a real crash scene, debris litters the roadway. In your body, the cholesterol spills out, infiltrates the arteries, and builds up into plaque. (See Figure 6.9.)

And like a real accident scene that draws the attention of rubber-neckers, your body sends platelets to the scene, which gather around the "injury," forming a blood clot. (See Figure 6.10.) This further "clogs traffic"—blood flow.

This process of "crashing" LDL buses continues over time and vascular disease develops, leading to a heart attack or stroke. (See Figure 6.11.)

Vascular disease (heart attack or stroke) is a very frightening disease when it strikes you or someone you love. You can take charge of your health and reduce your risk of developing vascular disease by altering your lifestyle, which includes diet and physical activity.

Figure 6.9

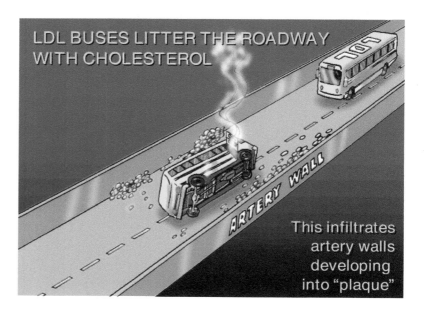

Figure 6.10

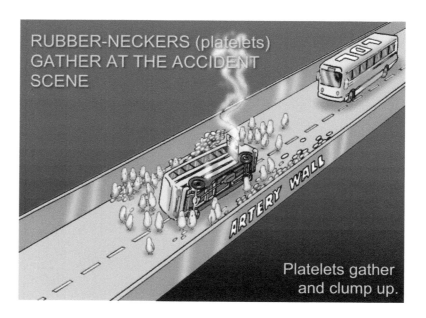

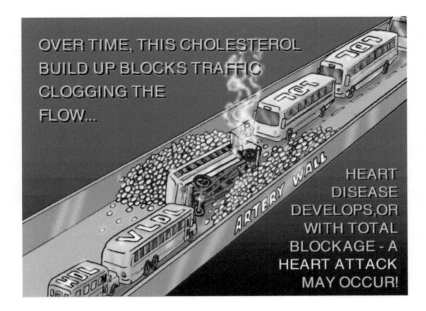

OVER TIME, THIS CHOLESTEROL BUILD UP BLOCKS TRAFFIC CLOGGING THE FLOW...

HEART DISEASE DEVELOPS, OR WITH TOTAL BLOCKAGE - A HEART ATTACK MAY OCCUR!

Figure 6.11

HEART DISEASE RISK FACTORS—ARE YOU AT RISK?

Let's take a look at the risk factors that predispose a person to increased chances of suffering from atherosclerosis and a heart attack or stroke. These factors are characteristics—some are lifestyle related, such as smoking, and some you can't do anything about, such as genetics and gender—that influence your risk of heart disease.

Coronary Heart Disease Major Risk Factors

- Cigarette Smoking
- Increasing Age
- Heredity/Race
- Male Gender
- Physical Inactivity

- Hypertension*
- Low HDL*
- High LDL*
- Diabetes*
- Obesity (abdominal body fat)*
- "Atherogenic" diet (diet high in saturated fat, low in fruits, vegetables and whole grains)*

* Indicates risk factors that are responsive to dietary intervention.

In addition to these major risk factors, there are others that may contribute to a person's coronary heart disease risk. Indicators of inflammation, specifically a blood marker called C-reactive protein, suggest there is a greater likelihood that inflammation is underway in artery walls. This in turn contributes to more LDL becoming oxidized, leading to plaque build-up.

Stress in high levels may also contribute indirectly to heart disease risk. Personal stress may be economic or job related, or stress may otherwise aggravate an existing risk factor, such as stimulating overeating, which causes obesity.

Nutrition Bite

Although men are generally at greater risk for developing heart disease, it is still the leading cause of death among women.

Metabolic Syndrome

Risk for coronary heart disease is great for people with **metabolic syndrome**. Two dominant factors characterize this condition:

- Abdominal obesity: a waist circumference of > 35 inches for women and > 40 inches for men
- Insulin resistance (above normal blood glucose indicating insulin is losing its effectiveness in processing carbohydrates)

As mentioned in Chapter 4 (and also covered more in Chapter 7), excess blood glucose promotes blood vessel damage and thus increases heart disease risk. Obesity in turn elicits insulin resistance.

Other characteristics of metabolic syndrome:

- Hypertension
- High fasting blood triglyceride levels
- Low HDL levels

There is a high prevalence of metabolic syndrome in the U.S. An estimated 50 million Americans have it, and of these, a growing number are teenagers and children. Genetic predisposition plays a role for many people of Hispanic, Native American, and African descent.

Total Cholesterol and Lipoprotein Levels

Let's now focus on high total blood cholesterol as a risk factor as well as levels of LDL and HDL cholesterol. When scientists look at population data to determine what level of cholesterol presents a risk for heart health, the information looks like the graph in Figure 6.12.

Circulating cholesterol levels below 200 mg/dL are considered healthy and levels above this value are risky. The specific numbers and associated risks look like the following:

< 200mg/dL	desirable blood cholesterol level
200–239 mg/dL	borderline high blood cholesterol
> 240 mg/dL	high blood cholesterol

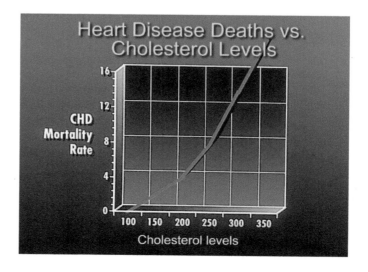

Figure 6.12

Recall that not all the lipoproteins are damaging to artery walls, so it is helpful to tease out LDL cholesterol levels (which can be measured with a lipoprotein screen). Here are LDL levels that are considered optimal to high risk:

< 100 mg/dL	optimal
100–129 mg/dL	above optimal
130–159 mg/dL	borderline high risk
160–189 mg/dL	high risk
> 190 mg/dL	very high risk

For HDL, the scavenger or "good" cholesterol carrier, low levels are risky and high levels are good. Research suggests that low HDL levels are as strong a risk for heart disease as total cholesterol levels.

< 40 mg/dL	low levels → high risk
≥ 60 mg/dL	high levels → low risk

Bottom line: You should know your numbers for total, LDL and HDL cholesterol, so you can assess your risk for heart disease.

THE ROLE OF DIET—FAT, CHOLESTEROL, FIBER, AND MORE

The connection between diet and heart disease risk is very strong. You can modify several of the major risk factors, such as high LDL and high blood pressure, by making changes in your diet along with increasing physical activity. Here are several of the major dietary factors:

Diet and Heart Disease Connection

- Total dietary fat
- Type of dietary fat (saturated, trans, monounsaturated, omega-3s)
- Cholesterol intake
- Fiber intake (soluble)
- Fruit, vegetable, and whole grains

Total Fat Intake

Your total fat intake, typically expressed as a percentage of calories, has an impact on blood cholesterol levels and heart disease risk. Many studies that examine fat intake in different countries have shown a positive correlation between fat intake and heart disease risk. (See Figure 6.13.)

In countries such as the United States and England where total fat intake and saturated fat intake combined is approximately one-third of the calories, risk for heart disease is high. In countries with low fat and saturated fat intakes, such as Korea and Egypt, heart disease risk is significantly lower.

FAT CONSUMPTION AND HEART DISEASE RISK

COUNTRY	% FAT CALORIE INTAKE	
USA	34%	high risk
England	38%	
Germany	38%	
Egypt	15%	low risk
China	18%	
Korea	10%	

*Exception: East African tribes, Eskimos
High fat/cholesterol diet → low risk

Figure 6.13

Two major exceptions to these observations are certain populations—native Eskimos and East African tribes. Native Eskimos, for example, consume nearly 60 percent of their calories in the form of fat (whale blubber and fatty fish), yet they have very low rates of heart disease attributed to high omega-3 intake. Tribes in Africa eat only animal products—meat, milk, and blood—yet their risk for heart disease is also very low despite a higher fat intake. Researchers attribute this to their genetics, very active lifestyle, and the profile of fats in the grassland-raised animals they consume.

Types of Fat

Saturated Fat: (for example, butter, lard, margarine, meats, and full-fat dairy products) When saturated fats are the major source of fat in the diet, lipoprotein transport is effected, which in turn leads to elevated circulating cholesterol levels. This is NOT to say that saturated fat is cholesterol, but instead that it indirectly impacts cholesterol levels, specifically clearance from the circulation.

- High saturated fat intake elevates LDL levels.
- This, in turn, increases heart disease risk.
- Trans fats also raise LDL levels and lower HDL and therefore heart disease risk.

ADVICE: **Reduce intake of saturated fat to less than 10 percent of total calories. Trans fat should be avoided.**

Monounsaturated Fat: (for example, olive oil, avocado, peanut oil, and canola oil) When monounsaturated fats are a major source of fat in the diet, lipoprotein transport is positively affected.

- Monounsaturated fats can lower total cholesterol levels (when substituted for saturated fats).
- Monounsaturated fats can lower LDL levels.
- Monounsaturated fats are neutral to HDL levels. (This is good news because these are the scavenger lipoproteins that help to lower heart disease risk.)

ADVICE: **Consume about 10 percent or more of your calories as monounsaturated fats.**

Polyunsaturated Fat: (for example, sunflower, soybean, safflower, and corn oils and nuts, and nut oils) When polyunsaturated fats are a major source of fat in the diet, lipoprotein transport is affected both positively and negatively.

- Polyunsaturated fats can lower total cholesterol when substituted for other fats in the diet.
- Polyunsaturated fats can lower LDL levels.
- Polyunsaturated fats can also lower HDL levels.

ADVICE: **Because polyunsaturated fats have a dual effect, it's best to limit intake to no more than 10 percent of total calories.**

Note: Omega-3 fats from seafood have a positive impact on heart health and it's recommended to eat seafood twice a week.

Cholesterol Intake

We learned from Chapter 5 that cholesterol has a variety of crucial roles in the body (sex hormone precursor, for example), but that cholesterol is NOT an essential nutrient because we can make it (in the liver) and make enough to meet our needs. Cholesterol is found in animal products such as eggs, cheese, meats, milk, fish, and other meats.

But does eating cholesterol mean that blood cholesterol levels are impacted? For most of the population, about 80 percent, homeostasis is in effect. That is, when we take in dietary cholesterol, our livers make less to keep things in balance. However for about 20 percent of the population, due to genetics or other lifestyle factors, the liver keeps pumping out cholesterol despite high levels in the diet. The end result is increased levels of total cholesterol and, particularly, high levels of LDL.

Thus, overall, the advice for the population is to moderate cholesterol intake because many foods rich in cholesterol may also be high in total fat and saturated fats. In Chapter 12, our discussion of the 2015 Dietary Guidelines examines dietary patterns focusing on plant-based foods (fruits, vegetables, beans, whole grains) that lessen risk for various diet-related chronic diseases including heart disease. Following this pattern of eating will lead to an overall lower cholesterol intake, but the impact on heart disease risk is more about various components in these foods that have heart-healthy properties.

ADVICE: **Consume less than 300 milligrams of cholesterol per day (Daily Value for cholesterol).**

Dietary Fiber Intake

You also learned in Chapter 3 that fiber, specifically water-soluble fiber, helps to lower heart disease risk. Now it's time to take a closer look. Water-soluble fiber can lower blood cholesterol levels by binding bile (made from cholesterol and involved in fat digestion) and cholesterol (from food) in the intestinal tract, and therefore block cholesterol absorption and even effectively "drains" some of the cholesterol from the body. Here's how water-soluble fiber works. When you eat a meal with cholesterol along with a water-soluble food source (beans, fruit, and oats), the fiber attracts cholesterol, blocking its absorption (as noted by the dashed arrow from the intestines), taking the cholesterol into the stool. (See Figure 6.14.)

Nutrition Bite

Beans such as black, navy, and pinto beans are a great source of water-soluble fiber. Studies show including a daily serving of beans helps to lower blood cholesterol levels.

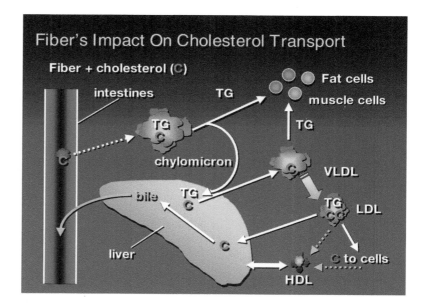

Figure 6.14

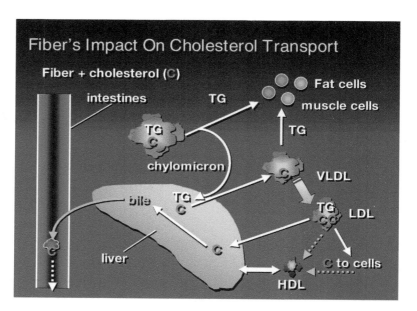

Figure 6.15

Water-soluble fiber also attracts bile, which ultimately comes from the liver (made from cholesterol). (See Figure 6.15.) The bile-fiber combo heads to the stool (as noted by the dashed arrow in the intestines), effectively taking away some of the body's cholesterol. The end result is lowering of blood cholesterol levels. In fact, eating more foods rich in water-soluble fiber is a very effective way to lower moderately elevated levels of blood cholesterol (200–250 mg/dL range).

ADVICE: **Eat adequate fiber (both types) by meeting the Daily Value of 25 grams.**

DIETARY RECOMMENDATIONS TO REDUCE YOUR RISK FOR HEART DISEASE

Now let's put all this advice together in the "Dietary Guidelines for Prevention and Treatment of Heart Disease" from the American Heart Association.

These guidelines are for all people over the age of 2.

- Total dietary intake of fat should be less than 25–35 percent of total calories.
- Saturated fat intake should be less than 10 percent of total calories (trans fat included).
- Dietary cholesterol intake should be less than 300 milligrams per day.
- Meet the Daily Value for fiber of 25 grams per day.
- Sodium intake should be less than 1,500 milligrams of sodium (this will be discussed in Chapter 8).
- Limit alcohol intake.
- Achieve a healthy weight.
- Physical activity—30 minutes or more most days a week.

When you complete your Diet Project, you will compare your intake of calories from total fat and saturated fat and see where you stand. Also, you will make comparisons with the Daily Value for fiber (25 grams) and cholesterol (300 milligrams).

Computing Recommended Intake of Fat and Saturated Fat

From these guidelines, you can determine your recommended fat and saturated fat intake (or figure out anyone's) in grams per day based on your calorie intake.

Expect this type of calculation on the exam. Being knowledgeable about this may help you advise your folks or other friends about limiting their fat intake for better heart health.

EXAMPLE: A friend interested in reducing his risk for heart disease eats 2,500 calories per day. What is his recommended fat and saturated fat intake?

Recommendations: less than 25–35 percent calories as fat
less than 10 percent calories as saturated fat

To calculate **total fat intake**, multiply the 35 percent recommendation by the total number of calories in your friend's diet:

2,500 calories × 0.35 = 875 calories

Convert this number to grams of fat by dividing this number by the physiological fuel value for fat:

875 calories divided by 9 calories/gram = 97 grams

Your friend should eat less than 97 grams of fat per day
for better heart health.

To calculate **saturated fat intake**, multiply the 10 percent recommendation by the total number of calories in your friend's diet:

2,500 calories × 0.10 = 250 calories

Convert this number to grams of saturated fat by dividing this number by the physiological fuel value for fat:

250 calories divided by 9 calories/gram = 28 grams

Your friend should eat less than 28 grams of saturated fat per day
for better heart health.

DAILY VALUE FOR FAT AND SATURATED FAT AND USING FOOD LABELS

The Daily Value for fat and saturated fat used on the Nutrition Facts food label are based on the dietary recommendations to reduce heart disease risk. Since the Daily Values are based on a 2,000-calorie diet, similar calculations from page 133 can be applied. This is just what the Food and Drug Administration did in establishing the Daily Value for fat and saturated fat. (See Figure 6.16.)

The daily value for total fat represents less than 30 percent fat calories and less than 10 percent fat calories from sataurated fat. You should commit these numbers to memory for the exam but also for future reference so that you can quickly compute what percent of the Daily Value a food provides for fat or saturated fat. This way you can decide whether that food makes good sense in relation to the rest of your daily intake.

Let's put these Daily Values to work and interpret a food label.

Compute the percent Daily Value for fat and saturated fat using information from a food label (grams of total fat and saturated fat per serving). (See Figures 6.17 and 6.18.)

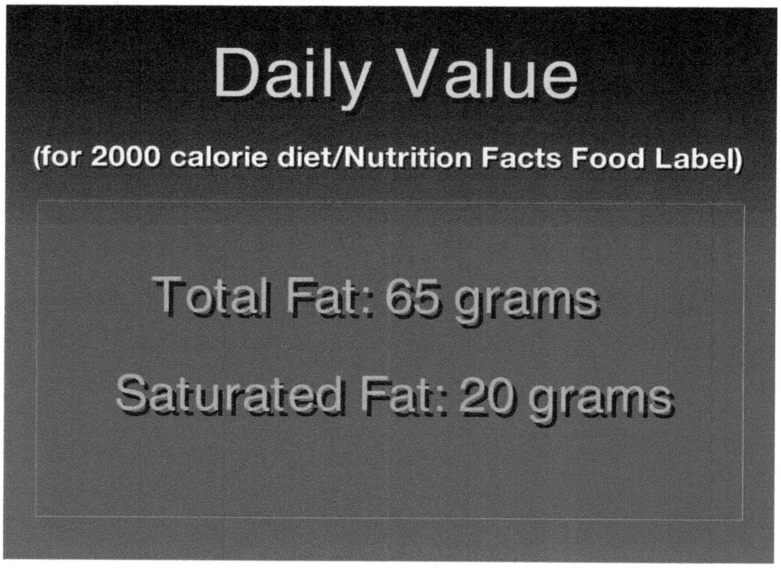

Daily Value

(for 2000 calorie diet/Nutrition Facts Food Label)

Total Fat: 65 grams

Saturated Fat: 20 grams

Figure 6.16

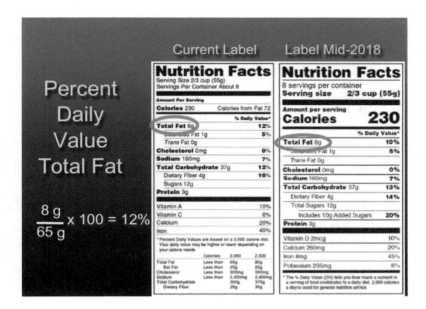

Figure 6.17

With knowledge about heart disease under your belt, you should feel confident about the dietary recommendations to reduce risk and why. Additionally, recognizing a person's risk factors should also become second nature: for example, high blood cholesterol level, inactive, smoker, and so on. Finally, make sure you feel comfortable about computing recommended fat and saturated fat intake (or budget) for a person given their calorie intake.

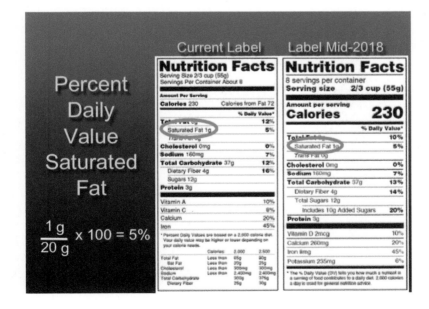

Figure 6.18

Quiz Yourself

6

CHAPTER

1. List a good food source of:

   • Cholesterol _____

   • Polyunsaturated fat _____

   • HDL _____

   • Fat type that raises blood cholesterol levels _____

2. Which of the following statement(s) concerning dietary fats and cholesterol is/are true?

   a. Consumption of diets containing a high level of saturated fatty acids is associated with a high level of blood cholesterol.

   b. All food fats that contain a high proportion of saturated fatty acids (40 percent or more), either naturally occurring or produced by hydrogenation, are major sources of dietary cholesterol.

   c. Reducing the proportion of dietary energy (calories) provided as fat and reducing the saturated fatty acid content of the diet will tend to reduce the blood cholesterol level.

   d. a + c are true.

   e. All the above (a through c) are true.

3. Which lipoprotein is thought to protect against cardiovascular disease?

   a. Low Density Lipoproteins (LDL)

   b. Very Low Density Lipoproteins (VLDL)

   c. High Density Lipoproteins (HDL)

   d. Triglycerides (TG)

4. Your friend has asked you if his daily fat intake of 92 grams and saturated fat intake of 33 grams meet recommendations to reduce risk of heart disease. His daily intake is 2400 kcal. Is he following recommendations? (SHOW WORK)

5. What specific dietary recommendations would you give to someone inter-ested in lowering his or her risk for cardiovascular disease?

_____

_____

_____

6. What is metabolic syndrome?

_____

_____

_____

7. A blood cholesterol level of 245 mg/dL is considered healthy.

   a. true
   b. false

8. A dietary intake of 245 mg/day for cholesterol is in keeping with recommendations.

   a. true
   b. false

9. Low HDL levels (< 40 mg/dL) reflect a greater risk for heart disease.

   a. true
   b. false

OBESITY, WEIGHT CONTROL, AND EATING DISORDERS— THE FACTS

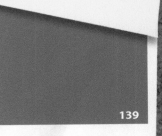

Although heart disease is referred to as the single leading cause of death in the United States, another ailment is plaguing our nation—obesity. In this chapter, we discuss the issue of energy imbalance, along with another related issue—eating disorders. At the onset, many of you may already have some views on obesity—its causes and the best ways to lose weight. We also have prejudices regarding obesity, such as beliefs that obese people are "lazy" and that excess weight is an issue of overeating. I urge you to read this chapter and engage in the course material with an open mind. Obesity is a complex condition with no simple solutions. Additionally, obesity prevention is paramount because much of our nation is either obese or overweight, and this negatively impacts our nation with rising health-care costs due to obesity-related health problems.

OBESITY STATISTICS

Take a quick look around on a crowded street or in a busy shopping mall, and you will notice that most people are overweight or even obese. The statistics are telling:

- Approximately two-thirds of adult men and women are obese or overweight based upon BMI (Body Mass Index, defined in the next section).
- Roughly 10 percent of pre-school age children are obese as well as 20 percent of kids ages 6 to 11 years old.
- By teen years, 20 percent are obese with an 80 percent likelihood that they will become obese as adults.

Chapter Objectives

In this chapter, we will cover the following:

- A healthy weight for you
- Body fat distribution and fat cell development
- Control of food intake—the body's defense against weight loss

- Obesity causes—why energy balance becomes skewed
- Weight loss—the options: what works and what to avoid
- Eating disorders—prevalence and health risks

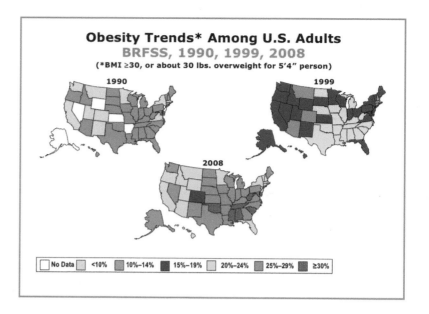

Figure 7.1

As evident from Figure 7.1, the prevalence of obesity among adults has dramatically increased over the past several decades. This figure shows the percent of the population by state that is obese. From 1990 to 2008, the prevalence of obesity has more than doubled in some states according to the U.S. Surgeon General's office and Centers for Disease Control. Since 2008, the rate of overweight and obesity (defined using a tool called Body Mass Index—page 143) has continued to increase. Currently two-thirds of the adult population is either overweight or obese. The rising obesity rate has profound implications on healthcare costs, and about $190 billion per year is spent on obesity-related health problems. Extreme obesity may also cut an individual's life span short by an estimated 12 years or more.

HEALTHY BODY WEIGHT—IS YOURS?

As an adult, your current body weight reflects in part your energy balance and fat stores. As you learned in Chapter 3, your energy intake (from fat, carbohydrate and protein) is balanced with your energy output (as BMR, activity and TEF) as shown in Figure 7.2.

Over time, if calorie intake equals output, then fat stores (just like your savings account in the bank) remain constant. And when you step on a bathroom scale, a steady body weight over that same period of time reflects this.

For many American adults, however, body weight (fat stores) are not steady. An increase in energy or fat stores occurs over time when energy balance is skewed: intake exceeds output. (See Figure 7.3.) This occurs several ways:

- when calorie intake increases and exceeds current caloric expenditure;
- when caloric intake is constant but caloric output decreases; or
- when both occur—caloric intake increases and caloric output decreases.

Regardless of how, the end result of excess calories in the body means the energy becomes stored as fat. This registers as a gain of body weight.

Our task now is to define how much fat, or using another measure such as body weight, is too much and presents health problems.

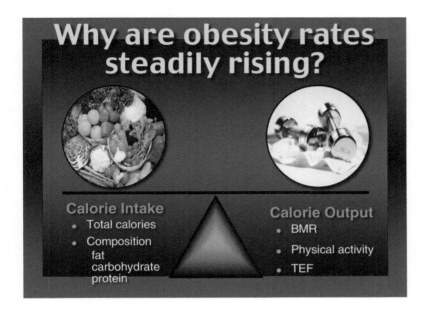

Figure 7.2

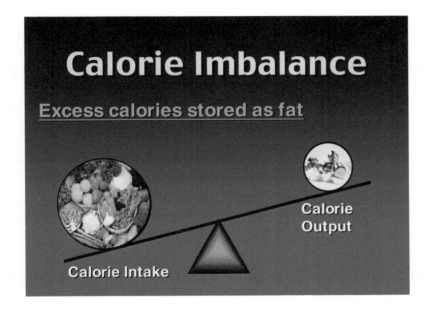

Figure 7.3

Defining Obesity

Culture, influenced by the latest imagery from TV, movies and the Internet, defines desirable body size in part. But science can define best the association between body weight and good health and the connection between body weight poor health and disease risk. Obesity is defined as excess body fat that contributes to adverse health effects.

As you can see in Figure 7.4, there is an association between increasing body weight and an increase in death rate. There are several methods used for obesity classification that either directly or indirectly assess body fat stores and, in turn, potential health problems. Here are two common methods used to assess weight status that determine if someone is overweight or obese.

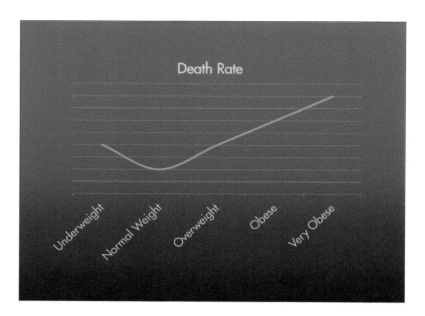

1. Body Fat

Determining what proportion (percentage) of a person's body weight is fat gets to the heart of the matter:

> Obese   25% body fat for men
> 35% body fat for women

Several techniques are in use to determine the proportion of body weight that is fat.

- **Skin-fold thickness technique** uses calipers to measure body fat through measurement of subcutaneous (underneath the skin) fat. This technique requires the individual to be skilled in using the calipers. Repeat measurements should be taken by the same technician to avoid error.
- **Underwater-weighing** or the hydrostatic technique measures body weight based upon the principle that fat floats (because fat weighs less than water). The greater the difference between what you weigh in water compared to what you weigh out of water, the greater the body fat content.
- **Bioelectrical impedance technique** involves passing a very small electrical current through the body, with body fat determined based on transmission of the electrical current. Fat conducts electricity poorly due to its low water content while muscle transmits the current well.
- **DXA (Dual-energy X-ray)** assesses body fat content by passing a very light x-ray over the body. Each tissue type, such as muscle and fat, absorbs the x-rays differently, allowing accurate measurement of the percent of body fat.

All of these, as well as other techniques, involve measurement error so that the value determined is an approximation.

Urban Myth

Myth: "Losing weight and achieving 0% body fat is healthy."

Not only is losing enough body fat to register 0% impossible, having no body fat would also be deadly. Since cell membranes have fat as part of their structure and some body fat stores are necessary for reproductive function (particularly in women), some body fat is essential for good health.

2. Body Mass Index (BMI)

The BMI measures a ratio of body weight to height that correlates well to body fat levels (even though BMI is **NOT** a direct measure of body fat).

> Obese   BMI equal to or more than 30

This technique involves computing a ratio of body weight to height. As shown in Figure 7.5, height is measured in meters and then squared.

As revealed in numerous research studies, there is an association between BMIs 25 and above with health problems, such as heart disease, stroke, and diabetes. Additionally, a person who is overweight experiences a much greater risk for becoming obese than a healthy-weight individual. Figure 7.5 shows normal, overweight, and obese BMIs.

What Is Your BMI?

Use the chart in Figure 7.6 to determine where your current body weight falls.

You can also use the graph in Figure 7.7 and plot what weight range is healthy for your height. Note there is no gender differentiation. Women, though, should be at the lower range of the healthy weight range for height and men toward the upper healthy weight range for height. (See Figure 7.7.)

While the BMI is fairly consistent in predicting obesity, the BMI may erroneously determine obesity for individuals who have large amounts of muscle mass. Athletes, such as muscular rugby or football players, may have BMIs in the high 20s or even over 30 and still be lean.

As you can see from our discussion, defining obesity is not quite black and white. There is "gray" around the definition and each of us should be assessed individually for health risks associated with our body weight and body fat levels.

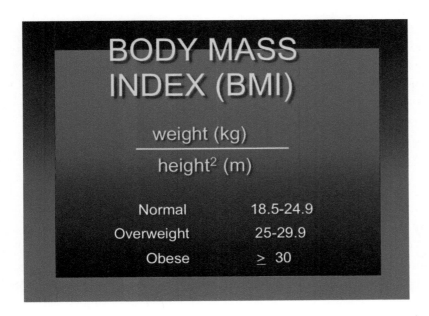

Figure 7.5

OVERWEIGHT AND OBESE CUT OFF POINTS		
HEIGHT	BMI OF 25 OVERWEIGHT	BMI OF 30 OBESE
Inches	Pounds	Pounds
58	119	147
60	128	153
62	136	164
64	145	174
66	155	186
68	164	197
70	174	207
72	184	221
74	194	233
76	205	246

Figure 7.6

In the BMI chart below, mark the square where your height and weight cross. The color of the square will show you if you are a healthy weight, overweight, or obese.

BMI	Healthy Weight						Overweight					Obese								
	19	20	21	22	23	24	25	26	27	28	29	30	31	32	33	34	35	36	37	38
Height	Weight (in pounds)																			
4'10"	91	96	100	105	110	115	119	124	129	134	138	143	148	153	158	162	167	172	177	181
4'11"	94	99	104	109	114	119	124	128	133	138	143	148	153	158	163	168	173	178	183	188
5'0"	97	102	107	112	118	123	128	133	138	143	148	153	158	163	168	174	179	184	189	194
5'1"	100	106	111	116	122	127	132	137	143	148	153	158	164	169	174	180	185	190	195	201
5'2"	104	109	115	120	126	131	136	142	147	153	158	164	169	175	180	186	191	196	202	207
5'3"	107	113	118	124	130	135	141	146	152	158	163	169	175	180	186	191	197	203	208	214
5'4"	110	116	122	128	134	140	145	151	157	163	169	174	180	186	192	197	204	209	215	221
5'5"	114	120	126	132	138	144	150	156	162	168	174	180	186	192	198	204	210	216	222	228
5'6"	118	124	130	136	142	148	155	161	167	173	179	186	192	198	204	210	216	223	229	235
5'7"	121	127	134	140	146	153	159	166	172	178	185	191	198	204	211	217	223	230	236	242
5'8"	125	131	138	144	151	158	164	171	177	184	190	197	203	210	216	223	230	236	243	249
5'9"	128	135	142	149	155	162	169	176	182	189	196	203	209	216	223	230	236	243	250	257
5'10"	132	139	146	153	160	167	174	181	188	195	202	209	216	222	229	236	243	250	257	264
5'11"	136	143	150	157	165	172	179	186	193	200	208	215	222	229	236	243	250	257	265	272
6'0"	140	147	154	162	169	177	184	191	199	206	213	221	228	235	242	250	258	265	272	279
6'1"	144	151	159	166	174	182	189	197	204	212	219	227	235	242	250	257	265	272	280	288
6'2"	148	155	163	171	179	186	194	202	210	218	225	233	241	249	256	264	272	280	287	295
6'3"	152	160	168	176	184	192	200	208	216	224	232	240	248	256	264	272	279	287	295	303
6'4"	156	164	172	180	189	197	205	213	221	230	238	246	254	263	271	279	287	295	304	312

Figure 7.7

BODY FAT DISTRIBUTION AND FAT CELL DEVELOPMENT

Determining if a person is overweight or obese represents part of the story. It is also important to determine where excess fat is located because certain profiles of body fat distribution present greater health risks than others. Additionally, understanding the nature of a fat cell is also important in deciphering obesity and health-related issues.

Both men and women have gender specific sites for fat storage, as shown in Figure 7.8.

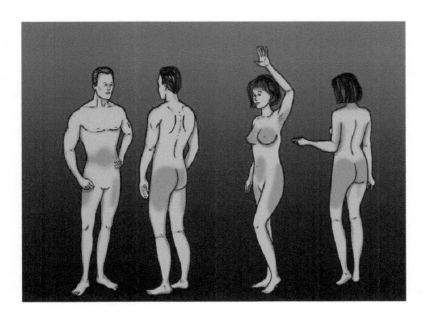

Figure 7.8

These fat depot sites are normal and reflect our "cave person" origins. In prehistoric times, survival meant getting through lean times when food was scarce and environmental conditions were tough. To ensure survival, humans evolved efficiency at storing fat (energy stores) when food was scarce. As a result, scientists suggest that men and women developed gender-specific sites of fat storage that allowed for survival. Women stored body fat in thighs, hips, and buttocks to ensure reproduction and men stored fat in locations such as the trunk region, which allowed for greater mobility.

Lower- and Upper-Body Obesity

With these gender-specific fat depot sites in mind, now let's look at excess fat gained in these regions and subsequent health risks that develop. There are two general types of body fat distribution seen in people, and more dramatically in obese people: lower- and upper-body obesity. (See Figure 7.9.)

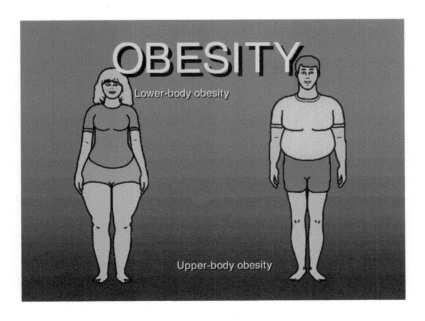

Figure 7.9

Lower-Body Obesity

- This type is sometimes called "pear-shaped" or "gynoid" obesity.
- Excess fat is stored in the hip and thigh region.
- This fat distribution is more common in women (based on gender-specific fat depot sites; seen in Figure 7.8).
- Research suggests that fat in this region is more resistant to weight loss, perhaps a throwback to early human times when women needed to maintain fat stores for pregnancy and breast-feeding.
- This type of fat distribution, by itself and in the absence of other health factors, such as high blood pressure, blood cholesterol, or waist measurement, does not pose a significant health risk.

Upper-Body Obesity

- This type is sometimes called "apple-shaped" or "android" obesity.
- Excess fat is stored in the abdominal/trunk area sometimes referred to as a "beer belly."
- This fat distribution is more common in men (based on gender-specific fat depot sites). But following menopause and drop in estrogen levels, women tend to store excess body fat in the abdomen region and develop upper-body obesity.
- This type of fat distribution is associated with a greater risk of health problems such as cardiovascular disease, diabetes, high blood pressure, and certain types of cancer. As shown in Figure 7.10, the location of this body fat—**visceral** fat—that is underneath the abdominal muscle wall, is near organs such as the liver and heart. As a result, this stored body fat appears to directly impact blood fat levels, insulin resistance, and blood pressure.

Determining Upper-Body Obesity

A simple measurement of the waist circumference determines upper-body obesity.

- Using a tape measure that is flexible, measure your waist just above the belly button, but below the last rib.

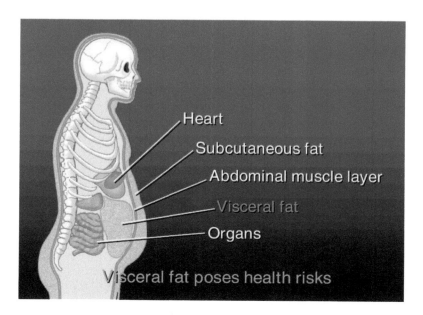

Figure 7.10

A waist measurement of >40 inches for men and >35 inches for women indicates abdominal obesity. Remember from the last chapter, large waist size characterizes metabolic syndrome.

Health Risks Associated with Obesity

Our discussion of body fat distribution brings us to summarize health problems associated with obesity in general. Obese individuals tend to be at greater risk for a variety of health problems including:

- Cardiovascular disease (heart disease)
- High LDL cholesterol
- Low HDL cholesterol
- High blood glucose (insulin resistance)
- Hypertension (high blood pressure)
- Diabetes (Type 2)
- Certain types of cancer (uterine, breast, colon, and prostate)
- Osteoarthritis (joint trouble due to the excess body weight)
- Emotional disturbances (many obese individuals experience discrimination, issues of low self-esteem, and subsequent feelings of depression)
- Pregnancy complications

While these health risks appear in adults, obese children and teens can also suffer from some of these conditions.

Fat Cells and Their Development

Fat is stored as triglyceride in cells called **adipose cells**. As shown in Figure 7.11, an adipose cell has a fat storage compartment, which can expand to hold more triglyceride or contract as triglyceride comes out of storage for energy use. Thus, when energy intake exceeds expenditure, triglyceride storage increases and fat cells expand. As you'll learn in the next section, the number of adipose cells may increase if more storage sites are needed.

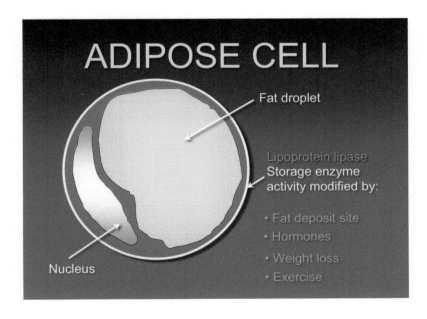

Figure 7.11

Enzymes that sit at the surface of the adipose cell are involved in the storage and release of triglyceride inside fat cells. An enzyme vital to the storage of triglyceride is called **lipoprotein lipase** or **LPL** for short. This enzyme's activity is influenced by several factors, which in turn means that adipose cells have varying capacity to store fat (an important issue when understanding obesity).

- Research studies show that LPL is more active at certain **fat depot sites** than others. Adipose cells in the hip and thigh region appear to have more active LPL than elsewhere in the body for women. On the other hand, LPL activity is greater in the abdomen region for men. This is in keeping with how women and men differ in fat storage sites.
- **Hormonal and metabolic** changes, such as during pregnancy, also influence the activity of LPL. When a woman becomes pregnant, LPL activity goes up in adipocytes from the breasts, hips, and other sites in order to store more fat. This ensures energy stores for the developing baby and breast-feeding and makes sense, especially thinking back to our early ancestors who often went without food during scarce times.
- Following **weight loss**, LPL activity goes up, which means the adipose cell WANTS to store fat, filling the fat cell back up despite your efforts and desires for lasting weight loss. This may seem contrary to what you want, but again think back to what makes sense in terms of our early ancestors and their survival. Someone who lost weight would need to restock energy stores so that they could survive another situation of low energy intake such as a famine. So increasing LPL activity in response to weight loss ensures a return of adequate fat reserves.
- **Exercise** also impacts LPL levels. When a person is physically active, their muscles need the triglycerides for fuel and their fat cells can do without. Thus, LPL activity at fat cells decline while this same enzyme that exists at muscle cells increases to meet energy demands at the muscle. This helps to explain why people who exercise routinely have less body fat (smaller fat cells) than folks who don't exercise.

Fat Cell Development

Understanding when and under what circumstances fat cells are made and change in size helps us to understand the development and prevention of obesity. The number of adipose cells *normally* increases during periods of growth. There are believed to be two periods of cell number increase, which are sometimes termed "critical periods."

1. **Fetal development to early childhood years:** Fat cells increase in number and fill with fat during the last few months of fetal development and up until the pre-school years.
2. **Puberty (approximately ages eleven to fourteen years):** Scientists believe that fat cell numbers again increase and then level off if a person maintains energy balance. If a young teen gains excess body fat, there may be an increase in the number of fat cells. Now consider that these new fat cells "want" triglyceride energy reserves to fill them. More fat cells translate to greater body fat levels. Obese teens run the risk of about a 70 to 80 percent chance of being obese as adults. Thus, considering the current trend in obesity rates among youth, health professionals encourage preventing excessive weight gain during the teen years.

Although the fat cell number is considered to be stable during adulthood, evidence from research shows that the adipose number may increase when weight gain stimulus is sufficient. During pregnancy, for example, when desirable weight gain of 25 to 35 pounds is dramatically exceeded, the fat cell number may increase. Also, during a period of extreme inactivity such as an injury, when a large amount of weight gain may occur, the fat cell number may increase. The significance of this is that **once a fat cell is made, it does not go away**. Considering that fat cells "want" to be filled with triglyceride for energy reserves, the more adipose cells a person has, most likely the more body fat they have. **With weight loss, fat cells shrink but they do not go away.**

Adipose development is summarized in Figure 7.12.

It is important to emphasize that, with weight loss, fat cell number does not change, and with excess weight gain earlier in life, adipose cell number is most likely increased and these cells are there to stay. (See Figure 7.13.)

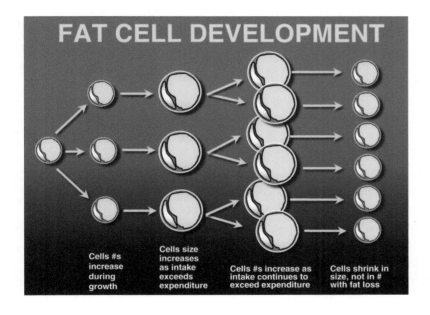

Figure 7.12

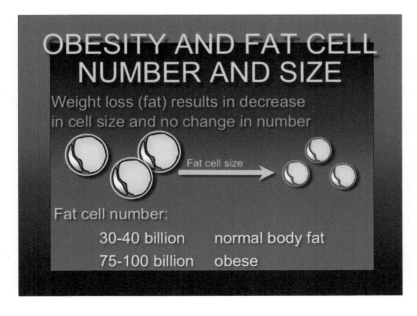

Figure 7.13

Liposuction

Is there a way to get "rid" of adipose cells? A surgical procedure called liposuction removes fat (adipose cells) from specific areas. While this is not specifically a treatment for obesity, it has become a popular way to "sculpt" the body and lessen fat in certain areas such as the thighs (bulges around the hips) or the tummy. This procedure may temporarily reduce fat in specific locations, but according to research may also result in a regain of body fat with filling of fat cells elsewhere and the creation of new fat cells.

FOOD INTAKE CONTROL

Before we can better understand the complexities of why obesity develops, we need to discuss the basics about why we eat—termed **food intake control**. We initiate the action of eating and cessation of eating for a variety of internal and external reasons or factors. Consider that each of us on average eats about 900,000 to over 1 million calories per year. This intake of calories, if you recall, is balanced with calorie output, as shown in Figure 7.2.

In energy balance, or weight maintenance, intake is balanced with output. This is actually quite an accomplishment considering being off by 50 or so calories per day (that is, intake greater than output of about half a small cookie each day) translates to about a one or two pound weight gain per year. Over the past decade, the average weight gain is about one to two pounds, suggesting most are "off" by about 50 or so calories daily. Thus, small errors in energy balance can spell weight gain over time and the development of obesity.

People who keep their weight steady are in energy homeostasis. But because most Americans are gaining weight and not balancing energy intake with output, let's take a look at why some people balance energy intake with energy output, while others do not. What follows are the many factors—both internal and external—that influence our food intake control.

Internal Factors of Food Intake Control

Many factors that are internal, that is, within the body, impact food intake control. Internal factors include brain centers, blood metabolites, and other signals that stimulate the body to eat, feelings of **hunger**, or that signal the body to not eat, feelings of **satiety**. These signals may stimulate food intake or satiety over the short term—within hours or minutes—or may signal eating or not eating over the long term—days or weeks.

There is a general theme around the control of food intake that has profound implications in relation to obesity. **The body is designed to defend against weight loss.** Remember, this response comes from our prehistoric ancestors who needed to survive times of scarce food supply. So rather than "being satisfied" at a lower weight or body fat level, signals designed for survival kick in and prompt eating over the short and long term to ensure adequate energy stores. Here are several internal factors that influence food intake control.

Central Nervous System

Brain centers—There are several regions in the brain that respond to signals from the body including small proteins, such as **ghrelin** or hormones, like insulin. One brain center called the **hypothalamus** responds to blood metabolites and hormones that signal to stimulate or suppress eating.

Brain chemicals—Serotonin, a chemical produced in the brain that exerts feeling of calmness, has been shown to influence eating.

Peripheral Factors

Hormones—Insulin, sex hormones, and others impact food intake control. For example, in the brain, insulin signals the brain and food intake is increased. During puberty, the female hormone estrogen prompts fat cells in the hip and thigh region to fill indirectly, stimulating increases in energy intake.

Fat mass and fat cell size—A hormone released by fat cells called **leptin** signals the brain (as shown in Figure 7.14) that fat stores are adequate and this modulates or lessens eating and stimulates BMR to help steady fat stores. If fat cells have shrunk due to weight loss, leptin levels decrease and food intake increases so as to fill fat stores back up.

Stomach signals—The stomach sends out its own signals such as the small protein called ghrelin. This hormone triggers eating as levels of ghrelin rise immediately prior to eating. Ghrelin levels also decline after a meal. But for some obese people, ghrelin levels stay elevated after eating, suggesting an explanation as to why some report "always feeling hungry." Also, the intestinal tract releases its own signals, one called CCK, and tells the brain in response to eating that you're full or satiated.

Exercise—While this may at first appear as an external factor, exercise initiates a series of internal changes that impact food intake. On a short-term basis, an exercise session (particularly an intense one) inhibits food intake most likely because of a brief rise in body temperature. Over the long term, food intake increases with regular exercise but a person typically has less body fat, smaller fat cells, and the

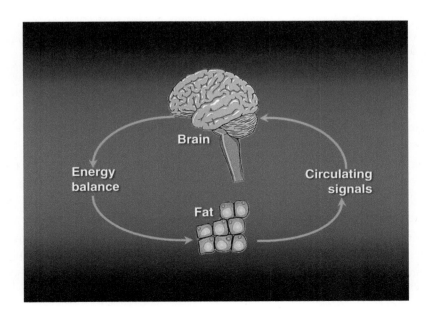

Figure 7.14

body has the ability to burn fat at muscle cells more effectively compared to a sedentary state. With exercise training, LPL activity at the muscle increases, while decreasing at adipose sites.

Conditions or Diseases That May Alter Food Intake

Pregnancy and breast-feeding—Eating changes with pregnancy; hunger levels may fluctuate due to changing hormone levels and fat gain occurs serving as energy reserves for pregnancy and breast-feeding. The hormones produced to maintain lactation (breast-feeding) stimulate food intake so that a woman has significant energy intake to contribute to breast milk production.

Obesity—The condition of obesity itself is known to impact food intake regulation, perhaps because of altered leptin levels, other signals to the brain, such as ghrelin, and to the brains' ability to respond to these signals. This altered response may be a consequence of obesity or a genetic predisposition.

Eating disorders—Discussed in a later section of this chapter, eating disorders anorexia and bulimia are characterized by abnormal eating patterns and behaviors. Brain chemical levels, such as serotonin levels, may be altered in a person with bulimia for example, which in turn impacts food intake. All food intake control in eating disordered individuals is believed to be both behaviorally and genetically rooted.

Cancer—With certain types of cancer, such as stomach or intestinal cancers, eating declines as the disease spreads. Additionally, cancer treatments are notorious for suppressing the appetite.

Psychological disturbances—Clinical depression and other psychological disturbances are often accompanied by changes in food intake. These are believed to have biological origins such as alterations in brain chemical levels.

External Factors

Various factors in our environment also impact our feelings of hunger and satiety. With external factors, our own personal experiences come into play as we respond based on childhood experiences, for example, in making decisions to eat certain foods. Here are a few external factors.

Time of day—Often we eat based on the "clock"—that is, when it is noon, we often decide it is time for lunch rather than basing the decision to eat on true feelings of hunger.

Temperature—the external temperature may stimulate hunger as with cold temperatures. This is believed to help build fat reserves in preparation for winter when food was scarce in early human evolution. Warmer temperatures suppress feelings of hunger (think of a very hot day and how you don't really feel like eating, especially a large meal).

Eating cues—We each respond to eating cues or visual signs of food, such as all-you-can-eat buffets, food courts, and other eateries. Studies show that when people are given a variety of foods to choose from, such as with a buffet, that they eat more compared to offerings of a few foods. Also, the larger the portion size we

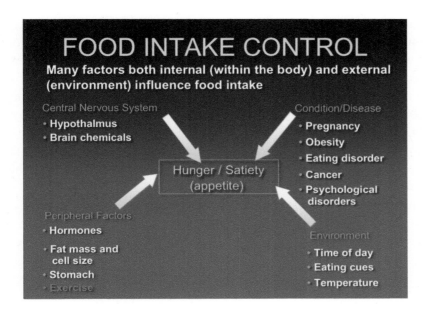

Figure 7.15

are served, generally the more we eat. Both of these are throwbacks to early human times when variety was important to ensure a good nutrient intake and that eating more when more food was available helped boost fat reserves for leaner times.

Food intake control is summarized in Figure 7.15.

OBESITY CAUSES—WHY ENERGY BALANCE BECOMES SKEWED

With your understanding of food intake control and the basic premise that the body is designed to defend against weight loss, let's now take a look into the many causes of obesity. Perhaps at the start of this chapter you had in mind a single "reason" for obesity—eating too much? Being lazy? By now though, you understand the complexities of how the body is designed to preserve fat stores, build up energy reserves to survive periods of famine or low energy intake, and ultimately, put fat "away for a rainy day."

When energy balance is skewed and the body puts excessive fat away (although contrary for optimal health), obesity develops. There are many reasons or causes behind why obesity develops in a given individual. Here are several proposed causes or theories behind obesity development.

Calorie imbalance: This may sound simple, but eating excess calories when calorie output is constant, means excess is converted to and stored as fat. An energy gap of approximately 50 to 100 calories daily can lead to a one to two pounds of weight gain per year and over 20 years, 10 to 20 pounds, and ultimately obesity develops. This increase in calorie intake may be very subtle and occur with lifestyle changes. A change in jobs for example where food is available at break time, or a change in work or sleeping habits that means more time exposed to your kitchen or another eating environment.

Inactivity: Expending fewer calories due to a decline of physical activity while caloric intake stays constant results in excess calories converted to and stored as fat. As with calorie imbalance above, an energy gap of about 100 calories daily results in a few pounds weight gain per year, and over time obesity develops. This decline in physical activity and subsequent reduction in calories burned may be very subtle, such as in the greater use of labor-saving devices—TV remote controls, automatic garage door openers, and the like. A falloff in physical activity may also occur with a change in lifestyle—new job, starting a family, or even forced inactivity due to an injury. Inactivity can explain much of the rise in obesity in children, teens, and adults over the past few decades.

Genetic influence: A genetic predisposition to put away fat more efficiently or to burn fewer calories (BMR or TEF) while not adjusting caloric intake results in excess calories that are converted to fat and stored. Obesity develops over time, and perhaps may be more likely to occur during childhood and teen years. Some examples of genetic influence include a form of leptin that does not "connect" well with the brain, thus eating behavior is not well regulated in relation to fat stores, as shown in Figures 7.16 and 7.17. Another example may be that a person has a lower than expected TEF (energy needed to digest and assimilate food) thus fewer calories are burned and without caloric intake compensation, excess fat storage occurs and obesity develops over time. How efficiently a person converts excess calories to body fat also has genetic origins as research studies with identical twins have shown.

Set point: This theory of obesity centers on the number of adipose cells a particular individual possesses and the average size of these cells. Consider a person who has 80 billion adipose cells, perhaps due to weight gain during teen years. Since fat cells prefer to be filled to a certain size (recall that fat cells are designed to serve as energy reserves and not shrink away to nothing), this person would have more body fat (obesity) compared to a person with 25 billion adipose cells. This suggests that a person with a high adipose cell number is "doomed" to be obese. As will be discussed in the next section, exercise can overcome this by encouraging

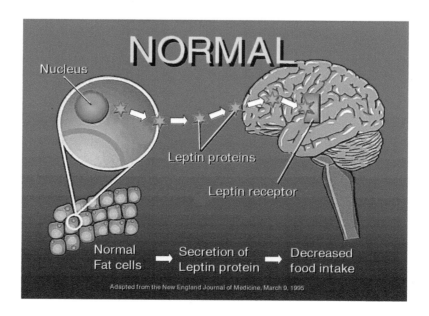

Figure 7.16

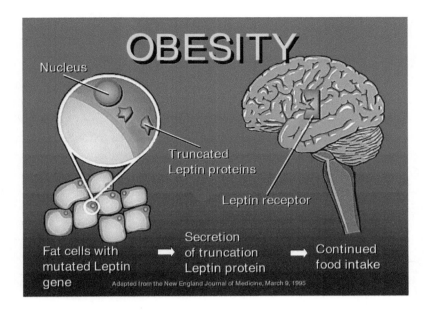

Figure 7.17

fat cells to "accept" being smaller as the muscles become the site where fat goes and gets used as a fuel source.

"Thrifty" metabolism: Along the lines of genetic influence, a "thrifty" metabolism or a lower than expected BMR would mean that person conserves or uses less energy than another person of equal body size. Thus, without reducing caloric intake, excess calories would accumulate (converted to fat) fat stores would increase and obesity would develop over time.

Diet composition: The composition of a person's diet over the long run may have an impact on obesity development. Studies show that eating a high-fat diet, compared to an equal calorie diet with a greater carbohydrate content, can lead to excess weight gain. How can this be if calorie intake is the same? When excess calories are consumed as fat, this is efficiently stored as body fat (not much to do in taking food fat and storing it in fat cells). But for excess calories eaten as protein or carbohydrate, there must first be a conversion to triglyceride in the liver and this must then be shipped to fat cells via lipoproteins. This metabolic work costs some calories so carbohydrate and protein are stored less efficiently as body fat compared to dietary fat's conversion. Additionally, diet patterns that are rich in fiber from fruits, vegetables, and whole grains are associated with lower BMI and smaller waist circumference.

Meal patterns: Some research suggests that the pattern of eating, specifically skipping meals, may have an influence in the development of obesity. Skipping meals, such as breakfast and lunch, may lead to overeating at the next meal. This, of course, would then lead to excess calories stored as fat. In an effort to lose weight, some people skip meals, inadvertently ending up eating more because they become ravenous. It's important to point out that eating in the evening does not necessarily lead to weight gain and obesity. If you balance calories in against calories out, then your weight stays steady even if you eat late into the evening. If you overeat, more calories in than calories out, then weight gain occurs, regardless of when you take in the excess calories.

Nutrition Bite

Sumo wrestlers of Japan practice a specific eating pattern of large meals a few times a day to induce weight gain. Many sumo wrestlers are morbidly obese with BMIs over 40.

WEIGHT LOSS OPTIONS—WHAT WORKS, WHAT TO AVOID

At this point in our obesity discussion, you undoubtedly see the complexities to this condition. This carries over to the treatment of obesity. Perhaps through your own personal experience, you recognize the difficulty in losing weight and then maintaining it. We are a nation obsessed with weight loss, despite the fact that over 65 percent of the population is obese or overweight, suggesting we are not successful with our efforts.

Why is it that weight loss efforts by most people using diet plans, such as the low-carb/high-protein diets, weight loss supplements, such as fat "burners" and appetite suppressants, and other gimmicks, such as skin patches that claim to help boost calorie burning, don't work? An estimated 85 percent of those who try these types of obesity treatment regain their lost weight and often then some.

In this section, we take a look at obesity treatment—what works and what to avoid. Much can be learned from individuals who have lost weight *and* kept this weight off for extended periods of time—several years of more. Bluntly put, it's relatively easy to lose weight; the trick is keeping it off and this requires lifestyle changes. So let's take a look at what works—a successful obesity treatment program.

The three key components to a successful program:

1. **Reduced energy diet**
2. **Behavior modification**
3. **Physical activity or exercise**

Since 1994, researchers from the University of Colorado and Brown Medical School have been compiling information about "successful losers" as part of the National Weight Control Registry (NWCR). Over five thousand participants have lost an average of 65 pounds and have kept it off for more than five years. Researchers tracked both how these participants have lost weight as well as how they have kept it off and learned that controlling calories, monitoring eating behaviors and routinely exercising all are common elements of success. Figure 7.18 shows a few of the common characteristics among NWCR members.

Let's take a look at each of these components in more detail.

1. Reduced Energy Diet

Calorie intake must be less than calorie output for weight loss to occur. An energy deficit forces fat out of storage for fuel use, and in turn, body fat decreases. Creating this calorie deficit involves:

- **Consuming a diet that meets nutrient needs (protein, fiber, vitamins, and minerals) except for energy.** Excluding food groups, such as fruits and grains to avoid carbs (high-protein diets) means missing out on fiber and other essential nutrients (such as vitamins).
- **Meeting individual tastes and habits.** Setting up a diet plan that meets the person's individual food preferences is important for compliance during the weight loss phase and important in the long term for weight maintenance. Forbidding certain foods, such as sweets or making a person eat foods that they

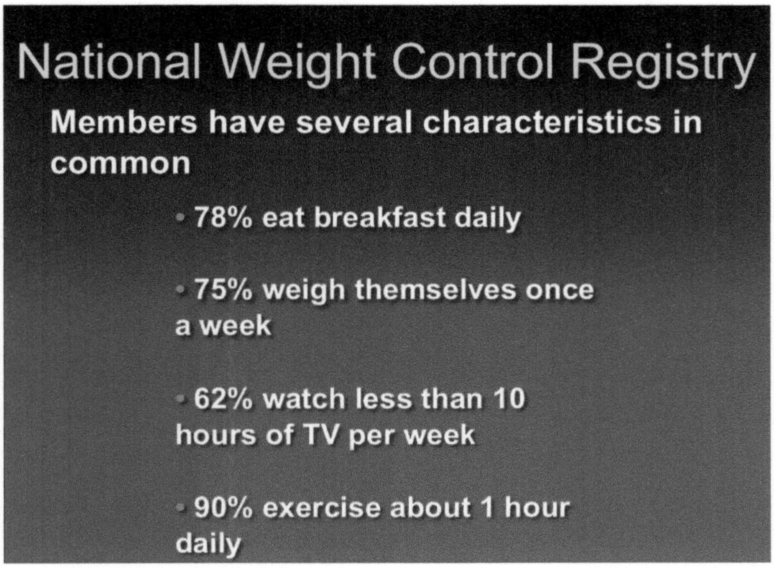

National Weight Control Registry

Members have several characteristics in common

- 78% eat breakfast daily
- 75% weigh themselves once a week
- 62% watch less than 10 hours of TV per week
- 90% exercise about 1 hour daily

Figure 7.18

don't care for often results in failure when the individual reverts to overeating their favorite foods and excluding "good-for-you" foods that they don't like.

- **Designing a plan that minimizes fatigue and hunger.** Creating a large energy deficit can leave a person feeling weak and very hungry. Not only does this hamper a person's ability to function, but can easily lead to diet failure when they find it difficult to fight ravenous hunger pangs. Additionally, severe calorie restriction leads to a loss of muscle mass as well as body fat since the body is forced to make carbohydrate out of protein tissue to fuel the brain. Instead of rapid weight loss, losing about a half pound to no more than two pounds per week can avoid this problem and is the recommended safe rate of weight loss. This translates to a calorie gap of about 250 to 1,000 calories per day. (This energy gap can also be created by exercise as well as cutting back on calorie intake, or a combination of the two.)

2. Behavior Modification

Changing current eating behavior leads to decreased calorie intake and the establishment of new eating behavior conducive to weight loss and maintenance.

- **Changing eating behavior.** This involves tracking current eating habits through the use of a detailed food diary. In this log, a person writes down not only what they eat and the amount, but also the time it took to eat the meal or snack, associated activities such as watching TV, mood, and hunger level. Through the assistance of a professional skilled in behavior modification, the diary is then evaluated for patterns such as rapid eating pace or munching mindlessly on snacks while watching TV.
- **Understanding response to environmental cues.** Also through the diary, a person can track which environmental cues trigger eating, such as being alone or TV viewing. Understanding response to these environmental triggers helps a person see what aspects of their environment should be changed to assist in weight loss and maintenance.

- **Cognitive restructuring.** Step-by-step behavior is modified, such as techniques to slow eating pace, finding alternative activities to TV viewing, or moving the TV from the eating area. Each of these steps is unique for individuals based on their own eating behaviors.

    Behavior modification works well for mildly overweight individuals. Once weight is lost, returning to the food diary every so often helps keep a person on track with their new habits.

3. Physical Activity

Increasing caloric expenditure through purposeful physical activity while keeping caloric intake the same (or decreasing it) creates an energy deficit that leads to fat loss. Beyond this benefit, there are many other health benefits attributable to increasing physical exercise.

- **Food intake control.** Perhaps the most important outcome of regular physical activity is better food intake control. This means that the body is better able to balance intake with output. Studies show that people who exercise regularly eat more than people who don't, but that exercisers have less body fat. Thus, exercise must allow the body to better balance in and out. On a short-term basis, exercise (especially intense forms such as an interval running workout) blunts appetite, thus decreasing calorie intake soon after exercise.
- **Body weight, fat loss, and lean tissue preservation.** Exercise specifically helps with fat loss. Triglycerides are pulled out of fat cells for use as fuel by the muscles. Also, exercise stimulates lean tissue or muscle to develop—tone and increase in size. This means a person can lose fat but preserve lean mass and get a sleeker look which cutting calories alone won't do. Also, an increase in muscle or lean tissue increases the number of calories burned at rest since this tissue costs more for the body to maintain than fat tissue.
- **Increased metabolism.** Exercise boosts the BMR so that a person is burning more calories at rest (see Chapter 3). This may be an extra 25 to 50 calories per day or perhaps more. In the long run, this means burning more calories compared to when your "body" was sedentary and this helps not only with weight loss, but with weight maintenance.
- **Weight maintenance.** Studies show that people who exercise keep lost weight off better than people who just diet or restrict calories. Much of what we have discussed thus far suggests that our bodies were designed to be physically active.
- **Improved sense of well-being.** Exercise has been shown to improve mood and sense of self. Often, people who are overweight or obese have low self-esteem. With the addition of physical activity, self-esteem improves. Dieting alone as a way to lose weight does not have this benefit.
- **Chronic disease prevention.** Regular exercise has a variety of health benefits, including lowering risk for heart disease, certain forms of cancer, improving blood sugar control and symptoms of diabetes, lowering high blood pressure, and boosting bone mineral density, which protects against osteoporosis. All these benefits and more are something that dieting alone can't do!

Combined, these three key components—reduced energy diet, behavior modification, and exercise—are essential in successful weight loss and maintenance.

Obesity Treatments with Poor Outcomes

Many different weight loss options are available—diet books, supplements, even surgery. While some people find success with a particular program, most attempt and fail. Here's a rundown on a few options with words of caution.

Very low-calorie diets. Often administered through a physician or another type of medically supervised facility, very low-calorie diets restrict energy intake to about 300 to 800 calories daily. Obese individuals with health problems should be medically supervised and monitored to prevent heart or kidney trouble. Also, participants should be counseled to make lifestyle changes in activity and eating habits to avoid regaining lost weight. These programs may be successful if well supervised, but often people don't stick with the program because these diets are very restrictive (usually liquid formulas) and monotanous.

Special formulas or products. These types of weight loss programs are centered on a product (or product line) that replaces real food. As with low-calorie diets, these are very restrictive and limit a person's ability to eat in "real" situations, such as with family and at social outings.

Extremes in macronutrient restriction. Weight loss programs that omit carbohydrate or fat generally don't work in the long run because they are very restrictive and people find them difficult to stick with in the long term. While people may find short-term success, long-term weight maintenance is poor with these diets. Additionally, they often lack in meeting essential nutrient needs, which is problematic in the long run.

Surgery. Several surgical procedures are used in treating severe obesity. Physicians may opt to recommend bariatric surgery for a person whose immediate health is greatly compromised by their excess weight. Surgery is indicated for individuals with a BMI of 40 and above as well as for people with a BMI of > 35 who also have health problems, such as diabetes and hypertension. Physicians generally do not recommend bariatric surgery for teens or individuals over 55 years old. Gastric bypass, as shown in Figure 7.19, involves bypassing most of the stomach and the

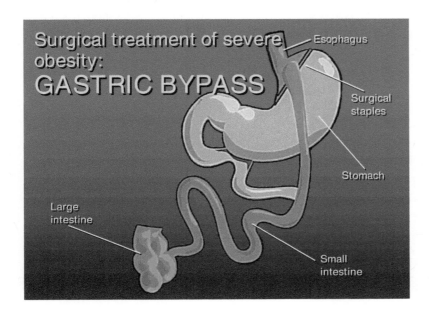

Figure 7.19

top portion of the small intestines and reconnecting the intestines to the top part of the stomach. This prevents foods from being digested and absorbed, which means most calories (along with nutrients) don't enter the body. Dramatic amount of weight is lost but there are potentially severe health problems and these patients must be monitored closely.

The more common and safer bariatric surgery is called gastric band or "lap band" procedure, which essentially limits the size of the stomach so very little food can fit. The band, as shown in Figure 7.20, can be tightened to make the stomach capacity smaller. Eating too much food creates discomfort so the person eats less and loses weight. These and other surgical procedures may be expensive and may not be covered by medical insurance. While some people do find success with obesity surgery, it requires changes in lifestyle as well as including the incorporation of exercise.

Drug therapy. Several drugs have been used in the treatment of obesity, but unfortunately, none with much success. Altering a level of a brain chemical through drug treatment may change eating behavior, but as we have learned, it is not the only factor in controlling calorie intake and obesity development. One drug currently used, called Orlistat by prescription or an over-the-counter version called Alli®, blocks fat absorption. As a result, a low-fat diet must be eaten in conjunction with drug therapy to avoid intestinal trouble due to malabsorption of fat. For the most part, drugs have a very modest effect and must be used in conjunction with lifestyle changes, including the addition of increased physical activity.

EATING DISORDERS—PREVALENCE AND PROBLEMS

Beyond obesity, there are other situations where energy balance is skewed—eating disorders. An estimated 10 million females and 1 million males suffer from the two eating disorders, **anorexia nervosa** and **bulimia**. The number of males with eating disorders may be much larger as there may be a greater stigma for men to report. These serious conditions are believed to have their origins in dieting, or restrictive eating, combined with environmental issues such as family life and participation

Nutrition Bite

Dietary supplements, such as those purchased on the Internet promoted as weight loss aids, are not clinically tested—that is, unlike prescription obesity drugs, dietary supplements sold as weight loss aids are not proven to work nor is their safety guaranteed.

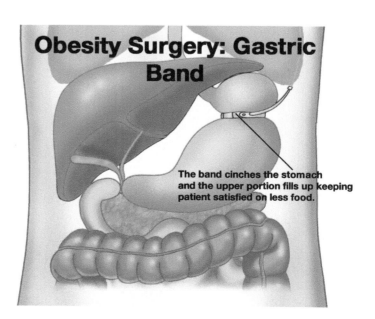

Figure 7.20

in weight-conscience sports. In fact, reports suggest that close to 15% of athletes struggle with either disordered eating patterns or diagnosed eating disorders. In this section, we discuss these two conditions and their related nutritional problems.

Anorexia Nervosa

This eating disorder is characterized by self-induced starvation and typically afflicts young women—mostly teenagers. About 5 to 10 percent of those with anorexia are male, though these numbers appear to be on the rise as more boys and men become overly concerned about their body images. Another characteristic of someone with anorexia is that she often comes from an affluent family and exhibits signs of perfectionism. Other criteria for those suffering from anorexia:

- Below or less than 85 percent of expected healthy body weight.
- Intense fear of becoming fat even though she is underweight for her age and height.
- Distortion of body image (unable to determine rationally that she is underweight). (See Figure 7.21.)
- Loss of a regular menstrual cycle—amenorrhea—for at least three months or more.

Anorexia sufferers deny their hunger and it is not clear if regulatory mechanisms for food intake control become "damaged" with starvation or that a person may be susceptible to anorexia since this eating disorder appears to run in certain families.

Bulimia

This eating disorder is characterized by recurrent episodes of binge eating and purging, or other methods to rid the excess calories. Bulimia is believed to afflict approximately 5 to 25 percent of college-aged females. Males also suffer from bulimia, especially men involved in weight-restrictive sports, such as wrestling and

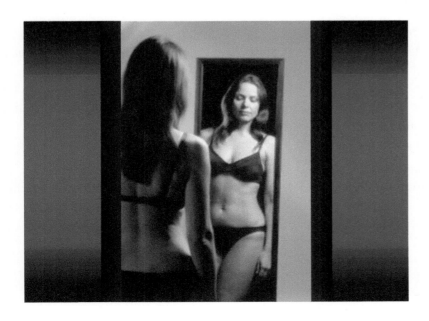

Figure 7.21

crew, even though cases appear to be underreported. Bulimia most likely gets its start when a person diets or restricts eating in an effort to lose weight. She often forbids herself to eat certain foods, lasting several days and then "giving in" and overeating on that food, such as cookies or ice cream. Extreme guilt follows, and she restricts again, only to succumb later. Over weeks and months, a cycle begins of restricting, binging, and soon she tries methods such as vomiting or the use of laxatives to rid her body of the excess food and calories. Here are some specific diagnostic characteristics of a person with bulimia.

- Eating large amounts of food in a short or discrete period of time. Binges may be 1,000 to over 10,000 calories of food—usually sweets. Binges are often planned and carried out in privacy.
- A feeling of no control during the binge, which is followed by feelings of extreme guilt.
- Purging type of behavior follows the binge, such as vomiting (self-induced with use of fingers down the throat or medication that induces vomiting), use of laxatives or diuretics (cause increase in urine output to reduce bloated feelings), periods of fasting and/or excessive exercise.
- Binging and purging behavior must occur twice a week for at least three months for bulimia to be diagnosed. (But as you might imagine, a person doesn't "wake up" one day and become bulimic. Instead, this disorder develops over time as a person continues the dieting and binging cycle.)

Nutritional Problems Associated with Eating Disorders

Anorexia—Since this is basically malnutrition brought on by starvation, many of the same symptoms are seen as in a person who is malnourished from a poor country.

- Protein deficiency and related problems (see Chapter 2)
- Calcium deficiency and related bone problems (stress fractures and early osteoporosis—covered in Chapter 8)
- Zinc and iron deficiency (anemia and poor immune health are often seen in anorexia sufferers)
- Vitamin deficiencies (with little food being eaten, various vitamin needs are not met and related symptoms are seen)
- Fine hair covers body—lanugo or peach fuzz like hair grows on the back, face, and arms as the body tries to stay warm (with starvation, the BMR drops so heat production is reduced and a person is often chilled or cold much of the time, dressing in layers of warm clothing)

Treatment for anorexia involves a team approach with psychiatrists, family therapists, physicians, and dieticians. The longer a person suffers from this eating disorder the harder it is to treat. Anorexia sufferers have a high rate of suicide deaths and death from organ failure.

Bulimia—With intermittent caloric restriction and overeating, the nutritional problems are generally less severe compared with anorexia.

- Loss of potassium due to heavy vomiting (in extreme cases, this may result in heart failure)
- Loss of fat-soluble vitamins when laxatives are abused (this decreases their absorption)
- Erosion of teeth enamel due to acid in vomit

Bulimics are treated with much more success when structured eating is implemented to avoid swings (dieting and binging). Also, therapy with antidepressant medication may be helpful to many sufferers because this eating disorder may have origins in altered levels of brain chemicals.

Quiz Yourself

7

CHAPTER

1. What time period(s) during the life span of humans are fat cell numbers normally increasing?

   a. third trimester of fetal development through the first year of life

   b. adolescent growth spurt (12–14 years of age)

   c. 20–25 years of age

   d. a and b above

2. Body fat distribution as measured by _____ is used as an indicator of abdominal obesity and subsequent health risks.

   a. height-to-weight ratio

   b. percent body fat

   c. waist circumference

   d. desirable body weight

3. With weight loss resulting in a decrease of body fat, fat cell size _____ and fat cell number _____. (Choose the best combination.)

   a. increases / decreases

   b. decreases / decreases

   c. unchanged / decreases

   d. decreases / unchanged

4. The Body Mass Index (BMI) can be used as an indicator of obesity. The BMI is:

   a. a ratio of body fat to age

   b. a ratio of weight to height (kg/m^2)

   c. a ratio of waist to hip measurement

   d. a ratio of body fat to body weight

   e. none of the above

5. A sound weight loss program should include:

   1. _____

   2. _____

   3. _____

6. Choose one of the components in question 5 and describe why this should be included in a weight loss program (include how this component contributes to weight loss and its benefits).

    _____

    _____

    _____

    _____

    _____

7. There are several theories for the cause of obesity. Describe how each of the following theories may lead to obesity in an individual.

    Inactivity: _____

    _____

    Fat cell size (fat mass): _____

    _____

    Genetic predisposition: _____

    _____

8. What is bulimia? How does dieting (restrictive eating) contribute to the development of this condition?

    _____

    _____

    _____

    _____

    _____

9. List one internal factor and one external factor that influences food intake control.

    Internal _____

    External _____

MINERALS—FROM BONES TO HORMONES—THE WORK HARD NUTRIENTS

8

Now that we've covered the first three classes of nutrients, actually the macronutrients protein, carbohydrate, and fat, it's time for the micronutrients. First up: minerals. This class of nutrient is the simplest. Minerals are elemental substances such as iron, calcium, and sodium. While simple elements, the roles of minerals are far reaching, as we will see—from bone structure to the delicate workings of hormones.

MINERALS—THEIR ORIGIN AND PATH THROUGH THE FOOD CHAIN

Let's define minerals as a nutrient category:

- Minerals are elemental substances other than carbon, hydrogen, oxygen, and nitrogen. Thus, they are inorganic. (In chemistry terminology, this means without carbon. For example, water is inorganic, but carbohydrate is organic.) Minerals are also single elements that keep their chemical identities and do not change in the body in the same way that we saw with protein, carbohydrate and fat.
- Minerals represent about five to six percent of your total body weight. Mineral content of the body varies with gender and race. Males generally have a greater mineral content (due to a greater skeletal mass). For people of Asian, Caucasian, and Hispanic descent, mineral composition is just below five percent of body weight, while those of African descent or blacks have a great mineral content of about six percent (primarily due to greater bone/skeletal mass).
- Minerals are essential nutrients and the body is unable to make them; thus, food (and water) is the only source.

Chapter Objectives

This chapter will cover several important minerals; however, not all of them will be covered because there are some 20 of nutritional significance. For each mineral, the following will be covered:

- The mineral's function
- Consequence of the mineral's deficiency (specifically related to its function)

- Issues of the mineral's bioavailability
- Food sources of the mineral
- Relationship of the mineral to specific health issues, such as bone health or heart disease

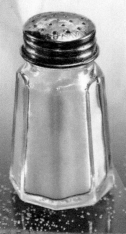

- Minerals function in a regulatory and/or structural role, but minerals do not provide energy. (What nutrients do provide energy?)
- Minerals originate from rocks and make their way into water, soil, and eventually plants, animals, and then us.

The Path of Minerals Through the Food Chain

An estimated four billion years ago when the earth formed, minerals were integrated into the earth's crust. Over time, they have made their way into water, as water trickles over and through layers of rock in the earth. Rocks and water become part of soil; then plants take up water and use minerals from the soil for their needs. Animals then eat the plants and drink the water. Finally, we drink the water, eat plants, and also eat animal products such as meat and milk. Thus, we get the minerals "directly" from the earth as shown in Figure 8.1.

With this in mind, you can see that a particular plant growing on mineral-deficient soil (such as the mineral iodine) would then lead to deficient intake of this mineral for the animals and people of this land. This is particularly true for people living in isolated areas, such as high in the Andes mountains of South America or in parts of Asia who eat only locally grown vegetables, fruits, grain, and animals existing in mineral-deficient soils. It is not necessary for us, however, to worry whether our neighborhood soil is mineral deficient or replete since we eat foods grown all over the United States and other countries.

There are two major classifications of minerals, which are based upon their presence in the body (as a percentage of body weight) and the amount required in our diets.

Major (Macro) Minerals

- present in the body at levels greater than 0.01 percent of the body weight
- required in amounts greater than 100 milligrams per day
- function in both structural and regulatory roles

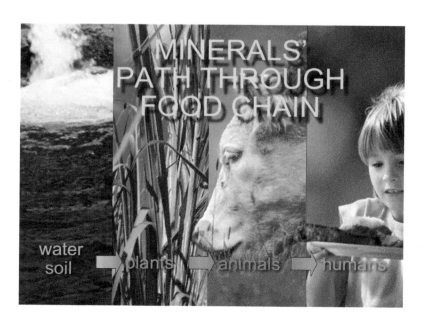

Figure 8.1

Some of the major minerals include calcium, phosphorous, sodium, potassium, magnesium, and chloride. In this course, we cover in detail calcium, sodium, and potassium. Although the others are just as vital in the diet, these three have particular health significance to you.

Trace (Micro) Minerals

- present in the body at levels less than 0.01 percent of the body weight (all the trace minerals added together would fit into a soup spoon!)
- required in amounts less than 50 milligrams per day
- function primarily in regulatory roles since their presence in the body is in such small amounts

Some of the trace minerals present in you and food include iron, zinc, copper, selenium, fluoride, iodine, and manganese. In this course, we cover iron, zinc, iodine, and fluoride. As with the major minerals, these select trace minerals have a particular relevance to you.

BIOAVAILABILITY

The concept of bioavailability is important in the discussion of minerals. Bioavailability is the amount or proportion (percentage) of a nutrient and, in our case, mineral that is available for absorption. Recall from earlier chapters that when we eat protein, carbohydrate, or fat, we are able to absorb about 90 to 95 percent of the nutrient (Chapter 3). The remaining 5 to 10 percent is undigested and unabsorbed, ending up in the stool. Thus, the bioavailability for protein, carbs, and fat is about 90 to 95 percent. For minerals, however, the numbers are quite different. Most minerals range in bioavailability from under 5 percent in the case of iron from foods like spinach, to over 60 percent for sodium from foods like snack crackers. The reason, in part, for minerals' range of bioavailability stems from their chemically "charged" character. Minerals, such as calcium and iron, possess a positive

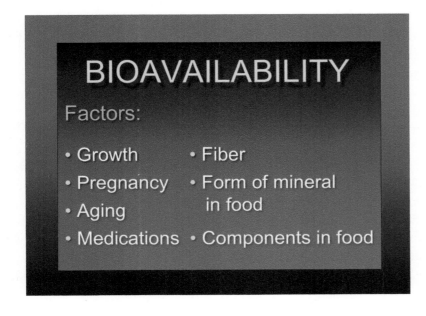

Figure 8.2

chemical charge, meaning that these minerals can attract other compounds, such as negatively charged minerals and proteins. This, in turn, impacts their absorption through the intestinal tract wall, and minerals may form stable compounds not easily absorbed.

Several factors can increase or decrease a specific mineral's bioavailability. Throughout our discussion of minerals, take note of these factors and their significance for that particular mineral. Many of these bioavailability factors may have personal significance and may contribute to poor mineral status for you.

Taking Bioavailability into Account in Setting Nutrient Requirements

Knowing that iron bioavailability from spinach is low, does this mean that we need to eat 10 to 20 times that amount to meet our needs? Look back to the notes on the RDA in Chapter 1. Several factors were mentioned that went into determining the RDAs for the nutrients. For example, issues of gender, physiological state (lactation, for example), and age are taken into account when setting nutrient requirements. The nutrient's bioavailability is also taken into account. Thus, for iron, the RDA is set knowing that about 10 percent of this mineral is absorbed on average from most foods. The RDA for various minerals, both major and trace, are set with issues of bioavailability in mind. As we cover each mineral, you will see that for some minerals, bioavailability factors can be significant.

MAJOR MINERALS

As each of these minerals are covered, keep in mind the function and how its deficiency relates to the mineral's role. Also, consider bioavailability factors, and how this may influence the requirement for the specific mineral. While memorizing the specific RDA is not necessary, you should recognize differences in need based on prominent factors, such as age, and, of course, learn about some good food sources.

Calcium

Perhaps the most famous of minerals, calcium plays both structural and regulatory roles. This mineral accounts for about 2% of your body weight or roughly 3 pounds.

Function

- **Structure:** Approximately 99 percent of the body's calcium is found in your teeth and bones. Bone formation starts with a protein latticework of collagen fibers (much like a trellis that roses climb upon), which is then overlaid with a calcium-phosphorous salt called hydroxyapatite. Your bones undergo constant remodeling by two types of cells called osteoblasts (building or construction cells) and osteoclasts (the breakdown or demolition cells). These two bone cell types work together over time to determine bone growth and bone changes. You can build bone mineral content or density (calcium) during your younger years until about ages 25 to 30. Typically after this time, calcium is lost from the bones and as we'll see with calcium deficiency, this speeds up with a calcium-deficient diet and other lifestyle factors such as inactivity and smoking.

- **Regulatory:** The remaining 1 percent of calcium is found in body tissues performing roles such as in blood clot formation and in muscle and nerve cell impulse transmission. For example, the heart muscle must have the proper levels of calcium for normal heart function. Another regulatory role of this mineral is as part of the calcium-binding protein called calmodulin. This protein mediates many cellular processes such as cell division and cell secretions. Emerging research also suggests that calcium may play a role in the prevention of diseases, such as cancer and high blood pressure.

Deficiency

Can you imagine the possibility of your heart stopping or your blood not clotting after a shaving nick if there was insufficient calcium in your system? These horrific consequences will not happen because maintenance of these regulatory roles is so vital to life. Remember the concept of homeostasis? Well, calcium homeostasis is a perfect example of many systems coming into play to maintain constant internal conditions (tissue levels of calcium). Essentially, your body "robs" your bones of calcium to maintain regulatory roles. Here's how it works. Visualize your bones as a "bank" of calcium just like your savings account that you use to make such purchases as college tuition and a car. Your tissue levels of calcium represent the ready cash you have on hand. If you're low on cash, you take cash out of your savings to make purchases. Your body works the same way. If tissue levels dip slightly due to a low intake from the diet, then the body responds by withdrawing calcium from your bones through the osteoclasts (much like an ATM machine that allows you to withdraw cash). In addition to this, other systems work to boost tissue levels back to normal. (See Figure 8.3.)

Calcium homeostasis is achieved three ways:

1. The bioavailability of calcium goes up in times of need (when tissue levels take a dip). A signal is sent to the intestines—vitamin D, which is needed to make a protein carrier for calcium absorption to help boost bioavailability.

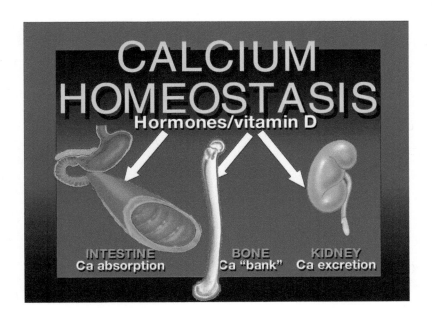

Figure 8.3

2. Hormones (released from the parathyroid gland) work on the excretion end and tell the kidneys not to excrete as much of this mineral in urine. The kidneys play a major role in the homeostasis of most major minerals (particularly sodium and potassium) in addition to calcium.

3. The osteoclast cells in the bone are stimulated by hormones to release calcium into the bloodstream.

Net result: Blood/tissue levels of calcium return to normal and vital calcium regulatory roles continue. But there is a price to pay. Over time, continued withdrawal of calcium from the bone without return "deposits" results in loss of bone mineral or calcium content. The results in children and adults differ.

Children: Calcium deficiency results in poor growth and bone mineralization. Mineral content of bone is low, and as a result, bones are soft and bow with the weight. This condition is called rickets, which we will discuss in more detail with vitamin D deficiency in Chapter 9.

Adults: Osteoporosis develops. This literally means "porous" bones and is characterized by weak bones with low mineral content. As shown in Figure 8.4, the cross section of a normal healthy bone looks like a sponge (with holes that allow for interchange with the circulation) but the osteoporotic bone looks lacy in appearance, much like a loofah pad with bigger holes and weak mineral structure.

Osteoporotic bones break easily, especially the bones in the spine, hip, and wrist. The spine or vertebral bones actually become so weak and fragile that they crush onto themselves, causing the person to shrink in size (lose height) and become slumped over. (See Figure 8.5.) This also causes great pain and severely limits motion and activity. Hip fractures and fractures of other bones due to osteoporosis put many older people in the hospital costing millions of dollars and severely limiting their mobility and often leading to secondary problems such as pneumonia and possible death.

The risk of developing osteoporosis is very high for women—about one in two will develop age-related mineral loss from bones and related fractures. Men also are at great risk later in life with about one in four suffering from osteoporosis. Even though poor calcium intake is an important factor, there are several other factors

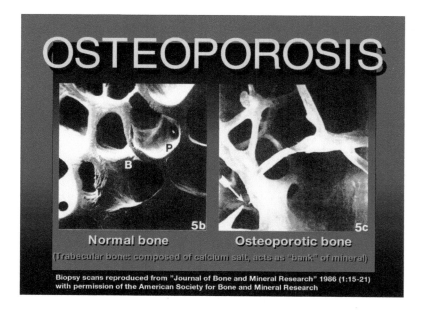

Figure 8.4

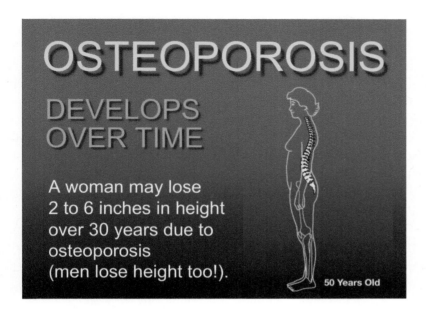

Figure 8.5

including lifestyle issues that impact bone density and bone health. Are you at risk for osteoporosis?

- **Risk increases with age.** The older a person is, the more they are at risk when calcium loss from the bone exceeds "deposits" in our later years.
- **Risk increases with long-term low-calcium intake.** If calcium intake is low during your formative (growth) years or during young adulthood, you have less calcium in your bone "bank" or in reserve to cover losses. Additionally, inadequate intake of calcium throughout a person's lifespan means greater loss from the bones in an effort to maintain regulatory roles in the body. Vitamin D intake also plays a role in osteoporosis risk as low intakes impact bone mineralization and calcium absorption.
- **Risk is greater for women than men.** Men generally have greater bone mineral density (content of calcium), thus a bigger savings account. Women also tend to live longer than men, thus signs of calcium loss from the bone eventually show up in these later years. And a woman tends to lose more calcium from bones as a result of hormonal changes. After menopause, when a woman's body ceases to make estrogen, bone loss is accelerated. This hormone helps maintain bone density, thus many women opt for estrogen replacement therapy post-menopause to help slow this loss. There are other medications used to help slow calcium loss and even encourage mineralization of bones.
- **Risk is greater in inactive people.** Physical activity, especially weight-bearing exercises, such as weight lifting and brisk walking help build denser bones.
- **Smoking and heavy alcohol consumption speed mineral loss from the bone.**
- **There is also evidence that a high intake of sodium from processed foods and caffeine may accelerate bone mineral loss in some people.** This relationship of calcium bone loss with high caffeine intake is genetically based and may pose a risk for osteoporosis for some people.

So ask yourself again—are you at risk for developing osteoporosis? Check your calcium intake on your Diet Project to see how your intake ranks with requirement. (See question #8 in this chapter's quiz.)

Bioavailability Issues

Calcium bioavailability is about 30 percent for adults. However, during times of greater needs such as pregnancy (forming skeletal mass of a newborn and building reserves for lactation) bioavailability boosts to about 50 percent. During teen years and other times of rapid growth, bioavailability also goes up to about 50 percent. Vitamin D is also needed for calcium absorption, thus factors that alter status of this vitamin may impair calcium bioavailability (more in Chapter 9). Bioavailability of calcium is decreased in the presence of particular food factors—phytate (phytic acid) found in whole grains and oxalate (oxalic acid) found in leafy green vegetables—they bind to calcium in the stomach and small intestine, and decrease calcium's absorption.

Requirement

Calcium requirements are listed in Figure 8.6 for various age groups. Note that the requirement for a woman who is pregnant or lactating is not greater. Since bioavailability goes up for this mineral in these conditions, this required level is considered sufficient. Additionally, calcium needs increase with age for women, reflecting the impact of menopause on calcium loss from bones.

Food Sources

A variety of food sources are listed in Figure 8.7. Calorie for calorie, non-fat dairy products, such as non-fat yogurt, are the best sources of this mineral. There are many calcium-fortified foods including orange juice and other fruit juices, breakfast cereals, and even milk boosted with extra calcium.

Issues of Calcium Supplementation and Excess

The real threat of developing osteoporosis has many people, particularly women, selecting calcium-fortified foods and taking calcium supplements. Supplements of this mineral may be a wise decision for many people who do not eat dairy products or eat other good sources of calcium. If you are considering a calcium supplement, keep a single dose to no more than 500 milligrams and take it with food. To ensure

CALCIUM REQUIREMENTS		
INDIVIDUAL		**AI RDA** **MG/DAY**
Child	1–3 years	700 mg
	4–8 years	1,000 mg
Child/teen	9–18 years	1,300 mg
Adult	19–50 years	1,000 mg
	51 + years male	1,000 mg
	51 + years female	1,200 mg
(pregnancy, lactation—same as age group)		

Figure 8.6

CALCIUM (Ca)

4. Food sources

Dairy, milk-1 cup	300 mg
Cheese, 1.5-2 oz.	300-400 mg
Yogurt, plain 8 oz.	450 mg
Meat, grain	poor
Tofu, 4oz.	150 mg
Black strap molasses-1T	150 mg
Broccoli, cooked 1 cup	100 mg
Salmon, canned 3oz.	180 mg
Tortilla, two 6" corn	100 mg
Fish sauce, 2T	50 mg

Phytate (grains), oxalate (greens) decreases bioavailability

Figure 8.7

maximum calcium absorption, take it with a meal that is not rich in calcium. There is no need to purchase fancy supplements—calcium carbonate is effective and inexpensive. Avoid supplements of bone meal or oyster shell because these may have small amounts of heavy metals, such as mercury, which may present toxicity problems over the long term.

Should you be concerned about taking too much calcium? It's best to avoid excessive calcium supplementation because this can hamper the absorption of another mineral, iron. The Safe Tolerable Upper Limit (UL) for calcium is 2,500 milligrams per day. As shown in Figure 8.8, you can come close to this amount in just one meal if you go overboard taking supplements and eating calcium-fortified and calcium-rich foods.

Urban Myth

Myth: "Calcium needs are easily met by drinking 'hard' tap water."

"Hard" water refers to the mineral salts dissolved in water that typically come from a well or underground source (table water). The level of calcium (and other minerals), however, is not sufficient to meet your needs (about 10% of calcium RDA is in a liter of water).

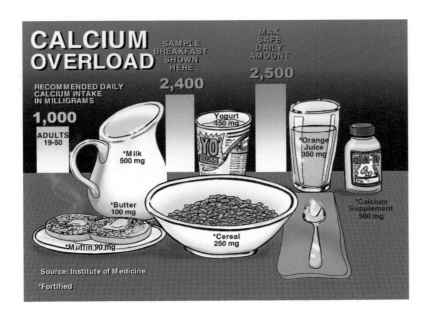

Figure 8.8

Sodium and Potassium

These two major minerals are covered together because they work closely together in regulating fluid balance and other roles. Sodium (better known as a component of table salt sodium chloride) is a notorious culprit in high blood pressure. However, both sodium and potassium play a role in healthy blood pressure regulation.

Function

Sodium and potassium are called electrolytes, simply a term used to describe minerals that dissolve in water and can form or carry an electrical charge (because they are positively charged atoms).

- **Both minerals are crucial in the regulation of fluid homeostasis.** The distribution of sodium and potassium differs in and outside the cell as shown in Figure 8.9. A majority of the sodium (chemically abbreviated Na$^+$ in the Periodic Table of Elements) is located outside the cell, called extracellular; potassium is located intracellular or inside the cell (chemically abbreviated K$^+$). Recall from Chapter 1 that two-thirds of the body water is intracellular and one-third is extracellular. This set distribution must be maintained for proper cellular function and metabolic reaction, and it is the division of sodium outside the cell and potassium inside the cell that ensures this fluid balance. These two minerals work in concert not only to aid in fluid balance but also maintenance of healthy blood pressure (blood is mostly water).
- **Both minerals serve in the transmission of nerve impulses.** It is again their distribution in and outside the cell that allows for nerve function. Movement of these positively charged elements across cell membranes allow for nerve impulse transmission from one cell to the next.

As with calcium, the kidneys along with several hormones maintain the homeostasis of both sodium and potassium. For example, excess sodium intake would result in hormonal signals to the kidneys to rid the excess in the urine.

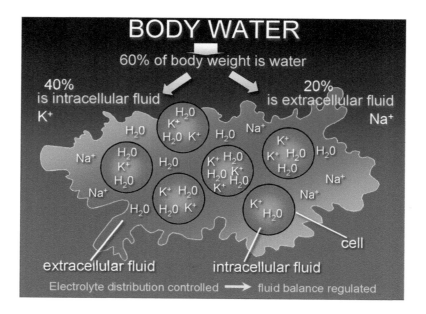

Figure 8.9

Deficiency

Lack of these minerals would rarely occur as a result of poor dietary intake since both are very plentiful in our diets. However, a low potassium intake relative to sodium intake may be an issue for some people and contribute to the development of high blood pressure (discussed later.)

The more likely possibility of a deficiency of either mineral results from a sudden loss of body fluids. This may occur with heavy sweating, which is primarily a loss of extracellular fluid, thus sodium is also lost (taste your sweat next time you're finished with a tough workout). Also, bouts of vomiting and diarrhea, which occur with food poisoning, the flu, or with an eating disorder, cause the loss of both potassium and sodium.

Symptoms of sodium or potassium deficiency include a drop in blood pressure, which gives you a light-headed, dizzy feeling. Also, muscle weakness and cramping along with nausea occur. During long bouts of exercise, such as running a marathon, drinking copious amounts of plain water can lead to a dilution of sodium in the circulation called hyponatremia. This condition can be life-threatening and requires medical attention. As a result, marathon runners slowly jogging are most likely sweating less than faster runners and are cautioned not to over-hydrate so as to avoid hyponatremia.

Bioavailability Issues

Both sodium and potassium are very bioavailable in the diet—over 60 to 80 percent. Excess intake and regulation of levels in the body occurs through the monitoring of fluid levels by a series of hormones and the action of the kidneys to excrete excess or hold on to either mineral if needed.

Requirement

While we often refer to the requirement as "the RDA," it is actually the Adequate Intake or "AI" because insufficient data exist for us to determine the RDA for sodium and potassium.

- Sodium: 1,500 milligrams daily (less for people over 50 years old)
- Potassium: 4,700 milligrams daily

Note that potassium intake should be about three times that of sodium. However, due to our intake of sodium from processed foods (added salt and other forms of sodium), our intake of sodium easily reaches 3,000 to over 5,000 milligrams daily. This coupled with the fact that processed foods are very low in potassium and that our intake of potassium-rich foods—fruits, vegetables, and juices—is low, our intake of potassium is overshadowed by sodium. Health professionals and researchers note that this disparity contributes to the development of high blood pressure, a major risk factor for heart disease. Additionally, a majority of people with hypertension and about a fourth of those with healthy blood pressure are "salt sensitive." With increasing salt (sodium) intake from processed foods and the use of the saltshaker, blood pressure levels rise as the body struggles to regulate fluid levels. For this reason, the 2015 Dietary Guidelines (Chapter 12) recommends consuming less than 2,300 milligrams of sodium daily in an effort to promote healthy blood pressure in the population. Also in an effort to promote healthy blood pressure, the Daily Value for sodium used on food labels is set at 2,300 milligrams.

As a result of this relationship between these minerals to heart health, the Food and Drug Administration has set Daily Values on food labels for both minerals.

- Sodium: 2,400 milligrams (a value not to exceed)*
- Potassium: 3,500 milligrams (a value to try and achieve, if not go beyond)

*The Institute of Medicine recommends lowering this value to 1,500 mg as many adults suffer from hypertension and heart disease. (Recall that hypertension is a major risk factor for heart disease.)

Food Sources

As a general rule, processed foods are loaded with sodium and fresh, unprocessed foods are loaded with potassium. This makes sense because potassium is found inside of cells (fruit and vegetables cells included). When you cut or process fruits and vegetables, you break open cells and potassium is lost in the rinsing and preparation of the foods. Typically, salt or other forms of sodium are added in the processing for taste and preservation of the foods. This explains why a fresh tomato has virtually no sodium and a few hundred milligrams of potassium. When you make that tomato into tomato sauce or ketchup, virtually all the potassium is lost during the processing while oodles of sodium is added. It's no wonder Americans consume so much unnecessary sodium, which may be contributing to hypertension, while at the same time getting little potassium, which also is contributing to high blood pressure.

Figure 8.10 shows how processed and fresh foods compare on sodium and potassium.

TRACE MINERALS

As a reminder, these minerals are called "trace" because they are present in the body in such small amounts and their requirements are also quite small—less than 50 milligrams daily. The trace minerals function primarily in regulation rather than structure as the major minerals do. Again, bioavailability issues reign supreme for

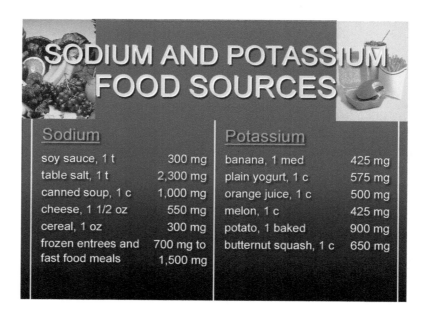

Sodium		Potassium	
soy sauce, 1 t	300 mg	banana, 1 med	425 mg
table salt, 1 t	2,300 mg	plain yogurt, 1 c	575 mg
canned soup, 1 c	1,000 mg	orange juice, 1 c	500 mg
cheese, 1 1/2 oz	550 mg	melon, 1 c	425 mg
cereal, 1 oz	300 mg	potato, 1 baked	900 mg
frozen entrees and fast food meals	700 mg to 1,500 mg	butternut squash, 1 c	650 mg

Figure 8.10

trace minerals. This issue may be of significance for you personally because your iron or zinc status and intake may be compromised by bioavailability factors.

Iron

Although one of the most abundant minerals in the earth's rocks and soils, iron deficiency ironically is the most common nutrient deficiency worldwide.

Function

- **As a regulatory mineral, iron is most noted for its ability to carry oxygen.** In the red blood cell, iron is part of an oxygen-carrying protein called hemoglobin. As the blood cell moves to the lungs, it picks up oxygen as you breathe, and this gas binds to iron (abbreviated by Fe in Figure 8.11). The blood cell then travels through your body and delivers the oxygen to cells for its use in energy metabolism. (Recall that fats and carbohydrates are broken down aerobically to release energy.) In the muscle cell, another oxygen-carrying protein called myoglobin, which also contains iron, actually picks up the oxygen from the blood cell to transfer it inside the cell for energy metabolism.
- **Iron also serves as a co-factor in several enzyme reactions involved in energy metabolism.** Iron plays a vital role in the actual release of energy from carbohydrates, fats, and protein.

Deficiency

Before we get into problems with inadequate iron (diet or losses from the body), there are a few things to establish about iron. The body treats this mineral much like a precious gem. Once inside the body, it tries hard not to lose it.

- The body does this by not losing much iron (if any) in the urine and other excretions.
- Blood cell iron is recycled; that is, when a blood cell dies (1 percent do every day), the iron is plucked out and reused.

Nutrition Bite

Muscle cells that get a lot of "action," such as leg muscles, have more myoglobin, hence more iron. This is why dark meat poultry (leg meat) contains more iron and is darker in color than white meat poultry (chest from the bird).

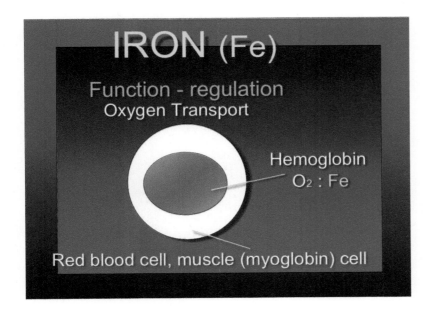

Figure 8.11

- Additionally, the body has the ability to change iron absorption in the small intestine. Thus, bioavailability changes as a reflection of need.
- The body has the ability to store extra iron in storage proteins called ferritin and hemosiderin.

Iron deficiency can result from poor diet or from losses of iron from the body such as blood losses. Iron deficiency results in low iron stores and low levels of hemoglobin. This is called iron-deficiency anemia. Anemia means "sick blood" and as you will see with other nutrient deficiencies, anemia may result. It is important to note that iron-deficiency anemia has specific characteristics. The blood has poor oxygen-carrying capacity, thus a person feels tired and very fatigued with exertion, such as exercise. Other symptoms include a smooth tongue (cells on the surface are unable to regrow properly), and in some cases spooned finger nails, as shown in Figure 8.12.

Fingernail Analysis

While spooned fingernails may be a sign of iron deficiency anemia, alterations to fingernail growth and appearance are an unlikely consequence of diet problems. Some Internet sites offer fingernail analysis. Beware not to fall prey to such an inaccurate assessment of your diet adequacy. Fingernails may become ridged, split, and flake as a result of detergents and exposure to other environmental factors. Your fingernails' composition and appearance is not a window to your diet adequacy. Instead, take a good look at your Diet Project assignment and see how you fared with your intake of protein, vitamins, and minerals.

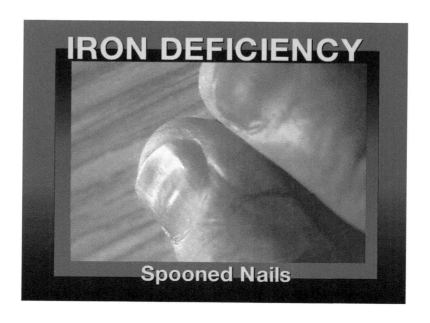

Figure 8.12

Those at risk for iron deficiency include those who are rapidly growing, such as infants and children. Also, women who are in their childbearing years are at risk because of the amount of blood (iron) that is lost due to menstruation. Unfortunately, iron deficiency anemia is far too common worldwide. Researchers believe that about one in three individuals, young and old alike, are anemic, making iron deficiency the most common nutrient inadequacy worldwide.

Bioavailability

Several factors can alter the bioavailability of iron, including (1) your iron status, (2) the form of iron in the food, and (3) meal composition or food factors.

1. **Iron status—How great is your need for iron?**

   Iron entry into the body through absorption via the small intestine is controlled and Figure 8.13 illustrates how need for iron impacts bioavailability. (Compare this to calcium, sodium, and other major minerals where excretion through the kidneys is mechanism for major mineral homeostasis.)
   - *Poor iron status:* Sites for absorption are empty, which signifies that iron stores are on the low side. Many women and children are in this situation. End result: Iron absorption or bioavailability gets a boost, hence more iron is absorbed from food.
   - *Good iron status:* Sites for absorption are mostly full, which signifies good iron stores. Most men are in this situation. End result: Iron absorption is reduced.

2. **Form of iron in food—meat versus nonmeat foods**

   There are two forms of iron related to the particular state of the iron—heme and non-heme iron.
   - **Heme** iron is the form of iron found only in meats (red meat, poultry, fish) and blood (clotted blood is eaten in some Asian cultures). The iron is bound to the proteins hemoglobin and myoglobin. This form of iron has good bio-availability—about 20 to 30 percent is available for absorption.

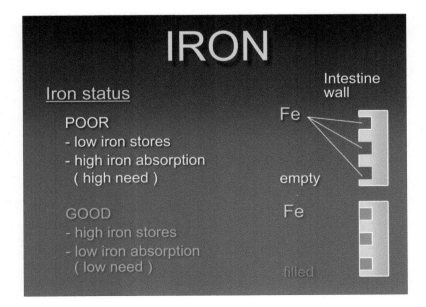

Figure 8.13

- **Non-heme** iron is found in plants, such as beans, grains, and green leafy vegetables. About 40 to 60 percent of the iron in meat is non-heme iron as well (this simply means iron is not bound to hemoglobin). The bioavailability of this iron form is much lower—less than 5 percent up to about 10 percent.

3. **Meal composition or food factors**

   A variety of factors in foods can either increase or decrease the bioavailability of non-heme iron. Numbers given here are for non-heme iron in a breakfast cereal.

   - Vitamin C (from berries, oranges, peppers, or a supplement) increases the bioavailability from 10 percent to about 20 percent.
   - A protein factor exists in meat that increases the bioavailability of non-heme iron eaten at the same meal (e.g., the non-heme iron both in the meat and in other foods, such as beans at that same meal).
   - Oxalate (found in greens such as spinach and Swiss chard) and phytates (in whole grains) reduce iron bioavailability by tightly binding with the iron in the intestine and preventing its absorption. This can greatly impact iron status for a person who avoids meats and relies on greens and a significant amount of whole grains as their major source of iron.
   - Extreme intakes of fiber about 50 grams or more (remember that the Daily Value for fiber is 25 grams) can decrease iron bioavailability by binding with the iron at that meal making this mineral unavailable for absorption.
   - Tannins, which are compounds found in coffee, tea, and red wines, decrease iron bioavailability by tightly binding together.

Requirement

The requirement for iron, shown in Figure 8.14, illustrates that women have a greater need due to higher losses of this mineral with regular menstruation.

Remember that iron's low bioavailability is taken into account in establishing the RDA for this mineral, but additional consideration is given for vegetarians whose intake of phytate, oxylate, and fiber is most likely high, reducing iron bioavailability. The RDA for pregnant women is so high that a supplement is required

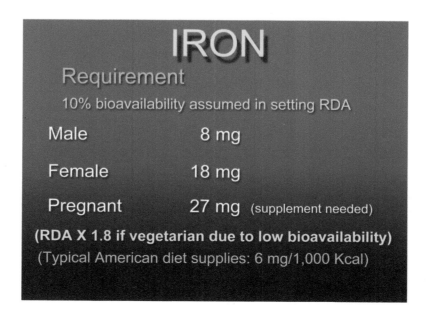

IRON
Requirement
10% bioavailability assumed in setting RDA

Male	8 mg
Female	18 mg
Pregnant	27 mg (supplement needed)

(RDA X 1.8 if vegetarian due to low bioavailability)
(Typical American diet supplies: 6 mg/1,000 Kcal)

Figure 8.14

to meet this need. Also note that the typical American diet supplies about 6 milligrams of iron for every 1,000 calories. Thus, women often don't meet their need for iron with their calorie intake that usually falls below 2,000 calories daily.

Food Sources

Iron in foods exists as either heme or non-heme. Recall that flesh and blood are heme iron sources (but not milk, even though it is an animal product). Whether you choose to eat meat or not, non-heme iron is your major source of iron in your diet. If you eat breakfast cereals regularly, your iron intake is most likely more than adequate since most cereals are iron-fortified. (See Figure 8.15.)

Toxicity

Getting too much iron in your body can spell trouble because your body has no active way to expel it—iron is stored, recycled, and little is lost from the body (compare this with sodium, for example, which excess is promptly excreted in the urine). Iron is a potent oxidant, which means it can cause some cellular damage. Therefore, excess iron should be avoided. Some people (about 1 in 250) have a genetic disorder called **hemochromatosis** where excessive iron is absorbed. This condition can cause serious damage to the liver, because excess iron is stored there, causing damage to tissue. Over time, iron builds up elsewhere and leads to liver cancer or failure. A person with this condition must avoid iron-fortified foods, such as breakfast cereal and must go in for blood-lettings (taking blood out) as a way to lower body iron stores.

Acute iron poisoning is a very serious problem in young children. A toddler who ingests vitamin or iron supplements can easily die of acute iron poisoning when the excess iron overwhelms the intestinal tract and enters the body and wreaks havoc. Remember to keep your vitamin supplements and other possible sources of iron in childproof containers and out of the reach of kids.

Finally, even if you think you are anemic due to poor iron intake, don't just take an iron supplement without the advice of a medical professional. Iron supplements can hamper the absorption of other minerals, such as zinc.

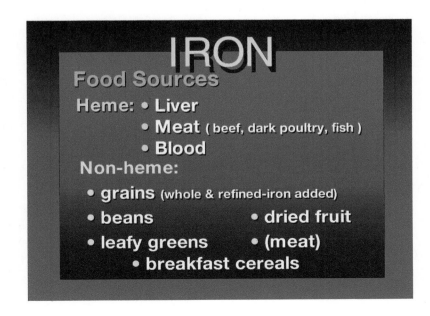

Figure 8.15

Zinc

Touted as the "male mineral," you'll find zinc added to supplements that claim to enhance sexual performance and fertility. Although zinc is involved in sperm production, among other things, claims about sexual performance have yet to be proven.

Function

This mineral operates as a regulatory nutrient and as an enzyme assistant or cofactor in many different enzyme-controlled reactions. A majority of these enzymes are involved in cell replication, the making of new cells. Thus, during periods of growth and development (pregnancy, childhood, puberty), zinc status is important. (See Figure 8.16.) Zinc also participates in immune function, but research has not shown conclusively that supplemental amounts of this mineral prevent illnesses, such as the common cold.

Deficiency

In the early 1960s, researchers in the Middle East discovered that men did not develop normally in terms of sexual maturation. Growth during puberty was hampered; secondary sexual characteristics, such as emergence of pubic hair and testicle enlargement did not occur. The diet of these men (women as well) was deficient in zinc because of a mostly vegetarian fare and a diet high in phytates (found in whole grains) since unleavened bread was a dietary staple.

Primary symptoms of zinc deficiency include:

- delayed sexual development—young adults appear to be in their childhood years
- impaired immune function (increased susceptibility to colds and flu)
- decreased taste perception (particularly seen in the elderly)
- reduced sperm count (although this has been produced experimentally, few cases of male infertility are due to poor zinc intake)

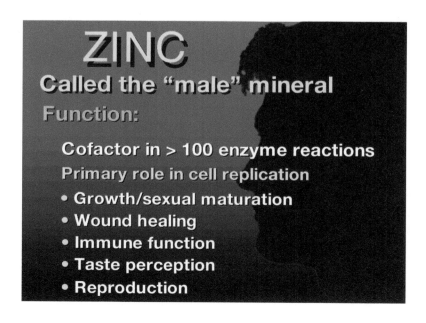

Figure 8.16

Bioavailability

As the researchers in the Middle East noted during the 1960s, zinc deficiency resulted from a low bioavailability of this mineral from unleavened bread. Unleavened bread is high in phytates because it is made from whole grains without leavening agents (yeast) so the phytate remains intact. Since 70 percent of the daily calories typically came from unleavened bread, zinc status was impacted as phytate reduces zinc's bioavailability.

In your diet, eating whole grains does not appreciably alter zinc bioavailability since you don't consume a majority of your calories from these foods. Most whole grain breads are made with yeast, which "deactivates" phytate and allows greater zinc bioavailability from whole grain breads.

Requirement

The RDA for zinc is shown in Figure 8.17. As for iron, zinc is not plentiful in the typical diets eaten by Americans (6 milligrams for every 1,000 calories). Zinc status may be marginal in the diets of people who take in few calories such as inactive women and the elderly.

Food Sources

Meats provide a very good and bioavailable (absorbable) source of zinc. Figure 8.18 shows several good food sources of zinc.

Iodine

Iodine is an excellent example of a mineral whose deficiency is linked to geographical location; that is, in areas where the soil is deficient in this mineral, and where people only eat locally grown food (plant and animal), iodine deficiency results.

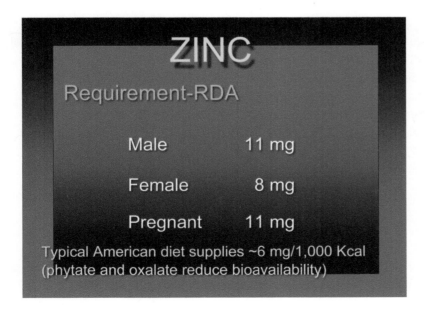

Figure 8.17

Food for Boosting Zinc Intake

Food	mg Zinc
Oysters (Eastern), 6 medium	77
Fortified Breakfast Cereal, 1 oz.	5–15
Beef, 3 oz. roasted	6.1
Turkey, dark 3 oz. roasted	3.8
Wheat germ, 2T	2.3
Garbanzo beans, 1/2 cup	1.3
Milk, 1 cup	1.0
Kidney beans, 1/2 cup	0.9

Figure 8.18

Function

Iodine is incorporated into the hormones made by the thyroid gland. This gland is located at the base of your neck and often during physical exams, your physician will ask you to swallow to perform a quick check on the size of your thyroid, which may reflect iodine deficiency as well as other diseases of the thyroid.

The thyroid hormones direct oxygen use by each and every cell in the body. Big job! Thus, thyroid hormones are vital in setting the energy use of the body. More specifically:

- energy use or Basal Metabolic Rate
- reproductive function
- growth

Deficiency

Inadequate intake of iodine comes from eating foods (both plant and animal products) that were grown or raised on iodine-deficient soils. Since in many poor, under-developed communities, people consume only food grown locally, iodine deficiency can readily develop. Iodine-deficient soil occurs in areas where there is lots of erosion such as in the mountains of Peru, or here in the United States within the Great Lakes region (northern Mideast.) Worldwide, iodine deficiency afflicts about 200 million people.

Iodine deficiency leads to the following:

- Inadequate intake of this mineral results in low levels of the iodine-containing thyroid hormones.
- The body senses this imbalance (recall homeostasis?) and sends a signal from the pituitary gland to make more thyroid hormone.
- In an effort to boost thyroid hormone production, the thyroid gland actually grows larger in size to trap more iodine from the blood.

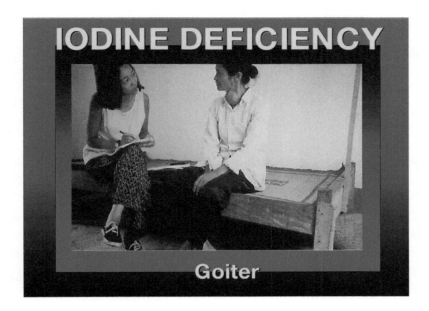

Figure 8.19

- This enlarged gland is called **goiter**. Goiter is shown in Figure 8.19. The Vietnamese woman on the right subsists on low-iodine intake from her locally grown foods.
- People with goiter also become sluggish and gain weight because their BMR has been lowered. In a small community, sluggish people can in turn impact the productivity of the community at large.
- A pregnant woman who becomes iodine deficient gives birth to an infant with **cretinism**, which is a permanent defect characterized by mental retardation, deafness, and blindness. This tragic outcome of pregnancy can also have an impact on the entire community suffering from iodine deficiency as an individual with cretinism requires care and resources, and thus, is not able to effectively contribute to the community in return.

Back in the early 1900s in the United States, iodine deficiency was determined to be the cause for goiter and the government implemented the first food fortification program with iodine fortification of table salt.

Requirement

The RDA for iodine is 150 micrograms, which is very easy to meet with a varied diet (i.e., food that is from various geographical locations—different parts of the United States and the world).

Food Sources

Iodine is present in most foods (dependent on soil and water content). In general, food grown closer to the ocean (coastal communities) have great iodine content because this mineral is in sea water and sea water's evaporation and eventual depositing as rain along the coast contributes to the iodine in the soil and water supply. Iodine also makes its ways into our food supply through the use of iodine-containing disinfectants used to clean machinery at restaurants, particularly fast-food eateries.

Fluoride

Chances are that you grew up using fluoridated toothpaste, or perhaps you were given fluoride pills to boost your intake in an effort to protect your teeth from tooth decay.

Function

- Fluoride is incorporated into bone and teeth structure through your system when this mineral is taken in drinking water or in pill form. This is particularly important for young children because it becomes a part of the tooth structure as it develops.
- When applied to the teeth topically as with toothpaste, mouthwashes, and even drinking water (which may contain fluoride) or during a fluoride treatment at the dentist's office, this mineral actually interchanges with tooth minerals and becomes incorporated into the enamel structure.
- Once part of the tooth structure, the fluoride helps the tooth become more resistant to decay that causes dental caries or cavities. Dental caries are caused by the action of bacteria-fermenting carbohydrate into acids that etch away at the enamel forming holes and divots that lead eventually to rotting of the teeth. Fluoride actually fights the action of the acid, thereby protecting the teeth.

Deficiency

- Some areas where there is naturally a low level of fluoride in the water supply (less than 1 part per million [ppm] or 1 milligram per liter of drinking water), there is a greater rate of dental caries.
- In those areas where the fluoride in the water supply is greater than 1 ppm, there is a lower rate of dental caries. (Water is the best way to get fluoride because food contains very little of this mineral.)
- Why is fighting tooth decay of such importance? Teeth that are riddled with cavities need dental care that many people cannot afford. Additionally, with many fillings as a result of cavities, these teeth are prone to other problems such as needing crowns or root canal work. This eventually may lead to missing teeth and denture work. Eventually with age the dentures don't fit and the person has a difficult time eating. This in turn may lead to life-threatening nutritional deficiencies. Bottom line: Get adequate fluoride when you are young and use fluoridated toothpaste all through your life to maintain healthy teeth.

Toxicity

For fluoride, getting too much does present a problem, even though only a cosmetic one. In areas where the fluoride is over several ppm, the condition fluorosis develops. This is characterized by chalky or mottled appearance to the enamel. In extreme cases, the teeth appear stained with mottled brown swirls. In this state, the teeth are very resistant to dental caries, but there are no health problems associated with fluorosis.

Children run the risk of mild fluorosis if they are given fluoride supplements and brush with fluoridated toothpaste (particularly if they don't rinse their mouth out and swallow the toothpaste). So it's important for caregivers to monitor a child's brushing activities.

Requirement

The Adequate Intake (AI) for fluoride is 4 milligrams daily.

Food Sources

Water can contain fluoride if the geographical location is such that it gets into the water supply from surrounding rocks; toothpaste and mouthwash contain fluoride if it has been added. Some drinking waters are fluoridated; that is, this mineral is added to the water supply to help the entire local community ward off dental caries. This costs about $1 per person per year and is a great way to protect against tooth decay. Not all local water supplies opt for this measure because some people express fear of adding a "chemical" to the water supply. Now that you know fluoride is an essential mineral that helps keep your teeth healthy for a lifetime, what do you think?

Quiz Yourself

8

CHAPTER

1. List a good food source for each nutrient.

   • Sodium _____

   • Calcium (nondairy) _____

   • Non-heme iron _____

   • Zinc _____

2. Which of the following statements about iron is NOT true?

   a. The RDA for iron is lower for women than for men.

   b. Iron absorption increases in a deficiency state.

   c. Iron is absorbed more effectively from animal flesh.

   d. Vitamin C, ascorbic acid, taken at the same time as iron, will increase iron absorption.

3. Which of the following statements does NOT describe the role of minerals in the body?

   a. They are important for growth.

   b. They make possible the transfer of nerve impulses.

   c. They are constituents of important body compounds.

   d. They provide 4 kcalories per gram.

   e. They help maintain water balance.

4. Sodium and potassium work closely together to regulate fluid balance.

   a. true

   b. false

5. Trace minerals, such as iron and zinc, are necessary in small amounts, approximately 10 grams daily (less than one-third of an ounce).

   a. true

   b. false

6. What organ plays a role in the homeostasis of most minerals?

   a. gall bladder

   b. pancreas

   c. liver

   d. kidneys

7. Define minerals and describe their path through the food chain.

_____

_____

_____

_____

8. Define osteoporosis.

_____

_____

_____

_____

List two factors that increase your risk and two factors that will decrease your risk for developing osteoporosis.

_____

_____

_____

_____

9. Define bioavailability and list factors that affect bioavailability.

_____

_____

_____

_____

VITAMINS—THE WONDROUS REGULATORY NUTRIENTS

9

With minerals under our belts, let's move on to the next group of micronutrients—vitamins. No doubt, you have heard about vitamins. Frequent news stories expound on the health benefits of vitamins; the Internet is loaded with websites selling various vitamin supplements; and perhaps, you take a vitamin supplement. This intriguing class of nutrient captures the interest of many such as health seekers, high-performance athletes, and those looking to defy aging. Vitamins work in the body as regulators that influence virtually everything from skin and bone health to the workings of energy metabolism and the immune system. In this chapter, we cover the wondrous work of vitamins and the truth behind some of the claims made about their "powers."

ROLES AND CLASSIFICATION OF VITAMINS

- As a class of nutrients, vitamins are organic substances. This means they contain the element carbon (unlike minerals that are inorganic).
- In the body, vitamins function as regulators. Vitamins DO NOT provide energy nor do they provide the body with structure.
- Each vitamin has a unique structure. That is, unlike protein or carbohydrates, vitamins do not have a common unit of structure, such as an amino acid.
- Vitamins needs differ among different species. For example, humans and other primates require vitamin C, but dogs and cats do not.
- Overall, vitamin requirements are small and range in the milligram or microgram quantity.
- Vitamins function in virtually all body cells, but they don't work together as a "complex" (this is despite what you may see on a bottle of vitamin supplements that reads "B complex").

Chapter Objectives

This chapter will cover many, but not all, of the 13 different vitamins. Specifically, we cover:

- Roles and classification of vitamins
  —Water-soluble vitamins
  —Fat-soluble vitamins
- Do you need a vitamin supplement?
- Dietary supplements—regulation and safety

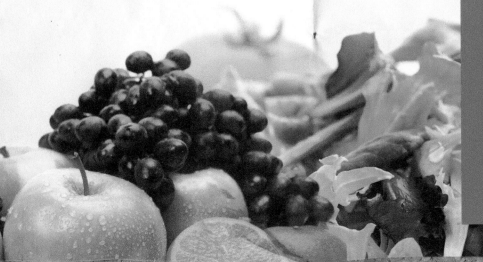

193

There are two classifications of vitamins based on their solubility in water. Due to a vitamin's particular chemical structure, it may "like" water and dissolve in it versus "dislike" water and prefer to be around fat (recall from Chapter 5 that fat and water don't mix). The two classifications of vitamins are water-soluble and fat-soluble.

Water-Soluble Vitamins

Characteristics of the water-soluble vitamin category (compare and contrast these with fat-soluble vitamins; see Quiz question #9):

- Water-soluble vitamins are found in the watery parts of the cells (inside compartments such as the mitochondria responsible for oxidation of carbohydrates and fats for energy).
- Turnover from the body is rapid, about 48 hours to several days. Therefore, your need for water-soluble vitamins is on a frequent basis.
- When consumed in excess, either from the diet or supplement, the body will maintain homeostasis and excrete the extra (either "whole" or in a broken-down form) in urine.
- Excess of water-soluble vitamins is not likely to be toxic.
- Water-soluble vitamins function as coenzymes, which means they facilitate enzyme action. Each water-soluble vitamin functions with one or more enzymes that allows a chemical reaction to occur.

The water-soluble vitamins covered in this chapter are listed in Figure 9.1.

Fat-Soluble Vitamins

- Since these vitamins are NOT soluble in water, they are found in the fatty parts of the body and cells, such as adipose tissue and cell membranes.
- Turnover within the body is very slow—over months. Therefore, the need is less frequent compared to water-soluble vitamins. (This difference becomes important when discussing deficiency of a vitamin—water-soluble deficiency can occur in several weeks on a poor diet, but it may take years to become deficient in some of the fat-soluble vitamins.)
- Excess of fat-soluble vitamins, whether from diet or a supplement, will stay in the body and be stored (in extreme cases of overdoing with a particular

Figure 9.1

WATER-SOLUBLE	
B VITAMINS	**VITAMIN C**
Thiamin (B_1)	Ascorbic acid
Riboflavin (B_2)	
Niacin (B_3)	
Pyrodoxine (B_6)	
Folate (folic acid)	
Vitamin B_{12}	

fat-soluble vitamin, the excess is deposited in fatty tissue). Thus, excess is NOT excreted in the urine.

- As a result, excess can be toxic and some fat-soluble vitamins, such as vitamin A, can even be fatal.
- Fat-soluble vitamins function in more general roles than the water-soluble vitamins. (They are not coenzymes.) The fat-soluble vitamins tend to "oversee" a system such as vitamin D, which is involved in the homeostasis of calcium and bone health.

The fat-soluble vitamins covered in this chapter are listed in the Figure 9.2.

Vitamins and the RDA

Throughout this book we have referred to the RDA (Recommended Dietary Allowances) and factors taken into account when establishing the RDA for a given nutrient. (For example, the quality of dietary proteins was taken into account in establishing the RDA for protein; see Chapter 2 for example.)

As a reminder, the RDA represents the recommended intake for many essential nutrients, such as protein, fiber, vitamins, and minerals meant to meet the needs of nearly all healthy people in the population. The RDA is not a minimum value, nor is it an average, but rather a safe and adequate intake that is meant to be averaged over several days.

Additionally, factors taken into account in establishing a given RDA include different age groups, pregnancy, and lactation. For minerals, issues of bioavailability are also considered. (Recall for the iron RDA, for example, that a 10 percent bioavailability from the diet is assumed.)

When it comes to vitamins, other considerations are factored in when establishing the RDAs. Many of the vitamins have chemical structures that make them unstable when exposed to heat, light, and even air. Thus, the RDA for many of the vitamins account for this issue of instability and the RDA reflects a greater value in accordance with this.

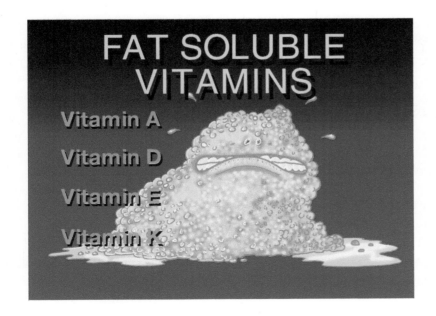

Figure 9.2

WATER-SOLUBLE VITAMINS

Before we get into each individual vitamin, let's take a look at the progression of water-soluble vitamin deficiency. You may have thought that you could develop deficiency problems within days of eating a vitamin-poor diet, when actually it takes several weeks.

Here's the progression of a water-soluble vitamin deficiency in a person who previously had been eating a diet with ample amounts of this particular vitamin.

Tissue saturation of the vitamin (which means the body fluids have an ample amount of the vitamin from diet)

Vitamin-deficient diet   ↓

Tissue levels of vitamin decline steadily

About 3 to 4 weeks   ↓

Biochemical lesion (enzyme activity decreases)

About 6 to 8 weeks   ↓

Clinical lesion (outward sign of deficiency—skin, tongue, etc. affected)

Following three to four weeks of a vitamin-deficient diet (very low amounts relative to requirement), you won't look any different and chances are you won't feel different (except perhaps some general fatigue). However, your cells will "look" different. A laboratory test could detect low activity of the enzyme that needs the particular vitamin which is deficient.

By six weeks or so, you will have an outward sign of deficiency. For water-soluble vitamins, common signs are:

- Skin disorders (dermatitis), such as cracking in the corner of the mouth, granular skin, darkening and peeling of the skin
- Intestinal tract trouble since these cells are high-turnover cells (smooth tongue, diarrhea)
- Muscle fatigue because the enzymes needed for energy metabolism become less effective (or not effective at all) in the absence of their vitamin helpers (coenzymes)

Vitamins

Vitamins were discovered around the beginning of the 1900s and got their name from "vital amine" (or vitamin) because nitrogen was associated with, what scientists thought at the time, a single vital substance that was not protein, carbohydrate, fat, or mineral. As each of these different compounds was discovered, they received names in the order of the alphabet. B vitamin was determined to be several different vitamins so they earned a numbering system that is still partially used today (e.g., vitamin B_6 and B_{12}).

For each of the water-soluble vitamins, we will cover:

1. Function
2. Deficiency problems (related to the vitamin's function)
3. Requirement
4. Food sources

Where Do the B Vitamins Work?

Most of the B vitamins are coenzymes in energy metabolism—the breakdown of carbohydrates, fats, and protein for fuel and in the manufacturing of glycogen, fat, and protein. Figure 9.3, as you may recall from Chapter 5, summarizes energy metabolism and indicates where some of the B vitamins operate. Seeing this may help you visualize how vital these B vitamins are for every cell's functioning.

Thiamin (Also Referred to as Vitamin B$_1$)

1. **Function:** Thiamin's basic function is regulatory and specifically works as a coenzyme in carbohydrate energy metabolism, as shown in Figure 9.4.
2. **Deficiency:** Thiamin deficiency appeared in populations that relied on grains, especially rice, for the bulk of their calories. In the 1800s, the process for refining grains—removing the coarse outer fiber and vitamin-rich hull—became widespread. The poorer people who had traditionally eaten brown rice (with the outer hull) began to eat white or "polished" rice as this was desirable since the more well-to-do people had long eaten hand-milled grains. But the wealthy also ate a varied diet and didn't rely on rice for a majority of their calories. (See Figure 9.5.) Since the poorer people ate about 80 percent of their calories as "polished" rice, thiamin deficiency developed, called **beriberi** (which means "I cannot, I cannot" in Sinhalese, a language

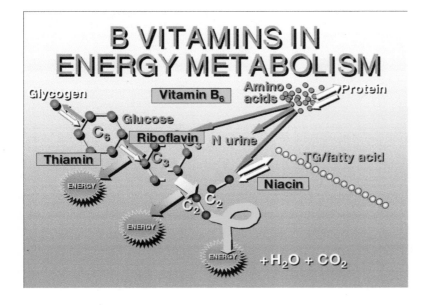

Figure 9.3

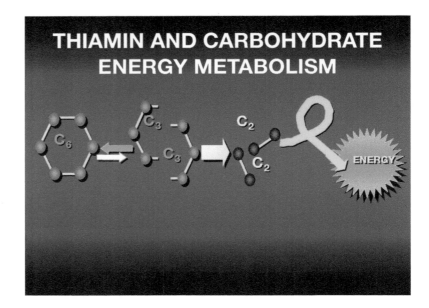

Figure 9.4

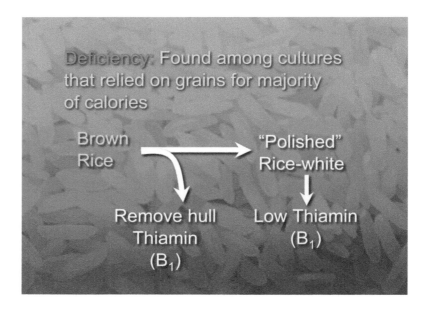

Figure 9.5

in Sri Lanka). Beriberi is characterized by muscle fatigue and nervous system dysfunction (these cells use carbohydrate for energy)—the people had trouble standing up and balancing (hence "I cannot get up"). Beriberi is also fatal and can result in heart failure.

Because beriberi was a problem, along with a few other B-vitamin deficiencies, the government implemented a grain enrichment program in the 1930s and 1940s to combat these problems. Now, by law, refined grain products have thiamin added back to whole grain levels (more on this in another section).

RDA FOR THIAMIN (B$_1$)	
19+ years male	1.2 mg/day
19+ years female	1.1 mg/day
Pregnancy	1.4 mg/day
Lactation	1.4 mg/day

Figure 9.6

3. **Requirement:** Listed in Figure 9.6 is the RDA for thiamin. While memorizing the numbers is not important, notice the milligram units and that women have greater needs when pregnant and lactating. The need for thiamin is based upon energy and carbohydrate intake—thus, a very active person who exercises quite a bit would take in more carbohydrate and therefore need more thiamin (but this increase in need can easily be met by food and does not require the use of supplements).

4. **Food sources:** Thiamin is found in many foods—meat, whole grains, beans, and liver being good sources. Pork is very high in thiamin. Food sources of thiamin are listed in Figure 9.7.

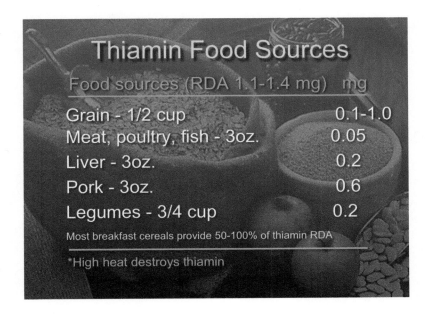

Thiamin Food Sources

Food sources (RDA 1.1-1.4 mg)   mg

Grain - 1/2 cup	0.1-1.0
Meat, poultry, fish - 3oz.	0.05
Liver - 3oz.	0.2
Pork - 3oz.	0.6
Legumes - 3/4 cup	0.2

Most breakfast cereals provide 50-100% of thiamin RDA

*High heat destroys thiamin

Figure 9.7

Riboflavin (Also Referred to as Vitamin B₂)

1. **Function:** Riboflavin's basic function is regulatory and it specifically serves as a coenzyme in carbohydrate energy metabolism. (See Figure 9.8.)
2. **Deficiency:** Riboflavin deficiency often occurs with other B-vitamin deficiencies and similar symptoms develop. The condition is called **ariboflavonosis** and is characterized by a smooth tongue, cracking at the corners of the mouth, and general fatigue.
3. **Requirement:** The requirement for riboflavin is listed in Figure 9.9.
4. **Food sources:** As shown in Figure 9.10, dairy products are a good source of riboflavin and for milk drinkers, this is the source of about half of the dietary riboflavin. Many foods, such as breakfast cereals, breads, and soymilk are either fortified (amounts added that are greater than what occurs in the food) or enriched (added back to original quantities) with riboflavin. Riboflavin is another B vitamin added back to refined grain products.

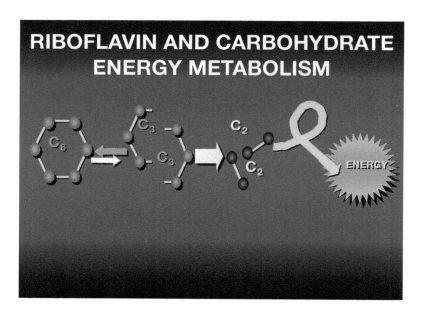

Figure 9.8

Figure 9.9

RDA FOR RIBOFLAVIN (B₂)	
19+ years male	1.3 mg/day
19+ years female	1.1 mg/day
Pregnancy	1.4 mg/day
Lactation	1.6 mg/day

RIBOFLAVIN (B₂) FOOD SOURCES	
FOOD SOURCES	mg
Milk – 1 cup	0.4
Soy milk	1.2
Meat – 3 oz.	0.15
Egg – 1	0.15
Dark green veggies	0.25
Whole grain	0.05/slice
Enriched grains	0.05/slice

1/2 intake from dairy products

*UV light destroys B₂

Figure 9.10

Niacin (Also Referred to as Vitamin B₃)

1. **Function:** Niacin's basic function is regulatory. Specifically, it works as a coenzyme in several reactions involved in the oxidation of carbohydrates, fats, and protein for fuel. Niacin also is a coenzyme in the building or making of fat. (See Figure 9.11.) Interestingly, our bodies can make some niacin from the amino acid tryptophan.
2. **Deficiency:** In the early 1900s, niacin deficiency was a killer disease in the southern United States. The diets of many poor people in this region consisted of just a few foods: refined corn grits, black-eyed peas, and salt pork (fatty

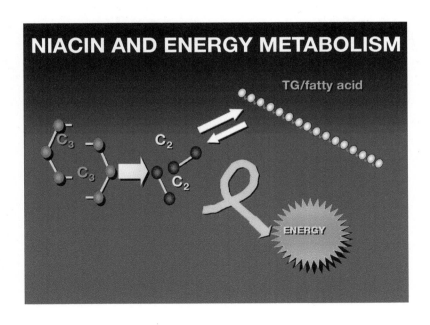

Figure 9.11

Pellagra

The mental disorder characteristic of pellagra was widespread and many mental institutions were built to handle the many thousands who suffered. At the time, the medical community did not realize that this disorder was caused by a lack of a nutrient in the diet. A physician, Dr. Goldberg, worked to show that pellagra was caused by the people's traditional diet and a dietary cure was soon developed.

pork with not much meat). This monotenous fare led to a serious disorder called **pellagra**, which was characterized by a dermatitis ("blackening" of skin exposed to light), diarrhea, dementia (severe mood swings and derangement), and then death. Notice that the symptoms are characteristic of water-soluble vitamin deficiency described earlier.

The traditional diet led to the niacin deficiency in three ways:

- The diet was very low in niacin.
- The niacin in corn is not very available for absorption (low bioavailability).
- The black-eyed peas are an incomplete protein and salt pork is low in protein. This presents a problem since the essential amino acid tryptophan can be converted to niacin in the body. It takes about 60 milligrams of tryptophan to make one milligram of niacin. Therefore, niacin is an essential nutrient that can be made by the body but not in sufficient amounts to meet needs.

Bottom line, these people were not getting enough or making enough niacin to meet their needs, and so pellagra developed. In the 1930s and 40s the government implemented the enrichment program for refined grains; niacin is another one of the B vitamins added back to grains after milling.

3. **Requirement:** The need for niacin, like thiamin, is based on energy needs. The requirement is listed in Figure 9.12.
4. **Food sources:** Niacin needs are easily met with a variety of foods. Good sources of niacin are listed in Figure 9.13.

RDA FOR NIACIN (B$_3$)	
19+ years male	16 mg/day
19+ years female	14 mg/day
Pregnancy	18 mg/day
Lactation	17 mg/day

Figure 9.12

NIACIN FOOD SOURCES

- Meat
- Fish
- Poultry
- Grains
- Cereals
- Beans
- Nuts

Figure 9.13

Vitamin B₆ (Also Referred to as Pyridoxine)

1. **Function:** Vitamin B₆'s basic function is regulatory. Specifically, it acts as a coenzyme in protein metabolism assisting the transfer of nitrogen from one amino acid to another. Vitamin B₆ is also involved in the breakdown of glycogen to glucose. (See Figure 9.14.)
2. **Deficiency:** Lack of vitamin B₆ causes similar water-soluble deficiency signs already discussed—diarrhea, skin changes, muscle fatigue. Anemia results because B₆ is also needed for the making of the hemoglobin protein found in red blood cells.
3. **Requirement:** The need for vitamin B₆ is related to protein requirement and intake. The RDA has been set at a level adequate for typical protein intakes of about 50 to 100 grams. The RDA for vitamin B₆ is listed in Figure 9.15. Notice that it increases in older people due to increased losses and turnover with aging combined with a poor intake.
4. **Food sources:** Food sources are listed in Figure 9.16. Whole grains are a good source, but not refined grains, because vitamin B₆ is not added back during the enrichment process.

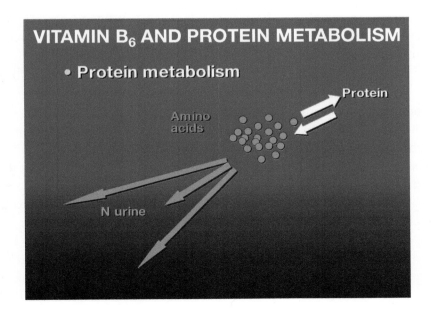

Figure 9.14

Figure 9.15

RDA FOR VITAMIN B$_6$		
19–50 years Male/female		1.3 mg/day
50+ years	female	1.5 mg/day
	male	1.7 mg/day
Pregnancy		1.9 mg/day
Lactation		2.0 mg/day

Figure 9.16

VITAMIN B$_6$ FOOD SOURCES	
FOOD SOURCES	mg
Meat, 3 oz.	0.1–0.9
Legumes, 1 cup	0.4
Banana, 1 medium	0.4
Green veggies, 1 cup	0.15
Whole grain breads	0.05/slice
Yeast, 1T	0.2

Vitamin B$_{12}$ and Folate (Also Called Folic Acid—The Chemical Form Used in Enrichment, Fortification, and Supplements)

These two B vitamins are discussed together since their roles are similar and they actually work together.

1. **Function:** These vitamins function as regulators and specifically work in the replication of genetic material (DNA and RNA) inside cells. Thus, they both play a crucial role in the growth and turnover of new cells. Vitamin B$_{12}$ also functions in the manufacturing of the covering around nerves called the myelin sheath.

2. **Deficiency:** Cells that turnover frequently in the body will be quickly affected by a deficiency of vitamin B$_{12}$ or folate. This includes red blood cells, which turnover or die at a rate of 1 percent each day, so they need to be replaced often.

    Anemia (sick blood) develops with deficiency of vitamin B$_{12}$ or folate. This form of anemia (different than iron-deficiency anemia) is characterized by large, immature blood cells. If a person is deficient in vitamin B$_{12}$, the nerves may also be damaged due to problems with myelin sheath formation and result in paralysis. This makes it imperative to determine the cause of anemia—vitamin B$_{12}$ or folate deficiency. Taking folate can mask a vitamin B$_{12}$ deficiency, which may ultimately lead to serious and permanent nerve damage.

Lack of folate pre-conception or during the first several weeks of pregnancy may lead to serious birth defects when cells are rapidly growing in the fetus. Studies show that taking folate before becoming pregnant and during pregnancy itself helps reduce the incidence of neural tube defects (a type of birth defect that involves the spinal cord and is often characterized by paralysis). For this reason, the government has added folate to the list of B vitamins added to refined grain products to improve intake in the general population. This will ensure that women will get adequate folate even if they are not planning a pregnancy. (About 50 percent of all pregnancies are unplanned and many women do not even know they are pregnant until a few weeks into the pregnancy when the spinal cord has developed.) Studies show that this fortification of grain products has helped significantly reduce the incidence of neural tube defects in the United States by an estimated 50 percent.

3. **Requirement:** The RDA for both vitamin B_{12} and folate are in the microgram quantity as shown in Figure 9.17. Notice the increased need for pregnant and lactating women. The need for vitamin B_{12} may increase with aging as the ability to absorb this vitamin declines due to a reduction in acid production.

4. **Food sources:** Good food sources of folate include: liver, citrus fruits, such as oranges and orange juice, and green leafy vegetables, such as spinach and asparagus. Grain products and breakfast cereals are fortified with folate (in the form of folic acid). Currently, the fortification of grains with folic acid is spurring debate about risks. Large population studies have revealed that an association may exist between folic acid excess and an increased risk for colon cancer in people with pre-cancerous polyps. Those at risk for colon cancer (diagnosis of polyps or family history) should be cautious about exceeding 100 percent fortification of folic acid in breakfast cereals, energy bars, and vitamin supplements.

   Good sources of vitamin B_{12} include most animal products—meats, fish, poultry, dairy, and vitamin B_{12}-fortified soymilk, soy products, and some breakfast cereals (see Figure 9.18).

Special Considerations for Vitamin B_{12}

This vitamin is unlike other water-soluble vitamins in several ways.

- Since vitamin B_{12} is a very large and fragile molecule, it needs some special care in the intestinal tract. The acid in the stomach can damage vitamin B_{12}. So to protect vitamin B_{12}, a special factor, called **intrinsic factor**, is manufactured by the stomach to bind with this vitamin and serve as protection and transport.

RDA FOR VITAMIN B_{12} AND FOLATE		
	B_{12}	FOLATE
19+ years Male/female	2.4 µg/day	400 µg/day
Pregnancy	2.6 µg/day	600 µg/day
Lactation	2.8 µg/day	500 µg/day

Figure 9.17

FOOD SOURCES	
VITAMIN B$_{12}$	**FOLATE (FOLATE ACID)**
Meats (all types)	Liver
Dairy	Citrus fruits
Eggs	Green leafy vegetables (spinach, broccoli, asparagus)
Seafood	
Fermented foods (miso, tempeh)	Beans (navy, garbanzo)
Fortified foods: soy milk, breakfast cereal (See Nutrition Facts food label)	Breakfast cereals (check Nutrition Facts food label)

Figure 9.18

This allows for absorption in the small intestine. A small group of people may genetically lack the ability to make this factor, and therefore need vitamin B$_{12}$ injections on a regular basis since they cannot absorb the vitamin.

- The mineral cobalt is part of vitamin B$_{12}$ structure, unlike other vitamins that don't have minerals as part of their chemical makeup.
- Vitamin B$_{12}$ is stored in the liver. If you eat a diet with sufficient amounts of this vitamin, you have about a year's supply stored. Recall that the other water-soluble vitamins are not stored.
- The distribution of vitamin B$_{12}$ in foods is unique—it is only found in animal products (meat, dairy, eggs, fish, etc.) and fermented foods. Fermented foods are those made with bacteria, such as miso (fermented soy) and generally are not adequate in B$_{12}$ content to meet needs.

Whole Grains, Refined Grains and Enrichment

Throughout our discussion of B vitamins, reference has been made to refined grains and the depletion or loss of nutrients. Let's take a look at the nutritional difference of whole grains compared to refined grains and how *some* of this disparity has been corrected.

Figure 9.19 shows a whole grain kernel, actually a seed of a plant, such as wheat or barley, which would grow into a new plant if allowed to sprout. So it makes sense that this whole kernel is rich in a variety of nutrients.

The outer layer—the bran layers or hull—contains water-insoluble fiber, B vitamins, and some minerals. The bulk of the kernel—what we eat and what feeds the developing plant—is starch (complex carbohydrate). The part that actually sprouts into a new plant is called the germ (rich in minerals and vitamins B and E). The germ also has a very small amount of polyunsaturated fats, which is why the vitamin E is there to protect these fats from oxidative damage due to sunlight or air.

If the germ is left with the grain during milling and made into flour or another grain item, the small amount of polyunsaturated fat may go "bad" or rancid due to its oxidation. This is the main reason why the germ is removed during processing to improve the shelf life of the grain product. In addition to shelf life, some people

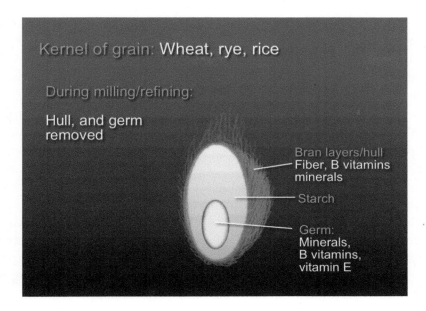

Figure 9.19

don't like the texture or taste of whole grain breads and other such products. Also, this dislike for whole grains is a bit of a throwback to when the peasants ate whole grain while the wealthy ate the refined grains.

As mentioned earlier in this chapter, during the 1800s, grain processors developed a way to refine grain—remove the coarse outer layers and the germ, leaving just the starch as shown in Figure 9.20. This starch could then be milled into flour and stored for long periods of time without going bad, which the public preferred. The downside—the whole grain had been stripped of many nutrients—fiber, B vitamins, vitamin E, and minerals, such as iron, zinc, and magnesium. As a result, many people by the late 1800s and 1900s had developed vitamin and mineral deficiencies, such as pellagra, beriberi, and iron-deficiency anemia.

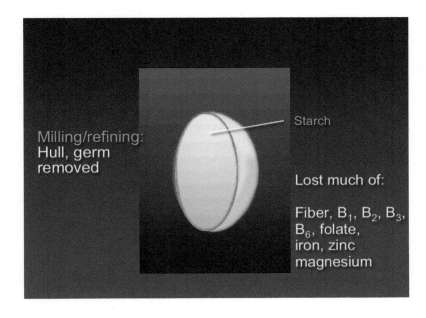

Figure 9.20

To combat these nutrient deficiencies, the government instituted the grain enrichment program. Under law, grain manufacturers are required to add thiamin (B_1), riboflavin (B_2), niacin (B_3), and iron at levels comparable to the unrefined whole grain. In 1998, folate was added to the list of enrichment nutrients. However, as shown in Figure 9.21 enriched refined grain products are not nutritionally comparable to whole grains because several nutrients are still lacking, including fiber, zinc, and other minerals and several vitamins. Additionally, unrefined grains also supply a wealth of protective compounds referred to generally as phytochemicals. Examples of such phytochemicals include lignans (a type of fiber), plant sterols, and fructooligosaccharides. Discussed in the next chapter, these compounds protect against cancer and other age-related diseases.

When you make grain choices in your diet, keep in mind that whole grain provides better nutrition than refined grain. So make an effort to use 100 percent whole wheat bread, brown rice, whole barley, and oats over their refined counterparts. Words or phrases such as "multigrain" or "Made with 9 whole grains" don't guarantee 100 percent whole grain. Look at the ingredient list for 100 percent whole grain, whole barley, oat, brown rice, and wheat. The 2015 Dietary Guidelines (Chapter 12) recommend that at least half of your daily grain servings are whole grain.

Vitamin C (Also Referred to as Ascorbic Acid)

1. **Function:** Vitamin C's basic function is regulatory. Specifically, it works in a chemical reaction to make the protein collagen. Recall from Chapter 2 that this protein has structural duties—collagen is the "glue" that holds your bones, connective tissue, lung tissue, blood vessels, and teeth together. Of the thousands of different proteins in your body (about 10,000 different ones), collagen makes up about 25 percent of your total body protein. (As you might guess, deficiency of vitamin C must have devastating consequences and it does.)

    Vitamin C also aids in iron absorption. Recall from Chapter 8 that iron's bioavailability is improved by the presence of vitamin C.

    Vitamin C also functions as an **antioxidant** in protecting fats—the liquid polyunsaturated fats—against oxidation (much like a fire extinguisher that

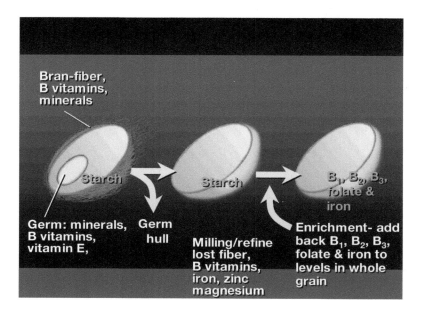

Figure 9.21

puts out small kitchen fires). Research shows that ample vitamin C intake over many years may lead to a lower risk of developing age-related diseases, such as cataracts, that are linked to oxidation of fats and other substances within the eye.

2. **Deficiency:** The deficiency of vitamin C actually impacted the exploration of the New World and the slave trade hundreds of years ago. The deficiency disease called **scurvy** was rampant among sailors on long voyages—many (about two-thirds) would die a hideous death of teeth falling out, hemorrhages under the skin, and painful joints and bones. Africans taken from their villages were brought on slave boats across the Atlantic Ocean and a good three-fourths would die from scurvy. This disease was not known on land because people ate fruits and vegetables that provided vitamin C.

   Scurvy is characterized by the following:

   * Painful, swollen, and bleeding gums result because the collagen is not being remade (remember protein turnover).
   * Teeth become loose and fall out.
   * Joints become painful and sore.
   * Bones become fragile. (Collagen is part of the bone matrix.)
   * Small hemorrhages form under the skin when blood leaks from the weakened blood vessels.
   * Eventually, scurvy is fatal.

3. **Requirement:** Vitamin C is a good example of a vitamin NOT required by all species. In fact, only humans, other primates, guinea pigs, fruit-eating bats, and trout are among the few animals that require vitamin C. The reason is that we lack the enzyme to make vitamin C from glucose (a very simple chemical reaction that we and the few other species cannot perform). Therefore, vitamin C is required in the diet.

   The RDA for vitamin C is listed in Figure 9.22. Notice that there is an additional 35 milligrams needed by people who smoke because this increases the breakdown of vitamin C in your system due to the oxidative stress.

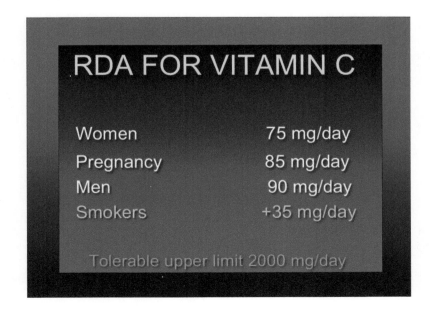

RDA FOR VITAMIN C	
Women	75 mg/day
Pregnancy	85 mg/day
Men	90 mg/day
Smokers	+35 mg/day
Tolerable upper limit 2000 mg/day	

Figure 9.22

There is a safe upper limit of 2,000 milligrams daily established for vitamin C, which is commonly taken in supplement form. Above this level, there may be adverse effects. Even though vitamin C is water-soluble, such large amounts may be detrimental. For example, at this level, the vitamin C may cause nausea, cramps, and an increased risk for the formation of kidney stones.

4. **Food sources:** Vitamin C is easily obtained from food. Many fruits, particularly citrus (oranges, grapefruit, tangerines) are excellent sources of this vitamin. Vegetables, such as peppers, tomatoes, and broccoli, are also very good sources as shown in Figure 9.23.

What about Vitamin C Supplements?

Many people opt to take vitamin C supplements in amounts well over the RDA, such as 500 or 1,000 milligram tablets in an effort to ward off diseases, such as cancer or to fend off the common cold. Research does suggest that getting ample vitamin C from the foods you eat may help lower your risk for age-related diseases. The scientific evidence for supplements, however, is not as compelling. This brings up the possibilities that the vitamin may interact with other substances, such as phytochemicals (non-vitamin compounds) in food to provide the health benefit rather than the vitamin C supplement alone. As for preventing or curing the common cold, research does not support that taking vitamin C on a regular basis prevents the cold virus. Studies also do not support that powdered vitamin C packets work in preventing colds or flu. If, however, you have a low vitamin C intake, this may weaken your immune system and make you more susceptible to getting a cold. Instead, taking vitamin C at the onset of a cold may help lessen the symptoms.

FAT-SOLUBLE VITAMINS

As described in the first section, fat-soluble vitamins are chemically different from water-soluble. This, in turn, influences fat-soluable vitamin turnover and storage in the body, and subsequently, the need and possible toxicity issues for these vitamins. As we cover the four fat-soluble vitamins, issues of storage and toxicity will be covered, which was not done for water-soluble vitamins (except vitamin B_{12}, which can be stored). Also note the functions of fat-soluble vitamins do not involve

---

Urban Myth

Myth: "Juicing a fruit or vegetable enhances the content of vitamins."

Juicing an orange or another fruit or vegetable typically separates the pulpy matter of the fruit or vegetable from the watery portion, which you drain off to drink. This process actually lowers vitamin content as not all the vitamins end up in the juice; some stay behind in the pulp (often discarded in this process).

Figure 9.23

VITAMIN C FOOD SOURCES	
FOOD SOURCES	**mg**
Milk, meat	0
Fresh fruit: kiwi, orange, strawberry, cantaloupe (1 cup)	40–100+
Orange juice, 6 oz.	90
Tomato, broccoli (1 cup)	40
Pepper (green, red, hot) (½ cup)	30–60+

a specific coenzyme duty, but rather function in a more general manner. Deficiency of fat-soluble vitamins progresses at a much different rate than water-soluble vitamins due to the storage and relatively slow turnover of fat-soluble vitamins. Consequently, it may take several years to become deficient, for example, in vitamin E.

Vitamin A

1. **Function:** Vitamin A's basic function is regulatory and specifically plays a role in several areas:

   - Vitamin A plays a role in the vision cycle—the ability to perceive light during low-light situations, such as dusk and dawn, or a dimly lit room. In the back of the eye, there are specialized cells that contain vitamin A, which is chemically modified when light comes in contact with these cells. This chemical modification in turn signals the brain of the presence of light.
   - Most of the body's vitamin A is involved in the maintenance of **epithelial** cells, which is the covering tissue in the body—skin, lining of the lungs, intestines, sinus cavities, urinary tract, and reproductive system. When totaled, epithelial cells account for a large surface area of the body.
   - Vitamin A is also involved in the growth of new bones, which occurs primarily at the ends where remodeling of the bones allows growth in length— a vital role for this vitamin during childhood and adolescence. Thus, during periods of growth, such as puberty and adolescence, adequate intake of this vitamin is crucial.

2. **Deficiency:** Several deficiency problems arise in response and may take months or years to develop depending upon the person's status (storage) of vitamin A prior to the inadequate diet.

   - **Night blindness** (related to the vision cycle), which is the inability to see in low-light situations (trouble driving at night, etc.).
   - **Xeropthalmia**—the surface of the eye or cornea sloughs off (the surface and inner eyelid are epithelial surfaces) and blindness occurs. In poor underdeveloped countries and communities, about 500,000 children go blind every year as a result of vitamin A deficiency. This is the number one cause of preventable blindness worldwide.
   - Infection of the lungs, skin, urinary tract, and other epithelial surfaces occurs when these surfaces are no longer maintained with a vitamin A deficiency. Bacteria and other pathogens invade the body and often a person dies from infection due to vitamin A deficiency.
   - Bone growth is halted with vitamin A deficiency and this leads to stunting of growth in children.

3. **Requirement:** Figure 9.24 illustrates vitamin A's structure as it is found in animal products, such as liver and milk. It is a ring structure with a long fatty-acid like chain attached. (This is why vitamin A is fat soluble.)

   In plants, there are pigment substances that give plants a yellow, orange, or red color called carotenes. There are some 400 different carotenes, and a few have what is called "vitamin A activity." As shown in Figure 9.25, carotenes look like two vitamin A units joined together. In fact, when you eat them, enzymes in the intestinal wall break carotene apart and vitamin A is formed. Not all carotenes are converted to vitamin A, and not all at the

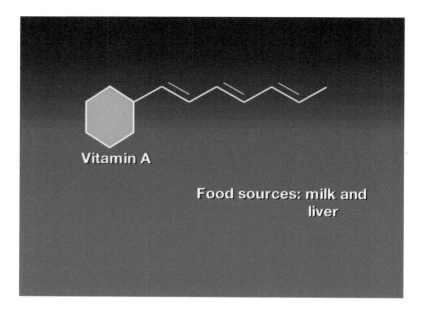

Figure 9.24

Figure 9.24

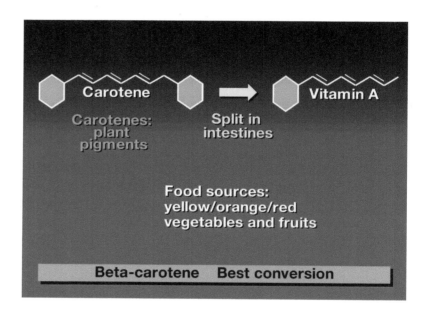

Figure 9.25

same efficiency. Beta-carotene (found in carrots, cantaloupe, and papaya, for example) is converted the best.

Plant food sources contain carotenes and animal sources contain vitamin A. In order to have a common "currency" when talking about vitamin A and its precursors like beta-carotene, we use a measurement called Retinal Activity Equivalent or RAE. Although these numbers are not to be memorized, 1 RAE = 1 microgram of retinol (animal vitamin A), 2 micrograms of beta-carotene from a supplement (converted more efficiently than from food), 12 micrograms of beta-carotene from food, and 24 micrograms of carotenes (other than beta-carotene).

With all of this said about vitamin A in animal products and carotenes in food, the requirement for vitamin A is expressed in RAE because you can meet your need from animal sources or plant sources, or both. The RDA for vitamin A is listed in Figure 9.26.

4. **Food sources:** Typically, about half of your vitamin A comes from animal sources (especially if you eat dairy products, which come fortified with vitamin A). Liver is an extraordinary source of vitamin A, as shown in Figure 9.27, because this organ is a site of storage for this vitamin.

5. **Toxicity and supplementation:** As a fat-soluble vitamin, vitamin A has some major toxicity concerns since excess from food or supplements stays in the body, which is either stored in the liver or tucked away in fatty tissue. Taken during pregnancy in large amounts (25 times the RDA), it can cause serious birth defects. At this level of intake, liver damage occurs along with swollen and painful gums.

For beta-carotene and other carotenes, there is no toxicity concerns (in terms of health) other than pigmentation of the skin, primarily an orange tinge to the palms and soles of the feet. This pigmentation develops when a person drinks copious amounts of carrot juice or takes beta-carotene supplements.

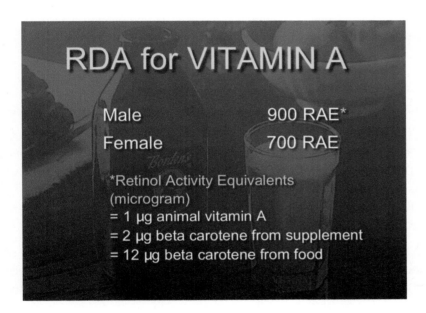

RDA for VITAMIN A

Male	900 RAE*
Female	700 RAE

*Retinol Activity Equivalents (microgram)
= 1 µg animal vitamin A
= 2 µg beta carotene from supplement
= 12 µg beta carotene from food

Figure 9.26

VITAMIN A FOOD SOURCES	
FOOD SOURCES	**RAE**
Liver (3 oz.)	9,000
Egg (1)	84
Milk (1 cup)	100
Orange–yellow fruit: Cantaloupe, apricot, papaya (1 cup)	100+
Orange–yellow vegetables: Carrot, butternut squash, pumpkin (1 cup)	300–1,000+

Figure 9.27

Vitamin A Toxicity

A person can experience acute toxicity (fatal) of vitamin A by consuming 1 million RAE, and this can be done through supplements or by eating the liver of a large animal that has stored a lot of this vitamin in preparation for a season of hibernation. Sadly, explorers to the North Pole killed a polar bear for food and ate the liver. As a result, a few of the explorers died from acute vitamin A poisoning (hypersloughing of the skin and other epithelial tissues).

As a side note, derivatives of vitamin A (Retin-A and Accutane) are used in the treatment of acne as well as the treatment of fine wrinkles (skin aging process). These vitamin A analogs cause the skin to slough off rapidly, revealing "fresh" skin. This new skin is very sensitive to UV sun exposure, making it more susceptible to sun damage. There is also a danger in taking oral vitamin A analogs (Accutane) for acne treatment because these can also cause severe birth defects. A woman using this medication should be on birth control to prevent pregnancy.

Vitamin D

1. **Function:** The basic function of this vitamin is regulatory, and it oversees the homeostasis of calcium metabolism:

   * Regulates calcium absorption in the intestinal tract through a protein carrier.
   * Directs the bones to mineralize (calcium-phosphorous salt called hydroxyapatite).
   * Regulates blood levels of calcium by directing the amount of calcium the kidneys excrete or retain.

   While we know vitamin D as a bone-building nutrient, there are several other roles for this hormone-like vitamin. Various cell types have receptors for vitamin D, allowing it to enter cells and participate with various roles in the cell growth's anti-inflammatory action. Toning down inflammatory responses in the body, especially those occurring chronically, may help lower the risk for diseases, such as diabetes and cancer.

2. **Deficiency:** Severe bone maladies were noted in children at the turn of the century in urban London, England. The city used coal for heat and fuel. This produced smoke, which clouded the sky and blocked UV light from the sun. The children, who also spent much of their time indoors, suffered from soft bones that bent under their bodyweight—a condition called **rickets**.

   Why might rickets—vitamin D deficiency—be tied into sunlight exposure? Vitamin D is actually much like a hormone. Your body can make this vitamin, and make enough to meet your needs given sufficient exposure to sunlight—about 30 minutes to hands and face per day for fair skin people and up to two hours for darker skin during the spring and summer months. Cholesterol is the building block for vitamin D and after a few chemical modifications, the first of which involves UV light, it becomes the vitamin as shown in Figure 9.28.

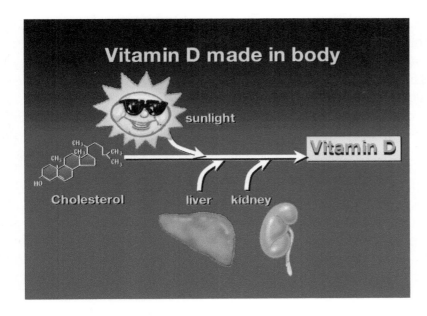

Figure 9.28

Rickets is characterized by:

- Soft bones that bow out or in (the long bones of the legs being most affected)
- Cartilage overgrows to compensate for lack of mineralized bone.
- The head of a young child becomes enlarged because the skull plates do not mineralize properly and migrate apart with cartilage filling in the gaps.

In adults, a type of rickets (osteomalacia) forms where the bones become soft. Elderly people who do not get enough sunlight exposure and inadequate vitamin D in their diet are likely to suffer. Additionally, their kidney and liver function may be compromised because of aging and medication use further aggravating the problem.

3. **Requirement:** Since exposure to sunlight varies, and many people also have dark skin, which in effect hampers the manufacturing of vitamin D (as does sun block, which is typically worn on the face and hands), this vitamin is deemed essential. The RDA has been determined as listed in Figure 9.29 and is

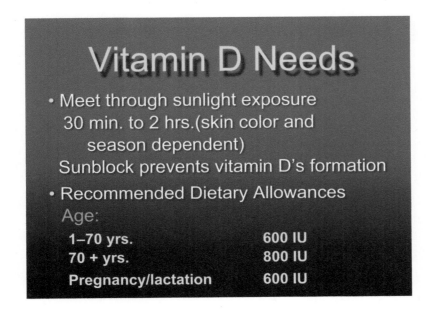

Figure 9.29

set to both prevent rickets as well as promote health. Note that need increases with age since the body's ability to manufacture this vitamin declines with age.

4. **Food sources:** Few foods are good sources of vitamin D. Primarily fatty fish, such as salmon and mackerel, are the best sources of vitamin D. (In the early 1900s, cod liver oil was used as a treatment for rickets and was later found to contain vitamin D.) Also, liver and eggs contain vitamin D. In the United States, milk is fortified with vitamin D as are some breakfast cereals. Mushrooms exposed to UV light also make vitamin D (look for presence on Nutrition Food Fact label).

5. **Toxicity:** At intake about three times the AI, vitamin D can be toxic in children since their bones are rapidly growing. Calcium levels in the blood increase and calcium is then deposited in soft tissue, such as organs. Overgrowth of bones in the face may occur, causing gross malformations.

Vitamin E

1. **Function:** The basic function of this vitamin is regulatory, and specifically, it acts as an antioxidant (like vitamin C and beta-carotene) protecting fatty acids with double bonds from oxidation. These fats reside in the cell membrane. So consider those cells exposed to oxygen (which can easily cause oxidative damage or rancidity of the fatty acid)—lungs, red blood cells, etc. Vitamin E actually rests on the cell membrane to protect these fats from oxidative damage. (See Fiure 9.30.)

   This brings up the impact of exercise on oxidative damage and need for vitamin E. During exercise, more oxygen is taken in to support the energy demands of the workout. This means the possibility of increased oxidative damage to polyunsaturated fatty acids in the membranes of muscle cells. Studies show that this does, in fact, occur, and that people who exercise may

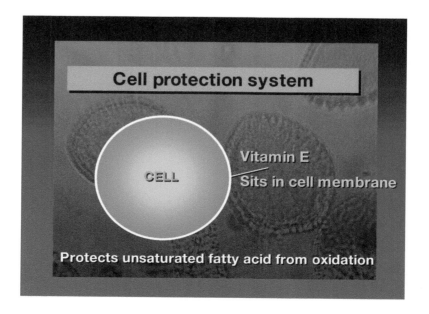

Figure 9.30

benefit from a greater intake of dietary antioxidants, such as vitamins E and C from foods.

2. **Deficiency:** True vitamin E deficiency is rare and is believed to take at least five to seven years to develop because this vitamin turns over very slowly. The consequence of vitamin E deficiency is a type of anemia called **hemolytic anemia** where the red blood cells break open because the cell membranes have been weakened as shown in Figure 9.31.

   A lifetime, marginal intake of vitamin E is believed linked to age-related ailments, such as cancer, heart, and Alzheimer's diseases. For example, with weakened cell membranes, carcinogens may be able to damage DNA more readily, leading to cancer. Many people take supplements of vitamin E in an effort to ward of these conditions. But research suggests that supplemental vitamin E may actually increase risk of cancer in those at risk, such as smokers.

3. **Requirement:** The requirement for vitamin E is based upon polyunsaturated fat intake. If a person has a very high intake of these fats (vegetable oils), vitamin E needs would increase.

   - The RDA for this vitamin is set at 15 milligrams daily for both men and women, and increases to 19 milligrams during lactation.

4. **Food sources:** Vitamin E comes from plant sources rich with polyunsaturated fats. (Recall that whole grains contain the germ with small amounts of these fats that need protection from oxidation so the plant has ingeniously put vitamin E there for that very reason.) Food sources are listed in Figure 9.32.

5. **Toxicity:** Out of the four fat-soluble vitamins, vitamin E appears to be the least toxic. The Tolerable Upper Safe Limit (UL) is set at 1,000 milligrams daily. Risks associated with excess vitamin E include bleeding (the blood does not clot as well) and flu-like symptoms. As mentioned previously, supplemental intake may increase cancer risk for those who are at risk for the disease.

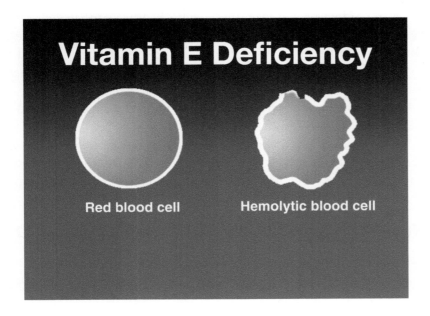

Figure 9.31

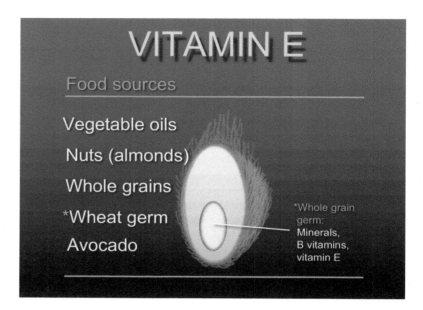

Figure 9.32

Vitamin K

1. **Function:** This vitamin functions as a regulatory nutrient and specifically:

   - Plays a role in several steps of blood clot formation
   - Participates in the mineralization of bone (specifically a modification of a bone protein)

2. **Deficiency:** Vitamin K deficiency is not common since some of our "intake" of this vitamin comes from the contribution of intestinal bacteria. These friendly microbes in our intestines make vitamin K, providing us a source of the vitamin even if our intake is low. Deficiency typically arises when a person has been taking antibiotics for an extended period of time (these medications kill infectious bacteria along with our beneficial intestinal bacteria).

   Also, certain people take anti-vitamin K drugs so that their blood will be less likely to clot. Can you guess whom? People with heart disease and narrowed arteries don't want their blood to clot in these clogged vessels so "thinner" blood is best. But as a result of the anti-vitamin K drug, these people may be at risk for reduced bone mineral density.

3 and 4. **Requirement and food sources:** The requirement and basic food sources are listed in Figure 9.33.

   At birth when you entered the world, your intestines were sterile or free of friendly bacteria. During the first few days of life, you got by with an injection of vitamin K given to all newborns to avoid the risk of bleeding.

DO YOU NEED A VITAMIN-MINERAL SUPPLEMENT?

After our two-chapter discussion of the micronutrients—minerals and vitamins—you may have the feeling that you might be in need of supplementation. Deficiency consequences sound devastating, and you may realize by now that your diet is not optimal. From your Diet Project forms, you can assess your typical intake and

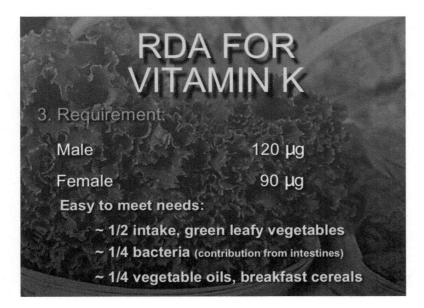

Figure 9.33

compare it to established requirements. This comparison may alert you to a less than adequate diet for one or more nutrients. Should you consider a supplement to boost your intake of the vitamins and minerals? As we will learn in Chapter 10, whole foods offer a wealth of phytochemicals in addition to vitamins and minerals. Research supports the fact that whole foods rather than supplements provide protection against age-related diseases, such as cancer, heart disease, and diabetes. This is one of the benefits of whole foods over supplements.

The Dietary Guidelines for Americans (Chapter 12) outlines a base diet that contains multiple servings of fruits, vegetables and whole grains along with other nutrient-dense foods, such as lean meats, beans, seafood and dairy, which supply sufficient amounts of the micronutrients. Additionally, our intake of many vitamins and minerals is more than adequate due to our consumption of vitamin- and mineral-fortified foods, such as breakfast cereals, energy bars, and beverages. There are times, however, when you may want to consider a supplement. Here are several considerations for use of a general multivitamin and mineral supplement that contains no more than 100 percent of the DRI for the micronutrients.

If your calorie intake is less than 1,500 calories daily (especially if you are female or elderly). At low-calorie intakes, it is challenging to meet your need for all the micronutrients. You must choose fruits, vegetables, whole grains, beans, lean meats, etc. This leaves little if any room for empty calorie foods such as candy or soda.

If you consume alcohol regularly and in excessive amounts. As discussed in the next chapter, alcohol effects nutrient status several ways, essentially putting you at risk for vitamin and mineral deficiencies.

If you are pregnant, or planning on becoming pregnant. Nutrient needs change and having good folate status is important for the prevention of certain birth defects. Also, iron needs rise so dramatically during pregnancy that a supplement is necessary.

If your eating habits are irregular or if you habitually make poor food choices. This perhaps fits your eating habits and hopefully by this point in the course you are interested in improving your food choices. In the event you do continue to eat irregularly, a multivitamin and mineral supplement helps fill in the gaps on those days when you eat poorly.

When choosing a multivitamin and mineral supplement, there are many choices such as high-priced brands to generic or store-name brands. Generally, these less expensive brands are made by some of the best supplement makers and are just as good as high-priced varieties. Unfortunately, as we will learn in the next section, the quality of supplements overall is poorly regulated so you can never be sure of what you are purchasing.

Dietary Supplements—Regulation and Safety

Vitamin pills, herbal preparation, and protein powders are just a few of the different dietary supplements sold in the United States. Currently, over 50,000 dietary supplements are for sale in the US alone. An estimated 50 percent of all Americans take one or more dietary supplements on a regular basis, leading to sales of $25 billion annually. What you may not be aware of are the laws that regulate the safety and efficacies of supplements are different than that that governs food. In fact, purchasing a dietary supplement is a "buyer beware" type of situation because the Food and Drug Administration does not strictly regulate this industry the same way that the food industry is controlled.

Let's first define a dietary supplement. (See Figure 9.34.)

The Food and Drug Administration, which is responsible for overseeing dietary supplements, states that they are intended to supplement the diets of some people, but not to replace the balance of the variety of foods important to a healthy diet.

The Dietary Supplement Health and Education Act (DSHEA) of 1994 has impacted the supplement industry and what manufacturers are able to state as claims on the label, in advertising and promotional materials including on the Internet. In accordance with DSHEA, supplement labels may carry "statements of nutritional support," which describes the effect of the ingredient on the body. This is called a "structure/function" claim. But label claims cannot make statements

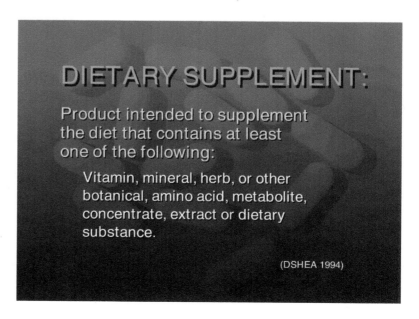

DIETARY SUPPLEMENT:

Product intended to supplement the diet that contains at least one of the following:

Vitamin, mineral, herb, or other botanical, amino acid, metabolite, concentrate, extract or dietary substance.

(DSHEA 1994)

Figure 9.34

that imply the supplements act as a drug or cure a disease. Examples of permissible and prohibited claims are shown in Figure 9.35.

Since the FDA has not evaluated manufacturers' claims, they must bear a disclaimer on the label as shown in Figure 9.36.

The manufacturer must be able to substantiate that "structure/function" statements are truthful, but they are NOT required to provide substantiation unless asked. So in other words, the FDA does NOT approve statements of nutritional support, but the FDA can object to them.

When considering a dietary supplement, there are some things you should consider, such as how to spot a fraudulent product. The following are some bogus claims that should alert you that the claims are most likely "too good to be true."

- "break through"
- "magical"
- "miracle cure"
- "new discovery"

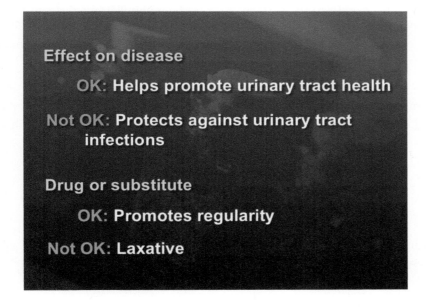

Figure 9.35

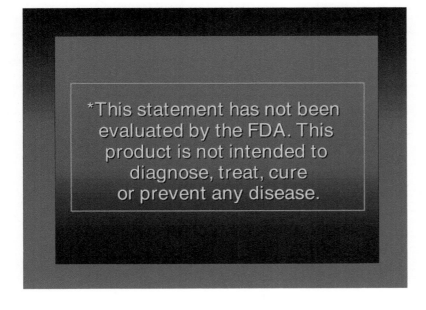

Figure 9.36

Here are several things to consider about supplements as it relates to potential health problems:

- Dietary supplements are NOT checked for quality and quantity of active ingredients. (This means you can't be sure what you are taking.)
- Some supplements may interact with prescriptions and over-the-counter medicines.
- Some supplements may increase complications during surgery (such as causing excessive bleeding).
- Many supplements have unsafe side effects. (Under the DSHEA of 1994 this is out of FDA's control.)

When you use the Internet for supplement information, here are some tips before you buy:

- Look for sites operated by the government, health organizations, or universities (FDA, American Heart Association, or National Institute of Health).
- Look for sites without advertisements (commercial sites promote their products).
- Question the source of the information (referenced with scientific journals, qualified author).

See pages 515–517 in the Appendix for more information on specific dietary supplements and up-to-date information on supplement recall. For more information, see Office of Dietary Supplements, National Institutes of Health http://ods.nih.gov

This is a suggested study aid for learning the function, deficiency, food source, etc. for the various vitamins and minerals—set up a table such as this recording information for each vitamin and mineral covered.

VITAMIN OR MINERAL	FUNCTION	DEFICIENCY	FOOD SOURCE	TOXICITY ISSUE	OTHER NOTES

Quiz Yourself

9

CHAPTER

1. List a good food source for each vitamin.

   - Vitamin C (non-citrus) _____
   - Niacin (B$_3$) _____
   - Beta-carotene _____
   - Vitamin B$_6$ _____
   - Folate _____
   - Vitamin B$_{12}$ _____
   - Vitamin E _____
   - Thiamin (B$_1$) _____

2. During the milling process of grain products, such as wheat, portions of the kernel are removed, which decreases the content of:

   a. B vitamins only
   b. B vitamins and zinc only
   c. B vitamins and fiber only
   d. B vitamins, iron, zinc, and fiber
   e. fiber and iron only

3. Therefore, grain products are enriched with

   a. B vitamins and fiber
   b. vitamin B$_6$, iron and fiber
   c. thiamin, riboflavin, niacin, and folate
   d. iron
   e. c and d above

4. Eating a diet deficient in water-soluble vitamins will result in clinical signs of vitamin deficiency in several weeks rather than years.

   a. true
   b. false

5. The effects of a deficiency of vitamin D are most readily observed in the

   a. muscular system
   b. epithelial tissue
   c. nervous system
   d. digestive system
   e. skeletal system

6. Which of the following micronutrients function as antioxidants protecting unsaturated fatty acids from oxidations?

   a. zinc and fluoride
   b. vitamin B_6, vitamin B_{12}, and folic acid
   c. calcium, potassium, and vitamin C
   d. vitamin C, vitamin E, and beta-carotene
   e. vitamin D, vitamin K, and vitamin E

7. This vitamin is needed for cell replication and a deficiency causes anemia. Adequate intake of this vitamin during pregnancy may help prevent birth defects.

   a. vitamin C
   b. vitamin B_{12}
   c. folate (folic acid)
   d. niacin (B_3)
   e. thiamin

8. Define vitamins and describe their function (include both categories).

   _____

   _____

   _____

9. Describe three ways the vitamin categories differ.

   _____

   _____

   _____

SPECIAL TOPICS THAT MAY SAVE YOUR LIFE!

10

We've covered all the nutrient classes and looked at the impact that some of these have on health and disease risk (fat intake and heart disease risk, for example). Now let's turn our attention to two special topics—alcohol and cancer. In the case of alcohol, consumption of this substance profoundly impacts a person's nutritional status. In our discussion, you will see how both in the short and long term, alcohol compromises health. Our discussion of cancer is an excellent way to tie in the various nutrients, their functions, and the roles they may play in the prevention of this often age-related disease.

Additionally, we will introduce the emerging topic of nutrigenomics—the interaction of food and genetics—to round out our discussion of diet and cancer along with the other diet-related diseases covered in earlier chapters.

NUTRITIONAL IMPACT OF ALCOHOL

According to a government survey, approximately 70 percent of young adults ages 18 to 25 years consume alcoholic beverages. And the survey showed this same age group had the highest rates of binge drinking (five or more drinks in a row in the last month) compared to other age groups. Risky drinking behavior tragically leads to a greater risk of traffic fatalities due to alcohol (51 percent of drivers ages 21 to 24 who died tested positive for alcohol). Besides posing a threat to themselves and others on the roads, consuming alcohol also poses health risks related to nutrition. Our discussion of alcohol first focuses on its metabolism and then on how this substance impacts nutritional status.

Chapter Objectives

In this chapter, we will cover:

- Impact of alcohol on nutritional status
- Role of diet on cancer risk
- Empty-calorie and nutrient-dense foods in the diet
- The influence of diet and chronic disease risk—nutrigenomics

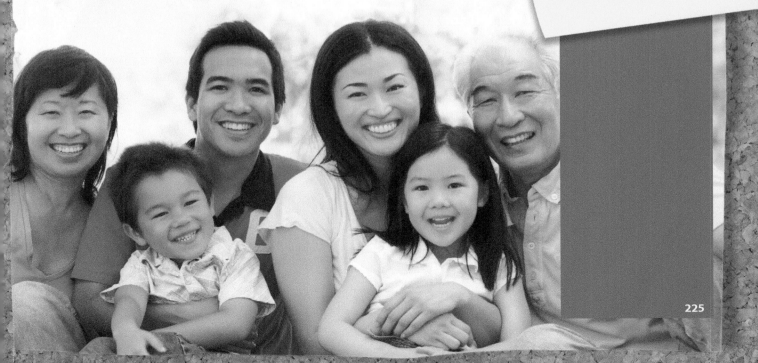

Alcohol and Its Metabolism

- Alcohol is a two-carbon molecule that is made from the fermentation of carbohydrates. Hops and barley (complex carbohydrates), for example, are fermented to make beer (with the aid of organisms such as yeast), which breaks down the carbohydrate to a two-carbon unit (similar to how glucose and fatty acids are broken down during their aerobic energy metabolism—recall from Chapters 4 and 5). Fruit, such as grapes, are fermented to make wine. Even though alcohol comes from carbohydrate—alcohol is NOT a carbohydrate. Contrary to what some people may think, alcohol is not a nutrient.

- Alcohol is small and a very simple molecule, thus it requires NO digestion. Unlike other substances we eat, alcohol can be absorbed through the stomach. If food is present, then the absorption through the stomach is slowed and the alcohol moves on to the small intestine for absorption (as shown in Figure 10.1). So, on an empty stomach, more alcohol enters your circulation, thereby impacting your brain and subsequently, motor function, speech, and judgment compared to drinking alcohol in conjunction with food.

- In the stomach lining, there is a small amount of an enzyme that can break down alcohol before it reaches the bloodstream (although this is not the primary way alcohol is metabolized in the body). Men possess a bit more of this enzyme in their stomach lining than women. Thus, at this first stage, less of the alcohol passes through into the circulation when a man has an alcoholic drink compared to a woman drinking the same amount of alcohol.

- The liver is the primary site for the metabolism or breakdown of alcohol, as shown in Figure 10.2. The enzyme, alcohol dehydrogenase, is responsible for converting alcohol (two-carbon unit) on to its way into the same two-carbon unit that is obtained from the breakdown of fats, carbs, and protein for fuel that then feeds into the TCA cycle (look back to Chapter 5 and Figure 5.26). Taking it through this cycle would break chemical bonds and release energy.

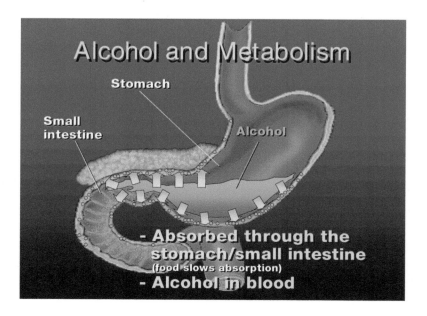

Figure 10.1

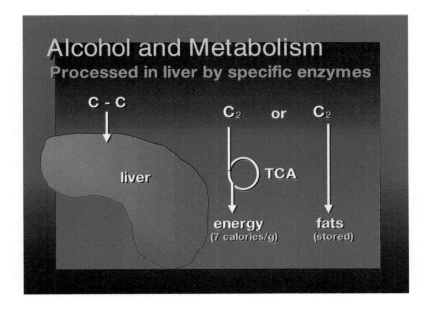

Figure 10.2

Alcohol—Men vs. Women

Men and women also differ in their ability to handle alcohol because of body composition differences. Since alcohol is water soluble, it "dissolves" in the blood and body water. Men have more body water than women (greater lean mass, less body fat—see Chapter 1), which means that for a man and woman of equal body size, the man has a greater volume of body water (blood included) to "dissolve" the alcohol. This means that after drinking the same of amount of alcohol, a woman would have a greater blood alcohol level compared to an equal-sized man.

Alcohol yields 7 calories per gram. The other option for alcohol is that, once converted to C_2 units, several can be "glued' together and a fatty acid can be made (which in turn leads to the making of a triglyceride or fat). This fat can then be shipped out of the liver and stored as body fat. **Thus, alcohol can be used as fuel or be converted to and stored as fat.**

- Most livers (or people) have the ability to process approximately 15 grams of alcohol per hour. This translates to one alcoholic drink per hour (12 ounces of beer, 5 ounces of wine, and 1.5 ounces of distilled spirits such as vodka). But this is just an estimate, because smaller people, particularly women, may not be able to process this much alcohol in one hour. Exceeding this intake would lead to elevated blood alcohol levels and the subsequent impact alcohol has on the brain (speech, inhibition level, coordination, etc.).

- Genetics also impacts the ability to process alcohol. Most notably, people of Asian descent have a decreased ability to process alcohol due to lack of proper enzyme to deal with alcohol. This means Asians feel the effects of alcohol more readily and also have discomfort (facial redness) due to the buildup of an alcohol by-product that is not processed normally.

- Another set of enzymes also break down alcohol called the "drug-metabolizing" enzymes (or cytochrome P450). These enzymes are also responsible for processing drugs such as painkillers and anesthesia. With chronic alcohol consumption (several drinks many days of the week), these enzymes adapt and can tolerate more alcohol and more drugs. This is why physicians ask about your alcohol use before going into surgery so as to know how much anesthesia to give. They don't want to under-dose and have you wake up on the operating table!

Impact of Alcohol on Liver Function

You can tell by this discussion that the liver is very busy processing alcohol each time a person takes a drink. But also recognize that the liver puts alcohol on the top of its priority list. This means the liver puts aside its regular duties such as building fluid balance proteins (Chapter 3) or the packaging of fat into lipoproteins (Chapter 5). The consequence on continued presence of alcohol can be devastating to liver function and overall body health.

- **The liver has a decreased ability to convert amino acids to glucose.** This means that during times without food, glucose levels will not be maintained well (part of the reason why some people feel hungry after a night of drinking). The brain, in turn, will not get the necessary carbohydrate (glucose) that it normally would have from the liver.
- **The liver's ability to produce proteins decreases.** The liver makes a host of regulatory proteins such as fluid balance proteins, coating proteins for lipoproteins, and transport proteins that move vitamins and other substances in the blood. The most important proteins affected are the lipoprotein "coats" that allow the lipoproteins to move through the watery environment of the blood. (Go back to Chapter 5 to get a feel for this again—recall that lipoproteins transport fat and cholesterol to cells.)
- **Fat accumulates in the liver and further disrupts liver function.** Without the protein coat, the fat and cholesterol droplets get "stuck" in the liver. This leads to fat accumulation in the liver, and eventually fatty liver and liver disease results, ultimately leading to death in many alcoholics.

Alcohol's Influence on Nutritional Status

Beyond alcohol's interference with liver function, this beverage also impacts nutritional status. Alcohol does this four ways:

1. **Ingestion:** When you drink alcohol, you most likely are not eating what you would have otherwise. This means you are "drinking" your calories rather than sitting down to a healthful meal. Also, alcohol can reduce your appetite. Thus, you may eat less food, particularly nutritious foods, such as fruits and vegetables.

    Most nutrients are impacted by reduced ingestion—protein, vitamins, and minerals.

2. **Absorption:** In the intestinal tract, alcohol reduces or impairs the absorption of many micronutrients. Those most impacted include thiamin, folate (alcohol

interferes with the conversion of folate to folic acid—the form the body uses), iron, and vitamin B_{12}. (The formation of Intrinsic Factor—made in the stomach—is interfered with by alcohol.)

3. **Metabolism:** Alcohol can actually alter the way a specific nutrient is handled or metabolized by the body. Several nutrients are "mishandled" because of alcohol, including vitamins D and A. (A healthy liver is needed for the proper metabolism of these vitamins.)

4. **Excretion:** Alcohol acts as a diuretic, which means it increases urine production. As a result, the kidneys are compromised in doing their job of filtering the blood. The result is an increased excretion of minerals zinc, potassium, calcium, and magnesium, along with folic acid.

Alcohol, Pregnancy and Birth Defects

As a general rule, women should avoid alcohol during pregnancy and breastfeeding. There is an association between consumption of alcohol during pregnancy, particularly during the first several weeks (often when a woman may not know she is pregnant) and fetal alcohol syndrome (FAS). Irreversible malformations of limbs and face and the central nervous system characterize this condition. Infants with FAS have higher mortality rates and behavioral and developmental problems their entire lives.

Empty Calories and Your Diet

It's a great time to bring up the concepts of **empty-calorie foods** and **nutrient dense foods**. Alcohol itself provides 7 calories per gram and no essential nutrients. (*Note:* Beer does contain small amounts of B vitamins and minerals, such as chromium, due to the brewing process. Red wine has bioactive compounds found in the skin of grapes that researchers have shown to have health benefits.) These calories then are "empty" in terms of overall contribution to your diet (see Figure 10.3 for calorie content of alcoholic beverages).

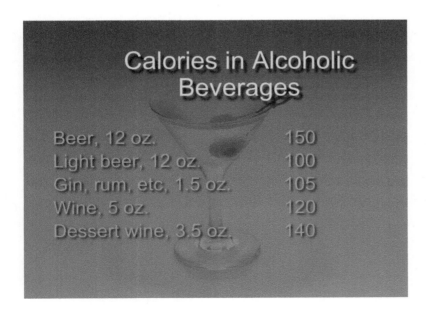

Calories in Alcoholic Beverages

Beer, 12 oz.	150
Light beer, 12 oz.	100
Gin, rum, etc, 1.5 oz.	105
Wine, 5 oz.	120
Dessert wine, 3.5 oz.	140

Figure 10.3

Empty-Calorie Food: This food (or beverage) provides little or nothing in the way of essential nutrients relative to the number of calories per serving.

Examples of empty-calorie foods include candy, chips, soda, and alcohol. Think back to your Diet Project and what you ate—what are a few empty-calorie foods in your diet? Consider the amount of empty-calorie foods you eat and what room is left for meeting your need for protein, fiber, and other essential nutrients. Figure 10.4 shows what most Americans consume in the way of empty calories.

Eating fewer empty calorie foods and replacing them with foods and beverages that have more to offer in the way of essential nutrients may make sense for you.

Nutrient-Dense Foods: These foods or beverages provide a good amount of one or more essential nutrients relative to the number of calories per serving. In Chapter 12, we address reducing the intake of added fats, sugars, and alcohol to improve health.

Examples of nutrient-dense foods include low-fat or non-fat dairy products, fruits, vegetables, and lean meats. Take a look at the three days you recorded your food intake as part of the Diet Project. Think about what nutrient-dense foods you currently eat and what nutrient-dense foods that you could also substitute for empty-calorie foods that you consume. For example, you could substitute a banana for a bag of chips with your lunch.

Health Benefits to Drinking?

Undoubtedly, you have heard that red wine or small amounts of alcohol may be "good" for you. The dangers of excessive alcohol consumption on health, such as disease and injury and including accidental death and suicide, outweigh possible health benefits. But it is worth noting that research studies do support moderate consumption (one or fewer drinks daily for women and two or fewer drinks for men) as beneficial for some individuals. Heart disease risk appears lower for those who drink moderately compared to abstainers. Compounds in red wine may have protective benefits for artery walls as well as keeping LDL from oxidizing. Also, alcohol helps raise HDL levels indirectly by impacting lipoprotein transport. Other studies show moderate consumers may have a lower incidence of Alzheimer's—an

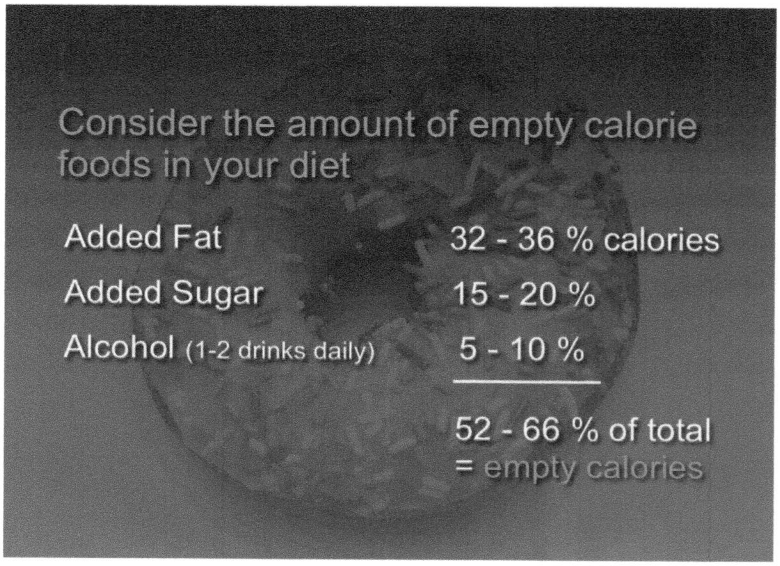

Consider the amount of empty calorie foods in your diet

Added Fat	32 - 36 % calories
Added Sugar	15 - 20 %
Alcohol (1-2 drinks daily)	5 - 10 %
	52 - 66 % of total = empty calories

Figure 10.4

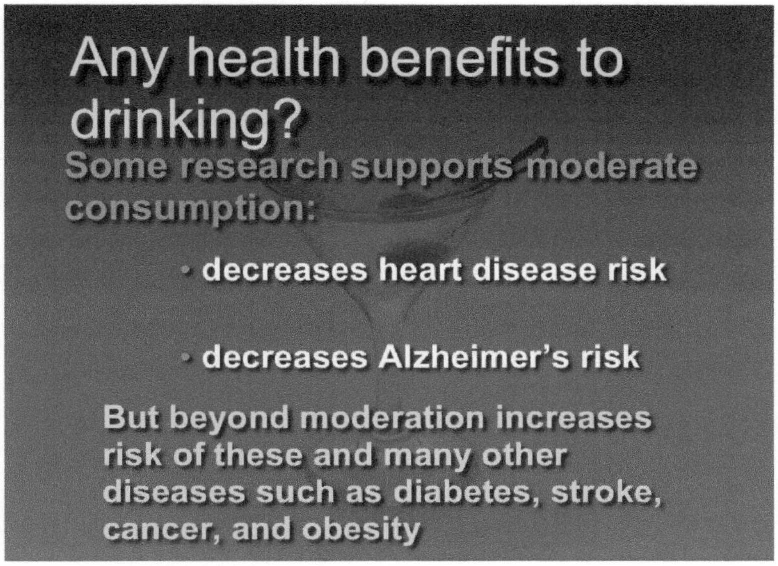

Figure 10.5

age-related disease resulting in decline of brain function. (See Appendix page 318 for more on alcohol, drink equivalents, and other important information about alcohol consumption from 2015 Dietary Guidelines.)

CHRONIC DISEASE—CANCER

In Chapter 6, we discussed the leading cause of death in the United States—heart disease. Cancer, another chronic, age-related disease, is a close number two on the list. Similar to heart disease, diet plays a major role in cancer risk (both increased and decreased). To get an understanding of cancer, let's take a look at its development on a cellular level. We'll use the development and progression of stomach cancer as our example.

- Cells in various organs and other tissues such as the stomach are constantly being replaced. A glitch can occur at some point when the genetic material called the DNA, which rests inside the nucleus of the cell, becomes altered or damaged. Referred to as **initiation** (shown in Figure 10.6), this alteration is caused by carcinogens (cancer-causing agents). Carcinogens can have dietary origins such as substances that form in food due to broiling or high-heat cooking. The cell now has a different or "bad" set of DNA, making it an altered cell that won't behave like a normal cell programmed now to make different proteins, use more nutrients or not "live" a normal life cycle of a cell.
- Given the right environment, this altered cell can grow (multiply) rapidly (shown in Figure 10.7)—referred to as **promotion**, this phase allows altered cells to quickly grow in numbers into cancer cells. High-fat diets and chronic alcohol consumption both act as cancer promoters to stomach cells.
- Once cancerous cells gain momentum, they take over an organ, such as the stomach by taking nutrients away from healthy cells, compromising that organ's ability to function normally. Additionally, the cancer cells can migrate through the circulation and spread to other parts of the body, referred to as **progression**. (See Figure 10.8.)

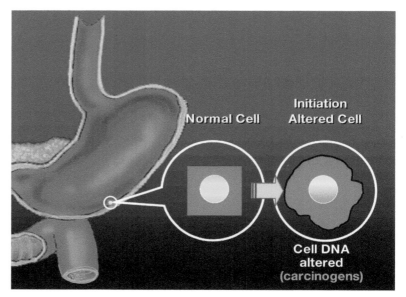

Figure 10.6

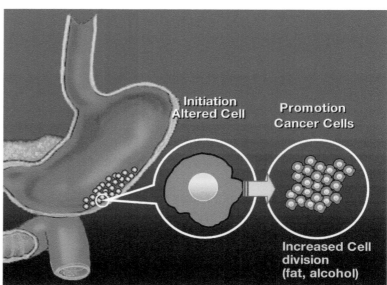

Figure 10.7

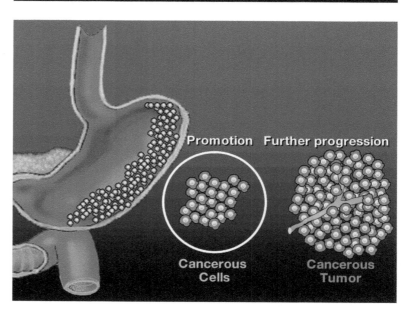

Figure 10.8

Role of Diet—Foods That Ward Off Cancer or That Increase Your Risk

The dietary link to cancer is very strong—research suggests that 30 to 60 percent of all cancers are preventable through diet modification. This diet-cancer prevention connection was demonstrated in a population research looking at prostate cancer risk in men from Japan and the United States. Prostate cancer risk is very low in Japan and researchers associate this with a traditional Eastern diet that includes several servings of soy foods weekly. When Japanese men move to the United States and adopt a Western diet (low soy food content, high in fat, low in fruits and vegetables), prostate cancer risk goes up and is comparable to American men of non-Japanese heritage. This suggests diet as a major factor rather than genetics.

Let's now take a look at specific factors in the diet that either increase or decrease cancer risk.

1. **Fat: ↑ risk**

   High-fat diets are linked to an increased risk of various cancers, such as cancer of the large intestine (colon), breast cancer, and prostate cancer. Fat-rich diets promote weight gain and obesity, which is a risk factor for cancer as excessive body fat levels promote cancer cell growth. Fat acts as a promoter and influences gene expression that in turn impacts cancer risk.

2. **Fiber: ↓ risk**

   A diet that is ample in whole grains, such as barley, whole wheat, and brown rice, along with fruits and vegetables, supplies plenty of fiber and is associated with a reduction of cancer risk, particularly of the large intestine. Fiber (recall from Chapter 4) helps speed the passage of waste, and this would in turn reduce the exposure time to potential carcinogens. Also, fiber bulks up the mass of material and dilutes carcinogens in the large intestine.

3. **Antioxidants (Vitamins C and E and beta-carotene) from foods: ↓ risk**

   A diet rich in these antioxidants found in fruits, vegetables (especially yellow-orange and green, leafy types), and whole grains (source of vitamin E) have been linked to a reduced cancer risk. These antioxidants are believed to protect cell membranes and cell nuclei from oxidative damage (caused by air pollution, cigarette smoke, etc.). This antioxidant protection helps ward off carcinogens and possible cancer initiation.

4. **Salt-cured, char-broiled, pickled, or smoked foods: ↑ risk**

   A diet that supplies these foods on a very regular basis (such as frequent or daily eating of barbeque meats, deli meats, and pickled foods) has been linked to increased cancer risk. These foods contain carcinogens. Char-broiled meats, for example, contain a carcinogen called heterocyclic amines or HAA for short (HAAs form when the protein in meat is burnt or cooked at high heat). Studies also show that diets high in red meats (beef primarily) are associated with cancer risk. You needn't worry though, if these foods are not a large part of your diet.

5. **Protective factors in food called phytochemicals: ↓ risk**

   Plants—like fruits, vegetables, and whole grains—contain an array of substances that protect the plant (a tomato growing on a vine, for example) from its environment—UV light, air pollution, insects, and microbes. These protective substances are called **phytochemicals** and when you eat a tomato, these substances go to work in you. Researchers have identified some 4,000 plus phytochemicals in fruits, vegetables, whole grains and other unsuspecting plant products, such as chocolate. Some phytochemicals actually block tumor growth; others halt or interfere with the initiation phase. Many of these phytochemicals have become popular for people to take as supplements. Isoflavones in soy foods, for example, are sold as supplements and people take them in hopes of reducing breast or prostate cancer risk. It's important to point out that research supports foods (soy foods) that supply isoflavones as cancer protection and not supplements. Researchers feel that isoflavones may interact with other items in food such as fiber or other nutrients to give the cancer protection benefit. Taking a supplement of isoflavones only gives you the one phytochemical, not the phytochemical in context with the whole food where the protection lies. Figure 10.9 shows some of the major phytochemical categories and food sources.

6. **Alcohol: ↑ risk**

   Studies show that drinking more than two alcoholic drinks per day increases cancer risk. Alcohol is a promoter and makes the environment more conducive for cancer cells to thrive. Adding smoking cigarettes to the "mix" with alcohol increases the risk for cancer exponentially. Smoke and substances in cigarettes are carcinogens. When combined, the two (cigarette smoking and drinking) become more dangerous than when alone.

7. **Mutagens: ↑ risk**

   Mutagens are substances that cause cells to mutate and more likely to turn into cancer cells. Some foods contain mutagens that are naturally present. Celery and mushrooms, for example, contain mutagens. However, these vegetables also supply protection against cancer with their phytochemical content. The cancer risk of naturally occurring mutagens is very low unless a person goes overboard and eats an excessive amount of a particular food (eating celery morning, noon, and night and drinking celery juice).

CAROTENOIDS	**FLAVONOIDS**	**ISOFLAVONES**	**INDOLES**
Red, orange, and deep green vegetables and fruits (cantaloupe, carrots, papaya) 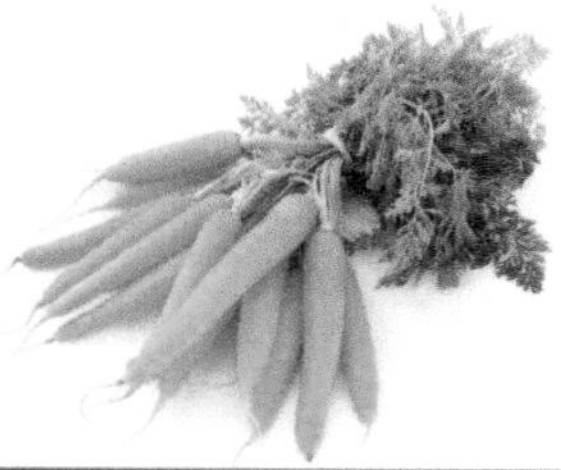	Deep red, blue, and purple vegetables and fruits (grapes, black tea, green tea, blueberries, soy products, whole wheat) 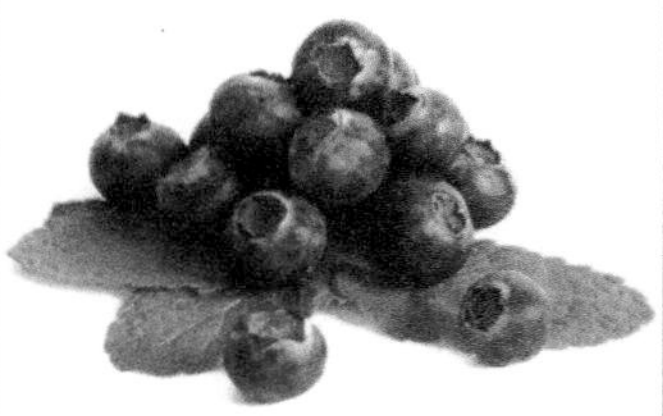	Soy and soy products, whole grains (tofu, soy milk, wheat berries) 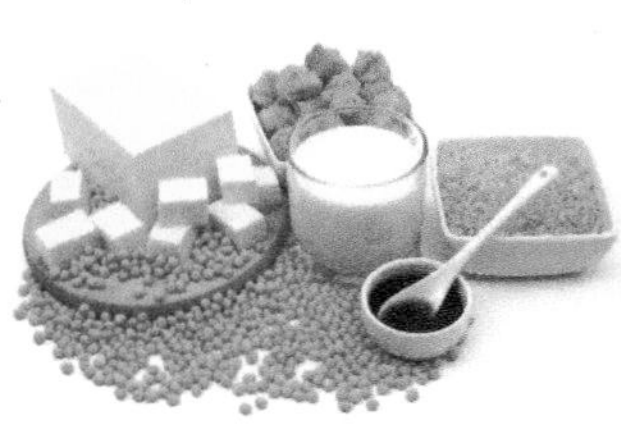	Cruciferous vegetables (garlic, leeks, onions, broccoli, cabbage, Brussels sprouts) 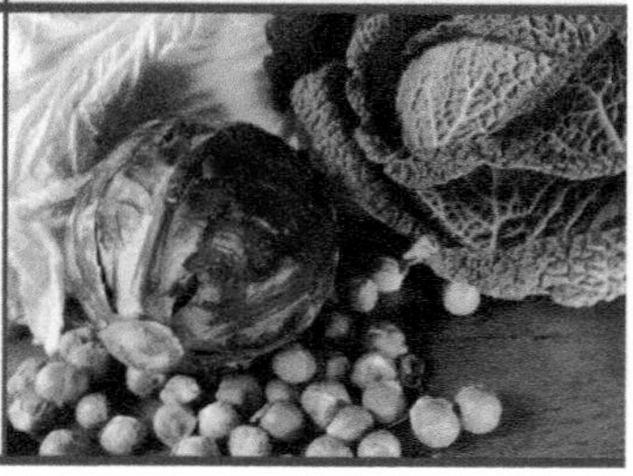

Figure 10.9

8. **Additives and pesticides: not a significant risk**

Some additives in foods do have carcinogenic potential, if consumed in large enough amounts. But the Food and Drug Administration strictly controls the use of additives and prohibits the use of those that represent a true cancer threat. Eating a varied diet helps lower even further this low risk from additives.

The same goes for pesticides that are used in traditional growing methods of fruits, vegetables, and whole grains. But this risk is very low. Since fruits, vegetables, and grains offer cancer-protection benefit, researchers feel that this very small risk is not worth worrying about.

Dietary Recommendations to Reduce Cancer Risk

After discussing these various factors that increase and decrease cancer risk, specific dietary recommendations can be made. These dietary recommendations are listed in Figure 10.10 and incorporate the major dietary components such as fat, fiber, fruits, vegetables, and other sources of protective factors that modify cancer risk.

After reviewing these, you should be prepared to tell a friend who is interested in lowering cancer risk what dietary modifications to make and why.

YOUR DIET, GENETICS AND HEALTH: NUTRIGENOMICS

By now, you have a good sense that what you eat impacts your health and risk for chronic diseases, such as cancer, heart disease, and diabetes. But, hypothetically, if your friend eats an identical diet to yours, his/her health and risks for the same chronic diseases would be different from yours. You, for example, may have a lower risk of developing type 2 diabetes while your friend may have a greater risk despite eating the same foods. Simply put, your genetics make a difference on how what you eat interacts with the expression of your genes. This is the study of a relatively new area or research called **nutrigenomics**—the interactions of genes and diet and the resulting affects on health and disease.

RECOMMENDATIONS TO REDUCE CANCER RISK

- Maintain a healthy body weight/avoid weight gain with age.
- Eat five or more servings of colorful fruits and vegetables daily.
- Choose whole grain over refined grains.
- Limit intake of salt-cured, smoked, and charbroiled foods, and reduce red meat intake.
- Consume alcoholic beverages in moderation.

Figure 10.10

Remember from Chapter 2 that the DNA is the genetic material that represents "instructions" for the body cells to make specific proteins. Each gene codes for a certain protein to be made or expressed. We each have about 25,000 different genes that are expressed (unique proteins that are made) and impact everything in your body from insulin action and lipoprotein transport (diabetes and heart disease) to fat storage and cell life span (obesity and cancer).

Over the past decade, nutrigenomic research studies have revealed that a person's diet—levels of fat, carbohydrate, and protein along with specific food components, such as plant pigments (e.g., lycopene in tomatoes) can act by turning "on" or "off" a gene expression. This, in turn, can impact health and/or the onset and progression of diseases. For example, studies show that some individuals produce greater levels of proteins (gene expression) involved in the inflammatory response. As described in Chapter 6, inflammation is central to the development of heart disease as well as other chronic ailments, such as Alzheimer's disease and periodontal disease. Dietary components, such as green tea and vitamin E from nuts, are known to reduce the production of pro-inflammaotry proteins, which in turn lessens the inflammatory process and disease risk.

The goal of nutrigenomic research is to identify gene expression involved in the disease process that is influenced by diet and determine an optimal diet, including specific foods that would optimize an individual's health. The notion of the "designer diet" is on the horizon. Health professionals already can genetically test for some diet-disease connections. The hope is that the process can be more complete and accessible so that we can each accurately determine what exact diet would be best for each of us based on our own genetics.

Quiz Yourself

10

CHAPTER

1. Define a nutrient-dense food.

   _____

   _____

   _____

2. List a food source for each of the following:

   • Empty-calorie food: _____

   • Nutrient-dense food: _____

3. The body's alcohol processing enzymes are found in the:

   a. stomach

   b. pancreas

   c. liver

   d. small intestine

4. Food additives are a major cause of cancer, producing effects greater than those associated with foods, which increase or decrease risk.

   a. true

   b. false

5. List the four ways alcohol impacts nutritional status and provide a nutrient affected for each.

   1. _____

   2. _____

   3. _____

   4. _____

6. What are phytochemicals? How do they help protect you from cancer?

   _____

   _____

   _____

7. Your friend is concerned about developing cancer and wants ways to lower their risk. Give five dietary recommendations to lower your friend's risk for cancer.

1. _____

2. _____

3. _____

4. _____

5. _____

NUTRITION AND ATHLETIC PERFORMANCE

As we wrap up our overview of introductory nutrition in these final chapters, applying what we've learned to certain groups of individuals helps solidify our new understanding of nutrition. In this chapter, we integrate and apply what we've learned about nutrition and its role in physical activity and performance. A person who participates in regular physical activity, which I refer to as an *athlete* (you don't have to compete to be an athlete!), has specific nutritional concerns. Undoubtedly, you've seen ads on the Internet or in magazines about special sports-related drinks, powders, and pills that claim to enhance athletic performance. Although many of these ads may be enticing, true nutritional issues for athletes focus more on the macronutrient needs (protein, carbohydrate, and fat) rather than special substances said to enhance performance. Certainly sport drinks and energy bars have their place in an athlete's diet, but a grasp of the basics goes a long way when setting up an eating plan for active people.

In this chapter, you will be pulling information from previous chapters and applying it to nutrition issues for athletes. From this, we develop practical recommendations about energy, carbohydrate, and protein needs, along with vitamins and minerals. Additionally, we also include issues regarding competition such as what to eat before exercise, what to eat after recovery, and how best to stay hydrated. With these topics and the additional sports nutrition articles in the Appendix, you may well find some practical dietary advice that will assist you in your efforts to stay healthy and fit.

Chapter Objectives

In this chapter, we will cover:

- Energy use during exercise—role of carbohydrate and fat
- Importance of carbohydrates for performance and recovery
- Water and sport drinks—what's best to drink and how much
- Performance-boosting aids—what works and what to avoid

ENERGY USE DURING EXERCISE— ROLE OF CARBOHYDRATE AND FAT

Determining an athlete's nutritional needs involves revisiting energy metabolism. In Chapter 5, we integrated energy metabolism of carbohydrate, protein, and fat. In this chapter, we'll take another look at energy metabolism, but in relationship to the impact of exercise. Think of the different types of physical activity you engage in— running, weight lifting, walking, bike riding, and kick boxing, to name a few. These activities

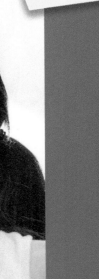

require differing efforts on your part and, in turn, require different proportions of carbohydrate and fat as fuel. Let's take a look at the energy expenditure for different types of exercise and then the types of fuel used during these activities.

Taking a look at the chart in Figure 11.1, you can see why an athlete requires more energy or calories per day than a person who is sedentary. Competitive athletes may need anywhere from 3,000 to over 5,000 calories daily compared to a typical inactive person who needs about 1,600 to 2,200 calories. Also notice that the weight-bearing exercises, such as running, burn more calories per hour than a non-weight-bearing activity. Moving your body against gravity requires more effort. In addition, men burn more calories than women for the same activity because they have more muscle mass and require more energy to support and move muscle than women who have a greater proportion of "inexpensive" fat tissue.

Fuel Sources

What are fuel sources in the body to support this activity? Recall from previous chapters that the energy nutrients are protein, carbohydrate, and fat. In your body, you can store both fat and carbohydrate but protein is not stored. Instead, body protein is functional tissue—serving a purpose. As review:

- **Carbohydrate:** Stored in the body as glycogen in the muscle and liver in limited quantities.
- **Fat:** Stored in virtually unlimited quantities throughout the body.
- **Protein:** Not stored in the body, but is functional tissue, such as muscles, organ protein, or enzymes (little of your energy needs come from protein—about 5 to 10 percent of total).

Inside a typical athlete, how much does all this represent in the way of calories? Since protein is not stored as energy and little is used as fuel, let's just look at stored carbohydrate and fat. Figure 11.2 shows the energy store of a fit, 70 kg (155 pound) man who has about 10 percent body fat. (Recall that 15 percent body fat is average or normal for a college-aged male.)

Energy expenditure during exercise (calories/hour)

	Male 170 lbs	Female 130 lbs
Bicycling (15 mph)	800	600
Running (8.5 min/mile)	925	700
Stair Climbing (machine med. effort)	485	370
Swimming (freestyle, moderate)	645	490
Walking (4 mph)	320	245

Figure 11.1

Body energy stores in 70 kg male (10% body fat)		
Body Fuel	Weight (kg)	Calories
Fat	7	63,000
Glycogen		
Liver	0.08-0.1	300-400
Muscle	0.3-0.4	1,200-1,600
Blood glucose	0.03	100

Figure 11.2

Fuel Use During Exercise

Let's go back to the integration of carbohydrate, fat, and protein energy metabolism to understand what fuel sources, and in what proportion they are used during various exercises. The diagram in Figure 11.3 (from Chapter 5) summarizes carbohydrate, fat, and protein energy metabolism. Since protein use for fuel is small, we'll ignore this for now. (However, protein fuel use can be an issue if glycogen stores have been depleted and no incoming carbohydrates are available—glucose must be made from protein to supply fuel for the brain.) This can occur during endurance exercise lasting more than a few hours.

What fuel sources are used during exercise, and under what conditions are certain fuels (specifically carbohydrate versus fat) preferred by the working muscles?

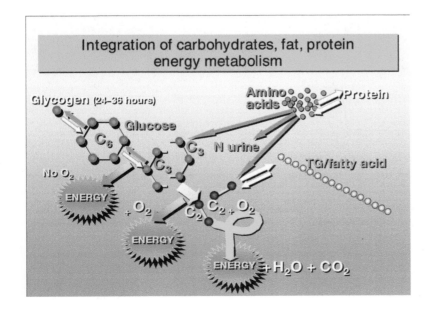

Figure 11.3

High-Intensity, Sprint Types of Activity

All muscle activity or work is driven or powered by a high-energy molecule called ATP. You have enough ATP in your muscles to last a few seconds for a burst of activity and then the ATP must be regenerated with the help of phosphocreatine. (More on creatine as a supplement to boost performance will be presented later in this chapter.) Even with this regeneration, you have less than 30 seconds worth of ATP. Your body then kicks into using glucose or C_6 anaerobically for fuel. Breaking down glucose without the presence of oxygen releases ATP (fuel) quickly and gives C_3 (see Figure 11.3).

Another name for this C_3 unit is lactic acid and if the amount of lactic acid produced exceeds what can be cleared by the muscle (and sent to the liver), the lactic acid accumulates. This along with an increasing acidity in the muscle contributes to fatigue during intense exercise (you know that "lead-like" feeling you may get as you do very intense exercise). This exclusive anaerobic use of glucose lasts up to about two minutes at which point the body can't keep up with the ATP demands and the lactic acid accumulation and must slow down to now use glucose and fat aerobically to regenerate ATP. (See Figure 11.4.)

Continuous, Endurance Types of Activity

For exercises lasting more than two minutes, aerobic use of both carbohydrate and fat occur. Glucose (C_6) is broken down completely to CO_2, H_2O, and energy (ATP) and fat is also broken down to these same end products. The amount or proportion of carbohydrate and fat used during exercise is dependent upon the intensity of that activity. The more intense exercise, such as hard running or an intense game of soccer, uses more energy per minute and a greater proportion of that energy is supplied by carbohydrate compared to less-intense exercises, such as walking or moderate cycling. During lower intensity exercises, less energy per minute is spent and a greater proportion of that fuel comes from fat. (See Figure 11.5.)

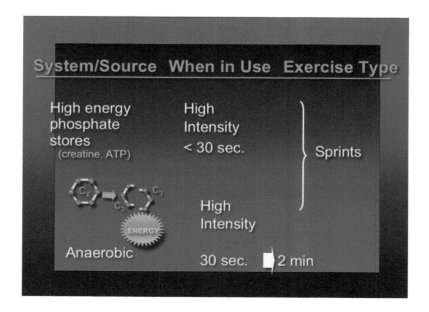

Figure 11.4

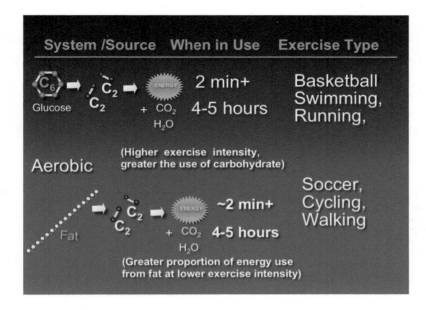

Figure 11.5

Figure 11.6 shows the use and site of fat and carbohydrate fuel stores. Fat (triglyceride) comes out of the fat cells as well as some triglyceride that is stored as small droplets in the muscle. Glycogen, which is stored in muscles, is used by that muscle for carbohydrate fuel.

What about "Fat-Burning" Exercises?

Perhaps you heard from a friend or on the Internet that certain exercises "burn" more body fat than others, so you'll lose more weight. Before you decide to buy into this idea, first let's go back—how is body fat lost? Recall from Chapter 7 on obesity and weight loss that calorie intake must be less than calorie output to lose body fat. You can do this by reducing the number of calories going in (what you eat), increasing the number going out (your activity), or a combination of both.

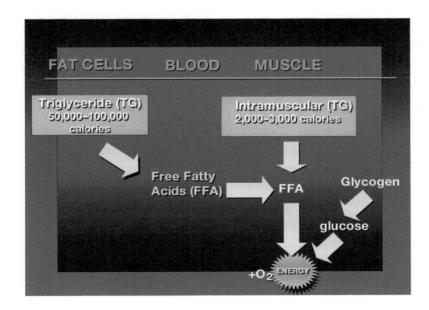

Figure 11.6

If you choose to boost your activity to lose weight, it actually makes no difference what you do in the way of activity—just do it! Burning calories by walking slowly or running fast both expend calories and ultimately, you will lose body fat if you end the day in a calorie deficit. Even though walking may burn proportionately more fat while fast running burns mostly carbohydrate and little fat, you readjust fuel burning during the rest of the day. Ultimately, creating a calorie deficit leads to fat loss as long as you don't compensate by filling in the energy gap by eating more food.

IMPORTANCE OF CARBOHYDRATES FOR PERFORMANCE AND RECOVERY

Now that we know the importance of both fat and carbohydrate as fuel sources during exercise, let's take a look at carbohydrates specifically since they are stored in limited amounts. As described above, a typical athlete stores approximately 2,000 calories of carbohydrate as glycogen in the muscles and liver. But fat is stored in a virtually "unlimited" supply. So, as you might expect, during continuous exercise, such as cycling or running (or a long game of soccer), glycogen stores are depleted, specifically in the muscles that do most of the work. This depletion of glycogen stores is illustrated in Figure 11.7.

Research studies have shown repeatedly that boosting glycogen stores through increasing dietary carbohydrate intake in turn raises glycogen stores and prolongs endurance. In short, if you increase the amount of carbs in your diet, you can run, cycle, swim, etc. for greater distances and longer times. Figure 11.8 illustrates results of scientific research and the relationship of dietary carbohydrate intake, muscle glycogen stores, and endurance performance.

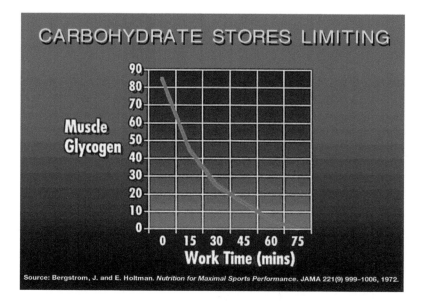

Figure 11.7

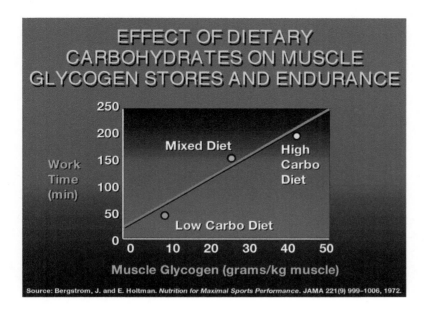

Figure 11.8

Researchers put a set of highly trained cyclists on a low-carbohydrate diet of about 40 percent carbohydrate calories (certainly not as low as an Atkins type diet). The cyclists ate this diet for several days and then showed up to the laboratory for testing. Their muscle glycogen levels (in calf muscle) were measured, and then they were asked to pedal at a set workload for as long as they could. The researchers noted that the cyclists could only pedal for 50 minutes. **Low carbs in the diet meant low glycogen levels and, in turn, poor endurance.**

The same cyclists were then put on another diet—about 55 percent of calories as carbohydrate for several days. The same muscle glycogen and endurance tests were performed. This time the cyclists had more glycogen in their calf muscles and could pedal 150 minutes at that same workload. **So more dietary carbohydrate and greater muscle glycogen stores meant better endurance.**

For a third time, the same cyclists were put through the test following a high-carbohydrate diet of 70 percent of the calories. Muscle glycogen stores were greater (but note not as dramatic an increase from the low to the medium carb diet, suggesting a limit to glycogen storage). The cyclists' endurance also improved, but as with muscle glycogen, not as dramatic an increase compared to the previous diet. But still, the relationship of increasing dietary carbohydrate, which increases muscle glycogen, and in turn endurance remains true.

From this research and countless other studies involving different types of athletes, exercise physiologists and sports nutrition professionals are able to make recommendations regarding carbohydrate intake for athletes (particularly endurance types). The Daily Value for carbohydrate is 300 grams (for a person eating a 2,000-calorie diet) and for athletes, 450 to 600 grams daily or about 50 to 65 percent of calories as carbohydrate is suggested. An athlete can also base his or her carbohydrate intake relative to body weight. Most athletes are recommended

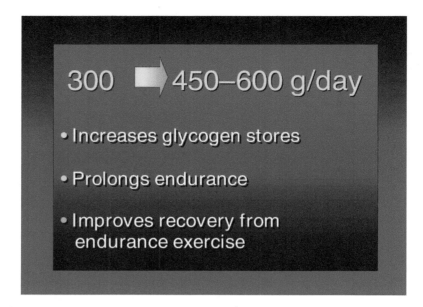

Figure 11.9

to consume between 3–10 g per kg body weight. This amount ensures recovery of glycogen stores following workouts so that another prolonged workout can be performed the next day.

Figure 11.9 summarizes the benefits of boosting carbohydrate intake for athletes.

So Where Does Protein and Fat Fit in the Diets of Athletes?

Recall from Chapter 2 that protein needs increase with exercise. This occurs for two reasons: (1) small amounts of protein are needed to repair damaged muscle proteins as a result of exercise (bumps and bruises along with tissue rebuilding following strength training exercise); and (2) the small amount of protein that is used as fuel during exercise can add up for an endurance-type athlete who is working out for a couple of hours or more daily. The amount of increase above the RDA of 0.8 grams/kg body per day is about 50 percent (or about 1.2 to 2.0 g/kg body weight daily). But this amount can easily be met through diet. Taking in about 15 percent of the total calories from protein from foods such as soy, fish, poultry, lean meats, low-fat dairy, and bean-grain combinations is recommended for athletes.

Fat is an important source of calories in an athlete's diet. Especially for those expending over 4,000 to 5,000 plus calories daily, a source of calorie-dense fat helps keep energy intake up because the sheer volume of food eaten becomes a challenge for some athletes. Healthful fats such as olive oil (in cooking or salads), avocados, nuts, and fish are good choices.

Figure 11.10 puts this all together in a recommended distribution of calories for athletes.

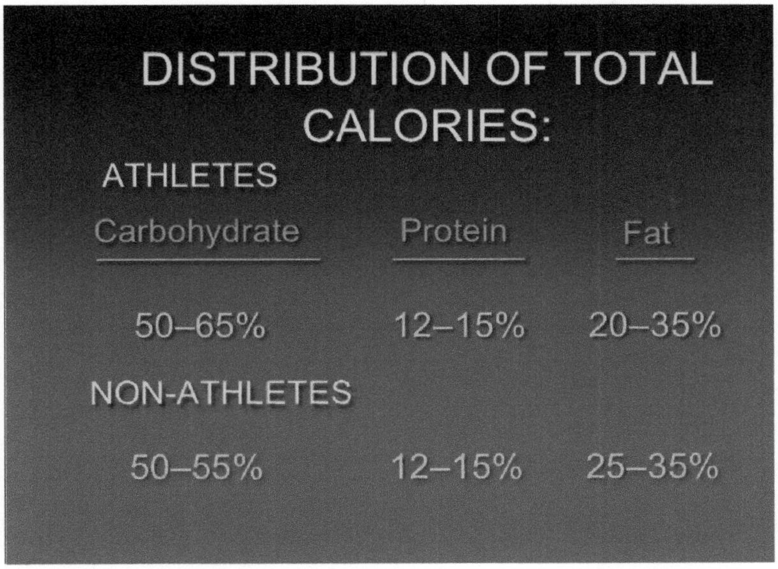

DISTRIBUTION OF TOTAL CALORIES:

ATHLETES		
Carbohydrate	Protein	Fat
50–65%	12–15%	20–35%
NON-ATHLETES		
50–55%	12–15%	25–35%

Figure 11.10

The following menu plans give you an idea of what an athletes (male and female) need to support 1 to 2 hours of daily training.

MALE ATHLETE

165 pounds
25 to 30 miles per week of running
2,800 calories daily

Day 1

Breakfast
2 hearty slices of whole wheat bread
   dipped in 1 egg, beaten
2 teaspoons trans-fat free margarine
3 tablespoons boysenberry syrup
1½ cups fresh fruit salad (apple, kiwi, banana)
1 cup fat-free milk

Snack
1 cup snap peas dipped in ½ cup plain,
   herb-seasoned yogurt

Lunch
Turkey wrap:
   1 whole wheat tortilla
   3 oz. roasted turkey slices
   ½ tomato, sliced
   1 tablespoon ranch dressing, low fat
   ½ cup shredded red cabbage
   1 oz. shredded jack cheese, reduced fat
1 cup vegetable juice
1 pear

Daily Amount of Food
From Each Group
2½ cups fruit
3½ cups vegetables
10 oz. equivalent grains
7 oz. equivalent meats/bean
3 cups dairy
3 teaspoons oil
462 discretionary calories
from added sugars and
additional fat

Snack
½ cup trail mix
8 oz. sports drink

Dinner
4 oz. grilled salmon topped with
   ½ cup mango salsa
1 cup mashed sweet potato
2 cups leafy greens with
   2 tablespoons olive oil dressing
Milkshake:
   1 cup low fat ice cream (8)
   ⅓ cup fat-free milk
   2 tablespoons chocolate syrup

FEMALE ATHLETE

130 pounds
25 to 30 miles per week of running
2,200 calories daily

Day 1

Breakfast
Buckwheat-blueberry pancakes
   3×3″ (½ cup blueberries)
2 tablespoons maple syrup
2 teaspoons soft margarine
2 tablespoons chopped almonds
½ cup diced apples with cinnamon
1 cup low-fat soy milk

Lunch
Lentil tomato chicken soup
1¼ canned lentil soup
½ cup canned diced tomatoes
2 oz. diced, cooked chicken
1 whole wheat roll
¾ cup radishes and snap peas
1 cup fat-free milk

Snack
1 small banana
8 oz. vegetable juice
1 oz. whole wheat pretzels

Dinner
1 low-fat frozen spinach lasagna
   1 cup noodles
   ½ cup ricotta cheese
   1 oz. mozzarella cheese
   ¾ cup cooked spinach
2 cups Romaine lettuce with:
   ½ cup tomato and cucumber slices
   2 tablespoons olive oil vinaigrette
1 oz. whole wheat sourdough bread
1 unsweetened beverage
½ cup ice cream with:
   2 tablespoons chocolate syrup
   1 cup strawberries

**Daily Amount of Food
From Each Group**
2 cups fruit
3 cups vegetables
7 oz. equivalent grains
6 oz. equivalent meats/bean
3 cups milk
6 teaspoons oil
290 discretionary calories
from added sugars and
additional fat

WATER AND SPORTS DRINKS—WHAT'S BEST TO DRINK AND HOW MUCH

As you probably know from personal experience, your fluid needs increase with exercise. How you meet that need, through drinking plain water, sport drinks, or other beverages such as soda, fruit juice, or fitness water, is often hotly debated. Let's first look at why fluid needs increase and then how best to meet that need.

Water is an absolutely essential nutrient and even more so for athletes:

- As you exercise, your muscles generate heat—recall that you burn some 100 calories for every mile of running—and this heat must be dissipated or you would literally "cook" your muscles and other proteins in the body. The body rids itself of this heat by releasing water onto the surface of the skin as sweat. As this sweat evaporates, the heat is "taken away." On average, you lose about a liter of water as sweat for every hour of continuous exercise. Evaporation of this liter takes away about 600 calories of heat.
- Water is also the medium that makes up the blood, which transports oxygen, carbohydrates, and other nutrients to hard-working muscles.
- With exercise, waste products are produced that must be transported out of cells via the circulation and excreted through the lungs (CO_2) or urine (metabolic waste). Again, we rely on body water to carry out this process.

As the body loses water due to sweating, several changes take place:

- A reduction of cardiac output (volume the heart pumps) as blood volume drops
- Drop in blood flow to the muscles and skin surface
- Reduction in sweat rate

With this loss of body water and compromise to several body systems, comes symptoms and consequences of **dehydration**, the loss of body fluids.

Some signs and consequences of dehydration due to sweating are heat accumulation in the body—you feel nauseous, fatigued, and experience loss of appetite; with declining cardiac function and increasing body temperature, performance is decreased; and you may feel flushed, light-headed, and suffer from muscle cramps.

Fluid replacement is key before, during, and after exercise to avoid dehydration and its consequences. Here are some fluid replacement guidelines:

- Drink about 2 cups of fluid prior to exercise (2–4 ml/lb of body weight)
- Drink ¼ cup to ¾ cup every 15 to 20 minutes during exercise. You may need less if you are exercising in a cooler climate or have a low sweat rate.
- Avoid sweat losses that exceed 2% of body weight (about 3 lbs or 48 oz. sweat loss for a 150-lb runner)

Nutrition Bite

Sweat rates are greater in endurance-trained athletes—marathon runners have been known to lose over 2½ liters of sweat per hour!

What's Best to Drink?

Water? Sports drink? Or what about the new fitness waters? Athletes must consider the amount of time they are working out and the intensity of that exercise to make a decision about what's best to drink. Carbohydrate stores become limiting after about 90 minutes to over two hours of continuous exercise. Low blood sugar levels, which result when liver glycogen stores run low, also become a limitation to performance. As just described, dehydration limits performance as well. Thus, during continuous exercise lasting about 90 minutes or more, taking in a source of both carbohydrate and water makes sense.

Research shows that sports drinks help replenish lost fluids and provide carbohydrate to prolong endurance. Most sports drinks consist of a carbohydrate source such as sucrose, glucose, or maltodextrin (a small complex carbohydrate) dissolved in water at the concentration of about 6 to 9 percent by weight (carbohydrate). This amount of carbohydrate allows for fluid absorption in the intestine while at the same time providing energy for exercising muscles. A higher concentration of carbohydrate would slow fluid absorption (as in fruit juices, energy drinks, fruit drinks, and sodas) and may cause sloshing in the stomach or even nausea if consumed during exercise. Most sports drinks also supply small amounts of minerals (electrolytes) that help replenish what's lost in sweat and assist in maintaining fluid balance and muscle contraction and encourage further drinking. Figure 11.11 lists some popular sports drinks.

During exercise, aim for replenishing lost fluids and carbohydrates by:

- Drinking ¼ to ¾ cup every 15 to 20 minutes
- Consuming 30 to 60 grams of carbohydrate every hour of continuous exercise (about 100 calories of carbohydrate per hour for exercise lasting 1–3 hours)
- Besides sport drink, also eating solid carbohydrate sources such as fruit, dried fruit, carbohydrate gels or chews (sold in grocery stores, sporting good stores, and online), or energy bars (check the label for carbohydrate content).
- Avoiding food with fat and protein because these are slow to digest and may cause stomach upset (additionally, fat and protein are not fuel sources in limiting supply during exercise). Some sport drinks contain protein, which a limited amount of research suggests certain amino acids may help delay fatigue during endurance exercises. See Figure 11.12 for a sample of what to eat and drink during a marathon run.

Urban Myth

Myth: "Eating a banana cures muscle cramps that occur during exercise."

Muscle cramping occurs for a variety of reasons, including overuse of the muscle (calf or thigh during running for example), dehydration as well as some individuals seem more prone to developing cramps during a long workout. Potassium (of which bananas are a good source) while an important electrolyte for fluid balance, does not cure cramping. Stopping your exercise, drinking fluids, and resting should alleviate the problem along with making sure you are well hydrated before exercise and are not restricting sodium.

COMPARING SPORTS DRINKS
(per 8-ounce serving)

	Calories	Protein (g)	Carbohydrate (g)	Fat (g)
Accelerade	80	9	15	0
Cytomax	50	0	13	0
Gatorade	50	0	14	0
Clif Quench	45	0	11	0
Powerade	50	0	14	0

Sports drinks are solution of 6–9% carbohydrate (glucose, fructose, sucrose, maltodextrins)

Figure 11.11

CARBOHYDRATE FEEDING SCHEDULE FOR A PROLONGED ENDURANCE EVENT

Mile 6	8 oz. sports drink
Mile 12	Carbohydrate gel
Mile 15	Apple slice, 8 oz. sports drink
Mile 17	Carbohydrate gel
Mile 21	8 oz. sports drink
Total CHO:	115 grams

Figure 11.12

What to Eat Before Exercise

While we're discussing how best to keep your body hydrated, you also may be curious about what's best to eat before a workout. Many athletes skip eating before they head off to a long practice or run several miles. Not a good decision. Your muscles are in need of carbohydrate energy, and your brain is also dependent upon glucose for fuel. Eating a few hours before you exercise helps to keep energy levels up and boosts your endurance. Here are some guidelines for pre-workout eating:

- Eat one to fours hours before you work out or compete. (Especially after a night's sleep, your body needs fuel.)
- Eat food high in carbohydrate—about 100 to 200 grams depending upon your body size and level of exercise (1–4 g carbohydrate/kg body weight one to four hours pre-exercise).
- Choose food with a moderate amount of protein and low in fat. (These slow digestion, but some is OK.)

Example meal: Two slices whole wheat bread spread with jam and peanut butter, one banana, and a cup of soymilk or low-fat milk.

What to Eat After Exercise

Following a workout, your body needs fuel and nutrients to recover and rebuild. Glycogen stores must be replaced, especially if you plan to workout the next day. Additionally, protein synthesis in the muscle steps up as muscle repair and new muscle proteins are built. Research studies show that refueling within thirty minutes to two hours following exercise optimizes recovery rather than waiting several hours to eat. Here are guidelines for post-workout eating:

- Eat a meal thirty minutes to two hours following exercise that lasts sixty minutes or more.
- Replace fluids lost as sweat—approximately 16 to 20 ounces of water or sports drink for every pound lost in sweat.

- Consume 0.7 gram carbohydrate/lb. of body weight during first two hours post-workout.
- Consume 20 to 25 grams of protein.
- Include foods that supply vitamins, electrolytes, and antioxidants (fruits, vegetables, whole grains).

PERFORMANCE BOOSTING AIDS—WHAT WORKS AND WHAT TO AVOID

Athletes strive for their best whether that's running fast, scoring goals, or making a quick tackle. Beyond staying hydrated, eating ample carbohydrates, and in general consuming a healthful diet, athletes often turn to supplements that claim to enhance performance. These aids, sometimes called ergogenic aids, which means work-enhancing aids, are available online, in grocery stores, and at sport shops. Recall from our discussion of dietary supplements in Chapter 9, the FDA regulation of these products are minimal and that claims made are for the most part, not substantiated. Here's a brief list of a few ergogenic aids:

Amino acids	Carnitine	Phosphate
Baking soda	Creatine	RNA/DNA
Bee pollen	Ginseng	Spirulina
Caffeine	Inosine	HGH (human growth hormone)

You now know that just because a supplement is sold, doesn't mean that it works or comes through on its claims. Many of these fall short on their performance claims, but a few have been shown through well-controlled scientific research to enhance performance. So how are you to know when you come across a potential supplement whether or not it lives up to its claims?

Here are some guidelines when evaluating a supplement:

- **Does the performance claim make sense?** That is, would it make sense for your body to adjust itself based on taking this substance or mixture? Remember homeostasis and the body's drive to stay constant internally.
- **What is the supporting evidence for the performance claim?** What supports the performance claim? Is it testimonials from athletes or scientific studies?
- **What is the consequence of taking the performance aid?** Are there any safety issues or concerns about the substance's legality (caffeine and other stimulants for example are banned in college and international competition).

When evaluating information online or in printed literature, it's important to determine the credibility of the source. Often manufacturers may give a "science-like" look to their product information when actually it is written by the supplement makers, and is not supported by unbiased scientific research.

Refer to the Office of Dietary Supplements from the National Institutes of Health for information about specific performance-enhancing aids. (See page 515 in Appendix.)

Quiz Yourself

1. During prolonged exercise body stores of _____ are depleted. These stores can be increased through a high dietary intake of _____ . (Choose the best combination.)

   a. protein / protein

   b. glycogen / protein or carbohydrate

   c. fat / carbohydrate

   d. glycogen / fat

   e. glycogen / carbohydrate

2. An athlete training daily and expending large amounts of energy should consume _____ grams of carbohydrate daily or approximately _____ of total calories. (Choose the best combination.)

   a. 100 grams / 40 percent

   b. 450 grams plus / 60 percent

   c. 200 grams / 45 percent

   d. 500 grams / $<$ 30 percent

3. Concerning fuel utilization, fats:

   a. are the main fuel for muscles while at rest and during light activity

   b. supply most of the energy for the brain

   c. supply most of the energy for high-intensity exercise

   d. provide more energy (calories) than an equal weight of carbohydrate

   e. both a and d

4. List two nutrients required/needed in greater amounts by athletes and why.

   1. _____   Why _____

   _____

   2. _____   Why _____

   _____

5. What is dehydration and why are athletes at increased risk for developing dehydration?

   _____

   _____

   _____

6. Dietary supplements sold to enhance athletic performance are tightly regulated by the FDA.

   a. true

   b. false

7. Give and example of a pre-exercise meal.

   _____

   _____

   _____

PULLING IT ALL TOGETHER—DIETARY GUIDELINES FOR AMERICANS AND FOOD LABELING

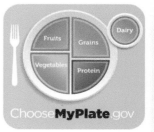

Choose **MyPlate**.gov

Take a moment and think about all that you have learned—from proteins, carbohydrates, and fats; to minerals, vitamins, and supplements; and obesity, cancer, and athletic performance. Immersing yourself in nutrition during this course has given you the knowledge to take charge of your health today and for a lifetime. In this chapter, we will pull together the concepts, principles, and facts from the previous eleven chapters and summarize them into guidelines for a healthy lifestyle. You can compare your food choices from the Diet Project you completed to the recommendations made here regarding optimal diet and health.

As you read this last chapter, think beyond the scope of this class and how the information you have learned can be incorporated into your daily life for better health.

DIETARY GUIDELINES—PRINCIPLES FOR HEALTHY EATING AND PHYSICAL ACTIVITY

The government, specifically the U.S. Department of Agriculture and Department of Health and Human Services, takes responsibility for making recommendations regarding diet and health. Every five years, these groups jointly issue a set of guidelines called the Dietary Guidelines for Americans 2015–2020.

Chapter Objectives

In this chapter, we will cover:
- Dietary Guidelines for Americans— principles for healthy eating patterns and physical activity
- MyPlate food guide.
- Using food labels for choosing an optimal diet

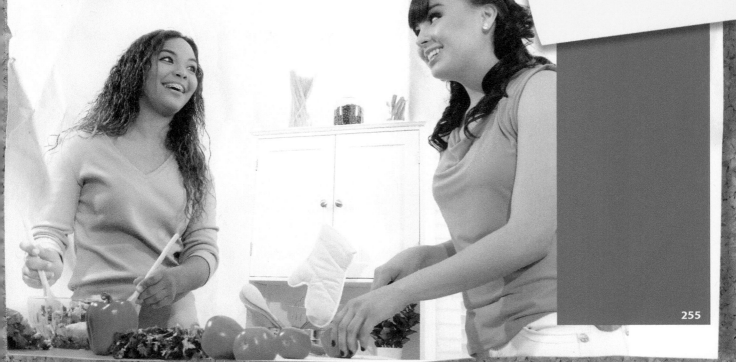

You can find in the Appendix (page 459) the "2015–2020 Dietary Guidelines Executive Summary" (http://health.gov/dietaryguidelines/2015/), along with a consumer summary (page 505). The Dietary Guidelines (DG) are key recommendations in the context of eating and physical activity patterns designed to promote overall health and a healthy body weight, as well as to reduce risk for chronic diseases related to diet and activity patterns. The DG 2015–2020 make a departure from the DG of 2010 and earlier by recognizing that healthy eating and activity patterns are not a rigid prescription of "eat this, not that" or "exercise this way but not that way." Instead, the current DG represent an adaptable framework in which people can select foods and activities they enjoy that fit in the context of cultural and social preferences.

The DG represent five simple Guidelines:

1. **Follow a healthy eating pattern across the lifespan.** All food and beverage choices matter. Choose a healthy eating pattern at an appropriate calorie level to help achieve and maintain a healthy body weight, support nutrient adequacy, and reduce the risk of chronic disease.

2. **Focus on variety, nutrient density, and amount.** To meet nutrient needs within calorie limits, choose a variety of nutrient-dense foods across and within all food groups in recommended amounts.

3. **Limit calories from added sugars and saturated fats and reduce sodium intake.** Consume an eating pattern low in added sugars, saturated fats, and sodium. Cut back on foods and beverages higher in these components to amounts that fit within healthy eating patterns.

4. **Shift to healthier food and beverage choices.** Choose nutrient-dense foods and beverages across and within all food groups in place of less healthy choices. Consider cultural and personal preferences to make these shifts easier to accomplish and maintain.

5. **Support healthy eating patterns for all.** Everyone has a role in helping to create and support healthy eating patterns in multiple settings nationwide; this includes at home, school, and work, and in communities.

We expand on these five Guidelines in this chapter and how you can follow them in your everyday food choices and physical activities.

The 2015–2020 DG were developed using a rigorous evaluation of the scientific evidence, which addresses a large number of specific diet and health related questions. Researchers as well as health and nutrition experts synthesized the evidence into specific recommendations. There is a requirement to update the Dietary Guidelines every five years to reflect current scientific and medical knowledge. A new set of updated Guidelines will be issued in the latter part of the year 2020. You can learn more about the process here:

http://health.gov/dietaryguidelines/2015/guidelines/introduction/
developing-the-dietary-guidelines-for-americans/

The DG are designed primarily to assist policymakers and health professionals in setting federal food, nutrition, and health programs, such as the National School Lunch Program and the School Breakfast Program. Thus, it is not expected that the public will wade through the details of the DG, but instead the DG have been translated into the MyPlate Food Guide (Figure 12.1 and page 505) and the Nutrition Facts Panel (page 278), which we have explored throughout the course.

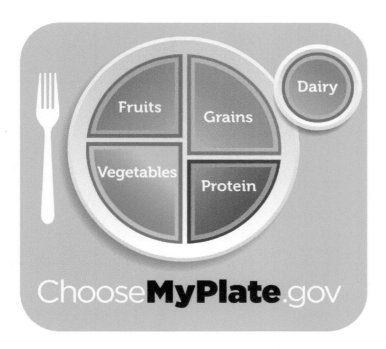

Figure 12.1

MyPlate is a Federal symbol that serves as a reminder to build healthy eating patterns by making healthy choices across the food groups. For more information about Dietary Guidelines implementation for the public MyPlate.gov

Before we get into each of the five Guidelines, let's look at three key rationales behind the DG. Keep each of these three rationales in mind as you think about the five Guidelines (and be prepared to write about this in the chapter quiz).

1. **Maintain a Healthy Weight**—Following the DG will encourage healthy body weight maintenance (as identified by BMI), curb adult weight gain, and prevent obesity.
2. **Promotion of Overall Health**—Following the DG will foster better health in the present by securing healthy eating patterns that meet needs for essential nutrients, prevent deficiency diseases, and promote optimal health.
3. **Prevention of Diet-related Chronic Diseases**—Following the DG will aid in lowering risks for a host of diet and inactivity-related ailments, including heart disease, diabetes, cancer, and osteoporosis. Figure 12.2 details the current prevalence of diet- and activity-related chronic diseases.

UNDERSTANDING THE DIETARY GUIDELINES

The DG uses a handful of terms throughout that must be defined here for better understanding of the DG's principles:

- Eating pattern—The combination of foods and beverages that constitute an individual's complete dietary intake over time. Often referred to as a "dietary pattern," an eating pattern may describe a customary way of eating or a combination of foods recommended for consumption. A specific example includes USDA Food Patterns.

Overweight and Obesity

- Currently over two-thirds of the population are overweight or obese.
- About one in three youths ages 2 to 19 years are overweight or obese.

Cardiovascular Disease

- 84 million Americans—35% of the population—have cardiovascular disease.
- 53% of the U.S. adult population (> age 20) has high total blood cholesterol (>200 mg/dl.).
- 8% of children ages 8 to 17 years have high total cholesterol levels.

Hypertension

- 29% of U.S. adults have hypertension.
- 27% of American adults have pre-hypertension—blood pressure numbers that are higher than normal, but not yet in the hypertension range.

Diabetes

- Approximately 14% of the population—ages 20 years and older have diabetes (Type 1 and Type 2) with nearly 90% of those having Type 2 diabetes.
- In children with type 2 diabetes, about 80% are obese.

Cancer

- Almost one in two men and women—approximately 41% of the population—will be diagnosed with cancer during their lifetime.
- Colon, breast, and prostate cancers (common cancer types in women and men) are related to diet and activity patterns.

Osteoporosis

- One out of every two women and one in four men ages 50 years and older will have an osteoporosis-related fracture in their lifetimes.
- About 85 to 90% of adult bone mass is acquired by the age of 18 in girls and the age of 20 in boys. Adequate nutrition and regular participation in physical activity are important factors in achieving and maintaining optimal bone mass.

Figure 12.2

- **Nutrient dense**—A characteristic of foods and beverages that provide vitamins, minerals, and other substances that contribute to adequate nutrient intakes. They may have positive health effects, with little or no solid fats and added sugars, refined starches, or sodium. Ideally, these foods and beverages also are in forms that retain naturally occurring components, such as dietary fiber. Nutrient-dense foods include all vegetables, fruits, whole grains, seafood, eggs, beans and peas, unsalted nuts and seeds, fat-free and low-fat dairy products, and lean meats and poultry—when prepared with little or no added solid fats, sugars, refined starches, and sodium. These foods contribute to meeting food group recommendations within calorie and sodium limits. The term "nutrient dense" indicates the nutrients and other beneficial substances in a food have not been "diluted" by the addition of calories from added solid fats, sugars, or refined starches, or by the solid fats naturally present in the food.

- **Variety**—A diverse assortment of foods and beverages across and within all food groups and subgroups selected to fulfill the recommended amounts without exceeding the limits for calories and other dietary components. For example, in the vegetables food group, selecting a variety of foods could be accomplished over the course of a week by choosing from all subgroups; this could include dark green, red, and orange vegetables, legumes (beans and peas), and starchy and other vegetables.

BASICS OF HEALTHY EATING AND PHYSICAL ACTIVITY PATTERNS

Let's take a closer look at Guidelines 1, 2, and 3:

1. **Follow a healthy eating pattern across the lifespan. All food and beverage choices matter. Choose a healthy eating pattern at an appropriate calorie level to help achieve and maintain a healthy body weight, support nutrient adequacy, and reduce the risk of chronic disease.**

2. **Focus on variety, nutrient density, and amount. To meet nutrient needs within calorie limits, choose a variety of nutrient-dense foods across and within all food groups in recommended amounts.**

3. **Limit calories from added sugars and saturated fats and reduce sodium intake. Consume an eating pattern low in added sugars, saturated fats, and sodium. Cut back on foods and beverages higher in these components to amounts that fit within healthy eating patterns.**

These three Guidelines emphasize healthy eating and activity patterns that balance with calorie intake to achieve a healthy weight throughout the lifespan.

A healthy eating pattern includes:

- A variety of vegetables from all of the subgroups—dark green, red and orange; legumes (beans and peas), starchy, and other
- Fruits, especially whole fruits
- Grains, at least half of which are whole grains
- Fat-free or low-fat dairy, including milk, yogurt, cheese, and/or fortified soy beverages
- A variety of protein foods, including seafood, lean meats and poultry, eggs, legumes (beans and peas), and nuts, seeds, and soy products
- Oils

At the same time, a healthy eating pattern limits certain components of foods and beverages:

- Saturated fats and *trans* fats, added sugars, and sodium.

The DG go further to recommend limits for the above as well as for alcohol. As we learned in Chapters 5 and 10, the intake of certain fats, sodium, and alcohol are of public health concern and can be linked with chronic diseases. Also, limiting added sugar intake is a must so that individuals can meet food group and nutrient needs for a given calorie intake.

PHYSICAL ACTIVITY GUIDELINES FOR AMERICANS RECOMMENDATIONS

Age	Recommendations
6 to 17 years	Children and adolescents should do 60 minutes (1 hour) or more of physical activity daily. • *Aerobic:* Most of the 60 or more minutes a day should be either moderate[a] or vigorous-intensity[b] aerobic physical activity, and should include vigorous-intensity physical activity at least 3 days a week. • *Muscle-strengthening:*[c] As part of their 60 or more minutes of daily physical activity, children and adolescents should include muscle-strengthening physical activity on at least 3 days of the week. • *Bone-strengthening:*[d] As part of their 60 or more minutes of daily physical activity, children and adolescents should include bone-strengthening physical activity on at least 3 days of the week. • It is important to encourage young people to participate in physical activities that are appropriate for their age, that are enjoyable, and that offer variety.
18 to 64 years	• All adults should avoid inactivity. Some physical activity is better than none, and adults who participate in any amount of physical activity gain some health benefits. • For substantial health benefits, adults should do at least 150 minutes (2 hours and 30 minutes) a week of moderate-intensity, or 75 minutes (1 hour and 15 minutes) a week of vigorous-intensity aerobic physical activity, or an equivalent combination of moderate- and vigorous-intensity aerobic activity. Aerobic activity should be performed in episodes of at least 10 minutes, and preferably, it should be spread throughout the week. • For additional and more extensive health benefits, adults should increase their aerobic physical activity to 300 minutes (5 hours) a week of moderate-intensity, or 150 minutes a week of vigorous-intensity aerobic physical activity, or an equivalent combination of moderate- and vigorous-intensity activity. Additional health benefits are gained by engaging in physical activity beyond this amount. • Adults should also include muscle-strengthening activities that involve all major muscle groups on 2 or more days a week.
65 years and older	• Older adults should follow the adult guidelines. When older adults cannot meet the adult guidelines, they should be as physically active as their abilities and conditions will allow. • Older adults should do exercises that maintain or improve balance if they are at risk of falling. • Older adults should determine their level of effort for physical activity relative to their level of fitness. • Older adults with chronic conditions should understand whether and how their conditions affect their ability to do regular physical activity safely.

[a] **Moderate-intensity physical activity:** Aerobic activity that increases a person's heart rate and breathing to some extent. On a scale relative to a person's capacity, moderate-intensity activity is usually a 5 or 6 on a 0 to 10 scale. Brisk walking, dancing, swimming, or bicycling on a level terrain are examples.
[b] **Vigorous-intensity physical activity:** Aerobic activity that greatly increases a person's heart rate and breathing. On a scale relative to a person's capacity, vigorous-intensity activity is usually a 7 or 8 on a 0 to 10 scale. Jogging, singles tennis, swimming continuous laps, or bicycling uphill are examples.
[c] **Muscle-strengthening activity:** Physical activity, including exercise that increases skeletal muscle strength, power, endurance, and mass. It includes strength training, resistance training, and muscular strength and endurance exercises.
[d] **Bone-strengthening activity:** Physical activity that produces an impact or tension force on bones, which promotes bone growth and strength. Running, jumping rope, and lifting weights are examples.

Source: Adapted from U.S. Department of Health and Human Services. *2008 Physical Activity Guidelines for Americans.* Washington (DC): U.S. Department of Health and Human Services; 2008. Available at http://www.health.gov/paguidelines. Accessed August 6, 2015.

Figure 12.3

- Consume less than 10% of calories per day from added sugars
- Consume less than 10% of calories per day from saturated fats
- Consume less than 2,300 milligrams (mg) per day of sodium
- If alcohol is consumed, it should be consumed in moderation—up to one drink per day for women and up to two drinks per day for men—and only by adults of legal drinking age

In addition to consuming a healthy eating pattern, all individuals in the U.S. should engage in regular physical activity. As noted in Chapter 7, the rates of obesity and overweight have steadily and alarmingly increased over the past decades in part due to a much lower level of physical activity. The following Physical Activity Guidelines for Americans from the U.S. Department of Health and Human Services provides types and prescribed amounts of physical activity needed each day for optimal health and healthy weight. Selecting a variety of enjoyable activities is encouraged; and a variety of online resources, including handouts and tracking device information, are available from:

www.healthfinder.gov

In summary, the goals for physical activity are:

- Adults need at least 150 minutes of moderate-intensity physical activity and should perform muscle-strengthening exercises on 2 or more days each week.
- Youths ages 6 to 17 years need at least 60 minutes of physical activity per day, including aerobic, muscle-strengthening, and bone-strengthening activities.

WHAT DOES A HEALTHY EATING PATTERN LOOK LIKE?

Determining what a healthy eating pattern may look like for you depends upon your calorie needs, which as we learned in Chapter 3 vary based upon age, sex, and physical activity level.

As you can see in Figure 12.4, calorie needs can vary dramatically based upon activity level for a given age, such as over 1,000 calories daily for an active teen male compared to his sedentary counterpart.

For simplicity, we will consider describing here a healthy eating pattern for a diet of 2,000 calories that meets the DG as well as the RDA for essential nutrients and the recommended distribution of calories from the macronutrients that we have covered in previous chapters. The Healthy U.S.-Style Healthy Eating Pattern shown in Figure 12.5 is for a 2,000-calorie diet, but you can retrieve 12 different calorie levels from *http://health.gov/dietaryguidelines/2015/guidelines/appendix-3/*

ESTIMATED CALORIE NEEDS PER DAY BY AGE, SEX, AND PHYSICAL ACTIVITY LEVEL

Gender	Age	Sedentary[a]	Moderately Active[b]	Active[c]
Males	2	1,000	1,000	1,000
	3	1,000	1,400	1,400
	4–5	1,200	1,400	1,600
	6–7	1,400	1,600	1,800
	8	1,400	1,600	2,000
	9	1,600	1,800	2,000
	10	1,600	1,800	2,200
	11	1,800	2,000	2,200
	12	1,800	2,200	2,400
	13	2,000	2,200	2,600
	14	2,000	2,400	2,800
	15	2,200	2,600	3,000
	16–18	2,400	2,800	3,200
	19–20	2,600	2,800	3,000
	21–25	2,400	2,800	3,000
	26–35	2,400	2,600	3,000
	36–40	2,400	2,600	2,800
	41–45	2,200	2,600	2,800
	46–55	2,200	2,400	2,800
	56–60	2,200	2,400	2,600
	61–65	2,000	2,400	2,600
	66–75	2,000	2,200	2,600
	76 and up	2,000	2,200	2,400
Females	2	1,000	1,000	1000
	3	1,000	1,,200	1,400
	4	1,200	1,400	1,400
	5–6	1,200	1,400	1,600
	7	1,200	1,600	1,800
	8–9	1,400	1,600	1,800
	10	1,400	1,800	2,000
	11	1,600	1,800	2,000
	12–13	1,600	2,000	2,200
	14–18	1,800	2,000	2,400
	19–25	2,000	2,200	2,400
	26–30	1,800	2,000	2,400
	31–50	1,800	2,000	2,200
	51–60	1,600	1,800	2,200
	61 and up	1,600	1,800	2,000

[a] Sedentary means a lifestyle that includes only the physical activity of independent living.

[b] Moderately Active means a lifestyle that includes physical activity equivalent to walking about 1.5 to 3 miles per day at 3 to 4 miles per hour, in addition to the activities of independent living.

[c] Active means a lifestyle that includes physical activity equivalent to walking more than 3 miles per day at 3 to 4 miles per hour, in addition to the activities of independent living.

[d] Estimates for females do not include women who are pregnant or breastfeeding.

Source: Institute of Medicine. Dietary Reference Intakes for Energy, Carbohydrate, Fiber, Fat, Fatty Acids, Cholesterol, Protein, and Amino Acids. Washington (DC): The National Academies Press, 2002.

Figure 12.4

HEALTHY U.S.-STYLE EATING PATTERN AT THE 2,000-CALORIE LEVEL, WITH DAILY OR WEEKLY AMOUNTS FROM FOOD GROUPS, SUBGROUPS, AND COMPONENTS

Food Group[a]	Amount[b] in the 2,000-Calorie-Level Pattern
Vegetables	2½ c-eq/day
Dark green	1½ c-eq/wk
Red and orange	5½ c-eq/wk
Legumes (beans and peas)	1½ c-eq/wk
Starchy	5 c-eq/wk
Other	4 c-eq/wk
Fruits	2 c-eq/day
Grains	6 oz-eq/day
Whole grains	≥ 3 oz-eq/day
Refined grains	≤ 3 oz-eq/day
Dairy	3 c-eq/day
Protein Foods	5½ oz-eq/day
Seafood	8 oz-eq/wk
Meats, poultry, eggs	26 oz-eq/wk
Nuts, seeds, soy products	5 oz-eq/wk
Oils	27 g/day
Limit on Calories for Other Uses (% of calories)[c]	270 kcal/day (14%)

[a] Definitions for each food group and subgroup are provided throughout the chapter and are compiled in Appendix 3.

[b] Food group amounts shown in cup (c) or ounce (oz) equivalents (eq). Oils are shown in grams (g). Quantity equivalents for each food group are defined in Appendix 3. Amounts will vary for those who need less than 2,000 or more than 2,000 calories per day. See Appendix 3 for all 12 calorie levels of the pattern.

[c] Assumes food choices to meet food group recommendations are in nutrient-dense forms. Calories from added sugars, added refined starches, solid fats, alcohol, and/or from eating more than the recommended amount of nutrient-dense foods are accounted for under this category.

Note: The total eating pattern should not exceed *Dietary Guidelines* limits for intake of calories from added sugars and saturated fats and alcohol and should be within the Acceptable Macronutrient Distribution Ranges for calories from protein, carbohydrate, and total fats. Most calorie patterns do not have enough calories available after meeting food group needs to consume 10 percent of calories from added sugars and 10 percent of calories from saturated fats and still stay within calorie limits. Values are rounded.

Figure 12.5

The U.S.-Style Eating Pattern is not the only way to eat while following the DG and in fact the DG point out as an example Mediterranean and Vegetarian Eating Patterns:

http://health.gov/dietaryguidelines/2015/guidelines/appendix-4/

http://health.gov/dietaryguidelines/2015/guidelines/appendix-5/

Before you jump into following one of the Healthy Eating Patterns, it is important to balance calories from foods and beverages with calories expended on metabolism and activity to maintain a healthy weight over time. Monitoring body weight and adjusting calorie intake as well as modifying how many calories burned in exercise are both important to achieving a healthy weight.

FOOD GROUPS

Vegetables

The recommended amount of vegetables for a 2,000 calorie diet is **2½ cups daily**, which includes all fresh, frozen, canned, and dried options in cooked or raw forms, as well as vegetable juice. In order to receive the nutritional and health benefits of vegetables, it is important to consume a variety from the following five groups. Also, limiting the use of added sodium (salt) and fats (cream, butter, or creamy sauces) used in preparation or found in ready-made vegetable side dishes will help keep the nutrient density of this group at its peak.

- **Dark-green vegetables:** All fresh, frozen, and canned dark green leafy vegetables and broccoli, cooked or raw: for example, broccoli, spinach, romaine, collard, turnips, and mustard greens.
- **Red and orange vegetables:** All fresh, frozen, and canned red and orange vegetables, cooked or raw: for example, tomatoes, red peppers, carrots, sweet potatoes, winter squash, and pumpkin.
- **Beans and peas:** All cooked and canned beans and peas: for example, kidney beans, lentils, chickpeas, and pinto beans. Legumes (beans and peas but not green beans and green or snap peas) are also rich in protein and can be counted into the protein food group as well)
- **Starchy vegetables:** All fresh, frozen, and canned starchy vegetables: for example, white potatoes, corn, and green peas.
- **Other vegetables:** All other vegetables, fresh, frozen, and canned, cooked or raw: for example, iceberg lettuce, green beans, and onions.

Key nutrients from vegetables: dietary fiber, a variety of minerals (potassium magnesium, iron, copper and manganese), an array of vitamins (vitamins A, C, E, and K, folate, vitamin B6, thiamin, niacin, and choline) and many different phytonutrients that have various health benefits as discussed in Chapter 10.

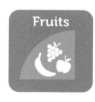

Fruit

A healthy-eating pattern of 2,000 calories includes a recommended **2 cups of fruit daily**, especially whole fruit. Whole fruits include fresh, canned, frozen, and dried forms. While 1 cup of 100% fruit juice does count as 1 cup of fruit, it is recommended that whole fruit be selected as fruit juices are typically much lower in fiber. And importantly, when consumed in excess, fruit juices can contribute to extra calories. For these reasons, at least half of the fruit consumed daily should be as whole fruit.

Key nutrients from fruits: dietary fiber, potassium, vitamins A and C, along with a wealth of phytonutrients.

Grains

A healthy-eating pattern of 2,000 calories recommends **6 ounce equivalents of grains daily** (with at least half coming from whole grains, see Figure 12.6). The grain group includes single grain foods such as rice, oatmeal, quinoa, and popcorn, as well as grains that are used as ingredients in breads, pasta, and cereals. Whole

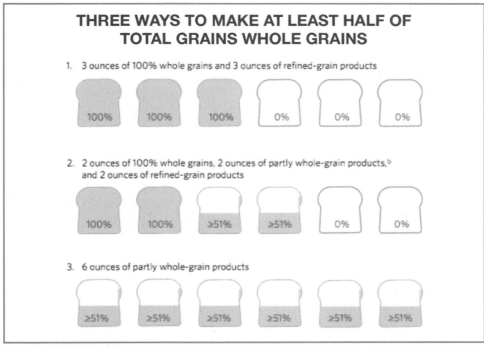

THREE WAYS TO MAKE AT LEAST HALF OF TOTAL GRAINS WHOLE GRAINS

1. 3 ounces of 100% whole grains and 3 ounces of refined-grain products

100% 100% 100% 0% 0% 0%

2. 2 ounces of 100% whole grains, 2 ounces of partly whole-grain products,[b] and 2 ounces of refined-grain products

100% 100% ≥51% ≥51% 0% 0%

3. 6 ounces of partly whole-grain products

≥51% ≥51% ≥51% ≥51% ≥51% ≥51%

From Dietary Guidelines for Americans 2010. Each one-ounce slice of bread represents a one-ounce equivalent of grains: one, one-ounce slice bread; one ounce uncooked pasta or rice; one-half cup cooked rice, pasta, or cereal; one tortilla (6 inches diameter); one pancake (5 inches diameter); one ounce ready-to-eat cereal (about one cup cereal flakes). The figure uses an example for a person whose recommendation is six ounces of total grains with at least three ounces from whole grains per day.

Figure 12.6

grains contain the entire kernel, which includes the bran and germ portions (as described in Figure 9.19.) When grains are refined, the bran layers and germ are removed. This means that dietary fiber, iron, and B vitamins are removed as well (see Chapter 9 for more.)

A food is a 100-percent whole-grain food if the only grains it contains are whole grains. One ounce-equivalent of whole grains has 16 g of whole grains. The recommendation to consume at least half of total grains as whole grains can be met in a number of ways.

The most direct way to meet the whole grain recommendation is to choose 100 percent whole-grain foods for at least half of all grains consumed. The relative amount of whole grain in the food can be inferred by the placement of the grain in the ingredients list. The whole grain should be the first ingredient—or the second ingredient, after water. For foods with multiple whole-grain ingredients, they should appear near the beginning of the ingredients list.

Many grain foods contain both whole grains and refined grains. These foods also can help people meet the whole grain recommendation, especially if a considerable proportion of the grain ingredients is whole grains. Another way to meet the recommendation to make at least half of grains whole grains is to choose products with at least 50 percent of the total weight as whole-grain ingredients. If a food has at least 8 g of whole grains per ounce-equivalent, it is at least half whole grains-Some product labels show the whole grains health claim or the grams of whole grain in the product. This information may help people identify food choices that have a substantial amount of whole grains.

Key nutrients from grains: dietary fiber, vitamins (thiamin, niacin, riboflavin, B6, vitamins A and E), minerals (iron, zinc, copper, magnesium, selenium, and manganese), and an array of phytonutrients.

Dairy

Instead of basing dairy recommendations on calorie level (intake), recommended serving numbers are based upon age due to the important nutrients supplied by dairy that are crucial for growth. Recommendations:

- **2 cup equivalents*** per day for children ages 2 to 3 years,
- **2½ cup equivalents*** per day for children ages 4 to 8 years, and
- **3 cup equivalents*** per day for adolescents ages 9 to 18 years and for adults.

Dairy includes fat-free and 1% dairy (milk, yogurt, cheese) or fortified soymilk (soy beverages) since these beverages are fortified with vitamins A and D along with calcium. It is important to look at the fat content of many dairy products, such as full fat milks and cheeses, which supply saturated fats and for some people should be limited. Also, some individuals who choose not to consume dairy due to lactose intolerance (see Chapter 4) or other reasons should look to other foods for calcium and vitamin D, as dairy is a critical source.

Key nutrients in dairy: protein, vitamins A, B12, and D, riboflavin, calcium, and choline.

Protein Foods

The 2,000-calorie Healthy-Eating pattern includes **5½ ounce equivalents** per day. Protein foods include all meats, poultry, seafood, eggs, nuts, seeds, and processed soy products. Meat and poultry should be lean or low fat. Beans and peas are considered part of this group, as well as of the vegetable group, but they should be counted in one group only. The goal is a variety of protein foods in their nutrient dense forms (roasted chicken rather than fried chicken for example.) The DG also make a specific recommendation to consume at least 8 ounce equivalents of seafood per week to ensure adequate intake of omega-3 essential fats.

The DG also specifically note that some groups of the population—men and male teens—over consume protein foods, which may push out other food groups such as vegetables and fruits. Also, the DG recognize that strong research evidence exists to show that a high meat diet and high intakes of processed meats (cured deli meats) are associated with increased chronic diseases such as CVD. For this reason, it is important to consider a variety of protein sources, including vegetable sources, and to take steps to limit sodium and saturated fats while balancing total calories to achieve a health weight.

Key nutrients in protein foods: protein, B vitamins, minerals (iron, selenium, zinc, and copper), and dietary fiber from plant protein sources. Nutrients provided by various protein foods differ, and this fact underscores the importance of variety in making protein food choice fit your health food pattern.

| \multicolumn{2}{c}{**MYPLATE FOOD GROUP SERVING SIZES**} |
Food Group	Equivalent

Grains	1 oz-equivalent:
	    1 slice bread
	    1/2 c cooked pasta, rice
	    1 c ready-to-eat cereal
	    1 small muffin
	    1/2 burger roll

Vegetable	1 cup-equivalent:
	    1 c cooked broccoli, carrots, green beans
	    2 c leafy greens (romaine lettuce, raw spinach)
	    1 c vegetable juice

Fruit	1 cup-equivalent:
	    1 c sliced fruit (strawberries, melon)
	    1/2 grapefruit
	    1 medium apple, pear

Milk	1 cup-equivalent:
	    1 c milk
	    1 c yogurt
	    1 c ice cream
	    1 1/2 oz hard cheese

Meat and Beans	1 oz-equivalent:
	    1 oz beef, pork, fish, poultry
	    1/4 c cooked lentils, pinto and other beans
	    1/4 c tofu
	    1 egg
	    1 T peanut butter
	    1/2 oz nuts and seeds

Figure 12.7

Oils provide a high percentage of mono-unsaturated and polyunsaturated fats while solid fats are saturated and/or contain trans fatty acids. Nuts, avocados, olives, and seafood provide oils in the diet, sources of omega fats, and vitamin E. In an effort to balance calories, people should reduce solid fat intake by replacing solid fats with small amounts of oils (canola, olive), and replace some meats with seafood, beans, nuts, and seeds.

ABOUT SEAFOOD

Seafood, which includes fish and shellfish, received particular attention in the 2010 Dietary Guidelines because of evidence of health benefits for the general populations as well as for women who are pregnant or breastfeeding. For the general population, consumption of about 8 ounces per week of a variety of seafood, which provide an average consumption of 250 mg per day of EPA and DHA, is associated with reduced cardiac deaths among individuals with and without preexisting CVD. Similarly, consumption by women who are pregnant or breastfeeding of at least 8 ounces per week from seafood choices that are sources of DHA is associated with improved infant health outcomes.

The recommendation to consume 8 or more ounces per week (less for young children) of seafood is for the total package of nutrients that seafood provides, including its EPA and DHA content. Some seafood choices with higher amounts of EPA and DHA should be included.

Strong evidence from mostly prospective cohort studies but also randomized controlled trials has shown that eating patterns that include seafood are associated with reduced risk of CVD, and moderate evidence indicates that these eating patterns are associated with reduced risk of obesity. As described earlier, eating patterns consist of multiple, interacting food components and the relationships to health exist for the overall eating pattern, not necessarily to an isolated aspect of the diet.

Mercury is a heavy metal found in the DG form of methyl mercury in seafood in varying levels. Seafood choices higher in EPA and DHA but lower in methyl mercury are encouraged. Seafood varieties commonly consumed in the United States that are higher in EPA and DHA and lower in methyl mercury include salmon, anchovies, herring, shad, sardines, Pacific oysters, trout, and Atlantic and Pacific mackerel (not king mackerel, which is high in methyl mercury). Individuals who regularly consume more than the recommended amounts of seafood that are in the Healthy U.S-Style Pattern should choose a mix of seafood that emphasizes choices relatively low in methyl mercury.

Some canned seafood, such as anchovies, may be high in sodium. To keep sodium intake below recommended limits, individuals can use the Nutrition Facts label to compare sodium amounts.

Women who are pregnant or breastfeeding should consume at least 8 and up to 12 ounces of a variety of seafood per week, from choices that are lower in methyl mercury. Obstetricians and pediatricians should provide guidance on how to make healthy food choices that include seafood. Women who are pregnant or breastfeeding and young children should not eat certain types of fish that are high in methyl mercury.

Figure 12.8

LIMITS ON CERTAIN FOOD COMPONENTS AS PART OF A HEALTHY EATING PATTERN

Following a 2,000 calorie Healthy-Style Eating Pattern with recommended servings of vegetables, fruits, grains, dairy, and protein eaten in their nutrient-dense forms (plain unsweetened/flavored yogurt versus sweetened fruit-flavored yogurt, for example) leaves a mere 270 calories for "extra foods." This means that added sugars, fats, and alcohol all must fit within the 2,000-calorie budget to maintain calorie balance and healthy weight. The trouble is that most foods Americans select (and which often are all that is available at some quick-stop eateries), are food choices with added calories from sugars and fats. To address this issue, the DG have set limits to help Americans stay within the healthy eating pattern.

Added Sugars

The DG Healthy Eating Pattern limits added sugars to **< 10% of the total calories per day**. This amounts to < 50 grams of added sugar for a 2,000 calorie diet. White sugar, high fructose corn syrup, corn syrup, corn syrup solids, honey, molasses, and maple syrup are many of the added sugars used in sodas, sports drinks, energy drinks, grain-based desserts, and fruit drinks that constitute almost 50 percent of the added sugar sources in our diets as noted in Figure 12.9 along with approximately 30% coming from snacks and sweets.

Figure 12.9 is a pie chart that shows the percentage of added sugars in the diet of the U.S. population ages 2 years and older that comes from different food categories: Beverages (not milk or 100% fruit juice) 47%; Snacks & Sweets 31%; Grains 8%; Mixed Dishes 6%; Dairy 4%; Condiments, Gravies, Spreads, Salad Dressings 2%; Vegetables 1%; Fruits & Fruit Juice 1%; Protein Foods: 0%.

An inset bar chart expands the Beverages (not milk or 100% fruit juice) category to depict the percentage of added sugars in the diet from different types of beverages: Soft Drinks 25%; Fruit Drinks 11%; Coffee & Tea 7%; Sport & Energy Drinks 3%; Alcoholic Beverages 1%.

Together, Soft Drinks, Fruit Drinks, and Sport & Energy Drinks are called Sugar-Sweetened Beverages, which comprise 39% of added sugars.

The purpose of the recommendation to limit added sugars within the healthy eating pattern is to make room for other key nutrients (dietary fiber, protein, vitamins, etc.) that promote optimal health and reduce chronic disease risk. The evidence that added sugars specifically cause chronic ailments such as diabetes is

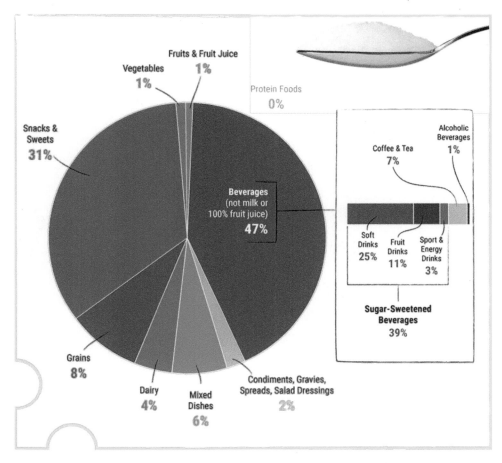

Figure 12.9

Food category sources of added sugars in the U.S. population ages 2 years and older

Data Source: What We Eat in America (WWEIA) Food Category analyses for the 2015 Dietary Guidelines Advisory Committee. Estimates based on day 1 dietary recalls from WWEIA, NHANES 2009–2010.

still under discussion, but what is known is that dietary patterns that supply lower amounts of added sugars (< 10% of calories) are associated with lower risk for various diet-related chronic diseases. There is room for added sugars in the diet, such as for sweet flavoring to otherwise tart foods, such as plain yogurt or tart fruits, for example. Careful label reading (ingredient lists) along with using the Nutrition Facts panel will help identify foods with added sugars.

Saturated Fats

The DG Healthy Eating Pattern limits saturated fats to **less than 10% of the total calories per day**, which amounts to < 20 grams of saturated fat for a 2,000 calorie eating plan. As we discussed in Chapter 6, replacing saturated fats in the diet with unsaturated fats is associated with lower levels of total cholesterol and LDL levels. Also, this switch in fat type is associated with a lower risk for heart attacks and related deaths.

As shown in Figure 12.10, the main sources of saturated fats in the diet are mixed dishes that contain cheese and/or meat along with burgers and sandwiches. Saturated fats are inherent in some foods, such as cheese and dairy (other than fat-free versions); and as long as fewer than 10% of the calories come from saturated

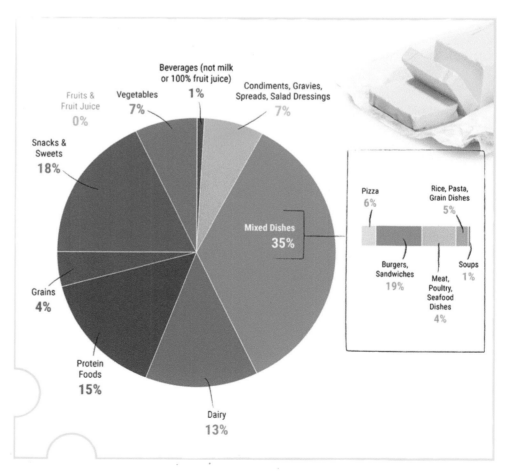

Figure 12.10

Food category sources of saturated fats in the U.S. population ages 2 Years and older

Data Source: What We Eat in America (WWEIA) Food Category analyses for the 2015 Dietary Guidelines Advisory Committee. Estimates based on day1 dietary recalls from WWEIA, NHANES 2009–2010.

fats, these foods can fit in a healthy eating pattern. However, saturated fats may be added to foods such as fried snacks and pastry items. These foods must be limited as they can contribute both excess calories and excess saturated fat in the diet.

Figure 12.10 is a pie chart that shows the percentage of saturated fats in the diet of the U.S. population ages 2 years and older that comes from different food categories: Mixed Dishes 35%; Snacks & Sweets 18%; Protein Foods 15%; Dairy 13%; Condiments, Gravies, Spreads, Salad Dressings 7%; Vegetables 7%; Grains 4%; Beverages (not milk or 100% fruit juice) 1%; Fruits & Fruit Juice 0%.

An inset bar chart expands the Mixed Dishes category to depict the percentage of saturated fats in the diet from different types of mixed dishes: Burgers, Sandwiches 19%; Pizza 6%; Rice, Pasta, Grain Dishes 5%; Meat, Poultry, Seafood Dishes 4%; Soups 1%.

Trans Fats

The DG recommend that synthetic sources of trans fats, such as partially hydrogenated oils (margarine and foods made with vegetable shortening) **be limited to as little as possible** in the diet for all ages of consumers. As covered in Chapter 6, trans fat intake is strongly associated with increased levels of circulating cholesterol and risk for CVD.

Dietary Cholesterol

The DG 2015–2020 do not give a specific numerical limit for cholesterol intake. Instead, they recommend that intakes be kept in check with a variety of plant and animal foods following the Healthy-Style Eating Patterns, which supply approximately 100 to 300 milligrams daily for all calorie levels. As noted later in this chapter, the Daily Value used in food labeling is **300 milligrams per day**.

Sodium

The DG recommend that sodium intake be limited to **less than 2,300 milligrams per day for adults**. We currently consume well above this limit at currently 3,440 milligrams (and tops 4,500 milligrams for those between the ages of 19 and 30). Scientific evidence shows a relationship between sodium intake and increased high blood pressure, a major risk factor for CVD. Figure 12.11 shows the various food categories and their contribution to sodium in the diet.

Figure 12.11 is a pie chart that shows the percentage of sodium in the diet of the U.S. population ages 2 years and older that comes from different food categories: Mixed Dishes 44%; Protein Foods 14%; Grains 11%; Vegetables 11%; Snacks & Sweets 8%; Dairy 5%; Condiments, Gravies, Spreads, Salad Dressings 5%; Beverages (not milk or 100% fruit juice) 3%; Fruits and Fruit Juice 0%.

A inset bar chart expands the Mixed Dishes category to show the percentage of sodium in the diet from different types of mixed dishes: Burgers, Sandwiches 21%; Rice, Pasta, Grain Dishes 7%; Pizza 6%; Meat, Poultry, Seafood Dishes 6%; Soups 4%.

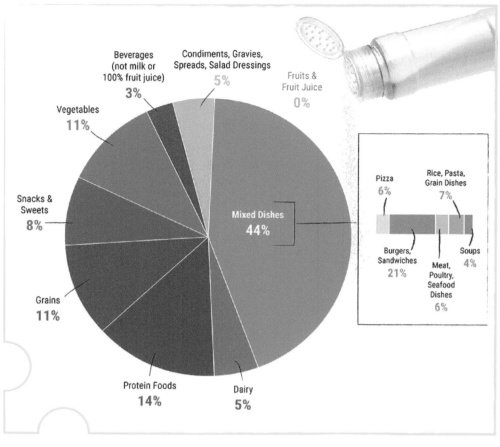

Figure 12.11

Food category sources of sodium in the U.S. population ages 2 years and older

Data Source: What We Eat in America (WWEIA) Food Category analyses for the 2015 Dietary Guidelines Advisory Committee. Estimates based on day 1 dietary recalls from WWEIA, NHANES 2009–2010.

Caffeine

Caffeine is not a nutrient; it is a dietary component that functions in the body as a stimulant. Caffeine occurs naturally in plants (e.g., coffee beans, tea leaves, cocoa beans, kola nuts). It also is added to foods and beverages (e.g., caffeinated soda, energy drinks). If caffeine is added to a food, it must be included in the listing of ingredients on the food label. Most intake of caffeine in the United States comes from coffee, tea, and soda. Caffeinated beverages vary widely in their caffeine content. Caffeinated coffee beverages include drip/brewed coffee (12 mg/fl oz), instant coffee (8 mg/fl oz), espresso (64 mg/fl oz), and specialty beverages made from coffee or espresso, such as cappuccinos and lattes. Amounts of caffeine in other beverages such as brewed black tea (6 mg/fl oz), brewed green tea (2-5 mg/fl oz), and caffeinated soda (1–4 mg/fl oz) also vary. Beverages within the energy drinks category have the greatest variability (3–35 mg/fl oz).

Much of the available evidence about caffeine focuses on coffee intake. Moderate coffee consumption (three to five 8-oz cups/day or up to 400 mg/day of caffeine) can be incorporated into healthy eating patterns. This guidance on coffee is informed by strong and consistent evidence showing that, in healthy adults, moderate coffee consumption is not associated with an increased risk of major chronic diseases (e.g., cancer) or premature death, especially from CVD. However, individuals who do not consume caffeinated coffee or other caffeinated beverages are not encouraged to incorporate them into their eating pattern. Limited and mixed evidence is available from randomized controlled trials examining the relationship between those energy drinks, which have high caffeine content and cardiovascular risk factors and other health outcomes. In addition, caffeinated beverages, such as some sodas or energy drinks, may include calories from added sugars, and although coffee itself has minimal calories, coffee beverages often contain added calories from cream, whole or 2% milk, creamer, and added sugars, which should be limited. The same considerations apply to calories added to tea or other similar beverages.

(Source: 2015 Dietary Guidelines)

HOW DO I "SHIFT" TO A HEALTHY EATING PATTERN?

Currently you may well not be following a healthy eating pattern. About three quarters of the population fall short on meeting recommendations for fruits, vegetables, dairy, and healthy oils. In addition, about two-thirds of the population is exceeding limits for added sugars, saturated fats, and sodium. In this section, we address this very issue of shifting from our current intake to a healthier eating pattern—the fourth Dietary Guideline.

> 4. **Shift to healthier food and beverage choices. Choose nutrient-dense foods and beverages across and within all food groups in place of less healthy choices. Consider cultural and personal preferences to make these shifts easier to accomplish and maintain.**

Figure 12.12 is a bar graph indicating the percentage of the U.S. population ages 1 year and older with intakes below the recommendation or above the limit for different food groups and dietary components.

- Vegetables: 87% have intakes below the goal;
- Fruit: 75% have intakes below the goal;
- Total Grains: 44% have intakes below the goal;
- Dairy: 86% have intakes below the goal;
- Protein Foods: 42% have intakes below the goal;
- Oils: 72% have intakes below the goal;
- Added sugars: 70% have intakes above the limit;
- Saturated fats: 71% have intakes above the limit;
- Sodium: 89% have intakes above the limit.

Knowing what changes to make and making changes to align with a healthy eating pattern is certainly overwhelming—at least the thought of it and deciding where to start! The idea with Dietary Guideline #4 is that there are many opportunities to make changes in food and beverage choices towards a healthier pattern and that these changes are aimed at being small, realistic, and, most importantly for you, shifts that you can sustain over time. Deciding not to "eat sweets any longer and instead snack on vegetables" is far from realistic or sustainable for most.

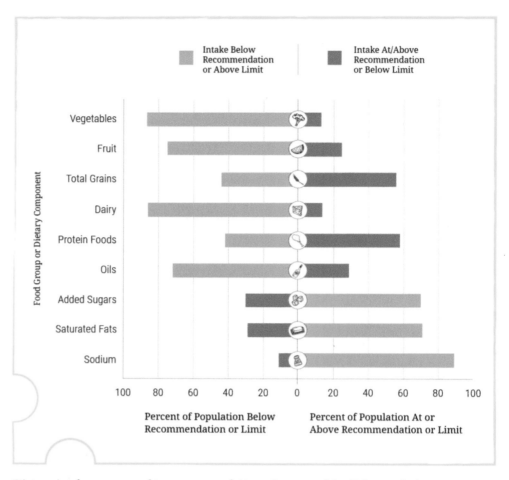

Figure 12.12

Dietary intakes compared to recommendations. Percent of the U.S. population ages 1 year and older that are below, at, or above each dietary goal or limit.

Note: The center (0) line is the goal or limit. For most, those represented by the orange sections of the bars, shifting toward the center line will improve their eating pattern.

Data Sources: What We Eat in America, NHANES 2007–2010 for average intakes by age-sex group. Healthy U.S.-Style Food Patterns, which vary based on age, sex, and activity level, for recommended intakes and limits.

Let's take a look at current intake for your age group (19 to 30 year olds) and consider some ideas for shifting towards a healthier eating pattern in each food group. This includes fruit, vegetables, grains, dairy, and protein foods, along with oils and items to limit (added sugars, solid fats, sodium).

Fruit

Currently both males and females ages 19 to 30 average approximately 1 of the 2 to 2½ cups of recommended fruit servings daily

A shift could include selecting whole fruit rather than packaged fruit "drink" that contains added sugar and much less fiber.

Vegetables

Males average 1¾ cups and females 1½ cups of vegetables daily—well under the recommended 2½ to 3 + cups (depending upon calorie needs.)

Increasing vegetable intake can be done at various eating opportunities during the day, such as opting for raw veggies for a snack with dip versus chips.

Grains

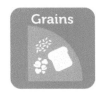

Grain intake by 19 to 30 year olds also falls off the mark. Total serving count is at the recommended amounts, but, out of the 6-ounce equivalents daily, fewer than 1 ounce is eaten as whole grain, with the rest as refined grains. So rather than getting most of one's grains as whole grains (brown rice, 100% whole grain cereal, or bread), we are instead consuming white bread and pasta and other highly refined grain foods low in fiber and other nutrients.

Shifting to whole grain choices could include selecting 100% whole grain bread for a sandwich rather than white or sourdough.

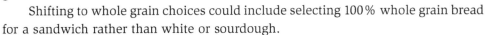

Dairy

Males (ages 19 to 30 years) average close to 2 cup equivalents and females only 1 cup—both below the recommended daily 3-cup equivalent for dairy.

A shift for you may look like drinking soy milk rather than soda at a meal or reaching for plain yogurt to top your fruit rather than a sweetened muffin.

Protein Foods

Males generally over consume (by approximately 10–15%) on protein foods ounce equivalents compared to what is recommended for their calorie level, while females meet recommendations. However, both males and females are at less than half their recommended seafood intake of 8 ounces per week and off the mark for plant protein sources as well.

A shift in protein foods could include substituting cooked fish (grilled or baked) for taco filling rather than fattier cuts of meat.

Oils

Limiting solid fats (saturated and trans) and shifting to vegetable oils is recommended. Both males and females consume over recommended levels of solid fats and too little of vegetable oils.

A shift to meeting recommendations could include cooking with vegetable oil (canola or olive oils) instead of stick margarine or butter.

Added Sugars

Shifting away from an average added sugar intake of almost 16% of the calories to less than 10% requires looking at foods and beverages in your diet that contain additional calories from added sugars. As noted in Figure 12.9, shifting from sugared beverages would be a good place to start. Consider reaching for plain water or fruit infused water rather than for a sweetened beverage

Sodium

Figure 12.11 illustrates the contribution of mixed dishes and other prepared foods to overall high sodium intake. Shifting to versions with lower sodium could include selecting fresh or frozen vegetables and meats (that do not have added sodium with sauces or other seasonings that contain sodium) or by selecting the version with lower sodium by using the Nutrition Facts label.

TRANSLATING THE DIETARY GUIDELINES INTO ACTION

This section addresses the fact that we all have a role in supporting healthy eating patterns—DG #5.

> **5. Support healthy eating patterns for all.** Everyone has a role in helping to create and support healthy eating patterns in multiple settings nationwide; this includes at home, school, and work, and in communities.

While DG #1 to #4 address food and activity patterns that promote health and reduce chronic disease risk, this DG addresses the fact that we all can and should play a part in supporting these efforts to adopt healthy eating and activity patterns. The details of this guideline focus on what policymakers and health professionals can do to support health patterns, but we need to recognize that we all can play a role by supporting healthy patterns in our own communities. Setting an example with your own food choices and lifestyle or getting involved with community activities and programs may in turn influence and support healthy patterns for all.

Ask yourself if your own education path (major in college) may provide an opportunity to influence change. For example, you may play a role in the design of a neighborhood that is creating more walking paths and parks for all in the community to utilize. Or as a psychology major, you may go on to assist people in making behavior changes that improve their health. The possibilities are endless and it's up to you to contribute.

Your Personal ChooseMyPlate

When you log on to *www.choosemyplate.gov*, you can get your own personalized eating plan linking on "SuperTracker." Here you can get personalized nutrition and physical activity plans, track your foods and activity and compare with recommendations and find a wealth of informaton including tips for healthy weight control. Check out *http://www.choosemypklate.gov/MyPlate-Daily-Checklist* for individualized eating plans (also in the Appendix and used for this chapter's quiz). Each plan designates the number of daily servings for each of the five food groups detailed above and the number of discretionary calories. See pages 510–514 for food plans for five different caloric intakes. These plans represent

MyPlate Daily Checklist available for 12 different caloric intakes (1,000 to 3,200 calories/day).

What are the serving sizes in each food group—for a whole grain or a vegetable for example? The serving sizes for each food group are listed in Figure 12.7. An ounce-equivalent (oz.-equivalent) is an amount of the food equal to one ounce (28 grams.) An important note about serving sizes: There is no standard definition for a serving size for a food group. You will find a serving size of grain listed as an oz.-equivalent (½ cup of breakfast cereal), but this is different from a serving size listed on a box of whole grain breakfast cereal (1 cup of breakfast cereal or two oz.-equivalents). As you select packaged foods, be sure to check the serving size listed on the package and compare it to your recommend food guide so as not to over-consume calories.

USING FOOD LABELS FOR HEALTHIER EATING

The primary goal behind the Nutrition Facts food label is to help you plan and choose foods that are part of a healthy diet based on the Dietary Guidelines for Americans and their principles of promoting general health and prevention of chronic disease. Now, at the end of the course we have a more complete "nutritional" view of food labels from when it was first brought up in Chapter 2.

The information on the Nutrition Facts food label is all about comparison—how does a serving of a specific food compare with reference intakes for total fat, saturated fat, protein, carbohydrate, fiber, and various vitamins and minerals. These reference intakes are the **Daily Values** that you have already learned about in previous chapters. The Daily Value is an intake that is recommended (and in some cases, such as fat, an intake not to exceed) based on a typical consumer eating a 2,000 calorie per day diet. Figure 12.14 shows the Daily Values used for comparison on food labels.

How to Read a Food Label

Let's take a "walk" through a Nutrition Facts food label (see Figure 12.13) and point out many of the important features.

- At the top portion of the label is information on the serving size ①. (See Figure 12.14.) This is important to note because what you serve yourself may in fact be two or more servings, which of course impacts the amount of calories, fat, and so on that you take in from this food.
- The midsection ② of the label presents information on the number of calories per serving along with the number of fat calories. This allows you a quick assessment of the food and a means of comparing this food to another.
- The amounts of fat, saturated fat, trans fat, cholesterol, and sodium per serving are listed ③ and this value is compared with the Daily Value for that nutrient. Remember from the Dietary Guidelines that these items are to be limited in the diet because of their connection with chronic disease. When the percent Daily Value is 5% or less this considered low and 20% or more is considered high.
- Amounts of carbohydrate, fiber, sugar (naturally occurring such as fruit sugar and lactose in milk, and added sugars such as in candy), and protein is presented.

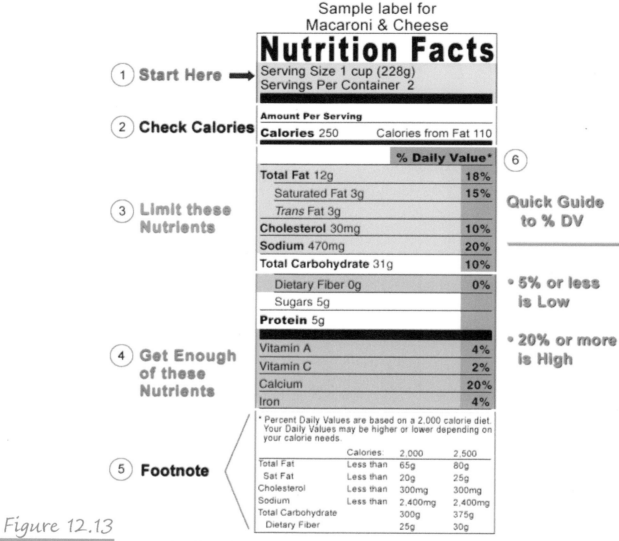

Figure 12.13

http://www.fda.gov/Food/LabelingNutrition/ConsumerInformation/ucm078889.htm

Daily Values

Fat	65 grams
Saturated fat	20 grams
Cholesterol	300 milligrams
Total carbohydrates	300 grams
Added sugar	50 grams
Fiber	25 grams
Sodium	2,400 milligrams
Protein	50 grams

Figure 12.14

These are compared to the Daily Value but note only for carbohydrate and fiber. The FDA does not require protein to be listed as a percent of Daily Value unless a claim is made on the package about the protein in the food. There is no Daily Value for sugar for comparison, but be aware that 4 grams of sugar is equivalent to a teaspoon.

• The FDA requires that four micronutrients—vitamins A and C and the minerals calcium and iron—be listed on the label as a percent of the Daily Value ④. If a food is fortified with other micronutrients, these too would be listed as percent Daily Value.

At the bottom of the label, room permitting, the Daily Values are listed along with adjusted amounts for a 2,500 calorie diet (footnote).

In Figure 12.15, the newly approved Nutrition Facts label contains many changes to assist consumers in choosing healthy food patterns:

① Serving size is listed prominently along with servings per container.

② Added sugars are separately listed as part of total sugars.

③ Four micronutrients—vitamin D, calcium, iron, and potassium—amounts as percent of Daily Value are noted as these nutrients are at risk for low intake in many Americans.

Putting the Dietary Guidelines for Americans, MyPlate, and Nutrition Facts food label all together in this way has perhaps given you a different perspective on these tools in planning a healthful diet.

Congratulate yourself—you now have a wealth of knowledge about your health and how diet plays a vital role for the promotion of a healthy body and general health and prevention of chronic diseases for a vital future.

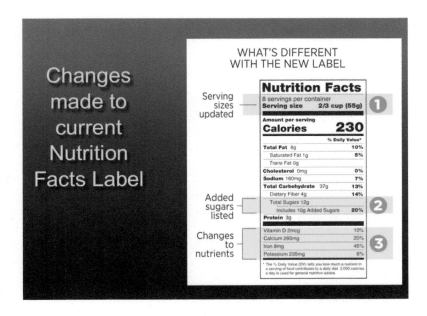

Figure 12.15

Quiz Yourself

12

CHAPTER

1. What are the three rationales behind the Dietary Guidelines for Americans?

   1. _____

   2. _____

   3. _____

2. What is a nutrient-dense food? Give five specific examples from each of the food groups.

_____

_____

_____

_____

_____

   1. _____

   2. _____

   3. _____

   4. _____

   5. _____

3. The Dietary Guidelines for Americans recommend at least 150 minutes of physical activity a week for adults.

   a. true

   b. false

4. Choose one of the leading diet-related chronic diseases (listed on page 258) that you feel may be an issue for you as you get older. Then identify food choices you currently make that may contribute to this disease and what shifts you currently can make to improve your healthy eating pattern.

Diet related chronic disease:

_____

Dietary choices you make that may contribute to your risk for this ailment (list at least two).

_____

_____

Identify two shifts you can make with your current eating pattern to improve your risk.

_____

_____

5. Choose one of the first three Dietary Guidelines from page 256 and describe how implementing this would meet the rationale behind the Dietary Guidelines noted in question 1 above.

_____

_____

_____

_____

_____

6. How many servings are recommended from each of the five food groups to meet your calorie intake?

Food Groups	_Recommended # of servings daily_
Grains	_____
Vegetables	_____
Fruits	_____
Milk	_____
Protein Foods (Meat & beans)	_____

Using the appropriate MyPlate Daily Checklist from the Appendix (pp. 510–514), fill in your food and beverage choices for yesterday. Then compare this to the five food groups and the recommended number of servings. Also, list the number of minutes you were physically active. How did you do? How would you shift your food and beverage choices for tomorrow to meet the goal for your calorie intake? How about your physical activity level? How would you shift this to reach your activity goal?

_____

_____

_____

_____

_____

_____

APPENDIX

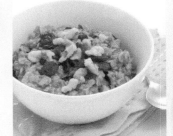

Nutrition 10
DIET PROJECT GUIDE

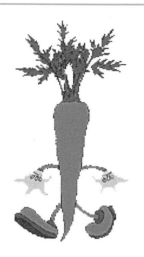 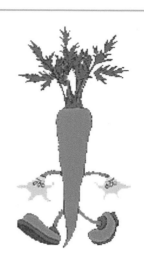 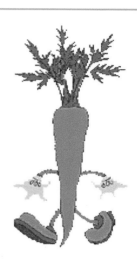

Important Dates to Remember

*Project Due Date _____

Late Due Date (for partial credit) _____

Projects Returned _____

**Re-Grade Submittal _____

*In class, or by 5 P.M. at TA office (no other location accepted)
**In class only! (no other location or time accepted)

Checklist for Turning In Your Diet Project

❏ **Food Record Forms for Three Days**   (pp. 295–299)

❏ **Summary and Comparison Forms**   (p. 301)

❏ **Calculations Page**   (p. 303)

❏ **MyPlate Daily Checklist**   (p. 307)

❏ **Unsealed Return Envelope**   (Distributed in Class on due date)
  with completed grade forms

HOW DOES *YOUR* DIET RATE?

Diet Project Guide Contents

BACKGROUND / INTRODUCTION

As you'll learn in class, the Recommended Dietary Allowances are the suggested levels of intake for a variety of essential nutrients. Because not everyone can possibly eat "perfectly" every day, they are meant to be averaged over several days' intake. Think of them as intake goals that you should be aiming for.

In keeping with the purpose of this class—putting nutrition knowledge into the context of personal health—you will record your diet for three days and then average the nutrient content from those three days. You will then compare your actual three-day average with the RDA goals and other dietary guidelines. This comparison will give you a idea of how good a job you are doing in meeting your body's needs for today and preventing chronic disease in years to come. Later, when you learn more about the functions of these nutrients and good food sources for them, you will understand their importance and be able to make choices that can improve your diet.

- To complete this project, you will need the following tools:
  —Your completed Food Record Pages (instructions will follow)
  —Food Composition Tables (starting on page 312 of the Appendix)
  —A calculator
- To get full credit for your project, you must submit (in the unsealed envelope provided in class):
  —Completed Food Record Pages for three days (extra Food Record form if needed)
  —Completed Calculation Page
  —Completed Summary and Comparison Forms and MyPlate Daily Checklist

If you have made several errors on your Diet Project, or you have omitted one or more of the required pages/forms, you will be given a "No Pass" grade. **IF** you correct these errors or omissions you get Dr. Applegate's or one of the Teaching Assistants' initials indicating corrections are correctly made, and **IF** you re-submit it by the deadline on the front page of this packet, you will still be able to get full credit. The TAs and Dr. Applegate are happy to look over your corrected Project to be sure you are on the right track—there is no reason not to get full credit, **if** you meet all the deadlines.

COMPLETING YOUR FOOD RECORD FORMS

STEP 1   **Record *everything* that you eat or drink (except water) for three consecutive days.** You must choose either Sunday, Monday, and Tuesday, or Thursday, Friday, and Saturday. We all tend to eat differently on the weekends, so including one weekend day will give you a better representation of your typical eating patterns. And please try to continue to eat as you usually would; being overly "good" (however you might define that) will not give you an accurate picture of your diet.

- **Don't record any nutrient supplements you might be taking (even though these are listed in the food tables).** This Project is your tool for discovering how well your food and beverage choices deliver the nutrients you need. (You may though record protein powders, nutritional bars and other supplement products that provide calories.)
- Place each food item on its own line. If you eat more items in one day than there are lines on the form, use the extra Food Record Form on page 305.
- When you are recording your food items, take careful note of the measure—cups, ounces, tablespoons, and teaspoons. Don't just write "bowlful" or "glassful" because not all bowls and glasses are the same size. It might be helpful to use kitchen measuring cups at first, until you can estimate with some accuracy. For items such as meat or cheese, remember that 3 oz. of cooked meat is about the size of an ordinary playing card, that one oz. of cheese is a cube about 1½ inches on a side, and that 4 oz. of raw meat usually cooks down to 3 oz., a medium size piece of fruit is about the size of a tennis ball. Also note that for household measures: 2 cups = 1 pint; 1 cup = 16 T; 2 T = 1 ounce, 3 t = 1 T; 8 ounces = 1 cup. (See Serving Size listing on page 287.)
- If you are eating most common frozen dinners or entrees or at a fast-food restaurant, write down the exact name of the item: *Healthy Choice* Chicken Chow Mein, *Taco Bell* Chicken Taco Supreme, *McDonald's* Big Mac, *Burger King* Whopper with cheese, etc. Enter drinks by the number of ounces they contain, not as "large" or "extra-large."
- Combination-type foods and drinks, such as casseroles or smoothies or mochas, present a challenge. Try to find out the types and amounts of ingredients that went into the casserole, and then estimate the share your serving represents (though many combination-type foods such as stews, soups and casseroles are listed in the food tables. For example, a casserole might be made from 12 oz. of penne pasta, 2 medium zucchini, a half-pound of ground turkey, and a 28-oz can of tomatoes. (Don't worry about entering spices or herbs.) If you ate one-fourth of this casserole, you would enter 3 oz. penne pasta, ½ medium zucchini, ~2 oz. of cooked ground turkey, and 7 oz. of canned tomatoes.

STEP 2   **Determine the nutrient values for each food item.** Use the Food Composition Tables found in the Appendix of this Reader starting on page 314, which have listings for most commonly consumed foods listed alphabetically. There are many categories, so look through the entire set of tables to find each food item. Categories include beverages, fast food (listed by restaurant), fish, fruits, grains (breads, pasta, rice), breakfast cereal, meals and dishes (including frozen, canned, and pizza), meats (including meat substitutes), nuts (peanut butter), poultry, sauces, snack foods, soups, sports products (energy bars, supplements, and sport drinks), and vegetables (fresh, canned & frozen). Find the food item that most closely matches the one on your Food Record. In some cases if the food item you recorded is not listed you may need to substitute, that is, choose the food item that most closely resembles, in terms of nutrient profile, what you ate.

Using a ruler or straight edge (to be sure you stay on the same line), record nutrient values for each item listed on the Food Record, calories, protein, carbohydrates, etc., paying attention to specific vitamin and mineral names as not all nutrient values listed in the tables will be recorded; phosphorus and potassium, for example.

- **DO NOT** use the Nutrition Facts Food Label from a food's packaging for nutrient information. While they are helpful in allowing consumers to compare food products, these labels don't serve our needs because they don't list all the nutrients we are interested in. Use the Food Composition Tables.
- Make careful note of the units and serving sizes. Don't write the food values for a loaf of bread when you only had *two slices!* What if the Table listing shows a serving of 1 cup of milk, but you actually consumed 2½ cups? You would then need to make the appropriate adjustment to all the food nutrient values given by multiplying them by 2.5.
- **If information is listed for an entire package or container, figure out what fraction of the container you ate and make appropriate adjustments such as, multiply by 0.25 if you ate ¼ of a whole pizza.**
- If a "—" is listed for the content of a particular nutrient, record it as "—" and assume a value of zero (0). The dash line means the information is not available.
- If you have eaten a food that is not in the Food Composition Tables (and you can't find an appropriate substitute), you can refer to the USDA web site *www.nal.usda.gov/fnic/ foodcomp/search* and enter your food item to obtain the nutrient profile. (Make appropriate adjustments based on serving size listed compared to what you ate.)
- Short names for some of the B vitamins may be listed: vitamin B_1 is thiamin, B_2 is riboflavin, and B_3 is niacin.

STEP 3   Total each column (except for the "amount" column) on each of your three Food Record Forms, and place the totals in the appropriate boxes at the bottom of the Forms.

HOW TO FILL OUT YOUR SUMMARY FORM

STEP 1   Transfer the Totals from each Food Record Form to the appropriate column. Be very careful to enter each item in its correct column.

STEP 2   Total each column. Total the nutrient values from your three days.

STEP 3   Find the average value. Divide the totals for each column by three to find your three-day average intake.

SERVING PORTIONS

Dana Wu Wassmer, MS, RD
Cosumnes River College

When I address the issue of serving size to my students, the first response I get is, "You've got to be kidding!" The next is the realization that they have been overeating for years. I mean, how were they to know that a serving size for a pancake is the size of a compact disc? Or that a serving of a baked potato is the size of a computer mouse? What? You too? So earlier this year when the Food and Drug Administration (FDA) announced that they are considering requiring food manufacturers to list the nutritional information for more realistic "portion" sizes on food packaging, it has been met with a mixed response.

A "portion" is the amount of food you decide to eat. For example, you eat one portion of meat, one portion of pasta, and one portion of cake. What is a portion to you may just be an appetizer to another. A portion size is not necessarily the same as a serving size since a serving size is the quantity designated by the food manufacturer. Also, a serving is not necessarily the recommended amount people should eat. However, they are to be considered a point of reference. The current serving size on food packaging was updated in the early 1990's. Before this, food manufacturers could call whatever size they wanted a "serving size." Typically, they would pick a serving size that would portray the nutrition information in the most appealing light (e.g., an unrealistically small serving size so the calorie numbers are low). Cereal companies often used this to their advantage and would typically choose one ounce as a serving size. One ounce is approximately the weight of 10 pennies. Visually, this is about ½–¾ cup of cold cereal. I don't know about you, but ½ cup of cereal would barely register in a colossal cereal bowl. But by choosing one ounce as the serving size, the calorie per serving is low (e.g., 90–100 calories per one ounce serving) leading many consumers to focus on the calorie level without really paying attention to the volume of food. Plus, it was almost impossible to compare products since the nutrition information displayed might be for different serving sizes.

Uniformity and realistic serving size were FDA's goal when they revamped the food label. The FDA utilized the survey data of Americans from the 1970–1980s to determine the typical eating habits and portion sizes for various foods. These portions became the standard serving sizes and were used on the updated food labels.

Unfortunately the method of establishing these serving sizes was flawed. The survey data was outdated and was based on self-reported intake. In this case, people were asked by researchers to keep a food record. However, when it comes to self-reporting, participants have a tendency to underestimate how much they eat. In addition, portion sizes have increased dramatically just in the past 20 years.

Twenty years ago, a portion size of a typical muffin was only 1.5 ounces (or 210 calories) or about the size of a hockey puck. Today, the muffin has more than doubled in size to 4.0 ounces (or 500 calories). A portion of a chocolate chip cookie was measured at 1.5 inches in diameter. Today, the cookie is 3.5 inch in diameter. The difference in size also means a difference of 220 calories. A bagel was 3-inches in diameter twenty years ago; today it is 6-inches. A large container of popcorn at the movie theater twenty years ago was 5 cups. Today, it is 11 cups. In addition, we have also created sizes bigger than large such as "jumbo," "king," or "super." Without a doubt, these examples confirm that our portions have been amplified, and not surprisingly, so have our bodies. Thus, the serving size of yesteryear does not reflect what is being consumed today.

There is also the designated serving size listed for each food group at mypyramid.gov. This is more of a recommended size for a serving and it comes with a recommended number of daily servings based on your age, gender, and activity level. For example, a recommended daily intake of 6–11 servings from the bread, cereal, and grain group does not mean eating 6–11 loaves of bread (even if they are made of whole grains). It means 6–11 servings where each serving is 1 slice of bread, 1 oz of cereal, or ½ cup of cooked pasta. That's right; HALF-a-cup of pasta is considered one serving. Looking at these recommendations, it is easy to see how you can eat excessive servings of pasta in one sitting.

If the FDA begins to require food companies to list the nutrition content based on realistic portions, many fear that people will get the wrong message. In seeing a food package printed with the information that one serving will provide 600 calories and that one serving is say, two cups, people may get the impression that they are supposed to eat two cups. Currently, a serving of chips on a food label is 1 ounce or about 11 individual Doritos chips. A more realistic portion of chips consumed by an average person is more like 30–40 chips in one sitting. (Many times it is the whole 9.5 ounce bag). If one ounce has 150 calories, then 30–40 chips would be 450–600 calories. That is a significant difference in calories. The FDA hopes that by listing "450" or "600" calories per serving, it would stop you and me from going in for another handful. Would the shock factor of seeing "600 calories per serving" be enough to make us walk away from a food? Or would you eat all 40 chips because the label says it is a serving? This is still being hotly debated.

Obviously the current serving size on food labels is not near the amount we actually eat. But the way the food is packaged leads us to think the amount is appropriate. Take for example Pop Tarts. These pastries come two to

Source: Weight-Control Information Network (WIN), a national service of the National Institute of Diabetes and Digestive and Kidney Disease (NIDDK), part of the National Institute of Health.

a package (four packages to a container). However, one serving is one pastry. I have a hard time envisioning that we would stop after eating one pastry and wrap up the remaining pastry for another day. Or how about a can of Progresso soup? A serving size is one cup. However, one can contains two servings. I guess Progresso expects you to share your soup every time you open a can. In addition, the size of our food portions have grown exponentially. When presented with more food, we tend to eat more.

Unfortunately, deciphering a serving from a food label may mean we need a food scale and measuring cup readily available. However, there are handy guidelines that we can use (without the use of scales and measuring tools) to assess if we are eating an appropriate serving. Below is a quick visual tool to use (from http://www.win.niddk.nih.gov/publications/just_enough.htm):

Serving Size	Everyday Objects
1 cup (a serving) of cereal or vegtable = a fist	
½ cup (a serving) of cooked rice, pasta, or potato = ½ baseball	
(A serving of) 1 baked potato = a fist	
1 medium fruit = a serving of fruit = a baseball	
½ cup of fresh fruit = a serving of fruit = ½ baseball	
1½ ounces of low-fat or fat-free cheese = 4 stacked dice	
½ cup of ice cream = ½ baseball	
2 tablespoons of peanut butter = a ping-pong ball	

Other tips include (from healthyeating.webmd.com):

- A deck of cards—a serving (3 ounces) of meat, fish, poultry or tofu
- The palm of your hand (just the palm, no fingers)—a serving of meat, fish or poultry
- A golf ball or large egg—one quarter cup of dried fruit or nuts
- One cassette tape—one (serving) slice of bread
- One hockey puck—one (serving) bagel, one muffin
- One tennis ball—about one half cup of ice cream
- A computer mouse—about the size of a small baked potato
- A compact disc—about the size of one serving of pancake or small waffle
- A thumb tip—about one teaspoon of peanut butter
- A check book—a serving of fish (approximately 3 oz.)
- One dental floss package—one brownie serving, one piece of chocolate serving

There are easy tools to make sure you are eating an adequate and not excessive serving. Keep these tips in mind when eating out. Restaurants are known for serving large portions. Many times the portions are sufficient to feed two (or more) adults. The supersized and value meals may seem like great deals, however, the only deal you get is a growing waist line. Use the tools like the ones listed above to moderate your portions. The FDA is attempting to provide us with more accurate information about what we are eating. However, it is still up to us to decide how much we are going to eat.

REFERENCES

Department of Health and Human Services, National Institutes of Health, National Heart, Lung, and Blood Institute. "Portion Distortion! Do You Know How Food Portions Have Changed in 20 Years?" 2010. 11 March 2010. http://hp2010.nhlbihin.net/oei_ss/PDII/pd2webtxt.htm

Neuman, William. "One Bowl = 2 Servings. F.D.A. May Fix That." 6 Feb. 2010. 11 March 2010. http://www.nytimes.com/2010/02/06/business/06portion.html.

Weight-control Information Network, National Institute of Diabetes and Digestive and Kidney Disease of the National Institute of Health, Department of Health and Human Services. "Just Enough for You: About Food Portions." June 2009. 11 March 2010. http://www.win.niddk.nih.gov/publications/just_enough.htm.

Zelman, Kathleen. "WebMD Portion Size Guide." 26 Nov. 2008. 11 March 2010. www.healthyeating.webmd.com.

COMPLETING YOUR CALCULATION PAGE

STEP 1   **Calculate your daily Energy and Protein Requirements.** Don't try to complete this portion of the page until we have covered these topics in class (see chapters 2 and 3). After that point, you will have all the information you need to complete Parts 1, 2, and 3.

STEP 2   **Calculate your Energy Intake Distribution. (Part 4)** Transfer the three-day average intakes (g/day) for carbohydrate, protein, and fat from the last line of your Summary Page to the appropriate lines in Part 4 of the Calculation Page. Convert these intakes from grams to kcalories by using the appropriate physiological fuel value. Finally, total these kcalories to determine your total calculated energy.

STEP 3   **Calculate your % Energy Distribution. (Part 5)** Using the kcalorie results that you calculated in Part 4, compute the relative percentages of your total calories coming from carbohydrate, protein, fat, and saturated fat.

HOW TO FILL OUT YOUR COMPARISON FORM

STEP 1   **Transfer your three-day average intakes from the last line of the Summary Form to the first line of the Comparison Form—EXCEPT for fat and saturated fat.** For these entries, use the "% kcal from fat" figure you computed in Part 5 (C_3) and "% kcal from saturated fat" (D_3) figure in Part 6 of the Calculation Page.

STEP 2   **Enter your daily Energy (E) and Protein (F) Requirements into the first two boxes of the "Standard" line of the Comparison Form.**

STEP 3   **Enter the appropriate set of RDAs/DRIs in the remaining boxes of the "Standard" row of the Comparison Form.** The RDAs/DRIs are on pages 292–293. RDAs/DRIs are listed for males, females, and by age—be sure you choose the set appropriate for you. Notice that some boxes have already been filled for you. These represent dietary recommendations set forth in the Dietary Guidelines for Americans 2010 for the prevention of chronic diseases. The values in this "Standard" row are the "goals" that you will make a comparison to your actual intake.

STEP 4   **Calculate what percent (%) of the "Standard" you are consuming.** To do this, you would divide your average intake by the Standard, and then multiply by 100 to get a percentage.

STEP 5   **Circle all nutrients for which your average daily intake was less than 100% of the standard.**

HOW TO FILL OUT YOUR MYPLATE DAILY CHECKLIST (pp. 307–308)

STEP 1   Transfer your intake for one of the week days you recorded (Monday, Tuesday, Thursday or Friday) in the center column listed "Write your food choices for each food group" being aware of each food group your food choices belong.

STEP 2   Record the amount of each food and beverage in measures that correspond to cups or ounce equivalents noted for each food group.

STEP 3   Check for combination foods such as pizza that fits into multiple groups—"grains" (crust) and "milk" (cheese) as well as vegetables (tomato sauce) and "protein" (ham).

STEP 4   Note your total number of servings in each food group and ask yourself if you reached your target number (identify "Y" or "N" in the second column).

STEP 5   Ask yourself if you successfully limited your intake of sodium (< 2,300 milligrams), saturated fat (< 20 grams) and added sugars (< 50 grams) per day. Take a look at your summary and comparison form for your daily sodium and saturated fat intakes. Added sugar intake was not determined so you can simply estimate. Circle "Y" or "N" as to whether you limited these items in your diet.

STEP 6   Recall the amount of physical activity such as jogging or bike riding you did for the day; now estimate for the week. Do you average at least 30 minutes a day (2½ hours per week)? Circle "Y" or "N."

STEP 7   Finally, identify one to two small changes you can make to improve your diet (such as drink more plain water rather than sweetened beverages) and boost your physical activity level (such as ride your bike to campus three days a week). List these changes in the "Track your MyPlate, MyWins" section at the bottom.

At the end of the quarter, you will have an opportunity to fill out this worksheet again and make a comparison to your current intake. Think about the benefits you have learned about increasing your intake of fruits and vegetables. Will you shift your pattern of foods to improve your health?

DIETARY REFERENCE INTAKES: RDA AND AI FOR VITAMINS

	Vitamin A (µg/d)[a]	Vitamin D (µg/d)[b,c]	Vitamin E (mg/d)[d]	Vitamin K (µg/d)	Vitamin C (mg/d)	Thiamin (mg/d)	Riboflavin (mg/d)	Niacin (mg/d)[e]	Folate (µg/d)[f]	Vitamin B_6 (mg/d)	Vitamin B_{12} (µg/d)	Choline (mg/d)[g]
Children												
1–3 y	300	15	6	30*	15	0.5	0.5	6	150	0.5	0.9	200*
4–8 y	400	15	7	55*	25	0.6	0.6	8	200	0.6	1.2	250*
Males												
9–13 y	600	15	11	60*	45	0.9	0.9	12	300	0.9	1.8	375*
14–18 y	900	15	15	75*	75	1.2	1.3	16	400	1.3	2.4	550*
19–30 y	900	15	15	120*	90	1.2	1.3	16	400	1.3	2.4	550*
31–50 y	900	15	15	120*	90	1.2	1.3	16	400	1.3	2.4	550*
51–70 y	900	15	15	120*	90	1.2	1.3	16	400	1.7	2.4	550*
>70 y	900	20	15	120*	90	1.2	1.3	16	400	1.7	2.4	550*
Females												
9–13 y	600	15	11	60*	45	0.9	0.9	12	300	1.0	1.8	375*
14–18 y	700	15	15	75*	65	1.0	1.0	14	400	1.2	2.4	400*
19–30 y	700	15	15	90*	75	1.1	1.1	14	400	1.3	2.4	425*
31–50 y	700	15	15	90*	75	1.1	1.1	14	400	1.3	2.4	425*
51–70 y	700	15	15	90*	75	1.1	1.1	14	400	1.5	2.4	425*
>70 y	700	20	15	90*	75	1.1	1.1	14	400	1.5	2.4	425*
Pregnancy												
14–18 y	750	15	15	75*	80	1.4	1.4	18	600	1.9	2.6	450*
19–30 y	770	15	15	90*	85	1.4	1.4	18	600	1.9	2.6	450*
31–50 y	770	15	15	90*	85	1.4	1.4	18	600	1.9	2.6	450*
Lactation												
14–18 y	1,200	15	19	75*	115	1.4	1.6	17	500	2.0	2.8	550*
19–30 y	1,300	15	19	90*	120	1.4	1.6	17	500	2.0	2.8	550*
31–50 y	1,300	15	19	90*	120	1.4	1.6	17	500	2.0	2.8	550*

Note: These are from the DRI reports (see www.nap.edu). RDAs are set to meet the needs of almost all (97%–98%) healthy individuals in a group. AI are more tentative values as insufficient research exists currently to set an RDS. Both RDAs and AIs may be used as goals for individuals.

Sources: Adapted from the *Dietary Reference Intake* series, National Academic Press. Copyright 1997, 1998, 2000, 2001, 2005, 2010 by the National Academy of Sciences. These reports may be accessed via www.nap.edu. Courtesy of the National Academies Press, Washington, D.C.

DIETARY REFERENCE INTAKES: RDA AND AI FOR MINERALS

	Calcium (mg/d)	Phosphorus (mg/d)	Magnesium (mg/d)	Iron (mg/d)	Zinc (mg/d)	Selenium (µg/d)	Iodine (µg/d)	Copper (µg/d)	Manganese (AI) (mg/d)	Fluoride (AI) (mg/d)	Chromium (AI) (µg/d)
Children											
1–3 y	700	460	80	7	3	20	90	340	1.2	0.7	11
4–8 y	1,000	500	130	10	5	30	90	440	1.5	1	15
Males											
9–13 y	1,300	1,250	240	8	8	40	120	700	1.9	2	25
14–18 y	1,300	1,250	410	11	11	55	150	890	2.2	3	35
19–30 y	1,000	700	400	8	11	55	150	900	2.3	4	35
31–50 y	1,000	700	420	8	11	55	150	900	2.3	4	35
51–70 y	1,000	700	420	8	11	55	150	900	2.3	4	30
>70 y	1,200	700	420	8	11	55	150	900	2.3	4	30
Females											
9–13 y	1,300	1,250	240	8	8	40	120	700	1.6	2	21
14–18 y	1,300	1,250	360	15	9	55	150	8909	1.6	3	24
19–30 y	1,000	700	310	18	8	55	150	900	1.8	3	25
31–50 y	1,000	700	320	18	8	55	150	900	1.8	3	25
51–70 y	1,200	700	320	8	8	55	150	900	1.8	3	20
>70 y	1,200	700	320	8	8	55	150	900	1.8	3	20
Pregnancy											
14–18 y	1,300	1,250	400	27	12	60	220	1,000	2.0	3	29
19–30 y	1,000	700	350	27	11	60	220	1,000	2.0	3	30
31–50 y	1,000	700	360	27	11	60	220	1,000	2.0	3	30
Lactation											
14–18 y	1,300	1,250	360	10	13	70	290	1,300	2.6	3	44
19–30 y	1,000	700	310	9	12	70	290	1,300	2.6	3	45
31–50 y	1,000	700	320	9	12	70	290	1,300	2.6	3	45

Note: These are from the DRI reports (see www.nap.edu). RDAs are set to meet the needs of almost all (97%-98%) healthy individuals in a group. AI are more tentative values as insufficient research exists currently to set an RDS. Both RDAs and AIs may be used as goals for individuals.

Sources: Adapted from the *Dietary Reference Intake* series, National Academic Press. Copyright 1997, 1998, 2000, 2001, 2005, 2010 by the National Academy of Sciences. These reports may be accessed via www.nap.edu. Courtesy of the National Academies Press, Washington, D.C.

NAME: _____   ID#: _____

Food Record Form *(Use one form for each day)*

Day and Date: _____

Food	Amount	Calories	Protein g	Carbohydrate g	Fiber g	Fat g	Saturated Fat g	Cholesterol mg	Vitamin A RE	Vitamin C mg	Thiamin mg	Niacin NE	Folate mcg	Vitamin B₁₂ mcg	Sodium mg	Potassium mg	Calcium mg	Iron mg	Zinc mg
Total																			

NAME: _____   ID#: _____

Food Record Form *(Use one form for each day)*

Day and Date: _____

Food	Amount	Calories	Protein g	Carbohydrate g	Fiber g	Fat g	Saturated Fat g	Cholesterol mg	Vitamin A RE	Vitamin C mg	Thiamin mg	Niacin NE	Folate mcg	Vitamin B12 mcg	Sodium mg	Potassium mg	Calcium mg	Iron mg	Zinc mg
Total																			

NAME: _____   ID#: _____

Food Record Form *(Use one form for each day)*

Day and Date: _____

Food	Amount	Calories	Protein g	Carbohydrate g	Fiber g	Fat g	Saturated Fat g	Cholesterol mg	Vitamin A RE	Vitamin C mg	Thiamin mg	Niacin NE	Folate mcg	Vitamin B12 mcg	Sodium mg	Potassium mg	Calcium mg	Iron mg	Zinc mg
Total																				

NAME: _____   ID#: _____

SUMMARY FORM

Day	Calories	Protein g	Carbohydrate g	Fiber g	Fat g	Saturated Fat g	Cholesterol mg	Vitamin A RE	Vitamin C mg	Thiamin mg	Niacin NE	Folate mcg	Vitamin B12 mcg	Sodium mg	Potassium mg	Calcium mg	Iron mg	Zinc mg
1																		
2																		
3																		
Total																		
Average daily intake (divide total by 3)		A_1	B_1		C_1	D_1												

COMPARISON FORM

Day	Calories	Protein g	Carbohydrate g	Fiber g	Fat % kcal	Saturated Fat % kcal	Cholesterol mg	Vitamin A RE	Vitamin C mg	Thiamin mg	Niacin NE	Folate mcg	Vitamin B12 mcg	Sodium mg	Potassium mg	Calcium mg	Iron mg	Zinc mg
Average daily intake (from above)	E^*	F^*			C_3^*	D_3^*												
Standard[a]			■	25g	30%	10%	300 mg							1500 mg	4700 mg			
Intake as percentage of standard[b]			■															

[a] Taken from RDA Tables. Be sure to use the appropriate gender and age RDAs.

* Use the calculation for your energy and protein requirements percent of calories as fat and saturated fat—from the Calculation Page.

[b] For example, if your protein intake was 50 g and the standard for a person your age was 46 g, then you consumed $(50/46) \times 100 = 109\%$ of the RDA.

Remember to circle values < 100% of standard. Check your values to make sure they *make sense!*

NAME: _____ ID# _____

1. Calculate your Basal Metabolic Rate (BMR)

> To convert weight from pounds to kilograms, divide weight in pounds by 2.2. For example, to convert 165 pounds to kilograms, divide 165 by 2.2 to get 75 kg:
> 165 lb ÷ 2.2 lb/kg = 75 kg

Sex: Male _____   Female _____

Body Weight (BW):   Pounds _____   Kg _____ (1 kg = 2.2 pounds)

Male: 1.0 kcal/kg•hr × BW (kg) × 24 hr/day = **BMR** = _____ **kcal/day**

Female: 0.9 kcal/kg•hr × BW (kg) × 24 hr/day = **BMR** = _____ **kcal/day**

2. Calculate your Daily Energy Requirement

Account for Activity: _____ × _____ = _____
                                                BMR $Activity\ level\ (see\ below)*$ $kcal\ for\ activity$

Thermic Effect of Food (TEF): _____ × 0.05 = _____
                                   $(BMR + kcal\ for\ activity)$ TEF

Energy Requirement: _____ + _____ + _____ = _____ ^{E} **kcal/day**
                         BMR $kcal\ for\ activity$ TEF $TOTAL$

> Transfer this number to the Comparison Form for your energy standard

ACTIVITY LEVEL BY ESTIMATION

Sedentary	30% of BMR	Moderate Activity	70% of BMR
Light Activity	50% of BMR	Strenuous Activity	100% of BMR

* For example, for Sedentary activity, enter .30 in the space for Activity level, for Light Activity, enter .50 in the space for Activity level, etc.

3. Calculate your Daily Protein Requirement

> Transfer this number to the Comparison Form for your protein standard

0.8 grams × _____ kg BW = _____ ^{F} grams protein/day

4. Calculate your Energy Intake Distribution

For each nutrient, use the average grams per day calculated on the Summary Form.

_____ ^{A_1} grams × 4 kcal/gram = _____ ^{A_2} **kcal Protein (P)**
$Protein$

_____ ^{B_1} grams × 4 kcal/gram = _____ ^{B_2} **kcal Carbohydrate (CHO)**
$Carbohydrate$

_____ ^{C_1} grams × 9 kcal/gram = _____ ^{C_2} **kcal Fat (F)**
Fat

Total Calculated Energy = _____ ^{D_2} **kcal/day**
                               $(P + CHO + F)$

Note: kcal = calories

5. Calculate your % Energy Distribution

Use the data from #4 above.

_____ ^{A_2} kcal P   ÷ _____ ^{D_2} total kcal × 100 = _____ ^{A_3} **% kcal from P**
                              $(P + CHO + F)$

_____ ^{B_2} kcal CHO ÷ _____ ^{D_2} total kcal × 100 = _____ ^{B_3} **% kcal from CHO**
                              $(P + CHO + F)$

_____ ^{C_2} kcal F   ÷ _____ ^{D_2} total kcal × 100 = _____ ^{C_3} **% kcal from F**
                              $(P + CHO + F)$

> Transfer this number to the Comparison Form for your average % kcal fat & % saturated fat

6. Calculate % kcal as Saturated Fat

_____ grams saturated fat × 9 kcal/g = (_____ kcal) ÷ (_____ total kcal **(from #4)**) × 100 = _____ % kcal
D_1 D_2 $Saturated\ Fat$ D_3

EXTRA FOOD FORM

NAME: _____

ID#: _____

Day: _____

(Use one form for each day)

Food	Amount	Calories	Protein g	Carbohydrate g	Fiber g	Fat g	Saturated Fat g	Cholesterol mg	Vitamin A RE	Vitamin C mg	Thiamin mg	Niacin NE	Folate mcg	Vitamin B12 mcg	Sodium mg	Potassium mg	Calcium mg	Iron mg	Zinc mg
Total																			

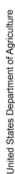

United States Department of Agriculture

MyPlate Daily Checklist

Find your Healthy Eating Style

Everything you eat and drink matters. Find your healthy eating style that reflects your preferences, culture, traditions, and budget—and maintain it for a lifetime! The right mix can help you be healthier now and into the future. The key is choosing a variety of foods and beverages from each food group—*and making sure that each choice is limited in saturated fat, sodium, and added sugars.* Start with small changes—**"MyWins"**—to make healthier choices you can enjoy.

Food Group Amounts for 2,000 Calories a Day

Fruits	Vegetables	Grains	Protein	Dairy
2 cups	**2 1/2 cups**	**6 ounces**	**5 1/2 ounces**	**3 cups**
Focus on whole fruits	**Vary your veggies**	**Make half your grains whole grains**	**Vary your protein routine**	**Move to low-fat or fat-free milk or yogurt**
Focus on whole fruits that are fresh, frozen, canned, or dried.	Choose a variety of colorful fresh, frozen, and canned vegetables—make sure to include dark green, red, and orange choices.	Find whole-grain foods by reading the Nutrition Facts label and ingredients list.	Mix up your protein foods to include seafood, beans and peas, unsalted nuts and seeds, soy products, eggs, and lean meats and poultry.	Choose fat-free milk, yogurt, and soy beverages (soy milk) to cut back on your saturated fat.

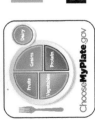

Limit

Drink and eat less sodium, saturated fat, and added sugars. Limit:

- Sodium to **2,300 milligrams** a day.
- Saturated fat to **22 grams** a day.
- Added sugars to **50 grams** a day.

Be active your way: Children 6 to 17 years old should move 60 minutes every day. Adults should be physically active at least 2 1/2 hours per week.
Use SuperTracker to create a personal plan based on your age, sex, height, weight, and physical activity level.
SuperTracker.usda.gov

MyPlate Daily Checklist

Write down the foods you ate today and track your daily MyPlate, MyWins!

Food group targets for a 2,000 calorie* pattern are:

Food group	Target	Write your food choices for each food group	Did you reach your target?
Fruits	**2 cups** 1 cup of fruits counts as • 1 cup raw or cooked fruit; or • 1/2 cup dried fruit; or • 1 cup 100% fruit juice.	_____ _____ _____ _____ _____	Y N
Vegetables	**2 1/2 cups** 1 cup vegetables counts as • 1 cup raw or cooked vegetables; or • 2 cups leafy salad greens; or • 1 cup 100% vegetable juice.	_____ _____ _____ _____ _____	Y N
Grains	**6 ounce equivalents** 1 ounce of grains counts as • 1 slice bread; or • 1 ounce ready-to-eat cereal; or • 1/2 cup cooked rice, pasta, or cereal.	_____ _____ _____ _____ _____	Y N
Protein	**5 1/2 ounce equivalents** 1 ounce of protein counts as • 1 ounce lean meat, poultry, or seafood; or • 1 egg; or • 1 Tbsp peanut butter; or • 1/4 cup cooked beans or peas; or • 1/2 ounce nuts or seeds.	_____ _____ _____ _____ _____	Y N
Dairy	**3 cups** 1 cup of dairy counts as • 1 cup milk; or • 1 cup yogurt; or • 1 cup fortified soy beverage; or • 1 1/2 ounces natural cheese or 2 ounces processed cheese.	_____ _____ _____ _____ _____	Y N

Limit:
• Sodium to **2,300 milligrams** a day.
• Saturated fat to **22 grams** a day.
• Added sugars to **50 grams** a day.

Y　N

Be active your way:

Adults:
• Be physically active at least **2 1/2 hours** per week.

Children 6 to 17 years old:
• Move at least **60 minutes** every day.

Y　N

MyWins — Track your MyPlate, MyWins

_____
_____

*This 2,000 calorie pattern is only an estimate of your needs. Monitor your body weight and adjust your calories if needed.

Center for Nutrition Policy and Promotion
January 2016
USDA is an equal opportunity provider and employer.

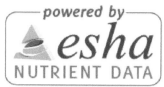

Food Name	Amount	Measure	Weight (g)	Calories	Protein (g)	Total Carb (g)	Dietary Fiber (g)	Total Fat (g)	Sat Fat (g)	Mono Fat (g)	Poly Fat (g)	Chol (mg)	Vit A (mcg RAE)	Vit D (mcg)
BEVERAGE AND BEVERAGE MIXES														
Carbonated Drinks														
Drink, lemonade, cnd, Country Time	1	Cup	247.20	90.00	0.00	23.00	0.00	0.00	0.00	0.00	0.00		0.00	
Soda, 7 Up	1	Cup	240.00	100.00	0.00	26.00	0.00	0.00	0.00	0.00	0.00	0.00	0.00	
Soda, club	1	Cup	236.80	0.00	0.00	0.00	0.00	0.00	0.00	0.00	0.00	0.00	0.00	
Soda, Coca Cola/Coke	1	Cup	246.00	102.67	0.00	26.67	0.00	0.00	0.00	0.00	0.00	0.00	0.00	0.00
Soda, Coca Cola/Coke, diet	1	Cup	239.50	1.00	0.00	0.08	0.00	0.00	0.00	0.00	0.00	0.00	0.00	0.00
Soda, cola	1	Cup	248.00	104.16	0.12	26.66	0.00	0.00	0.00	0.00	0.00	0.00	0.00	
Soda, cola Pepsi	1	Cup	240.00	100.00	0.00	27.33	0.00	0.00	0.00	0.00	0.00	0.00	0.00	
Soda, cola, diet Pepsi	1	Cup	240.00	0.00	0.00	0.00	0.00	0.00	0.00	0.00	0.00	0.00	0.00	
Soda, cola, diet, caff free Pepsi	1	Cup	240.00	0.00	0.00	0.00	0.00	0.00	0.00	0.00	0.00	0.00	0.00	
Soda, cola, diet, w/asp	1	Cup	236.80	2.37	0.24	0.24	0.00	0.00	0.00	0.00	0.00	0.00	0.00	
Soda, cream	1	Cup	247.20	126.07	0.00	32.88	0.00	0.00	0.00	0.00	0.00	0.00	0.00	
Soda, Dr Pepper	1	Cup	246.00	100.00	0.00	27.00	0.00	0.00	0.00	0.00	0.00		0.00	
Soda, ginger ale	1	Cup	244.00	82.96	0.00	21.40	0.00	0.00	0.00	0.00	0.00	0.00	0.00	
Soda, ginger ale, diet, Schweppes	1	Cup	246.70	0.00	0.00	0.00	0.00	0.00	0.00	0.00	0.00	0.00	0.00	
Soda, grape	1	Cup	248.00	106.64	0.00	27.78	0.00	0.00	0.00	0.00	0.00	0.00	0.00	
Soda, lemon lime	1	Cup	245.60	98.24	0.00	25.54	0.00	0.00	0.00	0.00	0.00	0.00	0.00	
Soda, lemon lime, dietSlice	1	Cup	240.00	2.67	0.00	0.67	0.00	0.00	0.00	0.00	0.00	0.00	0.00	
Soda, not cola/pepper, diet, w/sacc	1	Cup	236.80	0.00	0.00	0.24	0.00	0.00	0.00	0.00	0.00	0.00	0.00	0.00
Soda, orange	1	Cup	248.00	119.04	0.00	30.50	0.00	0.00	0.00	0.00	0.00	0.00	0.00	
Soda, pepper type, w/caff	1	Cup	245.60	100.70	0.00	25.54	0.00	0.25	0.17	0.00	0.00	0.00	0.00	
Soda, root beer	1	Cup	246.40	101.02	0.00	26.12	0.00	0.00	0.00	0.00	0.00	0.00	0.00	
Coffee and Substitutes														
Coffee, brewed, prep w/tap water	1	Cup	237.00	2.37	0.28	0.00	0.00	0.05	0.00	0.04	0.00	0.00	0.00	
Coffee, cappuccino, w/lowfat milk, double, tall Starbucks	1.5	Cup	244.00	110.00	8.00	11.00	0.00	3.50	2.50			15.00		
Coffee, cappuccino, w/whole milk, tall Starbucks	1.5	Cup	244.00	140.00	7.00	11.00	0.00	7.00	4.50			30.00		
Coffee, decaf, inst, prep w/water	1	Cup	179.00	3.58	0.21	0.77	0.00	0.00	0.00	0.00	0.00	0.00	0.00	
Coffee, espresso	1	Cup	240.00	21.60	0.02	3.67	0.00	0.43	0.22	0.00	0.22	0.00	0.00	0.00
Coffee, frappuccino, mocha, tall Starbucks	1.5	Cup	311.00	230.00	6.00	44.00	0.00	3.00	2.00			0.00		
Coffee, latte, iced, w/lowfat milk, double, tall Starbucks	1.5	Cup	392.00	90.00	7.00	10.00	0.00	3.00	2.00			15.00		
Coffee, latte, w/nonfat milk, double, tall Starbucks	1.5	Cup	367.00	120.00	12.00	17.00	0.00	0.50	0.00			5.00		
Coffee, latte, w/whole milk, double, tall Starbucks	1.5	Cup	366.00	210.00	11.00	17.00	0.00	11.00	7.00			45.00		
Coffee, mocha cappuccino, decaf, inst, dry pkt Maxwell House	1	Each	23.00	100.00	2.00	17.00	0.00	2.50	1.00			0.00	0.00	
Coffee, reg, inst, prep w/water	1	Cup	238.40	4.77	0.24	0.81	0.00	0.01	0.00	0.00	0.00	0.00	0.00	
Dairy Mixed Drinks and Mixes														
Drink, chocolate, dairy, rducd cal, w/asp, dry pkt, .75oz	1	Each	21.30	63.47	5.32	10.69	2.00	0.55	0.40	0.11	0.01	5.11	33.23	1.00
Drink, chocolate, dry mix	2.5	Teaspoon	21.60	75.38	0.71	19.50	0.95	0.67	0.40	0.22	0.02	0.00		
Drink, chocolate, prep f/dry mix w/milk	1	Cup	266.00	226.10	8.59	31.68	1.06	8.62	4.95	2.21	0.49	23.94	69.16	
Drink, strawberry, prep f/dry mix w/milk	1	Cup	266.00	234.08	7.98	32.72	0.00	8.25	5.08	2.36	0.30	31.92	69.16	2.66
Eggnog Darigold	0.5	Cup	128.83	180.00	3.00	22.00	0.00	9.00	5.00			70.00		0.00
Hot Cocoa, dry pkt Swiss Miss	1	Each	28.00	120.00	2.00	22.00	1.00	3.00	1.00			0.00	0.00	
Hot Cocoa, prep f/dry mix w/water	1	Cup	274.67	151.07	2.22	31.97	1.37	1.51	0.90	0.50	0.05	2.75		
Hot Cocoa, prep f/recipe w/milk	1	Cup	250.00	192.50	8.80	26.58	2.50	5.82	3.58	1.69	0.08	20.00	127.50	2.48
Hot Cocoa, rich chocolate, dry pkt Nestle	1	Each	28.00	112.00	1.30	24.24	0.67	1.11	0.29	0.35	0.27	1.68	0.00	1.96
Hot Cocoa, rich chocolate, w/o add sugar, dry pkt Nestle	1	Each	15.00	54.75	4.30	8.43	0.75	0.43	0.20	0.14	0.01	2.85	0.00	1.05

Vit E (mg)	Vit C	Vit B$_1$ Thia (mg)	Vit B$_2$ Ribo (mg)	Vit B$_3$ Nia (mg)	Fol (mcg)	Vit B$_6$ (mg)	Vita B$_{12}$ (mcg)	Sodi (mg)	Pota (mg)	Cal (mg)	Phos (mg)	Magn (mg)	Iron (mg)	Zinc (mg)	Caff (mg)	Alco (g)	Sol Fiber (g)	Insol Fiber (g)
	0.00							90.00							0.00	0.00	0.00	0.00
	0.00						0.00	50.00			45.00				0.00	0.00	0.00	0.00
0.00	0.00	0.00	0.00	0.00	0.00	0.00	0.00	49.73	4.74	11.84	0.00	2.37	0.02	0.24	0.00	0.00	0.00	0.00
0.00	0.00	0.00	0.00	0.00	0.00	0.00	0.00	5.33	2.46	7.38	36.00	2.46	0.07	0.02	30.67	0.00	0.00	0.00
0.00	0.00							4.00	12.00		18.00				31.00	0.00	0.00	0.00
0.00	0.00	0.00	0.00	0.00	0.00	0.00	0.00	9.92	2.48	7.44	32.24	2.48	0.05	0.02	24.80	0.00	0.00	0.00
	0.00						0.00	23.33		0.00	35.33		0.00		24.67	0.00	0.00	0.00
	0.00						0.00	23.33	5.33	0.00	27.33		0.00		24.00	0.00	0.00	0.00
	0.00						0.00	23.33		0.00	27.33		0.00		0.00	0.00	0.00	0.00
0.00	0.00	0.01	0.05	0.00	0.00	0.00	0.00	11.84	14.21	7.11	26.05	2.37	0.07	0.00	33.15	0.00	0.00	0.00
0.00	0.00	0.00	0.00	0.00	0.00	0.00	0.00	29.66	2.47	12.36	0.00	2.47	0.12	0.17	0.00	0.00	0.00	0.00
	0.00							35.00							27.20	0.00	0.00	0.00
0.00	0.00	0.00	0.00	0.00	0.00	0.00	0.00	17.08	2.44	7.32	0.00	2.44	0.44	0.12	0.00	0.00	0.00	0.00
	0.00							60.00							0.00	0.00	0.00	0.00
0.00	0.00	0.00	0.00	0.00	0.00	0.00	0.00	37.20	2.48	7.44	0.00	2.48	0.20	0.17	0.00	0.00	0.00	0.00
0.00	0.00	0.00	0.00	0.04	0.00	0.00	0.00	27.02	2.46	4.91	0.00	2.46	0.17	0.12	0.00	0.00	0.00	0.00
	0.00						0.00	23.33		0.00	0.00		0.00		0.00	0.00	0.00	0.00
0.00	0.00	0.00	0.00	0.00	0.00	0.00	0.00	37.89	4.74	9.47	0.00	2.37	0.09	0.12	26.05	0.00	0.00	0.00
0.00	0.00	0.00	0.00	0.00	0.00	0.00	0.00	29.76	4.96	12.40	2.48	2.48	0.15	0.25	0.00	0.00	0.00	0.00
0.00	0.00	0.00	0.00	0.00	0.00	0.00	0.00	24.56	2.46	7.37	27.02	0.00	0.10	0.10	24.56	0.00	0.00	0.00
0.00	0.00	0.00	0.00	0.00	0.00	0.00	0.00	32.03	2.46	12.32	0.00	2.46	0.12	0.17	0.00	0.00	0.00	0.00
0.02	0.00	0.03	0.18	0.45	4.74	0.00	0.00	4.74	116.13	4.74	7.11	7.11	0.02	0.05	94.80	0.00	0.00	0.00
	2.40							110.00		250.00			0.00		180.00	0.00	0.00	0.00
	2.40							105.00		250.00			0.00		90.00	0.00	0.00	0.00
0.00	0.00	0.00	0.03	0.50	0.00	0.00	0.00	3.58	82.34	5.37	7.16	8.95	0.11	0.00	1.79	0.00	0.00	0.00
0.00	0.48	0.00	0.42	12.50	2.40	0.00	0.00	33.60	276.00	4.80	16.80	192.00	0.31	0.12	168.00	0.00	0.00	0.00
	0.00							180.00		100.00			0.00		130.00	0.00	0.00	0.00
	1.20							100.00		250.00			0.00		180.00	0.00	0.00	0.00
	3.60							170.00		400.00			0.00		180.00	0.00	0.00	0.00
	3.60							170.00		400.00			0.00		180.00	0.00	0.00	0.00
	0.00						0.00	70.00	150.00	60.00			0.00				0.00	0.00
0.00	0.00	0.00	0.00	0.56	0.00	0.00	0.00	4.77	71.52	9.54	7.15	7.15	0.10	0.02	61.98	0.00	0.00	0.00
0.00	1.19	0.02	0.41	0.27	7.03	0.02	0.51	140.37	477.12	300.76	190.21	44.73	1.64	0.77	3.83	0.00		
0.01	0.15	0.01	0.03	0.11	1.51	0.00	0.00	45.36	127.66	7.99	27.65	21.17	0.68	0.33	7.78	0.00		
0.16	0.27	0.11	0.48	0.38	13.30	0.09	1.06	154.28	457.52	252.70	234.08	47.88	0.80	1.28	7.98	0.00		
0.27	2.39	0.09	0.42	0.22	13.30	0.10	0.88	127.68	369.74	292.60	228.76	31.92	0.21	0.93	0.00	0.00	0.00	0.00
	0.00							105.00		100.00			1.20		0.00	0.00	0.00	0.00
	0.00							130.00		40.00			1.08		0.00			
0.19	0.55	0.04	0.21	0.22	0.00	0.04	0.49	195.02	269.18	60.43	118.11	32.96	0.47	0.58	5.49	0.00		
0.08	0.50	0.10	0.45	0.33	12.50	0.10	1.05	110.00	492.50	262.50	262.50	57.50	1.20	1.58	5.00	0.00		
0.04	0.00	0.03	0.12	0.16	1.96	0.03	0.10	101.64	194.32	40.04	70.84	27.44	0.28	0.36	5.04	0.00		
0.01	0.41	0.06	0.22	0.18	5.85	0.05	0.45	142.05	288.15	123.45	135.00	27.00	0.39	0.60	15.75	0.00		

Food Name	Amount	Measure	Weight (g)	Calories	Protein (g)	Total Carb (g)	Dietary Fiber (g)	Total Fat (g)	Sat Fat (g)	Mono Fat (g)	Poly Fat (g)	Chol (mg)	Vit A (mcg RAE)	Vit D (mcg)
BEVERAGE AND BEVERAGE MIXES *(continued)*														
Hot Cocoa, w/asp add sod & vit A, prep f/dry w/water	1	Cup	256.00	74.24	3.23	13.93	1.28	0.59	0.01	0.19	0.02	0.00	35.84	
Hot Cocoa, w/marshmallows, dry pkt Nestle	1	Each	28.00	111.72	1.35	24.25	0.50	1.02	0.39	0.29	0.35	1.68	0.00	1.96
Instant Breakfast, chocolate malt, prep f/dry w/skm mlk Carnation	9	Fluid ounce	280.44	220.00	12.50	39.00	1.00	1.95	1.00			6.00		2.50
Instant Breakfast, milk chocolate, creamy, rtd, 10 fl oz can Carnation	10	Fluid ounce	314.00	220.00	12.00	37.00	2.00	2.50	1.00			10.00		2.51
Kefir, European	1	Cup	233.20	149.24	7.70	11.20	0.00	8.16						
Malt Beverage	1	Cup	236.80	87.62	0.50	19.06	0.00	0.28	0.06	0.04	0.13	0.00	0.24	
Malted Milk, chocolate, dry mix	3	Teaspoon	21.00	78.75	1.07	18.44	1.41	0.80	0.45	0.22	0.07	0.21	0.84	0.03
Malted Milk, chocolate, prep w/milk f/dry mix	1	Cup	265.00	225.25	8.93	29.68	1.33	8.72	4.99	2.19	0.55	26.50	68.90	
Malted Milk, chocolate, w/add nutrients, prep f/dry mix	1	Cup	265.00	222.60	8.90	28.94	1.06	8.64	4.95	2.17	0.54	26.50	903.65	
Malted Milk, natural, w/add nutrients, prep f/pwd w/milk	1	Cup	265.00	227.90	9.73	28.28	0.00	8.51	4.85	2.13	0.56	29.15	744.65	
Juice and Fruit Flavored Drinks														
Drink, breakfast, orange, prep f/pwd	1	Cup	248.00	121.52	0.00	31.37	0.25	0.00	0.00	0.00	0.00	0.00	190.96	
Drink, cherry, sug free, prep f/dry mix, 1/8 pkg Kool-Aid	1	Cup	237.00	5.00	0.00	0.00	0.00	0.00	0.00	0.00	0.00	0.00	0.00	
Drink, cherry, sug free, w/asp & Vit C, dry pkg Kool-Aid	1	Each	9.60	27.84	0.59	8.15		0.03						
Drink, cherry, unswtnd, dry pkg Kool-Aid	0.125	Each	0.50	0.00	0.00	0.00	0.00	0.00	0.00	0.00	0.00	0.00	0.00	
Drink, diet, kiwi strawberry Snapple	1	Cup	251.70	20.00	0.00	5.00		0.00	0.00	0.00	0.00	0.00		
Drink, fruit punch, cnd	1	Cup	248.00	116.56	0.00	29.69	0.50	0.01	0.00	0.00	0.01	0.00	4.96	
Drink, fruit punch, dry mix Crystal Light	0.5	Teaspoon	1.20	5.00	0.00	0.00	0.00	0.00	0.00	0.00	0.00	0.00	0.00	
Drink, fruit punch, prep f/fzn conc w/water	1	Cup	247.20	113.71	0.15	28.82	0.25	0.01	0.00	0.00	0.00	0.00	1.36	
Drink, fruit punch, sug free, low cal, rtd Crystal Light	1	Cup	241.00	5.00	0.00	0.00	0.00	0.00	0.00	0.00	0.00	0.00	0.00	
Drink, fruit, low cal	1	Cup	240.00	43.20	0.00	11.28	0.00	0.00	0.00	0.00	0.00	0.00	1.20	0.00
Drink, Island Punch Snapple	1	Cup	251.70	110.00	0.00	27.00		0.00	0.00	0.00	0.00	0.00		
Drink, lemonade, low cal, w/asp, prep f/pwd w/water	1	Cup	236.80	4.74	0.05	1.23	0.00	0.00	0.00	0.00	0.00	0.00	0.00	
Drink, lemonade, prep f/pwd w/water	1	Cup	264.00	102.96	0.00	26.85	0.00	0.00	0.00	0.00	0.00	0.00	0.00	
Drink, lemonade, sug free, low cal, rtd Crystal Light	1	Cup	241.00	5.00	0.00	0.00	0.00	0.00	0.00	0.00	0.00	0.00	0.00	
Drink, orange, cnd	1	Cup	248.00	126.48	0.00	31.99	0.00	0.02	0.00	0.00	0.01	0.00	2.48	
Gelatin, drinking, orange, prep f/pwd pkt w/water	1	Cup	240.00	117.60	10.80	18.48	0.00	0.48	0.05	0.09	0.22	0.00	0.00	
Juice Drink, citrus fruit, prep f/fzn conc w/water	1	Cup	248.00	124.00	0.45	30.23	0.25	0.12	0.00	0.00	0.00	0.00	2.48	
Juice Drink, cranberry apple, 10% juice Everfresh	1	Cup	236.40	120.00	0.00	31.00	0.00	0.00	0.00	0.00	0.00	0.00		
Juice Drink, cranberry apple, btld	1	Cup	244.80	173.81	0.17	44.33	0.24	0.12	0.00	0.00	0.00	0.00	0.37	
Juice Drink, cranberry apple, w/vit, low cal	1	Cup	240.00	45.60	0.24	11.28	0.24	0.00	0.00	0.00	0.00	0.00	0.36	0.00
Juice Drink, cranberry raspberry Snapple	1	Cup	251.70	120.00	0.00	29.00		0.00	0.00	0.00	0.00	0.00		
Juice Drink, fruit punch, prep f/fzn conc w/water	1	Cup	248.00	124.00	0.25	30.26	0.25	0.50	0.06	0.06	0.12	0.00	0.74	0.00
Juice Drink, grape, cnd	1	Cup	250.40	125.20	0.25	32.00	0.00	0.00	0.00	0.00	0.00	0.00	0.25	
Juice Drink, kiwi strawberry, rtd Snapple	1	Cup	244.00	117.12	0.24	28.79	0.00	0.00	0.00	0.00	0.00	0.00	0.00	
Juice Drink, Mango Madness Snapple	1	Cup	251.70	110.00	0.00	29.00		0.00	0.00	0.00	0.00	0.00		
Juice Drink, pineapple grapefruit, cnd	1	Cup	250.40	117.69	0.50	29.05	0.25	0.25	0.02	0.03	0.07	0.00	0.13	
Juice Drink, pineapple orange, cnd	1	Cup	250.40	125.20	3.26	29.55	0.25	0.00	0.00	0.00	0.00	0.00	2.50	
Juice Drink, raspberry peach Snapple	1	Cup	251.70	120.00	0.00	29.00		0.00	0.00	0.00	0.00	0.00		
Juice, Snapple Farms, apple juice Snapple	1	Cup	251.68	120.00	0.00	29.33		0.00	0.00	0.00	0.00	0.00		
Lemonade, pink, prep f/fzn conc w/water	1	Cup	247.20	98.88	0.25	25.96	0.00	0.05	0.01	0.00	0.03	0.00	0.25	0.00
Lemonade, white, prep f/fzn conc w/water	1	Cup	248.00	131.44	0.22	34.05	0.25	0.15	0.02	0.00	0.04	0.00	0.25	
Limeade, prep f/fzn conc w/water	1	Cup	247.20	103.82	0.10	26.13	0.00	0.02	0.00	0.00	0.00	0.00	0.12	

Vit E (mg)	Vit C	Vit B₁ Thia (mg)	Vit B₂ Ribo (mg)	Vit B₃ Nia (mg)	Fol (mcg)	Vit B₆ (mg)	Vita B₁₂ (mcg)	Sodi (mg)	Pota (mg)	Cal (mg)	Phos (mg)	Magn (mg)	Iron (mg)	Zinc (mg)	Caff (mg)	Alco (g)	Sol Fiber (g)	Insol Fiber (g)
0.08	0.26	0.05	0.28	0.22	2.56	0.06	0.33	227.84	540.16	120.32	179.20	43.52	1.00	0.69	2.56	0.00		
0.04	0.00	0.03	0.12	0.10	1.12	0.03	0.12	96.04	141.96	41.16	57.96	16.24	0.24	0.20	2.24	0.00		
6.82	30.00	0.38	0.43	5.00	100.00	0.50	1.50	264.00		500.00	250.00	100.00	4.50	3.75		0.00		
6.85	30.00	0.38	0.44	5.02	100.48	0.50	1.51	230.00	609.16	500.00	348.54	100.48	4.50	3.77		0.00		
								107.28	373.12		209.88	32.64	0.30		0.00	0.00	0.00	0.00
0.00	1.18	0.04	0.11	2.64	33.15	0.06	0.05	30.78	18.94	16.58	37.89	16.58	0.14	0.05	0.00	0.71	0.00	0.00
0.02	0.31	0.04	0.04	0.42	10.71	0.03	0.04	52.71	129.78	12.60	36.75	14.70	0.48	0.17	7.77	0.00		
0.16	0.27	0.14	0.49	0.69	23.85	0.12	1.11	159.00	455.80	259.70	241.15	39.75	0.56	1.09	7.95	0.00		
0.16	31.80	0.76	1.32	11.08	18.55	1.01	1.14	230.55	577.70	339.20	288.85	45.05	3.76	1.17	5.30	0.00		
0.32	27.56	0.73	1.21	10.58	15.90	0.86	1.06	190.80	530.00	325.95	283.55	39.75	3.60	1.09	0.00	0.00	0.00	0.00
0.00	73.16	0.00	0.22	2.54	0.00	0.25	0.00	9.92	59.52	126.48	47.12	2.48	0.02	0.02	0.00	0.00		
	6.00						0.00	5.00	0.00	0.00	0.00		0.00		0.00	0.00	0.00	0.00
	53.76						0.00	40.51	0.00	0.00			0.00		0.00	0.00		
	6.00						0.00	5.00	0.00	0.00			0.00		0.00	0.00	0.00	0.00
	0.00							10.00							0.00	0.00		
0.05	73.41	0.05	0.06	0.05	9.92	0.03	0.00	94.24	62.00	19.84	7.44	7.44	0.22	0.02	0.00	0.00		
	6.00						0.00	0.00	45.00	0.00					0.00	0.00	0.00	0.00
0.00	108.27	0.02	0.03	0.05	2.47	0.01	0.00	9.89	32.14	9.89	2.47	4.94	0.22	0.05	0.00	0.00		
	0.00							20.00	105.00	0.00	0.00		0.00		0.00	0.00	0.00	0.00
0.00	77.52	0.02	0.05	0.05	4.80	0.00	0.00	50.40	50.40	16.80	4.80	4.80	0.65	0.26	0.00	0.00	0.00	0.00
								10.00							0.00	0.00		
0.00	5.92	0.00	0.00	0.00	0.00	0.00	0.00	4.74	0.00	52.10	23.68	2.37	0.09	0.02	0.00	0.00	0.00	0.00
0.00	8.45	0.01	0.00	0.03	2.64	0.01	0.00	10.56	31.68	71.28	34.32	2.64	0.16	0.05	0.00	0.00	0.00	0.00
	0.00							20.00	160.00	0.00	0.00		0.00		0.00	0.00	0.00	0.00
0.05	84.57	0.01	0.01	0.08	9.92	0.02	0.00	39.68	44.64	14.88	2.48	4.96	0.69	0.22	0.00	0.00	0.00	0.00
0.00	89.04	0.00	0.00	0.00	0.00	0.00	0.00	57.60	4.80	4.80	0.00	2.40	0.00	0.05	0.00	0.00		
0.05	36.21	0.04	0.02	0.15	7.44	0.04	0.00	4.96	121.52	12.40	9.92	9.92	0.12	0.05	0.00	0.00		
								0.00							0.00	0.00	0.00	0.00
0.00	78.34	0.01	0.05	0.15	0.00	0.05	0.00	17.14	68.54	12.24	4.90	4.90	0.29	0.44	0.00	0.00		
0.00	76.80	0.00	0.05	0.14	0.00	0.05	0.00	4.80	64.80	16.80	7.20	4.80	0.14	0.10	0.00	0.00		
	0.00							10.00							0.00	0.00		
0.00	13.89	0.00	0.16	0.15	0.00	0.03	0.00	12.40	190.96	17.36	0.00	9.92	0.57	0.55	0.00	0.00		
0.00	40.06	0.02	0.03	0.17	2.50	0.04	0.00	2.50	82.63	7.51	10.02	7.51	0.25	0.05	0.00	0.00	0.00	0.00
	0.00							7.32		0.00			0.37		0.00	0.00	0.00	0.00
	0.00							10.00							0.00	0.00		
0.03	115.18	0.08	0.04	0.67	22.54	0.11	0.00	35.06	152.74	17.53	15.02	15.02	0.78	0.15	0.00	0.00		
0.08	56.34	0.08	0.05	0.52	22.54	0.12	0.00	7.51	115.18	12.52	10.02	15.02	0.68	0.15	0.00	0.00		
	0.00							10.00							0.00	0.00		
	0.00							26.67							0.00	0.00		
0.00	9.64	0.01	0.05	0.04	4.94	0.01	0.00	7.42	37.08	7.42	4.94	4.94	0.40	0.10	0.00	0.00	0.00	0.00
0.02	12.90	0.02	0.07	0.05	2.48	0.02	0.00	7.44	49.60	9.92	7.44	4.96	0.52	0.07	0.00	0.00		
0.00	5.93	0.00	0.01	0.02	2.47	0.01	0.00	4.94	22.25	7.42	2.47	2.47	0.02	0.02	0.00	0.00	0.00	0.00

Food Name	Amount	Measure	Weight (g)	Calories	Protein (g)	Total Carb (g)	Dietary Fiber (g)	Total Fat (g)	Sat Fat (g)	Mono Fat (g)	Poly Fat (g)	Chol (mg)	Vit A (mcg RAE)	Vit D (mcg)
BEVERAGE AND BEVERAGE MIXES *(continued)*														
Other Beverages														
Cocktail Mix, Bloody Mary, tabasco tomato, mild McIlhenny Company	8	Fluid ounce	242.00	55.66	2.18	11.86	0.97	0.00	0.00	0.00	0.00			
Drink, apple cider, spiced, inst, dry pkt Swiss Miss	1	Each	22.00	90.00	0.00	21.00	0.00	0.00	0.00	0.00	0.00	0.00	0.00	
Drink, energy, sugar free, can USDA SR-23 Red Bull	8.3	Fluid ounce	250.00	12.50	0.62	1.75	0.00	0.20				0.00	0.00	0.00
Drink, energy, zesty flax, dry mix Natural Ovens	1	Tablespoon	10.00	40.00	2.00	5.00	3.00	2.00	0.50		1.00	0.00	0.00	
Drink, sports, Powerade, lemon lime, rtd, svg USDA SR-23 Coca Cola	8	Fluid ounce	244.00	78.08	0.00	19.13	0.00	0.12	0.02	0.03	0.07	0.00	0.00	0.00
Teas														
Tea, brewed w/tap water	1	Cup	236.80	2.37	0.00	0.71	0.00	0.02	0.00	0.00	0.01	0.00	0.00	
Tea, chai, original, brewed w/water only Celestial Seasonings	1	Cup	236.80	0.00	0.00	0.00	0.00	0.00	0.00	0.00	0.00	0.00	0.00	
Tea, green, brewed Hain Celestial Group Celestial Seasonings	1	Cup	236.80	0.00	0.00	0.00	0.00	0.00	0.00	0.00	0.00	0.00	0.00	
Tea, green Snapple	1	Cup	251.70	100.00	0.00	25.00		0.00	0.00	0.00	0.00	0.00	0.00	
Tea, herbal, not chamomile, brewed	1	Cup	236.80	2.37	0.00	0.47	0.00	0.02	0.00	0.00	0.01	0.00	0.00	
Tea, lemon flvr, diet, w/sacc, inst, prep f/pwd	1	Cup	236.80	4.74	0.05	1.04	0.00	0.00	0.00	0.00	0.00	0.00	0.00	
Tea, lemon flvr, unswtnd, inst, prep f/pwd	1	Cup	238.00	4.76	0.01	0.95	0.00	0.00	0.00	0.00	0.00	0.00	0.00	
Tea, lemon flvr, w/sug & vit C, inst, prep f/pwd	1	Cup	259.00	88.06	0.26	22.01	0.00	0.03	0.01	0.00	0.02	0.00	0.00	0.00
Tea, sweet, can Lipton Brisk	1	Cup	259.00	70.00	0.00	18.00	0.00	0.00	0.00	0.00	0.00	0.00	0.00	
Tea, unswtnd, inst, prep f/pwd	1	Cup	236.80	2.37	0.07	0.40	0.00	0.00	0.00	0.00	0.00	0.00	0.00	
Water														
Water, btld, Perrier	1	Cup	236.56	0.00	0.00	0.00	0.00	0.00	0.00	0.00	0.00	0.00	0.00	
Water, tonic	1	Cup	244.00	82.96	0.00	21.47	0.00	0.00	0.00	0.00	0.00	0.00	0.00	
BEVERAGES, ALCOHOLIC														
Aquavit, 80 proof	1	Fluid ounce	27.80	64.22	0.00	0.00	0.00	0.00	0.00	0.00	0.00	0.00	0.00	
Beer, can/btl, 12 fl oz	12	Fluid ounce	356.40	139.00	1.07	10.76	0.00	0.00	0.00	0.00	0.00	0.00	0.00	
Beer, golden draft, each Anheuser-Busch	12	Fluid ounce	356.00	149.91	1.59	12.81		0.00	0.00	0.00	0.00	0.00		
Beer, Light Coors	12	Fluid ounce	352.90	105.00	0.70	4.99	0.00	0.00	0.00	0.00	0.00	0.00	0.00	
Beer, light, can/btl, 12 fl oz	12	Fluid ounce	354.00	102.66	0.99	5.17	0.00	0.00	0.00	0.00	0.00	0.00	0.00	
Beer, Light, each Anheuser-Busch	12	Fluid ounce	356.00	110.00	1.20	6.60		0.00	0.00	0.00	0.00	0.00		
Beer, non alcoholic Coors	12	Fluid ounce	352.90	72.99	0.79	14.20	0.00	0.00	0.00	0.00	0.00	0.00		
Brandy, 80 proof	1	Fluid ounce	27.80	64.22	0.00	0.00	0.00	0.00	0.00	0.00	0.00	0.00	0.00	
Gin, 80 proof	1	Fluid ounce	27.80	64.22	0.00	0.00	0.00	0.00	0.00	0.00	0.00	0.00	0.00	
Liqueur, coffee, 53 proof	1	Fluid ounce	34.80	116.93	0.03	16.29	0.00	0.10	0.04	0.01	0.04	0.00	0.00	
Mixed Drink, daiquiri, 6.8 oz can	1	Each	207.40	259.25	0.00	32.56	0.00	0.00	0.00	0.00	0.00	0.00	0.21	0.00
Mixed Drink, margarita USDA Survey Database	1	Each	77.00	169.65	0.05	10.78	0.06	0.09	0.01	0.01	0.03	0.00	0.16	0.00
Mixed Drink, martini, prep f/recipe	1	Fluid ounce	28.20	68.53	0.01	0.58	0.00	0.00	0.00	0.00	0.00	0.00	0.00	
Mixed Drink, pina colada, cnd, 6.8 fl oz	1	Each	221.68	525.38	1.33	61.18	0.22	16.85	14.57	0.98	0.30	0.00	2.22	
Mixed Drink, whiskey sour, 6.8 fl oz can	1	Each	209.44	249.23	0.00	28.06	0.21	0.00	0.00	0.00	0.00	0.00	2.09	
Alcohol, rum, 80 proof USDA SR-23	1	Fluid ounce	27.80	64.22	0.00	0.00	0.00	0.00	0.00	0.00	0.00	0.00	0.00	0.00
Alcohol, rum, 86 proof USDA SR-23	1	Fluid ounce	27.80	69.50	0.00	0.03	0.00	0.00	0.00	0.00	0.00	0.00	0.00	0.00
Tequila, 80 proof	1	Fluid ounce	27.80	64.22	0.00	0.00	0.00	0.00	0.00	0.00	0.00	0.00	0.00	
Vodka, 80 proof	1	Fluid ounce	27.80	64.22	0.00	0.00	0.00	0.00	0.00	0.00	0.00	0.00	0.00	
Wine, all table types	6	Fluid ounce	177.00	136.29	0.35	5.66	0.00	0.00	0.00	0.00	0.00	0.00	0.00	
Wine, cooler	1	Cup	226.67	113.02	0.26	13.45	0.07	0.05	0.01	0.00	0.01	0.00	0.16	0.00
CANDIES AND CONFECTIONS, GUM														
Candy Bar, 3 Musketeers, 2.13 oz bar	1	Each	60.39	251.20	1.93	46.38	1.09	7.79	3.93	2.59	0.27	6.64	9.06	
Candy Bar, 5th Avenue, 2oz bar	1	Each	56.70	273.29	4.98	35.54	1.76	13.60	3.77	6.01	1.92	3.40	7.94	
Candy Bar, almond chocolate, Golden Collection, 2.8oz pkg	1	Each	79.38	458.02	10.18	36.63	3.02	30.53	13.23	14.05	3.10	10.32		
Candy Bar, Almond Joy, 1.7oz	1	Each	48.19	230.85	1.99	28.68	2.41	12.98	8.48	2.54	0.57	1.93		
Candy Bar, Baby Ruth, 2.1 oz bar	1	Each	59.53	276.24	4.23	36.79	1.43	14.88	7.32	3.84	1.97	1.19		

Vit E (mg)	Vit C	Vit B$_1$ Thia (mg)	Vit B$_2$ Ribo (mg)	Vit B$_3$ Nia (mg)	Fol (mcg)	Vit B$_6$ (mg)	Vita B$_{12}$ (mcg)	Sodi (mg)	Pota (mg)	Cal (mg)	Phos (mg)	Magn (mg)	Iron (mg)	Zinc (mg)	Caff (mg)	Alco (g)	Sol Fiber (g)	Insol Fiber (g)
								1173.70		60.50		1.74			0.00	0.00		
	0.00							60.00	0.00			0.00			0.00	0.00	0.00	0.00
0.00	0.00	0.06	1.44	21.25	0.00	4.99	4.97	97.50	7.50	32.50	0.00	7.50	0.05	0.00	75.00	0.00	0.00	0.00
	0.00	0.15	0.17	2.00	40.00	0.20	0.60	2.00		60.00		40.00	1.08	2.25	0.00	0.00		
0.00	0.00	0.03	0.00	3.82	0.00	0.37	3.34	53.68	43.92	2.44	2.44	0.00	0.22	0.02	0.00	0.00	0.00	0.00
0.00	0.00	0.00	0.03	0.00	11.84	0.00	0.00	7.10	87.62	0.00	2.37	7.10	0.05	0.05	47.36	0.00	0.00	0.00
	0.00							0.00		0.00			0.00		30.00	0.00	0.00	0.00
	0.00							0.00	25.00	0.00			0.00		40.00	0.00	0.00	0.00
	0.00							10.00							18.00	0.00		
0.00	0.00	0.02	0.01	0.00	2.37	0.00	0.00	2.37	21.31	4.74	0.00	2.37	0.19	0.09	0.00	0.00	0.00	0.00
0.00	0.00	0.00	0.00	0.05	0.00	0.00	0.00	23.68	30.78	7.10	2.37	2.37	0.12	0.02	16.58	0.00	0.00	0.00
0.00	0.00	0.00	0.02	0.09	0.00	0.00	0.00	14.28	49.98	4.76	2.38	4.76	0.02	0.07	26.18	0.00	0.00	0.00
0.00	23.31	0.00	0.05	0.09	10.36	0.01	0.00	7.77	49.21	5.18	2.59	5.18	0.05	0.08	28.49	0.00	0.00	0.00
	0.00							50.00		0.00			0.00		5.00	0.00	0.00	0.00
0.00	0.00	0.00	0.00	0.09	0.00	0.00	0.00	7.10	47.36	7.10	2.37	4.74	0.05	0.02	30.78	0.00	0.00	0.00
0.00	0.00	0.00	0.00	0.00	0.00	0.00	0.00	2.37	0.00	33.12	0.00	0.00	0.00	0.00	0.00	0.00	0.00	0.00
0.00	0.00	0.00	0.00	0.00	0.00	0.00	0.00	9.76	0.00	2.44	0.00	0.00	0.02	0.24	0.00	0.00	0.00	0.00
0.00	0.00	0.00	0.00	0.00	0.00	0.00	0.00	0.28	0.56	0.00	1.11	0.00	0.01	0.01	0.00	9.29	0.00	0.00
0.00	0.00	0.02	0.09	1.83	21.38	0.16	0.07	14.26	96.23	14.26	49.90	21.38	0.07	0.04	0.00	12.83	0.00	0.00
							0.00	8.94							0.00	13.50		
		0.03	0.03	1.41				10.99	59.00	10.99					0.00	14.11	0.00	0.00
0.00	0.00	0.02	0.05	1.38	21.24	0.12	0.32	14.16	74.34	14.16	42.48	17.70	0.11	0.04	0.00	10.97	0.00	0.00
	0.00		0.08	1.64		0.18	0.00	9.00	90.00	11.00	139.01	17.09			0.00	15.30		
		0.03	0.07	1.41				10.00	54.01	19.00					0.00	1.78		
0.00	0.00	0.00	0.00	0.00	0.00	0.00	0.00	0.28	0.56	0.00	1.11	0.00	0.01	0.01	0.00	9.29	0.00	0.00
0.00	0.00	0.00	0.00	0.00	0.00	0.00	0.00	0.28	0.56	0.00	1.11	0.00	0.01	0.01	0.00	9.29	0.00	0.00
0.00	0.00	0.00	0.00	0.05	0.00	0.00	0.00	2.78	10.44	0.35	2.09	1.04	0.02	0.01	9.05	7.55	0.00	0.00
0.00	2.70	0.00	0.00	0.03	2.07	0.01	0.00	82.96	22.81	0.00	4.15	2.07	0.02	0.06	0.00	19.91	0.00	0.00
0.01	0.99	0.01	0.00	0.04	1.23	0.00	0.00	4.05	15.16	1.97	3.81	1.35	0.06	0.03	0.00	18.50		
0.00	0.00	0.00	0.00	0.01	0.00	0.00	0.00	0.85	4.51	0.28	0.56	0.56	0.01	0.00	0.00	9.56	0.00	0.00
0.07	3.33	0.04	0.01	0.23	13.30	0.04	0.00	157.39	183.99	2.22	79.80	13.30	0.07	0.44	0.00	19.95		
0.00	3.35	0.02	0.01	0.04	0.00	0.00	0.00	92.15	23.04	0.00	12.57	2.09	0.02	0.13	0.00	19.90		
0.00	0.00	0.00	0.00	0.00	0.00	0.00	0.00	0.28	0.56	0.00	1.39	0.00	0.03	0.02	0.00	9.29	0.00	0.00
0.00	0.00	0.00	0.00	0.00	0.00	0.00	0.00	0.28	0.56	0.00	1.11	0.00	0.01	0.01	0.00	10.01	0.00	0.00
0.00	0.00	0.00	0.00	0.00	0.00	0.00	0.00	0.28	0.56	0.00	1.11	0.00	0.01	0.01	0.00	9.29	0.00	0.00
0.00	0.00	0.00	0.00	0.00	0.00	0.00	0.00	0.28	0.28	0.00	1.39	0.00	0.00	0.00	0.00	9.29	0.00	0.00
0.00	0.00	0.00	0.03	0.13	1.77	0.04	0.01	10.62	148.68	14.16	23.01	15.93	0.62	0.10	0.00	16.46	0.00	0.00
0.01	4.05	0.01	0.02	0.10	2.69	0.03	0.01	19.04	102.23	12.83	14.77	11.93	0.62	0.13	0.00	8.82		
0.56	0.24	0.02	0.08	0.14	0.00	0.01	0.11	117.15	80.31	50.72	54.95	17.51	0.44	0.33	4.83	0.00		
1.53	0.23	0.08	0.05	2.21	20.41	0.06	0.10	127.58	196.75	41.39	79.95	35.15	0.68	0.64	2.84	0.00		
0.48	0.00	0.05	0.42	0.84		0.04	0.34	50.80	373.88	152.41	214.33	88.11	1.47	1.35		0.00		
0.01	0.34	0.01	0.07	0.23		0.03	0.06	68.44	122.42	30.84	53.98	31.81	0.61	0.39		0.00		
1.11	0.06	0.06	0.05	1.65	18.46	0.04	0.02	127.40	211.94	26.79	82.16	43.46	0.42	0.71	2.38	0.00		

Food Name	Amount	Measure	Weight (g)	Calories	Protein (g)	Total Carb (g)	Dietary Fiber (g)	Total Fat (g)	Sat Fat (g)	Mono Fat (g)	Poly Fat (g)	Chol (mg)	Vit A (mcg RAE)	Vit D (mcg)
CANDIES AND CONFECTIONS, GUM (continued)														
Candy Bar, Butterfinger, 2.16oz bar	1	Each	61.24	291.48	3.55	44.39	1.04	11.63	6.27	2.99	1.51	0.00		
Candy Bar, Caramello, 1.6oz bar	1	Each	45.36	209.56	2.81	28.94	0.54	9.61	5.77	2.40	0.29	12.25		0.00
Candy Bar, carob, 3oz bar	1	Each	85.05	459.27	6.93	47.87	3.23	26.67	24.68	0.41	0.25	2.55		
Candy Bar, Chunky, 1.25oz bar	1	Each	35.44	175.42	3.19	20.23	1.70	10.35	8.23	0.11	1.56	3.90		
Candy Bar, Crunch, 0.5oz USDA SR-23 Nestle	1	Each	14.20	71.00	0.71	9.51	0.27	3.69	2.27			1.85		
Candy Bar, Kit Kat, 1.625oz bar	1	Each	46.07	238.64	3.00	29.76	0.46	11.97	8.27	2.69	0.41	5.07	11.06	
Candy Bar, Krackel, 2.2oz bar	1	Each	62.37	319.33	4.13	39.89	1.37	16.58	9.93	3.90	0.36	6.86		
Candy Bar, Mars almond, 1.76oz bar	1	Each	50.00	233.50	4.05	31.35	1.00	11.50	3.63	5.35	1.99	8.50	7.50	
Candy Bar, milk chocolate, w/almonds, bites Hershey's Bites	17	Piece	39.00	214.50	3.81	19.89	1.40	13.93	6.78	5.61	0.94	7.41		
Candy Bar, Milky Way, 2.1oz bar	1	Each	59.53	251.83	2.68	42.69	1.01	9.59	4.64	3.58	0.36	8.33	10.72	
Candy Bar, Mounds, 1.9oz bar	1	Each	53.86	261.78	2.48	31.56	1.99	14.33	11.09	0.21	0.08	1.08	0.00	
Candy Bar, Mr. Goodbar, 1.75oz bar	1	Each	49.61	266.92	5.07	26.96	1.89	16.48	7.01	4.07	2.17	4.96	17.36	
Candy Bar, Nestle Crunch, 1.4 oz bar	1	Each	39.69	207.18	2.38	25.88	1.03	10.44	6.03	3.42	0.35	5.16		
Candy Bar, Skor, toffee bar, 1.4oz bar	1	Each	39.69	212.34	1.24	24.50	0.52	12.77	7.45	3.69	0.51	21.04		
Candy Bar, Snickers, 2oz bar	1	Each	56.70	264.79	5.17	36.64	1.42	10.86	4.17	4.67	1.53	7.94	22.11	
Candy Bar, Special Dark, sweet chocolate, 1.45oz bar	1	Each	41.11	218.28	2.28	24.42	2.67	13.32	7.89	2.11	0.18	2.06		
Candy Bar, Sweet Escapes, triple chocolate	1	Each	19.00	81.70	0.89	13.93	0.78	2.50	1.50	0.44	0.24	0.00	1.90	
Candy Bar, Symphony, milk chocolate, 1.5oz bar	1	Each	42.53	225.81	3.62	24.67	0.72	13.00	7.80	3.36	0.29	10.21		0.00
Candy Bar, Twix, caramel, 2oz bar	1	Each	56.70	282.93	2.61	37.18	0.62	13.83	5.05	7.60	0.48	2.84	14.74	
Candy, candy corn, prep f/recipe	10	Piece	10.80	40.39	0.00	10.09	0.00	0.00	0.00	0.00	0.00	0.00	0.00	
Candy, caramels	1	Piece	10.10	38.58	0.46	7.78	0.12	0.82	0.66	0.09	0.02	0.71	0.10	
Candy, chocolate cvrd, dietetic/low cal	1	Ounce-weight	28.35	163.01	3.57	12.05	1.02	11.17	6.21	3.10	1.23	5.95	15.59	
Candy, cotton Jays Foods	2.1	Ounce-weight	59.53	220.00	3.00	56.00		0.00	0.00	0.00	0.00	0.00		
Candy, fruit snacks, w/vit A C & E, pouch Farley Candy Company	1	Each	26.00	88.66	1.14	21.03		0.00	0.00	0.00	0.00	0.00		
Candy, Goobers, chocolate cvrd peanuts, 1.375oz pkg	1	Each	38.98	199.97	5.34	18.98	2.38	13.06	4.76	5.75	1.99	3.51	0.00	
Candy, gumdrops, sml, 1/2"	1	Each	3.20	12.67	0.00	3.16	0.00	0.00	0.00	0.00	0.00	0.00	0.00	
Candy, halavah, plain	1	Ounce-weight	28.35	132.96	3.54	17.15	1.28	6.10	1.17	2.32	2.40	0.00		0.00
Candy, hard, all flvrs, sml	1	Piece	3.00	11.82	0.00	2.94	0.00	0.01	0.00	0.00	0.00	0.00		
Candy, jellybeans, sml	10	Piece	11.00	41.25	0.00	10.29	0.02	0.01	0.00	0.00	0.00	0.00		
Candy, licorice Hershey Twizzlers	1	Each	9.00	30.00	0.00	7.00		0.00	0.00	0.00	0.00	0.00	0.00	
Candy, milk chocolate peanut, 1.67oz pkg	1	Each	47.34	244.30	4.48	28.62	1.61	12.42	4.89	5.21	1.99	4.26	12.31	
Candy, milk chocolate peanut, M&M USDA SR-23 Mars	0.25	Cup	42.50	218.88	4.07	25.70	1.57	11.11	4.32	3.44	1.47	3.40	9.35	0.00
Candy, milk chocolate, mini, 5oz pkg	1	Each	141.75	705.92	6.77	95.15	3.83	33.10	20.48	10.77	0.99	21.26		
Candy, Milk Duds Hershey	7	Each	21.00	90.00	1.00	15.00	0.00	3.50	1.00			0.00		
Candy, mints, After Eight	5	Piece	41.00	146.78	0.90	31.49	0.86	5.62	3.35	1.81	0.21	0.00	0.41	
Candy, peanut brittle, prep f/recipe	1.5	Ounce-weight	42.53	205.82	3.22	30.05	1.06	8.07	1.76	3.43	1.94	5.10	16.58	
Candy, peanut butter cups, .6oz single pkg Reese's	1	Each	17.01	87.60	1.74	9.42	0.61	5.19	1.83	2.23	0.95	1.02	2.89	
Candy, peanut butter cups, 1.6oz double pkg Reese's	1	Each	45.36	233.60	4.64	25.11	1.63	13.85	4.87	5.94	2.54	2.72	7.71	
Candy, peanuts, milk chocolate cvrd, pces	10	Piece	40.00	207.60	5.24	19.76	1.88	13.40	5.84	5.17	1.73	3.60	13.60	
Candy, Pieces, 1.6oz pkg Reese's	1	Each	45.36	225.44	5.65	27.15	1.36	11.24	7.45	2.02	0.85	0.00	0.00	
Candy, plain chocolate, 1.69oz pkg	1	Each	47.91	235.72	2.07	34.12	1.20	10.12	6.27	1.69	0.18	6.71	12.94	
Candy, plain chocolate, pces	10	Piece	7.00	34.44	0.30	4.98	0.18	1.48	0.92	0.25	0.03	0.98	1.89	
Candy, Raisinets, chocolate cvrd raisins, 1.58oz pkg	1	Each	44.79	184.55	2.11	31.89	2.28	7.12	3.29	2.66	0.85	1.79		
Candy, raisins, milk chocolate cvrd	1.5	Ounce-weight	42.53	165.85	1.74	29.04	1.79	6.29	3.74	2.02	0.22	1.28	10.21	
Candy, Rolo, caramels in milk chocolate, 1.91oz roll	1	Each	54.15	256.66	2.75	36.79	0.49	11.33	7.81	2.04	0.21	6.50	18.41	
Candy, Skittles, original bite size candies, 2.3oz pkg	1	Each	65.21	264.08	0.12	59.10	0.00	2.85	0.57	1.93	0.08	0.00	0.00	
Candy, Skittles, original, bite size, fun size USDA SR-23 Mars	1	Each	20.00	81.00	0.04	18.16	0.00	0.87	0.82	0.00	0.00	0.00	0.00	0.00
Candy, Sno Caps, sweet chocolate, box	1	Each	65.20	300.00	2.00	48.00	3.00	13.00	8.00			0.00	0.00	
Candy, Starburst, fruit chews, 2.07oz pkg	1	Each	58.68	232.39	0.23	49.59	0.00	4.87	0.73	2.09	1.83	0.00	0.00	
Candy, strawberry twists, 5 oz pkg	4	Piece	38.00	133.00	0.97	30.30	0.00	0.88	0.00			0.00	0.00	

Vit E (mg)	Vit C	Vit B₁ Thia (mg)	Vit B₂ Ribo (mg)	Vit B₃ Nia (mg)	Fol (mcg)	Vit B₆ (mg)	Vita B₁₂ (mcg)	Sodi (mg)	Pota (mg)	Cal (mg)	Phos (mg)	Magn (mg)	Iron (mg)	Zinc (mg)	Caff (mg)	Alco (g)	Sol Fiber (g)	Insol Fiber (g)
1.06	0.00	0.07	0.05	1.89	20.21	0.06	0.01	131.05	241.88	21.43	82.67	50.83	0.47	0.73	3.06	0.00		
0.10	0.77	0.02	0.18	0.52		0.02	0.29	55.34	154.68	96.62	68.04	19.05	0.49	0.43	1.81	0.00		
1.00	0.43	0.09	0.15	0.88	17.86	0.11	0.85	91.00	538.37	257.70	107.16	30.62	1.10	3.00	0.00	0.00		
0.53	0.11	0.03	0.14	0.67	7.80	0.04	0.13	18.78	189.24	50.68	73.71	25.87	0.44	0.65	10.28	0.00		
	0.07							21.30	43.31	14.20			0.10		4.26	0.00		
0.16	0.00	0.05	0.10	0.23	6.45	0.01	0.26	24.88	106.42	57.59	62.19	17.05	0.46	0.04	6.45	0.00		
0.05	0.50	0.03	0.12	0.16	3.74	0.02	0.36	122.25	202.70	98.54	76.72	8.11	0.66	0.31		0.00		
3.88	0.35	0.02	0.16	0.47	4.50	0.03	0.18	85.00	162.50	84.00	117.00	36.00	0.55	0.56	2.00	0.00		
0.15	0.70	0.03	0.15	0.24	6.24	0.03		28.86	183.69	85.80	88.53	23.01	0.58	0.52		0.00		
0.74	0.60	0.02	0.13	0.21	3.57	0.03	0.19	142.88	143.48	77.40	85.73	20.24	0.45	0.42	4.76	0.00		
0.10	0.38	0.00	0.00	0.00	0.00	0.00	0.00	78.10	172.91	11.31	0.00	0.00	1.13	0.00	9.16	0.00		
1.57	0.45	0.07	0.07	1.71	18.85	0.03	0.16	20.34	195.47	54.57	80.87	23.32	0.69	0.46	8.93	0.00		
0.44	0.12	0.13	0.22	1.57	31.36	0.16	0.15	52.79	136.53	67.08	80.17	23.02	0.20	0.57	9.53	0.00		
0.02	0.20	0.01	0.04	0.05	1.19	0.01	0.11	125.82	60.73	51.60	24.21	3.97	0.23	0.07		0.00		
0.85	0.00	0.03	0.07	2.04	15.31	0.05	0.09	129.28	183.14	59.54	107.73	40.82	0.68	1.42	4.54	0.00		
0.08	0.00	0.00	0.00	0.00	0.00	0.00	0.00	2.47	206.36	12.33	20.96	12.74	0.88	0.00	20.55	0.00		
0.17	0.00	0.01	0.02	0.09	1.71	0.00	0.03	30.02	67.45	99.94	25.27	12.35	0.43	0.22	2.28	0.00		
0.09	0.94	0.04	0.16	0.14		0.02	0.17	42.95	186.26	106.74	87.60	23.39	0.39	0.48	28.07	0.00		
1.10	0.23	0.07	0.11	0.43	10.77	0.01	0.16	109.43	107.16	51.03	61.80	18.14	0.46	0.57	1.70	0.00		
0.00	0.00	0.00	0.00	0.00	0.00	0.00	0.00	1.73	0.43	0.22	0.00	0.00	0.00	0.00	0.00	0.00	0.00	0.00
0.28	0.05	0.00	0.03	0.03	0.50	0.00	0.00	24.74	21.61	13.94	11.51	1.72	0.02	0.05	0.00	0.00		
0.83	0.40	0.06	0.13	0.64	7.37	0.04	0.24	30.90	171.80	85.90	94.12	28.35	0.41	0.77	2.55	0.00		
								0.00								0.00		
10.40	23.48							9.36								0.00	0.00	
0.99	0.00	0.05	0.08	2.03	3.12	0.08	0.11	15.98	195.69	49.51	115.38	46.39	0.52	0.85	8.58	0.00		
0.00	0.00	0.00	0.00	0.00	0.00	0.00	0.00	1.41	0.16	0.10	0.03	0.03	0.01	0.00	0.00	0.00		
0.81	0.03	0.12	0.03	0.81	18.43	0.10	0.01	55.28	53.01	9.36	172.08	61.80	1.28	1.23	0.00	0.00		
0.00	0.00	0.00	0.00	0.00	0.00	0.00	0.00	1.14	0.15	0.09	0.09	0.09	0.01	0.00	0.00	0.00	0.00	0.00
0.00	0.00	0.00	0.00	0.00	0.00	0.00	0.00	5.50	4.07	0.33	0.44	0.22	0.01	0.01	0.00	0.00		
	0.00							45.00		0.00			0.00		0.00	0.00		
1.21	0.24	0.05	0.07	1.94	17.99	0.04	0.08	22.73	164.29	47.82	110.31	35.98	0.54	1.14	5.21	0.00		
1.21	0.00	0.03	0.05	1.43	23.38	0.04	0.14	21.25	147.48	43.35	80.75	29.33	0.49	0.75	4.25	0.00		
1.35	0.85	0.07	0.32	0.35	7.09	0.04	0.43	96.39	415.33	164.43	235.31	65.21	1.74	1.49		0.00		
								40.00								0.00	0.00	0.00
0.16	0.00	0.02	0.02	0.12	0.41	0.01	0.00	4.92	68.88	9.43	23.37	18.45	0.63	0.24	8.20	0.00		
1.09	0.00	0.06	0.02	1.13	19.56	0.03	0.00	189.24	71.44	11.48	45.08	17.86	0.52	0.37	0.00	0.00		
0.03	0.05	0.03	0.02	0.76	8.51	0.02	0.10	53.41	58.34	13.27	27.39	10.55	0.21	0.22	3.06	0.00		
0.07	0.14	0.07	0.05	2.04	22.68	0.05	0.25	142.43	155.58	35.38	73.03	28.12	0.55	0.58	8.16	0.00		
1.38	0.00	0.05	0.07	1.70	3.20	0.08	0.18	16.40	200.80	41.60	84.80	38.40	0.52	0.96	8.80	0.00		
0.49	0.00	0.08	0.10	2.75	24.95	0.05	0.05	88.00	162.84	31.30	93.90	39.92	0.22	0.52	0.00	0.00		
0.53	0.24	0.03	0.08	0.10	2.87	0.01	0.16	29.23	97.26	50.31	54.62	16.29	0.53	0.53	5.27	0.00		
0.08	0.04	0.00	0.01	0.01	0.42	0.00	0.02	4.27	14.21	7.35	7.98	2.38	0.08	0.08	0.77	0.00		
0.47	0.09	0.04	0.10	0.18	2.24	0.05	0.09	16.13	230.24	48.38	64.50	20.16	0.53	0.35	11.20	0.00		
0.43	0.09	0.04	0.07	0.17	2.98	0.03	0.08	15.31	218.58	36.57	60.81	19.14	0.73	0.34	10.63	0.00		
0.48	0.49	0.01	0.06	0.02	0.00	0.00	0.15	101.80	101.80	78.52	38.45	0.00	0.23	0.00	1.62	0.00		
0.29	43.62	0.00	0.01	0.01	0.00	0.00	0.00	10.43	5.87	0.00	1.30	0.65	0.01	0.01	0.00	0.00	0.00	0.00
0.03	13.36	0.00	0.00	0.00	0.00	0.00	0.00	3.00	2.40	0.00	0.20	0.20	0.00	0.00	0.00	0.00	0.00	0.00
		0.03	0.03	0.18				0.00	21.10	0.00			1.08		22.62	0.00		
0.41	31.04	0.00	0.00	0.00	0.00	0.00	0.00	32.86	1.17	2.35	4.11	0.59	0.08	0.00	0.00	0.00	0.00	0.00
	0.00							109.06		0.00			0.19		0.00	0.00		

Food Name	Amount	Measure	Weight (g)	Calories	Protein (g)	Total Carb (g)	Dietary Fiber (g)	Total Fat (g)	Sat Fat (g)	Mono Fat (g)	Poly Fat (g)	Chol (mg)	Vit A (mcg RAE)	Vit D (mcg)
CANDIES AND CONFECTIONS, GUM *(continued)*														
Candy, Turtles, chocolate caramel pecans, 6oz pkg, Demet's	1	Piece	17.00	82.45	1.09	9.86	0.44	4.73	1.84	1.88	0.79	3.74		
Candy, York peppermint patty, sml, .5oz	1	Each	14.18	54.43	0.31	11.48	0.28	1.02	0.62	0.06	0.01	0.14		0.00
Chewing Gum, stick	1	Piece	3.00	7.41	0.00	1.98	0.07	0.01	0.00	0.00	0.00	0.00	0.00	0.00
Chewing Gum, sugarless	1	Piece	2.00	5.36	0.00	1.90	0.05	0.01	0.00	0.00	0.00	0.00	0.00	
Fruit Leather, cherry	1	Ounce-weight	28.35	104.89	0.15	22.68	0.40	1.70	0.68	0.88	0.00	0.00		
Fudge, chocolate, prep f/recipe	1	Piece	17.00	69.87	0.41	13.00	0.29	1.77	1.01	0.46	0.04	2.38	7.48	0.07
Fudge, vanilla, prep f/recipe	1	Piece	16.00	61.44	0.17	13.16	0.00	0.87	0.45	0.19	0.01	2.40	7.36	0.06
Marshmallows	4	Each	28.80	91.58	0.52	23.41	0.03	0.06	0.01	0.02	0.01	0.00	0.00	
Marshmallows, miniature Jet-Puffed	0.5	Cup	30.00	100.00	1.00	25.00	0.00	0.00	0.00	0.00	0.00	0.00	0.00	
CEREALS, BREAKFAST TYPE														
Cereal/Breakfast Bars														
Bar, cereal, Fiber One, oats & caramel General Mills Fiber One	1	Each	40.00	140.00	2.00	30.00	9.00	3.50	1.50			0.00	0.00	
Bar, cereal, Fiber One, oats & chocolate General Mills Fiber One	1	Each	40.00	140.00	2.00	29.00	9.00	4.00	1.50	1.50	0.50	0.00		
Bar, cereal, Fiber One, oats & peanut butter General Mills Fiber One	1	Each	40.00	150.00	3.00	28.00	9.00	4.50	2.00	1.50	0.50	0.00		
Cereals, Cooked and Dry														
Cereal, hot, apple spice Kashi Company	0.5	Cup	140.00	270.00	7.00	56.00	6.00	3.00				0.00	0.00	
Cereal, hot, Cream Of Rice, ckd w/water w/o salt	0.5	Cup	122.00	63.44	1.10	13.91	0.12	0.12	0.04	0.04	0.04	0.00	0.00	0.00
Cereal, hot, Cream Of Wheat, ckd w/water w/o salt	0.5	Cup	125.30	62.65	1.83	13.44	0.50	0.24	0.04	0.03	0.13	0.00	0.00	0.00
Cereal, hot, Cream Of Wheat, mix 'n eat, prep w/water f/pkt	1	Each	142.00	102.24	2.70	21.44	0.43	0.28	0.05	0.04	0.16	0.00	376.30	0.00
Cereal, hot, Malt-O-Meal, choc, ckd w/water & salt	0.5	Cup	120.00	61.20	1.80	12.96	0.48	0.12	0.02	0.03	0.02	0.00	0.00	0.00
Cereal, hot, Malt-O-Meal, plain, ckd w/water w/o salt	0.5	Cup	120.00	61.20	1.80	12.84	0.48	0.12	0.05	0.03	0.02	0.00	0.00	0.00
Cereal, hot, oat bran, prep w/water w/o salt Quaker Oats	0.5	Cup	109.50	47.08	2.22	8.20	1.86	1.04	0.18	0.34	0.40	0.00	1.10	0.00
Cereal, hot, oatmeal, apple spice, inst Nutrition for Women	1	Each	47.00	169.20	4.97	34.78	3.24	1.96	0.33	0.66	0.59	0.00	336.99	3.93
Cereal, hot, oatmeal, bkd apple, inst, prep w/water Quaker Oats	1	Each	177.00	169.92	3.58	34.43	3.19	1.96	0.34	0.68	0.57	0.00	368.16	
Cereal, hot, oatmeal, fruit & cream, inst, prep w/water Quaker Oats	1	Each	154.00	110.88	2.23	20.88	1.69	2.09	0.44	0.67	0.36	0.00	263.34	0.00
Cereal, hot, oatmeal, plain, inst, fort, prep w/water	1	Each	177.00	97.35	4.11	16.97	2.83	1.61	0.26	0.51	0.59	0.00	284.97	0.00
Cereal, hot, oatmeal, plain, quick, dry Quaker Oats	0.5	Cup	40.00	148.40	5.48	27.27	3.76	2.75	0.44	0.79	0.92	0.00	0.00	0.00
Cereal, hot, oatmeal, plain, unfort, prep w/water & salt	0.5	Cup	117.00	72.54	3.04	12.64	1.99	1.17	0.21	0.38	0.44	0.00	0.00	0.00
Cereal, hot, Ralston, ckd w/water & salt	0.5	Cup	126.50	67.04	2.78	14.17	3.04	0.38	0.07	0.05	0.18	0.00	0.00	
Grits, corn, white, quick, unenrich, ckd w/water & salt	0.5	Cup	121.00	72.60	1.70	15.73	0.24	0.24	0.04	0.06	0.10	0.00	0.00	0.00
Grits, hominy, white, quick, dry Quaker Oats	0.25	Cup	37.00	128.39	3.16	29.29	1.78	0.50	0.10	0.07	0.25	0.00	0.00	
Cereals, Ready To Eat														
Cereal, 100% Bran C.W. Post	0.33	Cup	29.00	83.23	3.68	22.68	8.29	0.61	0.09			0.00		0.00
Cereal, All-Bran Kellogg's Company	0.5	Cup	30.00	78.00	3.94	22.27	8.79	1.47	0.19	0.20	0.63	0.00	157.50	1.28
Cereal, bran, malted flour	0.33	Cup	29.00	83.23	3.68	22.68	8.29	0.61	0.09	0.09	0.32	0.00	225.04	0.00
Cereal, Cap'N Crunch	0.75	Cup	27.00	108.27	1.17	22.90	0.68	1.57	0.41	0.29	0.20	0.00	1.89	0.00
Cereal, Cheerios General Mills, Inc.	1	Cup	30.00	110.70	3.55	22.20	3.57	1.77	0.36	0.64	0.22	0.00	150.30	1.00
Cereal, Chex, corn General Mills, Inc.	1	Cup	30.00	111.90	2.10	25.80	0.60	0.27	0.06	0.06	0.10	0.00	137.10	0.00
Cereal, Chex, multi-bran General Mills, Inc.	1	Cup	49.00	165.62	3.43	41.16	6.37	1.23	0.25	0.30	0.54	0.00	116.62	0.89
Cereal, Chex, rice General Mills, Inc.	1.25	Cup	31.00	116.87	1.86	26.66	0.31	0.31	0.12	0.07	0.07	0.00	155.31	0.00
Cereal, Chex, wheat General Mills, Inc.	1	Cup	30.00	103.50	3.00	24.30	3.30	0.60	0.12	0.08	0.24	0.00	90.00	0.00

Vit E (mg)	Vit C	Vit B₁ Thia (mg)	Vit B₂ Ribo (mg)	Vit B₃ Nia (mg)	Fol (mcg)	Vit B₆ (mg)	Vita B₁₂ (mcg)	Sodi (mg)	Pota (mg)	Cal (mg)	Phos (mg)	Magn (mg)	Iron (mg)	Zinc (mg)	Caff (mg)	Alco (g)	Sol Fiber (g)	Insol Fiber (g)
	0.12	0.03	0.04	0.06	1.70	0.01	0.07	15.98	52.36	26.86	33.49	8.84	0.23	0.24	0.68	0.00		
0.00	0.00	0.00	0.01	0.12		0.00	0.00	3.97	15.73	1.56	0.00	8.93	0.13	0.11	1.42	0.00		
0.00	0.00	0.00	0.00	0.00	0.00	0.00	0.00	0.03	0.06	0.00	0.00	0.00	0.00	0.00	0.00	0.00		
0.00	0.00	0.00	0.00	0.00	0.00	0.00	0.00	0.14	0.00	0.40	0.00	0.00	0.00	0.00	0.00	0.00		
		0.00	0.00	0.00				55.57	45.64	6.52			0.08		0.00	0.00		
0.03	0.00	0.00	0.01	0.03	0.68	0.00	0.02	7.99	22.27	7.65	11.73	6.12	0.30	0.19	1.36	0.00		
0.02	0.00	0.00	0.01	0.01	0.16	0.00	0.01	8.16	7.36	5.44	4.48	0.48	0.00	0.02	0.00	0.00	0.00	0.00
0.00	0.00	0.00	0.00	0.02	0.29	0.00	0.00	23.04	1.44	0.86	2.30	0.58	0.06	0.01	0.00	0.00		
	0.00							30.00	0.00	0.00			0.08		0.00	0.00	0.00	0.00
	0.00							105.00		100.00			0.00		0.00	0.00		
	0.00							90.00		100.00			0.36			0.00		
	0.00							105.00		100.00			0.36		0.00	0.00		
		0.00	0.07	0.13	1.97	11.90	0.13		0.00	253.00	20.00	148.40		2.70		0.00	0.00	
0.02	0.00	0.00	0.00	0.49	3.66	0.04	0.00	1.22	24.40	3.66	20.74	3.66	0.24	0.20	0.00	0.00		
0.03	0.00	0.07	0.03	0.68	15.04	0.01	0.00	72.67	22.55	56.39	47.61	6.27	4.87	0.17	0.00	0.00		
0.01	0.00	0.43	0.28	4.97	100.82	0.57	0.00	241.40	38.34	19.88	19.88	7.10	8.09	0.24	0.00	0.00		
0.02	0.00	0.24	0.12	2.88	2.40	0.01	0.00	162.00	15.60	2.40	12.00	2.40	4.80	0.08	1.20	0.00		
0.01	0.00	0.24	0.12	2.88	2.40	0.01	0.00	1.20	15.60	2.40	12.00	2.40	4.80	0.08	1.20	0.00		
0.06	0.00	0.12	0.04	0.10	5.48	0.02	0.00	3.28	75.56	12.04	90.88	32.85	1.06	0.58	0.00	0.00		
5.31	0.38	0.33	0.38	4.49	156.98	0.78	1.34	315.84	137.24	397.62	133.48	36.19	7.08	0.86	0.00	0.00		
0.18	0.35	0.33	0.39	4.67	99.12	0.49	0.00	254.88	134.52	249.57	123.90	37.17	4.42	0.83	0.00	0.00		
0.12	0.15	0.24	0.28	3.34	70.84	0.35	0.02	144.76	78.54	90.86	83.16	23.10	3.17	0.49	0.00	0.00		
0.18	0.00	0.26	0.31	3.60	76.11	0.38	0.00	79.65	93.81	99.12	95.58	40.71	7.68	0.81	0.00	0.00		
0.28	0.00	0.22	0.05	0.33	12.80	0.04	0.00	1.20	143.20	18.80	183.20	108.00	1.86	1.28	0.00	0.00		
0.12	0.00	0.13	0.02	0.15	4.68	0.02	0.00	187.20	65.52	9.36	88.92	28.08	0.80	0.57	0.00	0.00	1.17	0.82
0.12	0.00	0.10	0.09	1.02	8.86	0.06	0.05	237.82	77.17	6.32	73.37	29.10	0.82	0.71	0.00	0.00		
0.02	0.00	0.02	0.01	0.24	1.21	0.03	0.00	269.83	26.62	0.00	14.52	4.84	0.24	0.08	0.00	0.00	0.20	0.04
	0.00	0.21	0.12	1.78	56.98	0.10	0.00	0.74	54.02	1.48	61.42	18.13	1.30	0.34	0.00	0.00		
	0.00	0.37	0.43	5.00	100.05	0.50	0.00	120.93	274.63	22.04	235.77	80.62	8.10	3.75	0.00	0.00		
0.38	6.00	0.68	0.81	4.44	393.00	3.60	5.64	72.60	306.00	116.70	345.00	108.60	5.28	3.72	0.00	0.00		
0.67	0.00	0.37	0.43	5.00	100.05	0.50	0.00	120.93	274.63	22.04	235.77	80.62	8.10	3.75	0.00	0.00		
0.25	0.00	0.43	0.48	5.71	420.12	0.57	0.00	202.23	54.00	4.05	45.09	15.12	5.16	4.28	0.00	0.00	0.22	0.45
0.11	6.00	0.54	0.50	5.76	200.10	0.66	1.43	213.30	208.80	121.50	132.30	39.30	10.32	4.62	0.00	0.00	2.28	1.29
0.05	6.00	0.38	0.43	5.01	200.10	0.50	1.50	287.70	24.90	99.90	21.60	8.40	9.00	3.75	0.00	0.00	0.00	0.60
0.15	5.39	0.33	0.38	4.46	356.23	0.45	1.32	321.93	189.63	89.18	178.36	53.41	14.46	3.33	0.00	0.00		
0.02	6.20	0.39	0.44	5.18	206.77	0.52	1.55	291.71	30.38	103.23	35.34	9.30	9.30	3.88	0.00	0.00	0.21	0.10
0.22	3.60	0.23	0.26	3.00	240.00	0.30	0.90	267.30	112.50	60.00	90.00	24.00	8.70	2.40	0.00	0.00	0.56	2.74

Food Name	Amount	Measure	Weight (g)	Calories	Protein (g)	Total Carb (g)	Dietary Fiber (g)	Total Fat (g)	Sat Fat (g)	Mono Fat (g)	Poly Fat (g)	Chol (mg)	Vit A (mcg RAE)	Vit D (mcg)
CEREALS, BREAKFAST TYPE *(continued)*														
Cereal, Cocoa Krispies Kellogg's Company	0.75	Cup	31.00	118.11	1.62	26.68	0.59	0.90	0.62	0.12	0.07	0.00	152.52	1.01
Cereal, Cookie Crisp Ralston Foods	1	Cup	30.00	116.70	1.20	26.40	0.45	0.90	0.18	0.44	0.21	0.00	143.10	1.00
Cereal, corn and oat, puffed, w/add sug	1.33	Cup	29.00	114.55	1.51	25.78	0.72	0.61	0.17	0.14	0.20	0.00	216.92	1.00
Cereal, corn flakes Kellogg's Company	1	Cup	28.00	101.08	1.85	24.39	0.70	0.17	0.05	0.03	0.09	0.00	127.68	1.06
Cereal, corn flakes, low sod	1	Cup	25.00	99.75	1.92	22.20	0.28	0.08	0.01	0.02	0.03	0.00	2.50	
Cereal, Cracklin' Oat Bran Kellogg's Company	0.75	Cup	55.00	224.95	4.57	39.27	6.44	8.03	2.31	4.57	1.16	0.00	252.45	1.12
Cereal, Crispix Kellogg's Company	1	Cup	29.00	109.33	1.97	24.94	0.14	0.23	0.06	0.06	0.12	0.00	142.97	1.00
Cereal, Crunchy Bran Quaker Oats	0.75	Cup	27.00	90.45	1.47	23.31	4.73	1.02	0.21	0.23	0.27	0.00	2.16	0.00
Cereal, Fiber One, Caramel Delight USDA SR-23 Big G Cereals	1	Cup	50.00	176.00	3.00	41.25	8.35	2.95	0.60	1.15	1.15	0.00		1.00
Cereal, Fiber One, honey clusters General Mills Fiber One	1	Cup	52.00	160.00	5.00	42.00	13.00	1.50	0.00	0.00	0.50	0.00		0.00
Cereal, Fiber One, Raisin Bran Clusters USDA SR-23 Big G Cereals	1	Cup	55.00	171.05	2.86	46.86	11.55	1.21	0.22	0.22	0.39	0.00		1.49
Cereal, Fiber One General Mills, Inc.	0.5	Cup	30.00	59.10	2.40	24.30	14.40	0.81	0.12	0.13	0.41	0.00	0.00	0.00
Cereal, Froot Loops Kellogg's Company	1	Cup	30.00	117.90	1.51	26.24	0.75	0.93	0.46	0.13	0.20	0.00	140.70	0.94
Cereal, Frosted Flakes, sugar Krusteaz	0.75	Cup	31.00	110.00	1.00	25.00	0.00	0.00	0.00	0.00	0.00	0.00		
Cereal, Frosted Mini Wheats, bite size Kellogg's Company	1	Cup	55.00	189.20	5.56	44.55	5.50	0.88	0.20	0.13	0.55	0.00	0.00	0.00
Cereal, Go Lean Kashi	0.75	Cup	40.00	113.60	10.44	23.20	7.84	0.76	0.16	0.16	0.44	0.00		
Cereal, Go Lean Crunch, honey almond flax USDA SR-23 Kashi	1	Cup	53.00	201.93	8.80	35.51	8.59	4.40	0.37	2.17	1.85	0.00	0.45	0.00
Cereal, Go Lean Crunch Kashi	1	Ounce-weight	28.35	106.88	4.97	19.26	4.31	1.64	0.13	0.91	0.60	0.00		
Cereal, Golden Grahams General Mills, Inc.	0.75	Cup	30.00	111.60	1.50	24.90	0.90	1.05	0.18	0.40	0.39	0.00	150.30	1.00
Cereal, granola, fruit, low fat Nature Valley	0.66	Cup	55.00	212.30	4.40	44.00	2.75	2.53	0.47	1.16	0.63	0.00	0.00	0.00
Cereal, granola, homemade, w/oats & wheat germ	0.5	Cup	61.00	298.90	9.07	32.30	5.25	14.86	2.77	4.66	6.53	0.00	0.61	0.00
Cereal, granola, tstd oats Nature Valley	0.5	Cup	56.50	254.81	5.96	37.22	3.62	9.96	1.31	6.67	1.92	0.00	0.00	
Cereal, Grape Nuts C.W. Post	0.5	Cup	58.00	208.22	6.26	47.15	5.05	1.10	0.23	0.20	0.67	0.00		1.00
Cereal, Heart to Heart Kashi	1	Ounce-weight	28.35	98.66	3.57	21.55	4.03	1.34	0.26	0.32	0.34	0.00	322.62	
Cereal, Honey Graham Oh!s Quaker Oats	0.75	Cup	27.00	110.97	1.07	22.62	0.57	2.00	0.54	0.36	0.19	0.00	177.12	0.00
Cereal, Just Right, crunchy nuggets Kellogg's Company	1	Cup	55.00	204.05	4.24	46.04	2.81	1.49	0.11	0.28	1.05	0.00	375.65	
Cereal, Kix General Mills, Inc.	1.33	Cup	30.00	113.10	1.80	25.80	0.90	0.60	0.15	0.16	0.20	0.00	152.40	1.06
Cereal, Life, plain Quaker Oats	0.75	Cup	32.00	120.00	3.17	24.99	2.11	1.40	0.26	0.48	0.45	0.00	0.64	0.00
Cereal, Lucky Charms General Mills, Inc.	1	Cup	30.00	114.00	2.10	24.90	1.50	1.14	0.24	0.25	0.29	0.00	150.30	1.00
Cereal, Nutri-Grain, wheat Nutri Grain	1	Ounce-weight	28.35	102.06	2.48	23.98	1.80	0.28	0.06	0.04	0.11	0.00	0.00	
Cereal, Oatmeal Crisp, w/almonds General Mills, Inc.	1	Cup	55.00	218.35	5.50	41.80	4.40	4.62	0.61	2.44	1.18	0.00	0.00	0.00
Cereal, Oatmeal Crisp, w/apples General Mills, Inc.	1	Cup	55.00	207.35	4.95	45.10	3.85	2.15	0.44	0.79	0.67	0.00	0.00	0.00
Cereal, Product 19 Kellogg's Company	1	Cup	30.00	99.90	2.31	24.90	0.99	0.42	0.09	0.12	0.21	0.00	214.20	0.98
Cereal, puffed rice Quaker Oats	1	Cup	14.00	53.62	0.98	12.29	0.20	0.13	0.04	0.03	0.05	0.00	0.00	0.00
Cereal, puffed rice, fort	1	Cup	14.00	56.28	0.88	12.57	0.24	0.07	0.02	0.01	0.02	0.00	0.00	0.47
Cereal, puffed wheat Kellogg's Company	1	Cup	15.00	49.80	1.37	12.27	1.71	0.24	0.05	0.12	0.08	0.00		
Cereal, puffed wheat, fort	1	Cup	12.00	43.68	1.76	9.55	0.53	0.14	0.02	0.02	0.07	0.00	0.00	0.40
Cereal, raisin bran	1	Cup	61.00	194.59	5.19	46.54	7.26	1.53	0.34	0.31	0.88	0.00	154.94	1.00
Cereal, raisin bran	1	Cup	56.00	210.00	4.00	45.00	6.00	1.50	0.00			0.00		
Cereal, Raisin Nut Bran General Mills, Inc.	1	Cup	55.00	209.00	5.16	41.45	5.06	4.40	0.77	2.36	0.88	0.00	0.00	0.00
Cereal, Raisin Squares, mini wheats Kellogg's Company	0.75	Cup	55.00	185.90	4.62	43.84	5.17	0.88	0.19	0.19	0.50	0.00	0.00	0.00
Cereal, Rice Krispies Kellogg's Company	1.25	Cup	33.00	118.80	2.29	28.03	0.13	0.36	0.13	0.09	0.13	0.00	153.12	1.02
Cereal, Shredded Wheat, bite size, frosted C.W. Post	1	Cup	52.00	183.04	4.06	43.58	4.99	0.99	0.16			0.00	0.00	0.00
Cereal, Shredded Wheat, spoon size C.W. Post	1	Cup	49.00	166.60	5.05	40.67	5.59	0.54	0.10			0.00	0.00	0.00
Cereal, Special K Kellogg's Company	1	Cup	31.00	117.49	6.98	22.01	0.74	0.48	0.11	0.12	0.25	0.00	230.33	1.25
Cereal, Tasteeos	1	Cup	24.00	94.32	3.07	18.98	2.54	0.67	0.23	0.17	0.18	0.00	317.76	0.00
Cereal, Total, wheat General Mills, Inc.	0.75	Cup	30.00	97.20	2.66	22.50	2.73	0.72	0.16	0.12	0.27	0.00	150.30	1.00
Cereal, Trix General Mills, Inc.	1	Cup	30.00	117.30	0.90	26.70	0.90	1.14	0.18	0.60	0.27	0.00	150.30	1.00

Vit E (mg)	Vit C	Vit B$_1$ Thia (mg)	Vit B$_2$ Ribo (mg)	Vit B$_3$ Nia (mg)	Fol (mcg)	Vit B$_6$ (mg)	Vita B$_{12}$ (mcg)	Sodi (mg)	Pota (mg)	Cal (mg)	Phos (mg)	Magn (mg)	Iron (mg)	Zinc (mg)	Caff (mg)	Alco (g)	Sol Fiber (g)	Insol Fiber (g)
0.08	15.00	0.46	0.70	4.96	197.47	1.02	2.15	196.85	61.07	39.68	31.62	11.78	6.88	1.49	1.55	0.00		
0.08	6.00	0.38	0.43	5.01	99.90	0.50	1.50	178.20	27.00	99.90	39.90	8.40	4.50	3.75	0.60	0.00		
0.06	0.00	0.37	0.43	5.00	100.05	0.50	1.50	215.47	34.80	4.93	26.97	10.73	2.70	1.50	0.00	0.00		
0.04	6.16	0.60	0.74	6.83	134.40	0.96	2.65	202.44	22.12	1.12	10.36	2.52	8.12	0.05	0.00	0.00		
0.04	0.00	0.00	0.04	0.10	8.25	0.02	0.00	2.50	18.25	10.75	12.25	3.25	0.56	0.07	0.00	0.00		
0.79	17.60	0.42	0.48	5.67	112.75	0.56	1.71	157.30	247.50	22.55	178.75	67.65	2.04	1.71	0.00	0.00		
0.04	5.80	0.55	0.61	6.99	279.85	0.70	2.09	209.96	37.70	6.09	26.39	7.25	8.12	1.45	0.00	0.00		
0.18	0.00	0.14	0.47	5.50	399.87	0.55	0.00	231.66	56.16	19.17	35.64	14.31	8.32	4.13	0.00	0.00	0.00	4.73
	6.00	0.40	0.45	5.00	100.00	0.50	1.50	226.00	131.50	100.00	100.00	32.00	4.50	3.75	0.00	0.00		
	0.00	0.38	0.43	5.00	100.00	0.50	1.50	280.00	320.00	100.00	100.00	32.00	4.50	3.75	0.00	0.00	3.00	10.00
	0.00	0.39	0.44	5.01	100.10	0.50	1.49	211.20	215.05	100.10	100.10	24.20	4.51	3.74	0.00	0.00		
0.21	6.00	0.38	0.43	5.01	99.90	0.50	1.50	128.70	232.20	99.90	150.00	60.00	4.50	3.75	0.00	0.00		
0.09	14.10	0.68	0.58	7.26	105.60	1.10	2.12	150.30	36.00	4.20	33.60	9.90	6.12	5.70	0.00	0.00		
	15.00							170.00	35.00	0.00			4.50		0.00	0.00	0.00	0.00
0.00	0.00	0.41	0.46	5.39	107.80	0.54	1.62	4.40	189.75	17.60	161.70	64.90	15.40	1.76	0.00	0.00		
0.24	0.00	0.14	0.06	1.30	25.60	0.13	0.00	66.00	370.40	56.00	190.00	66.00	2.00	0.28	0.00	0.00		
1.98	0.00	0.09	0.11	0.87	23.85	0.08	0.00	138.33	257.58	53.53	109.71	38.16	1.59	0.42	0.00	0.00		
0.51	0.00	0.02	0.09	0.09	0.57	0.00	0.00	109.15	160.46	24.66	60.39	23.53	1.00	0.26	0.00	0.00		
0.11	6.00	0.38	0.43	5.01	99.90	0.50	1.50	268.50	49.50	350.10	200.10	8.10	4.50	3.75	0.00	0.00	0.46	0.44
0.83	0.00	0.09	0.03	0.95	7.15	0.06	0.00	206.80	153.45	19.80	150.15	24.20	1.10	0.61	0.00	0.00		
3.59	0.73	0.45	0.18	1.29	50.63	0.19	0.00	13.42	327.57	47.58	278.77	106.75	2.59	2.51	0.00	0.00		
3.98	0.00	0.18	0.06	0.63	8.47	0.08	0.00	91.53	187.58	42.37	164.41	53.67	1.76	1.14			2.32	1.30
	0.00	0.38	0.42	5.00	99.76	0.50	1.50	353.80	178.06	19.72	138.62	58.00	16.20	1.20	0.00	0.00	2.78	2.27
11.60	25.80	0.15	0.06	0.53	343.60	1.74	5.16	0.85	85.05	15.31	24.95	85.05	1.85	1.30	0.00	0.00		
0.21	7.07	0.44	0.50	5.90	420.12	0.59	0.00	162.00	42.39	3.24	38.34	0.00	5.31	4.42	0.00	0.00		
1.47	0.00	0.39	0.44	5.01	102.30	0.50	1.49	337.70	121.00	14.30	106.15	34.10	16.23	0.88	0.00	0.00		
0.07	6.30	0.38	0.43	5.01	200.10	0.50	1.50	267.30	35.10	150.00	39.90	8.10	8.10	3.75	0.00	0.00	0.00	0.90
0.18	0.00	0.40	0.47	5.50	416.00	0.55	0.00	164.16	91.20	112.00	132.80	30.72	8.95	4.13	0.00	0.00	1.16	0.95
0.09	6.00	0.38	0.43	5.01	200.10	0.50	1.50	203.40	57.30	99.90	60.00	15.90	4.50	3.75	0.00	0.00	0.81	0.69
7.48	15.03	0.38	0.43	4.99	100.08	0.51	1.51	192.78	77.11	7.94	106.03	22.11	0.79	3.74	0.00	0.00		
1.90	6.05	0.37	0.42	5.01	100.10	0.50	1.49	236.50	184.25	19.80	150.15	59.95	4.51	3.74	0.00	0.00		
0.26	6.05	0.37	0.42	5.01	100.10	0.50	1.49	253.00	170.50	19.80	100.10	40.15	4.51	3.75	0.00	0.00		
13.50	61.20	1.50	1.71	20.01	399.90	2.07	6.00	207.00	50.10	4.80	39.90	15.90	18.09	15.30	0.00	0.00		
0.02	0.00	0.06	0.04	0.49	21.56	0.00	0.00	0.70	16.24	1.26	16.52	4.20	0.40	0.15	0.00	0.00	0.09	0.10
0.01	0.00	0.36	0.25	4.94	2.66	0.01	0.00	0.42	15.82	0.84	13.72	3.50	4.44	0.14	0.00	0.00	0.11	0.13
								0.45	71.10	6.00	63.15				0.00	0.00		
0.04	0.00	0.31	0.22	4.24	3.84	0.02	0.00	0.48	41.76	3.36	42.60	17.40	3.80	0.28	0.00	0.00		
0.41	0.43	0.39	0.44	5.19	103.70	0.52	1.55	361.73	372.10	29.28	258.64	82.96	4.64	1.55	0.00	0.00		
	6.00							320.00	300.00	40.00			18.00		0.00	0.00		
2.04		0.37	0.42	5.01	100.10	0.50	1.49	250.25	238.15	19.80	150.15	40.15	4.51	3.74	0.00	0.00		
0.36	0.00	0.39	0.44	5.17	103.95	0.52	1.60	3.30	264.55	21.45	155.65	43.45	15.40	1.54	0.00	0.00		
0.04	6.37	0.87	0.79	7.10	151.14	0.92	2.01	318.78	39.27	4.62	38.61	9.57	2.65	0.46	0.00	0.00		
	0.00	0.37	0.43	5.00	99.84	0.50	1.50	9.88	170.04	6.76	143.52	48.36	1.80	1.50	0.00	0.00		
	0.00	0.13	0.06	2.73	20.58	0.20	0.00	3.43	203.35	21.07	174.93	56.84	1.56	1.31	0.00	0.00		
4.74	20.99	0.53	0.59	7.13	399.90	1.98	6.05	223.51	60.76	9.30	67.89	19.22	8.37	0.90	0.00	0.00		
0.08	12.72	0.31	0.36	4.22	84.72	0.43	1.27	182.88	71.04	11.04	95.76	26.16	6.86	0.69	0.00	0.00	1.70	0.84
13.50	60.00	2.11	2.42	26.43	477.00	2.82	6.42	191.70	103.20	1104.00	88.80	39.30	22.35	17.46	0.00	0.00		
0.60	6.00	0.38	0.43	5.01	99.90	0.50	1.50	194.10	17.40	99.90	20.10	3.60	4.50	3.75	0.00	0.00	0.52	0.38

Food Name	Amount	Measure	Weight (g)	Calories	Protein (g)	Total Carb (g)	Dietary Fiber (g)	Total Fat (g)	Sat Fat (g)	Mono Fat (g)	Poly Fat (g)	Chol (mg)	Vit A (mcg RAE)	Vit D (mcg)
CEREALS, BREAKFAST TYPE (continued)														
Cereal, wheat, shredd, w/o sug & salt, spoon size	1	Cup	49.00	166.60	5.05	40.67	5.59	0.54	0.10	0.06	0.22	0.00	0.00	0.00
Cereal, Wheaties General Mills, Inc.	1	Cup	30.00	106.50	3.00	24.30	3.00	0.96	0.18	0.29	0.35	0.00	150.30	1.00
CHEESE AND CHEESE SUBSTITUTES														
Natural Cheeses														
Cheese, asiago, fresh, shredded Stella Foods	0.25	Cup	28.00	110.00	6.00	1.00	0.50	9.00	5.00			25.00		
Cheese, blue, 1" cube	1	Each	17.30	61.07	3.70	0.40	0.00	4.97	3.23	1.34	0.14	12.97	34.25	
Cheese, brick, 1" cube	1	Each	17.20	63.81	4.00	0.48	0.00	5.10	3.23	1.48	0.14	16.17	50.22	
Cheese, brie, 1" cube	1	Each	17.00	56.78	3.53	0.08	0.00	4.70	2.96	1.36	0.14	17.00	29.58	
Cheese, camembert, 1" cube	1	Each	17.00	51.00	3.37	0.08	0.00	4.12	2.59	1.19	0.12	12.24	40.97	0.05
Cheese, caraway	1	Ounce-weight	28.35	106.60	7.13	0.87	0.00	8.28	5.27	2.34	0.24	26.37	76.83	
Cheese, cheddar & monterey jack, shredded Sargento Food Inc.	0.25	Cup	28.00	110.00	7.00	1.00	0.00	9.00	5.00			30.00		
Cheese, cheddar, fancy, shredded Healthy Choice	0.25	Cup	28.00	50.00	8.00	1.00	1.00	1.50	1.00			5.00		
Cheese, cheddar, low sod, 1" cube	1	Each	17.30	68.85	4.22	0.33	0.00	5.65	3.59	1.59	0.17	17.30	45.67	
Cheese, cheddar, mild, shredded Sargento Fancy	0.25	Cup	28.00	110.00	7.00	1.00	0.00	9.00	5.00			30.00		
Cheese, cheddar, sharp Cracker Barrel	1	Ounce-weight	28.35	120.00	6.00	0.00	0.00	10.00	7.00			30.00		
Cheese, colby Kraft General Foods, Inc.	1	Ounce-weight	28.35	110.00	7.00	1.00	0.00	9.00	6.00			30.00		
Cheese, colby, low fat, 1" cube	1	Each	17.30	29.93	4.22	0.33	0.00	1.21	0.75	0.36	0.04	3.63	10.38	
Cheese, colby, slice, 1oz each	1	Each	28.35	111.70	6.74	0.73	0.00	9.10	5.73	2.63	0.27	26.93	74.84	
Cheese, edam	1	Ounce-weight	28.35	101.21	7.09	0.41	0.00	7.88	4.98	2.31	0.19	25.23	68.89	0.26
Cheese, feta, 1" cube	1	Each	17.00	44.88	2.41	0.70	0.00	3.62	2.54	0.79	0.10	15.13	21.25	
Cheese, fondue	2	Tablespoon	26.88	61.56	3.83	1.01	0.00	3.62	2.35	0.96	0.13	12.10	29.30	
Cheese, fontina, 1" cube	1	Each	15.00	58.35	3.84	0.24	0.00	4.67	2.88	1.30	0.25	17.40	39.15	
Cheese, four cheese, Mexican style, finely shredded Kraft General Foods, Inc.	0.33	Cup	32.00	120.00	7.00	1.00	0.00	10.00	7.00			30.00		
Cheese, goat, semi soft	1	Ounce-weight	28.35	103.19	6.11	0.72	0.00	8.46	5.85	1.93	0.20	22.40	115.38	
Cheese, gouda	1	Ounce-weight	28.35	100.93	7.07	0.63	0.00	7.78	4.99	2.19	0.19	32.32	46.78	0.07
Cheese, gruyere, 1" cube	1	Each	15.00	61.95	4.47	0.06	0.00	4.85	2.84	1.50	0.26	16.50	40.65	0.04
Cheese, Mexican, queso anejo, crumbled, cup	0.25	Cup	33.00	123.09	7.07	1.53	0.00	9.89	6.28	2.82	0.30	34.65	17.82	
Cheese, monterey jack, 1" cube	1	Each	17.20	64.16	4.21	0.11	0.00	5.21	3.28	1.51	0.15	15.31	34.06	
Cheese, monterey jack, hot pepper Land O'Lakes Incorporated	1	Ounce-weight	28.35	110.00	6.00	1.00	0.00	9.00	6.00			30.00		
Cheese, monterey, low fat, shredd	0.25	Cup	28.25	88.42	7.97	0.20	0.00	6.10	3.96	1.59	0.24	18.36	40.11	
Cheese, mozzarella, low moist, part skim Kraft General Foods, Inc.	1	Ounce-weight	28.35	80.00	8.00	1.00	0.00	5.00	3.50			15.00		
Cheese, mozzarella, part skm, shredded	0.25	Cup	28.25	71.75	6.86	0.78	0.00	4.50	2.85	1.27	0.13	18.08	35.88	0.04
Cheese, mozzarella, whole milk, slice, 1oz each	1	Each	34.00	102.00	7.54	0.74	0.00	7.60	4.47	2.23	0.26	26.86	60.86	
Cheese, muenster, 1" cube	1	Each	17.50	64.40	4.09	0.20	0.00	5.26	3.34	1.52	0.12	16.80	52.15	
Cheese, neufchatel	1	Ounce-weight	28.35	73.71	2.83	0.83	0.00	6.64	4.20	1.92	0.19	21.55	84.48	0.05
Cheese, parmesan, grated	1	Tablespoon	5.00	21.55	1.92	0.20	0.00	1.43	0.87	0.42	0.06	4.40	6.00	
Cheese, parmesan, hard, 1" cube	1	Each	10.30	40.38	3.69	0.33	0.00	2.66	1.69	0.78	0.06	7.00	11.12	0.08
Cheese, parmesan, shredded	1	Tablespoon	5.00	20.75	1.89	0.17	0.00	1.37	0.87	0.44	0.03	3.60	6.10	
Cheese, provolone, diced	0.25	Cup	33.00	115.83	8.44	0.70	0.00	8.79	5.63	2.44	0.25	22.77	77.88	
Cheese, ricotta, fat free Sargento Food Inc.	0.25	Cup	62.00	49.99	5.01	5.01	0.00	0.00	0.00	0.00	0.00	10.00	0.00	
Cheese, ricotta, part skim	0.25	Cup	62.00	85.56	7.06	3.19	0.00	4.90	3.05	1.43	0.16	19.22	66.34	
Cheese, ricotta, whole milk	0.25	Cup	62.00	107.88	6.99	1.88	0.00	8.04	5.15	2.25	0.25	31.62	74.40	
Cheese, romano, 100%, shredded Di Giorno	2	Tablespoon	5.00	20.00	2.00	0.00	0.00	1.50	1.00			5.00	0.00	
Cheese, roquefort, 3oz pkg	1	Ounce-weight	28.35	104.61	6.10	0.57	0.00	8.68	5.46	2.40	0.38	25.51	83.35	
Cheese, Swiss, 1" cube	1	Each	15.00	57.00	4.04	0.80	0.00	4.17	2.66	1.09	0.14	13.80	33.00	0.16
Cottage Cheese, 1% fat	0.5	Cup	113.00	81.36	14.00	3.07	0.00	1.15	0.73	0.33	0.04	4.52	12.43	
Cottage Cheese, 2% fat	0.5	Cup	113.00	101.70	15.53	4.10	0.00	2.18	1.38	0.62	0.07	9.04	23.73	
Cottage Cheese, 4% fat, lrg curd Knudsen	0.5	Cup	127.00	130.00	16.00	4.00	0.00	5.00	3.50			30.00		
Cottage Cheese, creamed, lrg curd, not packed	0.5	Cup	105.00	108.15	13.11	2.81	0.00	4.74	3.00	1.35	0.15	15.75	46.20	

Vit E (mg)	Vit C	Vit B₁ Thia (mg)	Vit B₂ Ribo (mg)	Vit B₃ Nia (mg)	Fol (mcg)	Vit B₆ (mg)	Vita B₁₂ (mcg)	Sodi (mg)	Pota (mg)	Cal (mg)	Phos (mg)	Magn (mg)	Iron (mg)	Zinc (mg)	Caff (mg)	Alco (g)	Sol Fiber (g)	Insol Fiber (g)
0.00	0.00	0.13	0.06	2.73	20.58	0.20	0.00	3.43	203.35	21.07	174.93	56.84	1.56	1.31	0.00	0.00		
0.19	6.00	0.75	0.85	9.99	200.10	1.00	3.00	217.50	111.00	0.00	99.90	32.10	8.10	7.50	0.00	0.00	1.02	1.98
	0.00							270.00		200.00			0.00		0.00	0.00		
0.05	0.00	0.01	0.06	0.17	6.23	0.03	0.21	241.33	44.29	91.34	66.95	3.98	0.05	0.46	0.00	0.00	0.00	0.00
0.05	0.00	0.00	0.06	0.02	3.44	0.01	0.22	96.32	23.39	115.93	77.57	4.13	0.07	0.45	0.00	0.00	0.00	0.00
0.04	0.00	0.01	0.09	0.06	11.05	0.04	0.28	106.93	25.84	31.28	31.96	3.40	0.08	0.40	0.00	0.00	0.00	0.00
0.04	0.00	0.00	0.08	0.11	10.54	0.04	0.22	143.14	31.79	65.96	58.99	3.40	0.06	0.40	0.00	0.00	0.00	0.00
0.14	0.00	0.01	0.13	0.05	5.10	0.02	0.08	195.61	26.37	190.80	138.91	6.24	0.18	0.83	0.00	0.00	0.00	0.00
	0.00							180.00		200.00			0.00		0.00	0.00	0.00	0.00
	0.00							220.00		100.00			0.00		0.00	0.00		
0.05	0.00	0.01	0.06	0.02	3.11	0.01	0.14	3.63	19.38	121.62	83.73	4.67	0.13	0.54	0.00	0.00	0.00	0.00
	0.00							180.00		200.00			0.00		0.00	0.00	0.00	0.00
	0.00		0.07					180.00	30.00	200.00	150.00		0.00	0.90	0.00	0.00	0.00	0.00
	0.00		0.10				0.24	180.00	15.00	200.00	150.00	0.00	0.00	0.90	0.00	0.00	0.00	0.00
0.01	0.00	0.00	0.04	0.01	1.90	0.01	0.09	105.88	11.42	71.79	83.73	2.77	0.07	0.32	0.00	0.00	0.00	0.00
0.08	0.00	0.00	0.11	0.03	5.10	0.02	0.24	171.23	36.00	194.20	129.56	7.37	0.22	0.87	0.00	0.00	0.00	0.00
0.07	0.00	0.01	0.11	0.02	4.54	0.02	0.43	273.58	53.30	207.24	151.96	8.50	0.12	1.07	0.00	0.00	0.00	0.00
0.03	0.00	0.03	0.14	0.17	5.44	0.07	0.29	189.72	10.54	83.81	57.29	3.23	0.11	0.49	0.00	0.00	0.00	0.00
0.06	0.00	0.01	0.05	0.05	2.15	0.02	0.22	35.48	28.22	127.95	82.25	6.18	0.11	0.53	0.00	0.08	0.00	0.00
0.04	0.00	0.00	0.03	0.02	0.90	0.01	0.25	120.00	9.60	82.50	51.90	2.10	0.04	0.52	0.00	0.00	0.00	0.00
	0.00		0.10					210.00	25.00	200.00	150.00		0.00	0.90	0.00	0.00	0.00	0.00
0.08	0.00	0.02	0.19	0.32	0.57	0.02	0.07	146.00	44.79	84.48	106.31	8.22	0.46	0.19	0.00	0.00	0.00	0.00
0.07	0.00	0.01	0.09	0.02	5.95	0.02	0.43	232.19	34.30	198.45	154.79	8.22	0.07	1.11	0.00	0.00	0.00	0.00
0.04	0.00	0.01	0.04	0.02	1.50	0.01	0.24	50.40	12.15	151.65	90.75	5.40	0.02	0.58	0.00	0.00	0.00	0.00
0.09	0.00	0.01	0.07	0.01	0.33	0.01	0.45	373.23	28.71	224.40	146.52	9.24	0.15	0.97	0.00	0.00	0.00	0.00
0.05	0.00	0.00	0.07	0.02	3.10	0.01	0.14	92.19	13.93	128.31	76.37	4.64	0.13	0.52	0.00	0.00	0.00	0.00
	0.00							140.00		200.00			0.00		0.00	0.00	0.00	0.00
0.06	0.00	0.01	0.10	0.03	5.08	0.02	0.24	159.33	22.88	199.16	125.43	7.63	0.21	0.85	0.00	0.00*	0.00	0.00
	0.00		0.07				0.36	200.00	20.00	200.00	150.00	0.00	0.00	1.20	0.00	0.00	0.00	0.00
0.04	0.00	0.01	0.08	0.03	2.54	0.02	0.24	174.87	23.73	220.91	130.80	6.50	0.07	0.78	0.00	0.00	0.00	0.00
0.06	0.00	0.01	0.10	0.04	2.38	0.01	0.78	213.18	25.84	171.70	120.36	6.80	0.15	0.99	0.00	0.00	0.00	0.00
0.05	0.00	0.00	0.06	0.02	2.10	0.01	0.26	109.90	23.45	125.47	81.90	4.72	0.07	0.49	0.00	0.00	0.00	0.00
0.26	0.00	0.00	0.06	0.04	3.12	0.01	0.08	113.12	32.32	21.26	38.56	2.27	0.08	0.15	0.00	0.00	0.00	0.00
0.01	0.00	0.00	0.02	0.01	0.50	0.00	0.11	76.45	6.25	55.45	36.45	1.90	0.05	0.19	0.00	0.00	0.00	0.00
0.02	0.00	0.00	0.04	0.02	0.72	0.00	0.12	165.01	9.48	121.95	71.48	4.53	0.08	0.29	0.00	0.00	0.00	0.00
0.04	0.00	0.00	0.02	0.01	0.40	0.01	0.07	84.80	4.85	62.65	36.75	2.55	0.04	0.16	0.00	0.00	0.00	0.00
0.08	0.00	0.01	0.11	0.06	3.30	0.02	0.48	289.08	45.54	249.48	163.68	9.24	0.18	1.07	0.00	0.00	0.00	0.00
	0.00							65.00		100.00			0.00		0.00	0.00	0.00	0.00
0.05	0.00	0.01	0.11	0.05	8.06	0.01	0.18	77.50	77.50	168.64	113.46	9.30	0.27	0.83	0.00	0.00	0.00	0.00
0.06	0.00	0.00	0.12	0.06	7.44	0.02	0.21	52.08	65.10	128.34	97.96	6.82	0.23	0.72	0.00	0.00	0.00	0.00
	0.00	0.00	0.00	0.00				70.00	0.00	40.00	40.00	0.00	0.00		0.00	0.00	0.00	0.00
0.22	0.00	0.01	0.17	0.21	13.89	0.04	0.18	512.85	25.80	187.68	111.13	8.50	0.16	0.59	0.00	0.00	0.00	0.00
0.06	0.00	0.01	0.04	0.02	0.90	0.01	0.50	28.80	11.55	118.65	85.05	5.70	0.03	0.66	0.00	0.00	0.00	0.00
0.01	0.00	0.02	0.19	0.14	13.56	0.08	0.71	458.78	97.18	68.93	151.42	5.65	0.16	0.43	0.00	0.00	0.00	0.00
0.02	0.00	0.03	0.21	0.16	14.69	0.09	0.80	458.78	108.48	77.97	170.63	6.78	0.18	0.47	0.00	0.00	0.00	0.00
	0.00	0.03	0.26				0.48	330.00	90.00	80.00	150.00		0.00		0.00	0.00	0.00	0.00
0.04	0.00	0.02	0.17	0.13	12.60	0.07	0.65	425.25	88.20	63.00	138.60	5.25	0.15	0.39	0.00	0.00	0.00	0.00

Food Name	Amount	Measure	Weight (g)	Calories	Protein (g)	Total Carb (g)	Dietary Fiber (g)	Total Fat (g)	Sat Fat (g)	Mono Fat (g)	Poly Fat (g)	Chol (mg)	Vit A (mcg RAE)	Vit D (mcg)
CHEESE AND CHEESE SUBSTITUTES *(continued)*														
Cottage Cheese, creamed, sml curd, not packed	0.5	Cup	112.50	115.88	14.05	3.02	0.00	5.07	3.21	1.45	0.16	16.88	49.50	
Cottage Cheese, creamed, w/fruit	0.5	Cup	113.00	109.61	12.08	5.21	0.23	4.35	2.61	1.17	0.14	14.69	42.94	
Cottage Cheese, fat free Breakstone's	0.5	Cup	124.00	80.00	13.00	6.00	0.00	0.00	0.00	0.00	0.00	5.00		
Cottage Cheese, nonfat, lrg curd, dry	0.5	Cup	113.00	96.05	19.52	2.09	0.00	0.47	0.31	0.12	0.02	7.91	10.17	
Cottage Cheese, nonfat, sml curd, dry	0.5	Cup	113.00	96.05	19.52	2.09	0.00	0.47	0.31	0.12	0.02	7.91	10.17	
Cream Cheese	2	Tablespoon	29.00	101.21	2.19	0.77	0.00	10.11	6.37	2.85	0.37	31.90	106.14	
Cream Cheese, fat free	2	Tablespoon	29.00	27.84	4.18	1.68	0.00	0.39	0.26	0.10	0.02	2.32	80.91	
Cream Cheese, light, soft Philadelphia	2	Tablespoon	32.00	70.00	3.00	2.00	0.00	5.00	3.50			15.00		
Cream Cheese, soft Philadelphia	2	Tablespoon	30.00	100.00	2.00	1.00	0.00	10.00	7.00			30.00		
Cream Cheese, w/chives, whipped Philadelphia	2	Tablespoon	21.00	70.00	1.00	1.00	0.00	6.00	4.00			20.00		
Cream Cheese, whipped Philadelphia	2	Tablespoon	21.00	70.00	1.00	1.00	0.00	7.00	4.50			25.00		
Process Cheese and Cheese Substitutes														
Cheese Food, American, cold pack	1	Ounce-weight	28.35	93.84	5.58	2.36	0.00	6.94	4.36	2.03	0.21	18.14	45.08	
Cheese Food, American, past, proc, 1.2oz slice Kraft General Foods, Inc.	1	Each	34.00	113.33	6.48	3.24	0.00	8.10	5.67			24.29		
Cheese Food, American, white, past, proc, rducd fat, sliceKraft Singles	1	Piece	21.00	50.00	4.00	2.00	0.00	3.00	2.00			10.00		
Cheese Food, monterey, past, proc, slice Kraft Singles	1	Piece	21.00	70.00	4.00	2.00	0.00	5.00	3.50			15.00		
Cheese Food, sharp, past, proc, slice Kraft Singles	1	Piece	21.00	70.00	4.00	1.00	0.00	6.00	3.50			20.00		
Cheese Product, past, proc, light Kraft General Foods, Inc.	2	Tablespoon	35.00	75.25	5.70	5.67	0.07	3.32	2.24			12.25		
Cheese Sauce, past, proc, squeezable Kraft General Foods, Inc.	2	Tablespoon	33.00	100.00	2.00	4.00	0.00	8.00	4.00			15.00		
Cheese Spread, American, w/disod phosphate, 5oz jar	1	Ounce-weight	28.35	82.21	4.65	2.48	0.00	6.02	3.78	1.77	0.18	15.59	50.75	
Cheese Substitute, mozzarella, 1" cube	1	Each	17.60	43.65	2.02	4.17	0.00	2.15	0.65	1.10	0.31	0.00	76.91	
Cheese Substitute, soy, American Panos Brands Soy Kaas	1	Slice	19.00	45.00	3.00	3.00	0.00	2.00	0.50	0.50	1.00	0.00		
Cheese, American, past, proc, w/disod phosphate, shredded	0.25	Cup	28.25	105.94	6.26	0.45	0.00	8.83	5.56	2.53	0.28	26.55	71.75	
Cheese, American, yellow, low fat, singles Healthy Choice	1	Piece	21.00	40.00	5.00	2.00	0.00	1.00	0.50			5.00		
Cheese, pimento, past, proc, shredded	0.25	Cup	28.25	105.94	6.25	0.49	0.03	8.81	5.55	2.52	0.28	26.55	70.06	
Cheese, Swiss, past, proc, w/disod phosphate, shredded	0.25	Cup	28.25	94.35	6.99	0.59	0.00	7.07	4.53	1.99	0.18	24.01	55.93	
DAIRY PRODUCTS AND SUBSTITUTES														
Creams and Substitutes														
Cream Substitute, hydrog veg oil & soy prot, liquid	1	Tablespoon	15.00	20.40	0.15	1.71	0.00	1.50	0.29	1.13	0.00	0.00	0.15	
Cream Substitute, pwd	1	Teaspoon	1.96	10.70	0.09	1.08	0.00	0.70	0.64	0.02	0.00	0.00	0.04	
Cream, half & half	2	Tablespoon	30.00	39.00	0.89	1.29	0.00	3.45	2.15	1.00	0.13	11.10	29.10	
Cream Substitute, cinnamon hazelnut flvr Dean Foods International Delight	1	Tablespoon	17.00	40.00	0.00	7.00	0.00	1.50	0.00			0.00	0.00	
Cream Substitute, cinnamon hazelnut flvr, fat free Dean Foods International Delight	1	Tablespoon	17.00	30.00	0.00	7.00	0.00	0.00	0.00	0.00	0.00	0.00	0.00	
Cream, whipping, heavy	2	Tablespoon	29.75	102.64	0.61	0.83	0.00	11.01	6.85	3.18	0.41	40.76	122.27	0.39
Cream, whipping, light	2	Tablespoon	29.88	87.25	0.65	0.88	0.00	9.24	5.78	2.72	0.26	33.17	83.37	
Creamer, non-dairy Carnation Coffee Mate	1	Tablespoon	17.00	20.00	0.00	2.00	0.00	1.00	0.00	0.50	0.00	0.00	0.00	
Creamer, non-dairy, Cafe Mocha flvr Carnation Coffee Mate	1	Tablespoon	17.00	40.00	0.00	5.00	0.00	2.00	0.00	1.00	0.00	0.00	0.00	
Creamer, non-dairy, cinnamon hazelnut flvr, fat free International Delight	1	Tablespoon	17.00	30.00	0.00	7.00	0.00	0.00	0.00	0.00	0.00	0.00	0.00	
Sour Cream, cultured	2	Tablespoon	28.75	61.52	0.91	1.23	0.00	6.03	3.75	1.74	0.22	12.65	50.89	
Sour Cream, imitation, cultured	2	Tablespoon	28.75	59.80	0.69	1.91	0.00	5.61	5.11	0.17	0.02	0.00	0.00	
Sour Cream, rducd fat, cultured	2	Tablespoon	30.00	40.50	0.88	1.28	0.00	3.60	2.24	1.04	0.13	11.70	30.60	

Vit E (mg)	Vit C	Vit B₁ Thia (mg)	Vit B₂ Ribo (mg)	Vit B₃ Nia (mg)	Fol (mcg)	Vit B₆ (mg)	Vita B₁₂ (mcg)	Sodi (mg)	Pota (mg)	Cal (mg)	Phos (mg)	Magn (mg)	Iron (mg)	Zinc (mg)	Caff (mg)	Alco (g)	Sol Fiber (g)	Insol Fiber (g)
0.04	0.00	0.02	0.18	0.14	13.50	0.08	0.70	455.62	94.50	67.50	148.50	5.62	0.16	0.42	0.00	0.00	0.00	0.00
0.05	1.58	0.04	0.16	0.17	12.43	0.08	0.60	388.72	101.70	59.89	127.69	7.91	0.18	0.37	0.00	0.00		
	0.00		0.26				0.48	440.00	150.00	80.00	150.00		0.00		0.00	0.00	0.00	0.00
0.00	0.00	0.03	0.16	0.18	16.95	0.09	0.94	14.69	36.16	36.16	117.52	4.52	0.26	0.53	0.00	0.00	0.00	0.00
0.00	0.00	0.03	0.16	0.18	16.95	0.09	0.94	14.69	36.16	36.16	117.52	4.52	0.26	0.53	0.00	0.00	0.00	0.00
0.09	0.00	0.00	0.06	0.03	3.77	0.01	0.12	85.84	34.51	23.20	30.16	1.74	0.35	0.16	0.00	0.00	0.00	0.00
0.00	0.00	0.01	0.05	0.05	10.73	0.01	0.16	158.05	47.27	53.65	125.86	4.06	0.05	0.26	0.00	0.00	0.00	0.00
	0.00		0.03				0.00	150.00	55.00	40.00	40.00	0.00	0.00	0.00	0.00	0.00	0.00	0.00
	0.00		0.03				0.00	100.00	40.00	20.00	40.00	0.00	0.00	0.00	0.00	0.00	0.00	0.00
	0.00		0.03					130.00	30.00	20.00	20.00		0.00	0.00	0.00	0.00	0.00	0.00
	0.00		0.03				0.00	85.00	25.00	0.00	20.00	0.00	0.00	0.00	0.00	0.00	0.00	0.00
0.19	0.00	0.01	0.12	0.02	1.42	0.04	0.36	273.86	102.91	140.90	113.40	8.50	0.24	0.85	0.00	0.00	0.00	0.00
	0.00		0.17				0.19	453.33	80.95	161.90	161.90	0.00	0.00	0.97	0.00	0.00	0.00	0.00
	0.00		0.10				0.24	320.00	60.00	150.00	100.00	0.00	0.00	0.60	0.00	0.00	0.00	0.00
	0.00		0.10				0.24	290.00	55.00	100.00	100.00	0.00	0.00	0.60	0.00	0.00	0.00	0.00
	0.00		0.07				0.12	300.00	25.00	100.00	100.00	0.00	0.00	0.60	0.00	0.00	0.00	0.00
	0.14		0.12				0.12	596.75	103.95	146.30	330.05	8.00	0.06	0.83	0.00	0.00		
	0.00		0.07				0.00	470.00	30.00	60.00	200.00	0.00	0.00	0.30	0.00	0.00	0.00	0.00
0.09	0.00	0.01	0.12	0.04	1.98	0.04	0.11	460.69	68.61	159.33	248.06	8.22	0.09	0.74	0.00	0.00	0.00	0.00
0.02	0.02	0.01	0.08	0.06	1.94	0.01	0.14	120.56	80.08	107.36	102.61	7.22	0.07	0.34	0.00	0.00	0.00	0.00
	0.00							180.00		150.00			0.00		0.00	0.00	0.00	0.00
0.08	0.00	0.01	0.10	0.02	2.26	0.02	0.20	420.64	47.74	155.94	144.92	7.63	0.05	0.80	0.00	0.00	0.00	0.00
	0.00	0.02	0.05	0.00				200.00		150.00			0.00		0.00	0.00	0.00	0.00
0.08	0.65	0.01	0.10	0.02	2.26	0.02	0.20	403.41	45.76	173.45	210.18	6.21	0.12	0.84	0.00	0.00		
0.10	0.00	0.00	0.08	0.01	1.69	0.01	0.35	387.02	61.02	218.09	215.26	8.19	0.17	1.02	0.00	0.00	0.00	0.00
0.12	0.00	0.00	0.00	0.00	0.00	0.00	0.00	11.85	28.65	1.35	9.60	0.00	0.00	0.00	0.00	0.00	0.00	0.00
0.01	0.00	0.00	0.00	0.00	0.00	0.00	0.00	3.55	15.92	0.43	8.27	0.08	0.02	0.01	0.00	0.00	0.00	0.00
0.10	0.27	0.01	0.04	0.02	0.90	0.01	0.10	12.30	39.00	31.50	28.50	3.00	0.02	0.15	0.00	0.00	0.00	0.00
	0.00							5.00		0.00			0.00		0.00	0.00	0.00	0.00
	0.00							5.00		0.00			0.00		0.00	0.00	0.00	0.00
0.32	0.18	0.01	0.03	0.01	1.19	0.01	0.05	11.31	22.31	19.34	18.45	2.08	0.01	0.07	0.00	0.00	0.00	0.00
0.26	0.18	0.01	0.04	0.01	1.20	0.01	0.06	10.16	28.98	20.62	18.23	2.09	0.01	0.07	0.00	0.00	0.00	0.00
	0.00							0.00	25.00	0.00			0.00		0.00	0.00	0.00	0.00
	0.00							5.00	30.00	0.00			0.00		0.00	0.00	0.00	0.00
	0.00							5.00		0.00			0.00		0.00	0.00	0.00	0.00
0.17	0.26	0.01	0.04	0.02	3.16	0.00	0.09	15.24	41.40	33.35	24.44	3.16	0.02	0.08	0.00	0.00	0.00	0.00
0.21	0.00	0.00	0.00	0.00	0.00	0.00	0.00	29.32	46.29	0.86	12.94	1.72	0.11	0.34	0.00	0.00	0.00	0.00
0.10	0.27	0.01	0.04	0.02	3.30	0.00	0.09	12.30	38.70	31.20	28.50	3.00	0.02	0.15	0.00	0.00	0.00	0.00

Food Name	Amount	Measure	Weight (g)	Calories	Protein (g)	Total Carb (g)	Dietary Fiber (g)	Total Fat (g)	Sat Fat (g)	Mono Fat (g)	Poly Fat (g)	Chol (mg)	Vit A (mcg RAE)	Vit D (mcg)
DAIRY PRODUCTS AND SUBSTITUTES *(continued)*														
Milks and Non-Dairy Milks														
Buttermilk, dried	1	Tablespoon	7.50	29.03	2.57	3.68	0.00	0.43	0.27	0.13	0.02	5.18	3.68	
Buttermilk, low fat, cultured	1	Cup	245.00	98.00	8.11	11.74	0.00	2.16	1.34	0.62	0.08	9.80	17.15	
Eggnog	1	Cup	254.00	342.90	9.68	34.39	0.00	19.00	11.29	5.67	0.86	149.86	114.30	
Eggnog, prep f/dry mix w/milk	1	Cup	272.00	258.40	7.97	38.62	0.00	8.21	4.63	2.09	0.51	29.92	70.72	
Milk Substitute, fluid, w/hydrog veg oil	1	Cup	244.00	148.84	4.27	15.03	0.00	8.32	1.87	4.88	1.19	0.00	0.00	
Milk Substitute, fluid, w/lauric acid oil	1	Cup	244.00	148.84	4.27	15.03	0.00	8.32	7.41	0.43	0.02	0.00	0.00	
Milk, 1%, prot fort, w/add vit A & D	1	Cup	246.00	118.08	9.67	13.58	0.00	2.88	1.79	0.83	0.11	9.84	150.06	2.46
Milk, 1%, w/add vit A & D	1	Cup	244.00	102.48	8.22	12.18	0.00	2.37	1.54	0.68	0.09	12.20	141.52	3.17
Milk, 2%, prot fort, w/add vit A, ckd	1	Cup	244.00	135.46	9.64	13.40	0.00	4.83	3.01	1.40	0.18	18.79		2.44
Milk, 2%, prot fort, w/vit D	1	Cup	246.00	137.76	9.72	13.51	0.00	4.87	3.03	1.41	0.18	19.68	0.62	2.46
Milk, 2%, w/add nonfat milk solids, not fortified	1	Cup	245.00	137.20	9.68	13.45	0.00	4.85	3.02	0.16	0.02	19.60	41.65	
Milk, 2%, w/add vit A & D Darigold, Inc.	1	Cup	245.00	130.00	8.00	13.00	0.00	5.00	3.00			20.00		2.50
Milk, almond, chocolate Pacific Foods of Oregon Pacific Natural Foods	8	Fluid ounce	245.00	102.36	1.49	18.70	0.94	2.85	0.00			0.00	25.00	2.50
Milk, almond, original, unsweetened Blue Diamond Almond Breeze	8	Fluid ounce	227.00	40.00	1.00	2.00	1.00	3.00	0.00			0.00		2.50
Milk, almond, vanilla Pacific Foods of Oregon Pacific Natural Foods	8	Fluid ounce	245.00	71.60	1.12	10.98	0.52	2.66	0.00			0.00	25.00	2.50
Milk, chocolate, cmrcl	1	Cup	250.00	207.50	7.92	25.85	2.00	8.48	5.26	2.48	0.31	30.00	65.00	2.50
Milk, chocolate, prep w/syrup	1	Cup	282.00	253.80	8.66	36.04	0.85	8.35	4.74	2.09	0.49	25.38	70.50	4.23
Milk, cond, swtnd, cnd	2	Tablespoon	38.25	122.78	3.03	20.81	0.00	3.33	2.10	0.93	0.13	13.00	28.30	
Milk, evaporated, w/add vit A, cnd	2	Tablespoon	31.50	42.21	2.15	3.16	0.00	2.38	1.45	0.74	0.08	9.13	35.28	
Milk, goat	1	Cup	244.00	168.36	8.69	10.86	0.00	10.10	6.51	2.71	0.36	26.84	139.08	0.73
Milk, Indian buffalo	1	Cup	244.00	236.68	9.15	12.64	0.00	16.81	11.22	4.36	0.36	46.36	129.32	
Milk, low fat, chocolate, cmrcl	1	Cup	250.00	157.50	8.10	26.10	1.25	2.50	1.54	0.75	0.09	7.50	145.00	2.50
Milk, nonfat/skim, prot fort, w/vit A	1	Cup	246.00	100.86	9.74	13.68	0.00	0.62	0.40	0.16	0.02	4.92	150.06	2.46
Milk, nonfat/skim, w/add vit A	1	Cup	245.00	83.30	8.26	12.15	0.00	0.20	0.13	0.05	0.01	4.90	149.45	2.54
Milk, nonfat/skim, w/add vit A, inst, dry pwd	1	Tablespoon	4.25	15.22	1.49	2.22	0.00	0.03	0.02	0.01	0.00	0.77	30.13	0.47
Milk, nonfat/skim, w/o add vit A, dry mix	1	Tablespoon	7.50	27.15	2.71	3.90	0.00	0.06	0.04	0.02	0.00	1.50	0.45	0.62
Milk, sheep	1	Cup	245.00	264.60	14.65	13.13	0.00	17.15	11.28	4.22	0.75	66.15	107.80	
Milk, whole, 3.25%	1	Cup	244.00	146.40	7.86	11.03	0.00	7.93	4.55	1.98	0.48	24.40	68.32	2.47
Milk, whole, dry pwd	1	Tablespoon	8.00	39.68	2.11	3.07	0.00	2.14	1.34	0.63	0.05	7.76	20.56	0.62
Rice Milk, original Imagine Foods	1	Cup	244.80	119.95	0.42	24.82	0.00	1.98	0.17	1.34	0.31	0.00	0.24	0.00
Rice Milk, vanilla Hain Celestial Group Rice Dream	8	Fluid ounce	248.00	130.00	1.00	28.00	0.00	2.00	0.00			0.00	0.00	0.00
Rice Milk, vanilla, enrich Hain Celestial Group Rice Dream	8	Fluid ounce	249.00	130.00	1.00	28.00	0.00	2.00	0.00			0.00		2.50
Soy Milk	1	Cup	245.00	127.40	10.98	12.08	3.19	4.70	0.57	0.94	1.88	0.00	75.95	0.98
Soy Milk, asrtd flvrs, light, w/add calc vit A & D USDA SR-23	1	Cup	243.00	114.21	5.10	20.02	1.70	1.56	0.08	0.09	0.98	0.00	148.64	2.92
Soy Milk, chocolate USDA SR-23	1	Cup	243.00	153.09	5.49	24.18	0.97	3.72	0.58	0.92	2.03	0.00	0.36	0.00
Soy Milk, chocolate, light, w/add calc vit A & D USDA SR-23	1	Cup	243.00	114.21	5.10	20.02	1.70	1.56	0.08	0.09	0.98	0.00	148.64	2.92
Soy Milk, chocolate, enrich Imagine Foods	1	Cup	244.00	201.73	6.72	35.54	0.96	3.36	0.48			0.00		2.40
Soy Milk, original, light Vitasoy Incorporated	1	Cup	228.30	90.00	4.00	15.00		2.00	0.00	0.50	1.00	0.00		
Yogurt														
Kefir, blueberry Springfield Creamery Nancy's	1	Cup	225.00	220.00	7.00	26.00	1.00	8.00	6.00			35.00		
Kefir, strawberry Springfield Creamery Nancy's	1	Cup	225.00	200.00	7.00	23.00	1.00	8.00	6.00			35.00		
Yogurt, banana, low fat General Mills Yoplait Thick & Creamy	1	Container	170.00	190.00	7.00	32.00	0.00	3.50	2.00			15.00		2.00
Yogurt, burstin' melon berry, tube General Mills Yoplait Go-Gurt	1	Each	64.00	80.00	2.00	13.00	0.00	2.00	1.00			5.00	0.00	
Yogurt, cool cotton candy, tube General Mills Yoplait Go-Gurt	1	Each	64.00	80.00	2.00	13.00	0.00	2.00	1.00			5.00	0.00	
Yogurt, fruit, low fat, 10g prot/8oz ctn	1	Each	226.80	231.34	9.91	43.21	0.00	2.45	1.58	0.67	0.07	9.07	22.68	
Yogurt, Greek, 0% FAGE USA FAGE Total	1	Cup	227.00	120.00	20.00	9.00	0.00	0.00	0.00	0.00	0.00	0.00	0.00	

Vit E (mg)	Vit C	Vit B₁ Thia (mg)	Vit B₂ Ribo (mg)	Vit B₃ Nia (mg)	Fol (mcg)	Vit B₆ (mg)	Vita B₁₂ (mcg)	Sodi (mg)	Pota (mg)	Cal (mg)	Phos (mg)	Magn (mg)	Iron (mg)	Zinc (mg)	Caff (mg)	Alco (g)	Sol Fiber (g)	Insol Fiber (g)
0.01	0.43	0.03	0.12	0.07	3.53	0.03	0.29	38.78	119.40	88.80	69.98	8.25	0.02	0.30	0.00	0.00	0.00	0.00
0.12	2.45	0.08	0.38	0.14	12.25	0.08	0.54	257.25	369.95	284.20	218.05	26.95	0.12	1.03	0.00	0.00	0.00	0.00
0.51	3.81	0.09	0.48	0.27	2.54	0.13	1.14	137.16	419.10	330.20	276.86	48.26	0.51	1.17	0.00	0.00	0.00	0.00
0.16	0.00	0.11	0.45	0.30	13.60	0.09	1.06	149.60	329.12	250.24	209.44	27.20	0.33	0.95	0.00	0.00	0.00	0.00
0.68	0.00	0.03	0.21	0.00	0.00	0.00	0.00	190.32	278.16	80.52	180.56	14.64	0.95	2.88	0.00	0.00	0.00	0.00
2.56	0.00	0.03	0.21	0.00	0.00	0.00	0.00	190.32	278.16	80.52	180.56	14.64	0.95	2.88	0.00	0.00	0.00	0.00
0.10	2.95	0.11	0.47	0.25	14.76	0.12	1.06	142.68	442.80	349.32	273.06	39.36	0.15	1.11	0.00	0.00	0.00	0.00
0.02	0.00	0.05	0.45	0.23	12.20	0.09	1.07	107.36	366.00	290.36	231.80	26.84	0.07	1.02	0.00	0.00	0.00	0.00
0.08	1.37	0.10	0.43	0.25	11.71	0.11	1.00	143.47	443.35	349.16	273.28	39.24	0.15	1.10	0.00	0.00	0.00	0.00
0.10	2.71	0.11	0.48	0.25	14.76	0.13	1.06	145.14	447.72	351.78	275.52	39.36	0.15	1.11	0.00	0.00	0.00	0.00
0.17	2.70	0.11	0.48	0.25	12.25	0.11	0.96	144.55	445.90	350.35	274.40	36.75	0.15	1.00	0.00	0.00	0.00	0.00
	1.20		0.45					125.00		250.00			0.00		0.00	0.00	0.00	0.00
	0.00		0.51					144.73	135.32	10.08			0.04			0.00		
10.07	0.00							180.00	190.00	200.00	40.00	16.00	0.36		0.00	0.00		
	0.00		0.51					141.16	143.56	7.37			0.00		0.00	0.00		
0.15	2.25	0.09	0.40	0.31	12.50	0.10	0.82	150.00	417.50	280.00	252.50	32.50	0.60	1.02	5.00	0.00		
0.14	0.00	0.11	0.47	0.39	14.10	0.09	1.07	132.54	408.90	250.98	253.80	50.76	0.90	1.21	5.64	0.00		
0.06	0.99	0.03	0.16	0.08	4.21	0.02	0.17	48.58	141.91	108.63	96.77	9.94	0.07	0.36	0.00	0.00	0.00	0.00
0.06	0.60	0.01	0.10	0.06	2.52	0.02	0.05	33.39	95.44	82.21	63.94	7.56	0.06	0.24	0.00	0.00	0.00	0.00
0.17	3.17	0.12	0.34	0.68	2.44	0.11	0.17	122.00	497.76	326.96	270.84	34.16	0.12	0.73	0.00	0.00	0.00	0.00
	5.61	0.13	0.33	0.22	14.64	0.06	0.88	126.88	434.32	412.36	285.48	75.64	0.29	0.54	0.00	0.00	0.00	0.00
0.05	2.25	0.10	0.42	0.32	12.50	0.10	0.85	152.50	425.00	287.50	257.50	32.50	0.60	1.02	5.00	0.00		
0.10	2.71	0.11	0.48	0.25	14.76	0.12	1.06	145.14	447.72	351.78	275.52	39.36	0.15	1.11	0.00	0.00	0.00	0.00
0.02	0.00	0.11	0.45	0.23	12.25	0.09	1.30	102.90	382.20	306.25	247.45	26.95	0.07	1.03	0.00	0.00	0.00	0.00
0.00	0.24	0.02	0.07	0.04	2.13	0.01	0.17	23.33	72.46	52.32	41.86	4.97	0.01	0.19	0.00	0.00	0.00	0.00
0.00	0.51	0.03	0.12	0.07	3.75	0.03	0.30	40.13	134.55	94.28	72.60	8.25	0.02	0.31	0.00	0.00	0.00	0.00
0.25	10.29	0.16	0.87	1.02	17.15	0.15	1.74	107.80	335.65	472.85	387.10	44.10	0.25	1.32	0.00	0.00	0.00	0.00
0.15	0.00	0.11	0.45	0.26	12.20	0.09	1.07	97.60	348.92	275.72	222.04	24.40	0.07	0.98	0.00	0.00	0.00	0.00
0.04	0.69	0.02	0.10	0.05	2.96	0.02	0.26	29.68	106.40	72.96	62.08	6.80	0.04	0.27	0.00	0.00	0.00	0.00
1.76	1.22	0.08	0.01	1.91	90.58	0.04	0.00	85.68	68.54	19.58	34.27	9.79	0.20	0.24	0.00	0.00	0.00	0.00
0.81	0.00							90.00		20.00			0.00		0.00	0.00	0.00	0.00
0.81	0.00						1.50	90.00		300.00	150.00		0.00		0.00	0.00	0.00	0.00
3.31	0.00	0.15	0.12	0.71	39.20	0.24	2.99	134.75	303.80	93.10	134.75	61.25	2.70	1.08	0.00	0.00	0.47	2.72
0.32	0.00	0.09	0.49	1.24	21.87	0.09	2.43	111.78	349.92	298.89	211.41	36.45	1.43	0.56	4.86	0.00		
0.02	4.13	0.05	0.64	1.25	26.73	0.19	1.70	128.79	347.49	60.75	123.93	36.45	1.17	0.83	4.86	0.00		
0.32	0.00	0.09	0.49	1.24	21.87	0.09	2.43	111.78	349.92	298.89	211.41	36.45	1.43	0.56	4.86	0.00		
4.83	0.00	0.14	0.07	0.77	57.64	0.12	2.88	153.70	336.22	288.19	240.16	57.64	1.73	0.58		0.00		
		0.09	0.07					95.00	125.00	80.00					0.00	0.00		
	6.00							120.00		250.00			0.00		0.00	0.00		
	21.00							110.00		250.00			0.36		0.00	0.00		
	0.00							100.00	310.00	300.00	150.00		0.00		0.00	0.00	0.00	0.00
	0.00		0.07					40.00	110.00	100.00	60.00		0.00		0.00	0.00	0.00	0.00
	0.00		0.07					40.00	110.00	100.00	60.00		0.00		0.00	0.00	0.00	0.00
0.05	1.59	0.08	0.40	0.22	20.41	0.09	1.07	131.54	442.26	344.74	269.89	34.02	0.16	1.68	0.00	0.00	0.00	0.00
	0.00							85.00		150.00			0.00		0.00	0.00	0.00	0.00

Food Name	Amount	Measure	Weight (g)	Calories	Protein (g)	Total Carb (g)	Dietary Fiber (g)	Total Fat (g)	Sat Fat (g)	Mono Fat (g)	Poly Fat (g)	Chol (mg)	Vit A (mcg RAE)	Vit D (mcg)
DAIRY PRODUCTS AND SUBSTITUTES *(continued)*														
Yogurt, Greek, 2% FAGE USA FAGE Total	1	Cup	227.00	150.00	19.00	9.00	0.00	4.50	3.00			15.00		
Yogurt, Greek, 2%, w/cherry FAGE USA FAGE Total	1	Container	150.00	140.00	10.00	19.00	0.00	2.50	1.50			5.00	0.00	
Yogurt, Greek, 2%, w/honey FAGE USA FAGE Total	1	Container	150.00	180.00	10.00	29.00	0.00	2.50	1.50			5.00	0.00	
Yogurt, Greek, w/honey & walnuts FAGE USA FAGE Total	1	Container	160.00	310.00	9.00	30.00	0.00	17.00	10.00			20.00		
Yogurt, plain, low fat, 12g prot/8oz ctn	1	Each	226.80	142.88	11.91	15.97	0.00	3.52	2.27	0.97	0.10	13.61	31.75	
Yogurt, plain, skim, 13g prot/8oz ctn	1	Each	226.80	127.01	13.00	17.42	0.00	0.41	0.26	0.11	0.01	4.54	4.54	
Yogurt, plain, whole milk, 8g prot/8oz ctn	1	Each	226.80	138.35	7.87	10.57	0.00	7.37	4.75	2.03	0.21	29.48	61.24	
Yogurt, soy, plain, 8oz ctn Silk	1	Each	170.10	90.00	3.75	16.50	0.75	1.88	0.00			0.00		
Yogurt, soy, vanilla USDA SR-23 Silk	1	Each	170.10	149.69	5.00	25.02	1.02	2.99	0.00			0.00	0.00	
Yogurt, vanilla, low fat, 8oz ctn	1	Each	226.80	192.78	11.18	31.30	0.00	2.84	1.83	0.78	0.08	11.34	27.22	
Yogurt, vanilla, nonfat, 8oz ctn	1	Each	227.00	206.56	11.62	39.70	0.00	0.37	0.24	0.10	0.01	3.65	4.06	0.06
DESSERTS														
Brownies and Bars														
Bar, wafer, w/peanut butter, chocolate cvrd, Nutty Bars Little Debbies	1	Each	57.00	312.36	4.56	31.46		18.70	3.59					
Brownie, dry mix Gold Medal	1	Ounce-weight	28.35	124.17	1.70	21.55	0.94	3.69	1.25	1.33	0.31	9.64		
Brownie, fudge, chewy, dry mix, svg Martha White	1	Ounce-weight	28.35	115.67	1.34	23.53		1.78	0.45					
Brownie, nut, w/o icing & nut topping Keebler Company Incorporated	1	Each	35.00	151.20	1.40	22.05	0.70	6.30	1.61			8.05		
Brownie, prep f/recipe, 2" square	1	Each	24.00	111.84	1.49	12.05	0.53	6.98	1.76	2.60	2.26	17.52	42.24	
Brownie, special dietary, prep f/dry mix, 2" square	1	Each	22.00	84.48	0.84	15.69	0.81	2.44	1.12	1.01	0.18	0.00	0.00	
Cakes														
Cake, angel food, cmrcl prep, 9" whl or 1/12 pce	1	Piece	28.35	73.14	1.67	16.39	0.43	0.23	0.03	0.02	0.10	0.00	0.00	
Cake, angel food, prep f/dry mix, tube, 10" whl or 1/12 pce	1	Piece	50.00	128.50	3.05	29.35	0.10	0.15	0.02	0.01	0.06	0.00	0.00	
Cake, Boston cream pie, cmrcl prep, 9" whl or 1/6 pce	1	Piece	92.00	231.84	2.21	39.47	1.29	7.82	2.25	4.18	0.93	34.04	22.08	
Cake, carrot, layer, w/cream cheese frosting, whl or 1/24pce Mrs. Smith's	1	Piece	76.00	300.00	3.00	35.00	1.00	16.00	4.00			20.00		
Cake, chocolate mousse, enchantment, 9" whl or 1/14 pce Mrs. Smith's	1	Piece	130.00	510.00	5.00	68.00	2.00	25.00	12.00			35.00		
Cake, chocolate, prep f/rec, w/o frosting 9" whl or 1/12 pce	1	Piece	95.00	340.10	5.03	50.73	1.52	14.34	5.16	5.74	2.62	55.10	38.00	
Cake, chocolate, w/chocolate icing, cmrcl prep 1/8th of 18oz	1	Piece	64.00	234.88	2.62	34.94	1.79	10.50	3.05	5.61	1.18	26.88	16.64	
Cake, coffee, cheese, 1/6 of 16oz	1	Piece	76.00	257.64	5.32	33.67	0.76	11.55	4.10	5.42	1.25	64.60	65.36	
Cake, coffee, cinnamon, w/crumb topping prep f/mix 8" or 1/8	1	Piece	56.00	178.08	3.08	29.57	0.67	5.38	1.04	2.16	1.77	27.44	19.60	
Cake, coffee, cinnamon, w/crumb topping, enrich, indv cake	1	Each	57.00	238.26	3.88	26.62	1.14	13.28	3.30	7.40	1.78	18.24	18.81	
Cake, coffee, fruit, 1/8	1	Piece	50.00	155.50	2.60	25.75	1.25	5.10	1.25	2.78	0.74	3.50	3.50	
Cake, Ding Dongs, w/cream filling, Hostess Ralston Foods	1	Each	80.00	368.00	3.12	45.36	1.84	19.36	11.04	3.99	1.20	13.60		
Cake, gingerbread, prep f/rec, 1/9 of 8" square	1	Piece	74.00	263.44	2.89	36.41	0.61	12.14	3.05	5.27	3.12	23.68	10.36	
Cake, krimpet, Kreme Krimpies, sponge cake w/filling TastyKake, Inc.	2	Each	57.00	230.00	2.00	37.00	0.00	8.00	1.50			40.00		
Cake, pineapple upside down, prep f/rec, 1/9th of 8" square	1	Piece	115.00	366.85	4.02	58.07	0.92	13.91	3.35	5.97	3.77	25.30	71.30	
Cake, pound, w/butter, cmrcl prep, 1/10 pce	1	Piece	30.00	116.40	1.65	14.64	0.15	5.97	3.47	1.77	0.32	66.30	44.70	
Cake, sponge, cmrcl prep, 1/12 of 16oz	1	Piece	38.00	109.82	2.05	23.22	0.19	1.03	0.30	0.36	0.17	38.76	16.72	
Cake, white, dry mix, 18.5 oz pkg	1	Ounce-weight	28.35	120.77	1.28	22.11	0.26	3.09	0.46	1.30	1.16	0.00		
Cake, white, w/o frosting, prep f/recipe, 9" or 1/12 pce	1	Piece	74.00	264.18	4.00	42.33	0.59	9.18	2.42	3.93	2.33	1.48	11.10	

Vit E (mg)	Vit C	Vit B₁ Thia (mg)	Vit B₂ Ribo (mg)	Vit B₃ Nia (mg)	Fol (mcg)	Vit B₆ (mg)	Vita B₁₂ (mcg)	Sodi (mg)	Pota (mg)	Cal (mg)	Phos (mg)	Magn (mg)	Iron (mg)	Zinc (mg)	Caff (mg)	Alco (g)	Sol Fiber (g)	Insol Fiber (g)
	0.00							75.00		150.00			0.00		0.00	0.00	0.00	0.00
	0.00							40.00		80.00			0.00		0.00	0.00	0.00	0.00
	0.00							40.00		80.00			0.00		0.00	0.00	0.00	0.00
	0.00							35.00		100.00			0.36		0.00	0.00	0.00	0.00
0.07	1.81	0.10	0.49	0.26	24.95	0.11	1.27	158.76	530.71	415.04	326.59	38.56	0.18	2.02	0.00	0.00	0.00	0.00
0.00	2.04	0.11	0.53	0.28	27.22	0.12	1.38	174.64	578.34	451.33	356.08	43.09	0.20	2.20	0.00	0.00	0.00	0.00
0.14	1.13	0.07	0.32	0.17	15.88	0.07	0.84	104.33	351.54	274.43	215.46	27.22	0.11	1.34	0.00	0.00	0.00	0.00
	0.00							22.50		525.00			0.68		0.00	0.00		
	29.94							20.41		299.38			1.45		0.00	0.00		
0.05	1.81	0.10	0.46	0.24	24.95	0.10	1.20	149.69	496.69	387.83	306.18	36.29	0.16	1.88	0.00	0.00	0.00	0.00
0.01	1.76	0.10	0.48	0.25	24.75	0.11	1.24	155.43	517.56	404.13	317.96	38.75	0.20	1.97	0.00	0.00	0.00	0.00
	1.14							127.11								0.00		
	0.00	0.04	0.05	0.37				83.63	100.08	6.80			0.85			0.00		
								140.05					1.10			0.00		
	0.00	0.09	0.07	0.60	7.35			101.50		9.41			0.35			0.00		
0.70	0.07	0.04	0.05	0.23	6.96	0.02	0.04	82.32	42.24	13.68	31.68	12.72	0.44	0.23		0.00		
0.00	0.00	0.02	0.03	0.22	9.46	0.00	0.01	20.68	69.08	2.64	11.44	1.32	0.30	0.03	0.44	0.00		
0.03	0.00	0.03	0.14	0.25	9.92	0.01	0.02	212.34	26.37	39.69	9.07	3.40	0.15	0.02	0.00	0.00	0.13	0.30
0.00	0.00	0.05	0.10	0.09	9.50	0.00	0.02	254.50	67.50	42.00	116.00	4.00	0.12	0.06	0.00	0.00	0.03	0.07
0.14	0.18	0.38	0.25	0.18	12.88	0.02	0.15	132.48	35.88	21.16	45.08	5.52	0.35	0.15	0.00	0.00		
								380.00								0.00	0.00	
								250.00								0.00		
1.51	0.19	0.13	0.20	1.08	25.65	0.04	0.15	299.25	133.00	57.00	100.70	30.40	1.53	0.66		0.00	0.35	1.17
0.01	0.06	0.02	0.09	0.37	10.88	0.03	0.09	213.76	128.00	27.52	78.08	21.76	1.41	0.44	7.42	0.00		
1.19	0.08	0.08	0.09	0.52	29.64	0.04	0.26	257.64	219.64	44.84	76.76	11.40	0.49	0.45	0.00	0.00	0.16	0.60
0.11	0.11	0.09	0.10	0.85	26.88	0.03	0.08	235.76	62.72	76.16	120.40	10.08	0.80	0.25	0.00	0.00	0.14	0.53
1.94	0.17	0.12	0.13	0.96	34.77	0.02	0.10	200.07	70.11	30.78	61.56	12.54	1.09	0.46	0.00	0.00	0.24	0.90
0.42	0.40	0.02	0.10	1.29	23.50	0.02	0.01	192.50	45.00	22.50	59.00	8.50	1.22	0.32	0.00	0.00	0.25	1.00
								240.80		3.20			1.84			0.00		
1.78	0.07	0.14	0.12	1.29	24.42	0.14	0.04	241.98	324.86	52.54	39.96	51.80	2.13	0.29	0.00	0.00		
	0.00							160.00		20.00			0.72		0.00	0.00	0.00	0.00
1.54	1.38	0.18	0.18	1.37	29.90	0.04	0.09	366.85	128.80	138.00	94.30	14.95	1.70	0.36	0.00	0.00		
0.20	0.00	0.04	0.07	0.39	12.30	0.01	0.08	119.40	35.70	10.50	41.10	3.30	0.41	0.14	0.00	0.00	0.04	0.11
0.09	0.00	0.09	0.10	0.73	17.86	0.02	0.09	92.72	37.62	26.60	52.06	4.18	1.03	0.19	0.00	0.00	0.05	0.14
0.25	0.09	0.07	0.06	0.30	25.80	0.01	0.05	188.24	33.17	54.43	95.54	3.12	0.40	0.13	0.00	0.00	0.06	0.20
0.09	0.15	0.14	0.18	1.13	28.12	0.02	0.06	241.98	70.30	96.20	68.82	8.88	1.12	0.24	0.00	0.00	0.12	0.47

Food Name	Amount	Measure	Weight (g)	Calories	Protein (g)	Total Carb (g)	Dietary Fiber (g)	Total Fat (g)	Sat Fat (g)	Mono Fat (g)	Poly Fat (g)	Chol (mg)	Vit A (mcg RAE)	Vit D (mcg)
DESSERTS *(continued)*														
Cake, yellow, w/chocolate icing, cmrcl prep, 1/8 of 18oz	1	Piece	64.00	242.56	2.43	35.46	1.15	11.14	2.98	6.14	1.35	35.20	21.12	
Cake, yellow, w/vanilla icing, cmrcl prep, 1/8 of 18oz	1	Piece	64.00	238.72	2.24	37.63	0.19	9.28	1.52	3.91	3.30	35.20	12.16	
Cheesecake, amaretto The Cheesecake Lady	1	Each	113.40	420.00	7.00	30.00	1.00	31.00	16.00			100.00		
Cheesecake, cmrcl prep, 1/6 of 17oz	1	Piece	80.00	256.80	4.40	20.40	0.32	18.00	7.94	6.91	1.28	44.00	113.60	
Cheesecake, no bake, prep f/dry mix, 1/12 of 9"	1	Piece	99.00	271.26	5.45	35.15	1.88	12.57	6.62	4.47	0.80	28.71	95.04	
Cupcake, snack, choc, w/buttercream icing & cream filling Tasty Baking Company Tastykake	3	Each	99.00	390.00	4.00	63.00	2.00	15.00	4.00			20.00	0.00	0.09
Muffin, coffee coffee, fzn Krusteaz	1	Each	57.00	229.14	3.53	28.50	1.14	11.17	2.04	3.35	5.78	41.04		
Cookies														
Cookie, anisette sponge, w/o lemon juice & rind 4" × 1 1/8" × 7/8	2	Each	26.00	94.90	2.76	15.52	0.26	2.37	0.88	1.07	0.41	94.90	43.42	
Cookie, biscotti, almond Perugina	1	Each	26.77	120.00	1.00	17.00	1.00	5.00	2.00			25.00	0.00	
Cookie, biscuit, shortbread, intl collection Pepperidge Farm	2	Each	27.00	140.00	25.00	5.00	2.00	7.00	5.00			17.00	0.00	
Cookie, bordeaux, distinctive Pepperidge Farm	4	Each	28.00	130.00	1.00	20.00	1.00	5.00	2.50	1.50	0.00	10.00	0.00	
Cookie, butter, enrich, cmrcl prep	5	Each	25.00	116.75	1.52	17.23	0.20	4.70	2.76	1.38	0.25	29.25	41.25	
Cookie, chocolate chip Archway Cookies	3	Each	27.00	130.00	1.00	17.00	0.00	7.00	2.00			10.00	0.00	
Cookie, chocolate chip, dry mix Arrowhead Mills, Inc.	1	Ounce-weight	28.35	113.40	1.42	22.68	0.00	2.12	0.72			0.00	0.00	
Cookie, chocolate chip, enrich, higher fat cmrcl lrg 3.5"-4"	1	Each	40.00	195.60	2.20	25.63	1.16	9.89	3.07	5.31	0.55	0.00	0.00	
Cookie, chocolate chip, fudge, big, homestyle Grandma's	1	Each	39.00	170.00	1.00	26.00	1.00	7.00	2.50			5.00	0.00	
Cookie, chocolate chip, lower fat, cmrcl prep	3	Each	30.00	135.90	1.74	21.99	1.08	4.62	1.14	1.83	1.39	0.00		
Cookie, chocolate chip, prep w/butter f/recipe 2 1/4"	2	Each	32.00	156.16	1.82	18.62	0.80	9.08	4.50	2.64	1.46	22.40	44.48	
Cookie, chocolate chip, refrig dough, svg, spooned f/roll	1	Each	29.00	128.47	1.28	17.81	0.43	5.92	1.95	3.02	0.63	6.96	5.22	
Cookie, chocolate chip, soft, cmrcl prep	2	Each	30.00	137.40	1.05	17.73	0.96	7.29	2.22	3.91	1.05	0.00		
Cookie, chocolate chip, special dietary, cmrcl prep, 1 5/8"	4	Each	28.00	126.00	1.09	20.55	0.45	4.70	1.17	1.89	1.41	0.00	0.28	
Cookie, chocolate sandwich, creme filled	3	Each	30.00	139.80	1.60	21.50	0.87	5.72	1.10	3.19	0.68	0.00		
Cookie, chocolate sandwich, creme filled, special dietary	3	Each	30.00	138.30	1.35	20.31	1.23	6.63	1.15	2.77	2.38	0.00	0.30	
Cookie, coconut macaroon, prep f/recipe, 2"	1	Each	24.00	96.96	0.86	17.33	0.43	3.05	2.70	0.13	0.03	0.00	0.00	
Cookie, fig bar	2	Each	32.00	111.36	1.18	22.69	1.47	2.34	0.36	0.96	0.89	0.00	2.88	
Cookie, fortune	3	Each	24.00	90.72	1.01	20.16	0.38	0.65	0.16	0.32	0.11	0.48	0.24	
Cookie, gingersnap	4	Each	28.00	116.48	1.57	21.53	0.62	2.74	0.69	1.50	0.38	0.00	0.03	
Cookie, graham, Goldfish Pepperidge Farm	19	Each	30.00	150.00	2.00	20.00	2.00	7.00	2.50			15.00	0.00	
Cookie, lemon nut crunch, old fash Pepperidge Farm	3	Each	31.00	170.00	2.00	18.00	2.00	9.00	2.00	4.50	1.50	5.00	0.00	
Cookie, marshmallow pie, chocolate coated .75" × 3"	1	Each	39.00	164.19	1.56	26.40	0.78	6.59	1.84	3.64	0.76	0.00	0.39	
Cookie, molasses, lrg, 3 1/2" to 4"	1	Each	32.00	137.60	1.79	23.62	0.32	4.10	1.03	2.28	0.55	0.00	0.00	
Cookie, oatmeal raisin, big, homestyle Grandma's	1	Each	39.00	160.00	1.00	26.00	1.00	6.00	1.50			5.00	0.00	
Cookie, oatmeal raisin, special dietary, cmrcl prep, 1 5/8"	4	Each	28.00	125.72	1.34	19.57	0.81	5.04	0.76	2.12	1.90	0.00	0.28	
Cookie, oatmeal, cmrcl prep, big, 3 1/2" to 4"	1	Each	25.00	112.50	1.55	17.18	0.70	4.53	1.13	2.51	0.64	0.00	1.25	
Cookie, oatmeal, prep f/recipe, 2 5/8"	2	Each	30.00	134.10	2.04	19.92	0.86	5.37	1.07	2.30	1.68	10.80	48.00	
Cookie, oatmeal, refrig dough, each	2	Each	32.00	135.68	1.73	18.91	0.80	6.05	1.53	3.37	0.83	7.68	1.28	
Cookie, Oreo chocolate sandwich Nabisco	3	Each	33.00	160.00	2.00	23.00	1.00	7.00	1.50			0.00		
Cookie, peanut butter bar TastyKake, Inc.	1	Each	43.00	240.00	2.00	18.00	1.00	11.00	3.00			5.00	0.00	
Cookie, peanut butter sandwich	2	Each	28.00	133.84	2.46	18.37	0.53	5.91	1.40	3.14	1.06	0.00	0.28	
Cookie, peanut butter sandwich, special dietary	3	Each	30.00	160.50	3.00	15.24	0.49	10.20	1.48	4.62	3.61	0.00	0.00	

Vit E (mg)	Vit C	Vit B₁ Thia (mg)	Vit B₂ Ribo (mg)	Vit B₃ Nia (mg)	Fol (mcg)	Vit B₆ (mg)	Vita B₁₂ (mcg)	Sodi (mg)	Pota (mg)	Cal (mg)	Phos (mg)	Magn (mg)	Iron (mg)	Zinc (mg)	Caff (mg)	Alco (g)	Sol Fiber (g)	Insol Fiber (g)
1.45	0.00	0.08	0.10	0.80	14.08	0.02	0.11	215.68	113.92	23.68	103.04	19.20	1.33	0.40		0.00	0.24	0.91
1.22	0.00	0.06	0.04	0.32	17.28	0.02	0.10	220.16	33.92	39.68	91.52	3.84	0.68	0.16	0.00	0.00	0.04	0.15
	0.00							260.00		80.00			1.80			0.00		
1.26	0.32	0.02	0.15	0.16	14.40	0.04	0.14	165.60	72.00	40.80	74.40	8.80	0.50	0.41	0.00	0.00		
1.09	0.50	0.12	0.26	0.49	29.70	0.05	0.31	376.20	208.89	170.28	231.66	18.81	0.47	0.46	0.00	0.00		
1.26	0.00	0.11	0.13	0.85	30.69	0.03	0.10	410.00	160.70	40.00	97.58	41.29	1.44	0.69	0.00	0.00		
	0.00							249.66	56.43	18.92	80.94		0.87		0.00	0.00		
0.33	0.00	0.08	0.11	0.55	20.02	0.03	0.20	38.22	29.38	12.22	44.98	3.12	0.93	0.29	0.00	0.00		
	0.00							45.00		0.00			0.36		0.00	0.00		
		0.00	0.00	0.00	0.00			0.50		0.00			0.00		0.00	0.00		
	0.00	0.08	0.68	0.80				95.00		0.00			0.36		0.00	0.00		
0.14	0.00	0.09	0.08	0.80	19.00	0.01	0.09	87.75	27.75	7.25	25.50	3.00	0.56	0.10	0.00	0.00	0.07	0.13
	0.00							70.00		0.00			0.72			0.00	0.00	0.00
	0.00	0.04	0.06	0.57				155.92	42.52	0.00			1.02			0.00	0.00	0.00
0.64	0.00	0.09	0.09	0.96	25.20	0.01	0.00	118.80	59.20	14.00	46.40	19.20	1.43	0.29	4.40	0.00		
	0.00							160.00		0.00			1.08			0.00		
0.54	0.00	0.09	0.08	0.83	21.00	0.08	0.00	113.10	36.90	5.70	25.20	8.40	0.92	0.21	2.10	0.00		
0.28	0.06	0.06	0.06	0.44	10.56	0.02	0.02	109.12	70.72	12.16	32.00	17.60	0.80	0.30		0.00		
0.68	0.00	0.06	0.06	0.57	16.53	0.01	0.02	60.61	52.20	7.25	20.01	6.96	0.66	0.14	2.61	0.00		
0.87	0.00	0.03	0.06	0.49	11.70	0.05	0.00	97.80	27.90	4.50	15.00	10.50	0.72	0.14	2.10	0.00		
0.30	0.00	0.10	0.06	0.79	15.12	0.01	0.00	3.08	55.72	12.88	30.52	5.88	0.98	0.13	2.24	0.00		
0.52	0.00	0.05	0.04	0.80	15.90	0.00	0.01	144.90	56.10	6.30	27.60	14.40	3.16	0.29	3.90	0.00		
0.55	0.00	0.16	0.09	1.19	21.60	0.01	0.01	72.90	88.50	29.40	60.00	7.80	1.42	0.17	0.90	0.00		
0.04	0.00	0.00	0.03	0.03	0.96	0.02	0.01	59.28	37.44	1.68	10.32	5.04	0.18	0.17	0.00	0.00		
0.21	0.10	0.05	0.07	0.60	11.20	0.02	0.03	112.00	66.24	20.48	19.84	8.64	0.93	0.13	0.00	0.00		
0.01	0.00	0.04	0.03	0.44	15.84	0.00	0.00	65.76	9.84	2.88	8.40	1.68	0.34	0.04	0.00	0.00		
0.27	0.00	0.06	0.08	0.91	24.36	0.03	0.00	183.12	96.88	21.56	23.24	13.72	1.79	0.16	0.00	0.00		
	0.00	0.09	0.07	0.80				150.00					0.72			0.00	0.00	
	0.00	0.06	0.03	0.40				60.00		0.00			0.36			0.00	0.00	
0.05	0.04	0.04	0.08	0.31	8.97	0.02	0.07	65.52	70.98	17.94	37.83	14.04	0.99	0.25	1.95	0.00		
0.04	0.00	0.11	0.08	0.97	28.48	0.03	0.00	146.88	110.72	23.68	30.40	16.64	2.06	0.14	0.00	0.00		
	0.00							250.00		100.00			1.08			0.00	0.00	
0.43	0.08	0.13	0.06	0.91	12.88	0.01	0.00	2.52	49.00	15.12	34.16	4.76	1.14	0.14	0.00	0.00		
0.06	0.12	0.07	0.06	0.56	14.75	0.02	0.00	95.75	35.50	9.25	34.50	8.25	0.64	0.20	0.00	0.00		
0.81	0.06	0.08	0.05	0.39	9.90	0.02	0.03	179.40	54.60	31.50	50.10	12.90	0.81	0.28	0.00	0.00		
0.82	0.00	0.07	0.04	0.60	11.20	0.01	0.01	94.08	47.04	9.92	33.28	8.96	0.68					
								220.00	60.00				0.72			0.00		
	0.00							110.00		0.00			0.72		0.00	0.00		
0.52	0.03	0.09	0.07	1.05	17.08	0.04	0.07	103.04	53.76	14.84	52.64	13.72	0.73	0.30	0.00	0.00		
1.72	0.00	0.10	0.04	1.58	16.20	0.02	0.00	123.60	88.20	12.90	46.20	15.30	0.77	0.31	0.00	0.00		

Food Name	Amount	Measure	Weight (g)	Calories	Protein (g)	Total Carb (g)	Dietary Fiber (g)	Total Fat (g)	Sat Fat (g)	Mono Fat (g)	Poly Fat (g)	Chol (mg)	Vit A (mcg RAE)	Vit D (mcg)
DESSERTS *(continued)*														
Cookie, peanut butter, big Grandma's	1	Each	39.00	190.00	2.00	22.00	1.00	9.00	2.00			5.00	0.00	
Cookie, peanut butter, cmrcl prep	2	Each	30.00	143.10	2.88	17.67	0.54	7.08	1.35	3.71	1.66	0.30	0.90	
Cookie, peanut butter, prep f/recipe, 3"	1	Each	20.00	95.00	1.80	11.78	0.40	4.76	0.89	2.17	1.45	6.20	27.40	
Cookie, peanut butter, refrig dough, each	2	Each	32.00	146.56	2.62	16.67	0.35	8.00	1.86	4.20	1.54	8.64	4.48	
Cookie, raisin, soft type	2	Each	30.00	120.30	1.23	20.40	0.36	4.08	1.04	2.29	0.53	0.60	2.40	
Cookie, shortbread, old fash Pepperidge Farm	2	Each	26.00	140.00	2.00	16.00	1.00	7.00	2.50	3.50	0.50	5.00	0.00	
Cookie, shortbread, pecan, cmrcl prep, 2"	2	Each	28.00	151.76	1.37	16.32	0.50	9.10	2.30	5.22	1.16	9.24	0.28	
Cookie, shortbread, plain, cmrcl prep, 1 5/8" square	4	Each	32.00	160.64	1.95	20.64	0.58	7.71	1.95	4.29	1.03	6.40	5.76	
Cookie, sugar wafer, creme filled, lrg, 3 1/2" × 1" × 1/2"	3	Each	27.00	137.97	1.11	18.93	0.16	6.56	0.98	2.79	2.47	0.00	0.00	
Cookie, sugar wafer, creme filled, special dietary	7	Each	28.00	140.56	0.87	18.48	0.49	7.20	1.07	3.06	2.72	0.00	0.00	
Cookie, sugar, bkd f/refrig dough, rolled	2	Each	30.00	145.20	1.41	19.68	0.24	6.93	1.77	3.90	0.87	9.60	3.60	
Cookie, sugar, cmrcl prep	2	Each	30.00	143.40	1.53	20.37	0.24	6.33	1.63	3.55	0.80	15.30	7.80	
Cookie, Thin Mints Little Brownie Bakers	4	Each	28.35	140.00	1.00	18.00	1.00	8.00	2.00			0.00	0.00	
Cookie, vanilla sandwich, creme filled, oval 3 1/8" × 1 1/4"	2	Each	30.00	144.90	1.35	21.63	0.45	6.00	0.89	2.53	2.27	0.00	0.00	
Cookie, vanilla wafer, golden, art flvr Keebler Company Incorporated	8	Each	31.00	147.25	1.61	21.61		6.05	1.11	3.53	0.52			
Cookie, vanilla wafer, higher fat	4	Each	24.00	113.52	1.03	17.06	0.48	4.66	1.18	2.66	0.58	0.00		0.03
Cookie, vanilla wafer, lower fat, lrg	5	Each	30.00	132.30	1.50	22.08	0.57	4.56	1.15	1.96	1.17	15.30	2.40	
Crackers, animal, 2oz box	1	Each	56.70	252.88	3.91	42.01	0.62	7.82	1.97	4.35	1.06	0.00	0.00	
Doughnuts														
Doughnut, buttermilk, glazed Entenmann's	1	Each	64.00	270.00	3.00	35.00	0.00	13.00	3.00			15.00	0.00	
Doughnut, cake, chocolate, glazed/sugared, med, 3"	1	Each	42.00	175.14	1.89	24.11	0.92	8.36	2.16	4.74	1.04	23.94	5.04	
Doughnut, cake, glazed/sugared, med, 3"	1	Each	45.00	191.70	2.34	22.86	0.67	10.30	2.67	5.71	1.31	14.40	1.35	
Doughnut, cake, w/chocolate icing, sml, 2"	1	Each	28.00	132.72	1.40	13.44	0.56	8.68	2.27	4.90	1.06	17.08	1.96	
Doughnut, cream puff, choc, custard filled, prep f/rec 3.5 × 2	1	Each	112.00	293.44	7.17	27.10	0.67	17.58	4.61	7.26	4.42	142.24	222.88	
Doughnut, cream puff, custard filled, miniature, prep f/rec	1	Each	23.00	59.34	1.54	5.27	0.09	3.57	0.85	1.50	0.96	30.82	32.66	
Doughnut, creme filled, 3 1/2" oval	1	Each	85.00	306.85	5.44	25.50	0.68	20.83	4.62	10.27	2.62	20.40	9.35	
Doughnut, French crullers, glazed, 3"	1	Each	41.00	168.92	1.27	24.39	0.49	7.50	1.91	4.28	0.94	4.51	0.82	
Doughnut, glazed, enrich, extra lrg, 5"	1	Each	122.00	491.66	7.81	54.05	1.46	27.82	7.09	15.70	3.54	7.32	4.88	
Doughnut, jelly filled, 3 1/2" oval	1	Each	85.00	289.00	5.02	33.15	0.77	15.90	4.12	8.69	2.02	22.10	14.45	
Doughnut, powdered sugar, mini TastyKake, Inc.	1	Each	11.83	48.32	0.67	6.66	0.17	2.00	0.42			4.17	0.00	
Frozen Desserts														
Frozen Dessert Bar, ice novelty, fruit, rducd cal, w/asp	1	Each	51.00	12.24	0.26	3.16	0.00	0.05	0.00			0.00	0.02	
Frozen Dessert Bar, orange, all nat, fat free Good Humor-Breyers	1	Each	52.00	50.00	0.00	13.00	0.00	0.00	0.00	0.00	0.00	0.00	0.00	
Frozen Dessert Bar, skim milk, dietary	1	Each	81.00	88.49	2.23	18.71	0.00	1.00	0.23	0.13	0.39	1.25	38.13	
Frozen Dessert Bar, tropical, no sug add, fat free Good Humor-Breyers	1	Each	45.00	25.00	0.00	5.00	0.00	0.00	0.00	0.00	0.00	0.00	0.00	
Frozen Dessert Pop, cherry Unilever Popsicle	1	Each	57.00	45.00	0.00	11.00	0.00	0.00	0.00	0.00	0.00	0.00	0.00	
Frozen Dessert Pop, double stick	1	Each	128.00	92.16	0.00	24.19	0.00	0.00	0.00	0.00	0.00	0.00	0.00	
Frozen Dessert Pop, grape CoolBrands Better For Kids Crayola	1	Each	36.00	25.00	0.00	7.00	0.00	0.00	0.00	0.00	0.00	0.00	0.00	
Frozen Dessert Pop, grape Unilever Popsicle	1	Each	57.00	45.00	0.00	11.00	0.00	0.00	0.00	0.00	0.00	0.00	0.00	
Frozen Dessert Pop, orange Unilever Popsicle	1	Each	57.00	45.00	0.00	11.00	0.00	0.00	0.00	0.00	0.00	0.00	0.00	
Frozen Dessert, Dibs, vanilla Nestle Dreyer's	26	Piece	104.00	380.00	4.00	30.00	1.00	27.00	17.00			25.00		
Frozen Dessert, vanilla Hain Celestial Group Rice Dream	0.5	Cup	92.00	150.00	0.00	23.00	1.00	6.00	0.50			0.00		
Frozen Dessert Sandwich, van choc chip Tofutti Brands, Inc.	1	Each	77.00	230.00	3.00	30.00	0.00	11.00	3.00			0.00	0.00	
Frozen Dessert Sandwich, vanilla Tofutti Brands, Inc.	1	Each	77.00	215.00	3.00	28.00	0.00	10.00	3.00			0.00	0.00	

Vit E (mg)	Vit C	Vit B₁ Thia (mg)	Vit B₂ Ribo (mg)	Vit B₃ Nia (mg)	Fol (mcg)	Vit B₆ (mg)	Vita B₁₂ (mcg)	Sodi (mg)	Pota (mg)	Cal (mg)	Phos (mg)	Magn (mg)	Iron (mg)	Zinc (mg)	Caff (mg)	Alco (g)	Sol Fiber (g)	Insol Fiber (g)
	0.00							200.00		0.00			0.72		0.00	0.00		
0.66	0.00	0.05	0.05	1.28	21.60	0.03	0.01	124.50	50.10	10.50	25.80	13.50	0.75	0.16	0.00	0.00		
0.76	0.02	0.05	0.04	0.70	11.00	0.02	0.02	103.60	46.20	7.80	23.20	7.80	0.45	0.17	0.00	0.00		
1.30	0.00	0.06	0.06	1.32	18.24	0.04	0.01	127.04	98.56	32.32	77.12	11.84	0.54	0.21	0.00	0.00		
0.67	0.12	0.06	0.06	0.59	9.60	0.02	0.01	101.40	42.00	13.80	24.90	6.30	0.69	0.10	0.00	0.00		
	0.00	0.06	0.03	0.80				105.00		0.00			0.36		0.00	0.00		
1.06	0.00	0.08	0.07	0.69	17.64	0.01	0.00	78.68	20.44	8.40	23.80	5.04	0.68	0.16	0.00	0.00		
0.11	0.00	0.11	0.11	1.07	22.40	0.03	0.03	145.60	32.00	11.20	34.56	5.44	0.88	0.17	0.00	0.00	0.21	0.37
0.53	0.00	0.03	0.05	0.66	14.04	0.00	0.00	39.69	15.93	4.86	15.12	2.97	0.53	0.10	0.00	0.00		
1.14	0.00	0.05	0.03	0.43	11.76	0.00	0.00	2.52	17.08	14.84	9.52	1.68	0.40	0.06	0.00	0.00		
0.06	0.00	0.05	0.04	0.72	21.00	0.01	0.02	140.40	48.90	27.00	56.10	2.40	0.55	0.08	0.00	0.00	0.09	0.15
0.08	0.03	0.07	0.06	0.81	15.90	0.02	0.06	107.10	18.90	6.30	24.00	3.60	0.64	0.13	0.00	0.00	0.09	0.15
	0.00							80.00		200.00					0.00	0.00		
0.48	0.00	0.08	0.07	0.81	15.00	0.01	0.00	104.70	27.30	8.10	22.50	4.20	0.66	0.12	0.00	0.00		
	0.00	0.05	0.03	0.47	13.02			119.66		11.16			0.74		0.00	0.00		
0.34	0.00	0.09	0.05	0.71	10.32	0.01	0.01	73.44	25.68	6.00	15.36	2.88	0.53	0.08	0.00	0.00		
0.07	0.00	0.08	0.10	0.93	18.00	0.02	0.04	93.60	29.10	14.40	31.20	4.20	0.71	0.11	0.00	0.00		
0.08	0.00	0.21	0.19	1.97	58.40	0.02	0.04	222.83	56.70	24.38	64.64	10.21	1.57	0.36	0.00	0.00		
	0.00							290.00		60.00			1.08		0.00	0.00	0.00	0.00
0.09	0.04	0.02	0.03	0.20	18.90	0.01	0.04	142.80	44.52	89.46	68.04	14.28	0.95	0.24	0.42	0.00	0.21	0.71
0.45	0.04	0.10	0.09	0.68	20.70	0.01	0.11	180.90	45.90	27.00	52.65	7.65	0.48	0.20	0.00	0.00	0.24	0.44
0.10	0.06	0.04	0.03	0.36	13.16	0.01	0.07	120.12	54.88	9.80	56.56	11.20	0.69	0.17	0.56	0.00	0.17	0.39
2.25	0.34	0.13	0.30	0.89	48.16	0.07	0.38	377.44	131.04	70.56	119.84	16.80	1.32	0.68	2.24	0.00	0.16	0.51
0.33	0.07	0.03	0.06	0.19	8.51	0.01	0.08	78.43	26.45	15.18	25.07	2.76	0.27	0.14	0.00	0.00	0.03	0.06
0.25	0.00	0.29	0.13	1.91	59.50	0.06	0.12	262.65	68.00	21.25	64.60	17.00	1.56	0.68	0.00	0.00	0.20	0.48
0.07	0.00	0.07	0.09	0.87	17.22	0.01	0.02	141.45	31.98	10.66	50.43	4.92	0.99	0.11	0.00	0.00	0.17	0.32
0.43	0.12	0.44	0.26	3.48	59.78	0.07	0.11	417.24	131.76	52.46	113.46	26.84	2.49	0.94	0.00	0.00	0.48	0.98
0.37	0.00	0.27	0.12	1.82	57.80	0.09	0.19	249.05	67.15	21.25	72.25	17.00	1.50	0.64	0.00	0.00	0.18	0.59
	0.00							58.32		3.33			0.06		0.00	0.00		
0.00	0.00	0.00	0.00	0.08	0.00	0.00	0.00	2.55	13.26	1.02	0.00	1.02	0.07	0.02	0.00	0.00	0.00	0.00
	4.80							5.00		0.00			0.00		0.00	0.00	0.00	0.00
0.07	0.63	0.03	0.11	0.06	3.38	0.03	0.24	43.90	107.23	81.05	65.36	9.25	0.04	0.26	0.00	0.00		
	2.40							0.00		0.00			0.00		0.00	0.00	0.00	0.00
	0.00							0.00		0.00			0.00		0.00	0.00	0.00	0.00
0.00	0.00	0.00	0.00	0.00	0.00	0.00	0.00	15.36	5.12	0.00	0.00	1.28	0.00	0.03	0.00	0.00	0.00	0.00
1.37	6.00							0.00		0.00			0.00		0.00	0.00	0.00	0.00
	0.00							0.00		0.00			0.00		0.00	0.00	0.00	0.00
	0.00							0.00		0.00			0.00		0.00	0.00	0.00	0.00
								65.00	100.00								0.00	
	1.20							100.00		20.00			0.72		0.00	0.00		
	0.00							155.00	4.00	0.00			0.00				0.00	0.00
	0.00							141.00	4.00	0.00			0.00				0.00	0.00

Food Name	Amount	Measure	Weight (g)	Calories	Protein (g)	Total Carb (g)	Dietary Fiber (g)	Total Fat (g)	Sat Fat (g)	Mono Fat (g)	Poly Fat (g)	Chol (mg)	Vit A (mcg RAE)	Vit D (mcg)
DESSERTS *(continued)*														
Frozen Dessert, carob Imagine Foods	0.5	Cup	92.00	150.00	1.00	24.00	2.00	6.00	0.50			0.00		
Frozen Dessert, ice novelty, Italian, restaurant prep	0.5	Cup	116.00	61.48	0.04	15.67	0.00	0.03	0.00	0.00	0.00	0.00	9.28	
Frozen Dessert, ice novelty, lime	0.5	Cup	99.00	126.72	0.40	32.27	0.00	0.00	0.00	0.00	0.00	0.00	0.00	
Frozen Yogurt Bar, carob coated	1	Each	41.00	100.18	2.02	12.87	0.35	4.66	3.75	0.55	0.09	0.91	18.07	
Frozen Yogurt Bar, chocolate coated	1	Each	41.00	109.04	1.32	11.84	0.10	6.73	5.34	0.81	0.16	0.64	17.34	
Frozen Yogurt, chocolate, low fat	0.5	Cup	96.50	109.65	5.05	20.84	1.50	1.88	1.18	0.56	0.06	4.81	11.89	
Frozen Yogurt, chocolate, soft serve, cup	0.5	Cup	72.00	115.20	2.88	17.93	1.58	4.32	2.61	1.26	0.16	3.60	31.68	
Frozen Yogurt, coffee, nonfat, soft serve, mix Haagen Dazs	0.5	Cup	95.00	110.00	5.00	22.00	0.00	0.00	0.00	0.00	0.00	3.00	0.00	
Frozen Yogurt, vanilla, soft serve	0.5	Cup	72.00	117.36	2.88	17.42	0.00	4.03	2.46	1.14	0.15	1.44	42.48	
Ice Cream Bar, chocolate & dark chocolate Haagen Dazs	1	Each	83.00	284.80	4.07	22.78	1.63	19.53	12.21			69.17		
Ice Cream Bar, cookie sandwich	1	Each	59.00	143.63	2.62	21.75	0.55	5.61	3.24	1.65	0.36	19.78	50.14	0.06
Ice Cream Bar, vanilla, chocolate coated	1	Each	91.00	280.00	3.00	24.00	0.00	19.00	14.00			20.00		
Ice Cream Bar, vanilla, dark chocolate coated, Eskimo Pie	1	Each	50.00	165.50	2.05	12.25		12.05	7.25			14.00		
Ice Cream Bar, vanilla, uncoated Haagen Dazs	1	Each	78.00	190.00	3.00	15.00	0.00	13.00	8.00			85.00		
Ice Cream Sandwich	1	Each	59.00	143.63	2.62	21.75	0.55	5.61	3.24	1.65	0.36	19.78	50.14	0.06
Ice Cream, butter pecan Ben & Jerry's	0.5	Cup	100.00	290.00	4.00	20.00	1.00	21.00	10.00			70.00		
Ice Cream, chocolate Haagen Dazs	0.5	Cup	106.00	270.00	5.00	22.00	1.00	18.00	9.90			115.00		
Ice Cream, chocolate, 3.5 fl oz indv pkg	1	Each	58.00	125.28	2.20	16.36	0.70	6.38	3.94	1.86	0.24	19.72	68.44	
Ice Cream, chocolate, light, no sugar add	3	Ounce-weight	85.05	129.28	3.01	21.60	0.77	4.88	3.07	0.79	0.45	13.61	63.79	
Ice Cream, chocolate Nestle Haagen Dazs	0.5	Cup	106.00	270.00	5.00	22.00	1.00	18.00	11.00			115.00		
Ice Cream, French vanilla, soft serve	0.5	Cup	86.00	190.92	3.53	19.09	0.60	11.18	6.43	3.00	0.39	78.26	139.32	
Ice Cream, strawberry, 3.5 fl oz indv pkg	1	Each	58.00	111.36	1.86	16.01	0.53	4.87	3.01	1.39	0.18	16.82	55.68	
Ice Cream, vanilla	0.5	Cup	66.00	132.66	2.31	15.58	0.47	7.26	4.48	1.96	0.30	29.04	77.88	0.57
Ice Cream, vanilla, light, 50% less fat	0.5	Cup	66.00	108.90	3.15	17.03	0.20	3.19	1.93	0.85	0.15	17.82	41.58	0.43
Ice Cream, vanilla, light, 50% less fat, soft serve	0.5	Cup	88.00	110.88	4.32	19.18	0.00	2.29	1.44	0.67	0.09	10.56	25.52	
Ice Cream, vanilla, light, no add sug, w/asp	0.5	Cup	65.00	100.75	2.58	13.93	0.46	4.84	2.63	1.21	0.48	17.55	55.90	
Ice Cream, vanilla, rich	0.5	Cup	74.00	184.26	2.59	16.50	0.00	11.99	7.64	3.30	0.50	68.08	134.68	0.81
Milk Shake, chocolate, fast food, 10 fl oz each	1	Each	208.00	264.16	7.07	42.64	3.95	7.70	4.81	2.24	0.29	27.04	54.08	1.80
Milk Shake, chocolate, thick, 10.6 fl oz	1	Each	300.00	357.00	9.15	63.45	0.90	8.10	5.04	2.34	0.30	33.00	54.00	3.00
Ice Cream, vanilla, light Unilever Ben & Jerry's	0.5	Cup	88.00	160.00	4.00	19.00	0.00	7.00	4.50			40.00		
Milk Shake, vanilla, thick, 11 fl oz	1	Each	313.00	350.56	12.08	55.56	0.00	9.48	5.90	2.74	0.35	37.56	78.25	
Sherbet, orange	0.5	Cup	74.00	106.56	0.81	22.50	2.44	1.48	0.86	0.39	0.06	0.00	7.40	
Sorbet, chocolate Haagen Dazs	0.5	Cup	105.00	120.00	2.00	28.00	2.00	0.00	0.00	0.00	0.00	0.00	0.00	
Sorbet, mango Haagen Dazs	0.5	Cup	113.00	120.00	0.00	31.00	1.00	0.00	0.00	0.00	0.00	0.00		
Sorbet, raspberry Haagen Dazs	0.5	Cup	105.00	120.00	0.00	30.00	2.00	0.00	0.00	0.00	0.00	0.00	0.00	
Fruit Desserts														
Cobbler, apple, fzn, whl or 1/18 pce Mrs. Smith's	1	Piece	126.00	280.00	2.00	42.00	2.00	12.00	2.50			0.00		
Cobbler, peach crumb, fzn Pet Ritz	1	Piece	123.00	230.00	2.00	38.00	1.00	7.00	3.00	3.00	1.00	5.00	0.00	
Strudel, apple	1	Piece	71.00	194.54	2.34	29.18	1.56	7.95	1.45	2.32	3.77	4.26	4.26	
Gelatin Desserts														
Gelatin Substitute, cherry gel, low prot, prep f/dry mix Kingsmill Foods Company, Ltd.	0.5	Cup	120.00	86.40	0.02	22.24		0.02						
Gelatin, lemon, prep f/dry mix Jell-O	0.5	Cup	140.00	80.00	2.00	19.00	0.00	0.00	0.00	0.00	0.00	0.00	0.00	
Gelatin, orange, snack cup Juicy Gels	1	Each	99.22	99.99	0.00	25.00	0.00	0.00	0.00	0.00	0.00	0.00	0.00	
Gelatin, orange, sug free, low cal, snack cup Jell-O	1	Each	92.00	10.00	1.00	0.00	0.00	0.00	0.00	0.00	0.00	0.00	0.00	
Gelatin, rducd cal, w/asp add minerals & vit C dry mix svg	1	Each	2.50	8.63	1.38	0.83	0.00	0.00	0.00	0.00	0.00	0.00	0.00	
Pastries and Sweet Rolls														
Croissant, cheese, sml	1	Each	42.00	173.88	3.86	19.74	1.09	8.78	4.46	2.73	1.00	23.94	85.68	

Vit E (mg)	Vit C	Vit B$_1$ Thia (mg)	Vit B$_2$ Ribo (mg)	Vit B$_3$ Nia (mg)	Fol (mcg)	Vit B$_6$ (mg)	Vita B$_{12}$ (mcg)	Sodi (mg)	Pota (mg)	Cal (mg)	Phos (mg)	Magn (mg)	Iron (mg)	Zinc (mg)	Caff (mg)	Alco (g)	Sol Fiber (g)	Insol Fiber (g)
	1.20							100.00		20.00			0.72		0.00	0.00		
0.00	0.59	0.00	0.01	0.83	5.80	0.00	0.00	4.64	6.96	1.16	0.00	0.00	0.11	0.04	0.00	0.00	0.00	0.00
0.00	0.99	0.00	0.00	0.01	0.00	0.00	0.00	21.78	2.97	1.98	0.99	0.99	0.16	0.02	0.00	0.00	0.00	0.00
0.22	0.30	0.02	0.09	0.19	4.48	0.04	0.18	37.51	125.26	73.32	52.61	7.76	0.21	0.46		0.00		
0.03	0.25	0.01	0.07	0.10	2.02	0.03	0.09	27.78	74.41	45.89	43.30	5.82	0.14	0.15	3.28	0.00		
0.06	0.64	0.05	0.19	0.22	10.44	0.05	0.44	56.49	310.70	149.82	150.05	37.66	0.85	1.02	2.89	0.00		
0.10	0.22	0.03	0.15	0.22	7.92	0.05	0.21	70.56	187.92	105.84	100.08	19.44	0.90	0.35	2.16	0.00		
	0.00							75.00		150.00			0.00		0.00	0.00	0.00	
0.08	0.58	0.03	0.16	0.20	4.32	0.06	0.21	62.64	151.92	102.96	92.88	10.08	0.22	0.30	0.00	0.00	0.00	0.00
	0.00		0.08					48.82	177.80	81.37	83.00		2.20			0.00		
0.07	0.27	0.03	0.12	0.18	4.83	0.03	0.18	36.37	122.38	60.02	63.68	12.67	0.28	0.43		0.00		
	1.20							75.00		100.00			0.36			0.00	0.00	0.00
								34.00		59.50						0.00		
	0.00							65.00		100.00			0.00		0.00	0.00	0.00	0.00
0.07	0.27	0.03	0.12	0.18	4.83	0.03	0.18	36.37	122.38	60.02	63.68	12.67	0.28	0.43		0.00		
	0.00							80.00		150.00			0.72		0.00	0.00		
	0.00	0.18	0.85	0.85				75.00	238.50	150.00	106.00		1.08			0.00		
0.17	0.41	0.02	0.11	0.13	9.28	0.03	0.17	44.08	144.42	63.22	62.06	16.82	0.54	0.34	1.74	0.00		
0.26	0.60	0.04	0.15	0.09	4.25	0.04	0.32	63.79	166.70	102.91	90.15	12.76	0.41	0.34	0.00	0.00		
	0.00							60.00		150.00			1.08			0.00		
0.52	0.69	0.04	0.16	0.08	7.74	0.04	0.43	52.46	152.22	112.66	99.76	10.32	0.18	0.45	0.00	0.00		
0.03	4.47	0.03	0.15	0.10	6.96	0.03	0.18	34.80	109.04	69.60	58.00	8.12	0.12	0.20	0.00	0.00		
0.20	0.40	0.02	0.16	0.08	3.30	0.03	0.26	52.80	131.34	84.48	69.30	9.24	0.06	0.46	0.00	0.00		
0.08	0.79	0.04	0.17	0.09	3.96	0.03	0.31	48.84	137.28	106.26	67.98	9.24	0.12	0.48	0.00	0.00		
0.05	0.80	0.04	0.18	0.10	4.40	0.04	0.45	61.60	194.48	138.16	106.48	12.32	0.05	0.47	0.00	0.00	0.00	0.00
0.19	0.59	0.02	0.08	0.05	2.60	0.02	0.34	62.40	127.40	88.40	48.75	5.85	0.12	0.20	0.00	0.00		
0.37	0.00	0.03	0.12	0.06	5.92	0.03	0.29	45.14	116.18	86.58	77.70	8.14	0.25	0.35	0.00	0.00	0.00	0.00
0.23	0.83	0.12	0.51	0.33	10.40	0.10	0.71	201.76	416.00	235.04	212.16	35.36	0.64	0.85	2.08	0.00		
0.15	0.00	0.14	0.67	0.37	15.00	0.08	0.96	333.00	672.00	396.00	378.00	48.00	0.93	1.44	6.00	0.00		
	0.00							60.00		150.00			0.36		0.00	0.00	0.00	0.00
0.16	0.00	0.09	0.61	0.46	21.91	0.13	1.63	297.35	572.79	456.98	359.95	37.56	0.31	1.22	0.00	0.00	0.00	0.00
0.02	4.29	0.02	0.07	0.06	5.18	0.02	0.09	34.04	71.04	39.96	29.60	5.92	0.10	0.36	0.00	0.00		
	0.00							70.00		0.00			1.08			0.00		
	12.00							0.00		0.00					0.00	0.00		
	2.40							0.00	55.70	0.00			0.00		0.00	0.00		
	0.00							260.00		0.00			0.36		0.00	0.00		
	6.00							170.00		0.00			0.00		0.00	0.00		
1.01	1.21	0.03	0.02	0.23	19.88	0.03	0.16	190.99	105.79	10.65	23.43	6.39	0.30	0.13	0.00	0.00		
								4.96	166.88		13.28				0.00	0.00		
	0.00							120.00	0.00	0.00	40.00		0.00		0.00	0.00	0.00	0.00
	0.00							40.00		0.00			0.00		0.00	0.00	0.00	0.00
	0.00							45.00	0.00	0.00	0.00		0.00		0.00	0.00	0.00	0.00
0.00	12.25	0.00	0.00	0.00	0.35	0.00	0.00	68.78	49.63	0.05	0.00	0.03	0.00	0.00	0.00	0.00	0.00	0.00
0.60	0.08	0.22	0.14	0.91	31.08	0.03	0.13	233.10	55.44	22.26	54.60	10.08	0.90	0.39	0.00	0.00	0.37	0.72

Food Name	Amount	Measure	Weight (g)	Calories	Protein (g)	Total Carb (g)	Dietary Fiber (g)	Total Fat (g)	Sat Fat (g)	Mono Fat (g)	Poly Fat (g)	Chol (mg)	Vit A (mcg RAE)	Vit D (mcg)
DESSERTS *(continued)*														
Danish, almond, 15oz ring or 1/8 pce	1	Piece	53.16	228.59	3.77	24.29	1.06	13.40	3.09	7.27	2.28	24.45	4.78	
Danish, apple cinnamon, enrich, lrg, 7"	1	Each	142.00	526.82	7.67	67.88	2.70	26.27	6.90	14.24	3.36	161.88	21.30	
Danish, apple cinnamon, enrich, med, 4 1/4"	1	Each	71.00	263.41	3.83	33.94	1.35	13.13	3.45	7.12	1.68	80.94	10.65	
Fritter, apple	1	Each	24.00	87.01	1.44	8.05	0.35	5.55	1.23	2.39	1.60	20.25	12.53	
Fruit Burrito, apple, sml	1	Each	74.00	230.88	2.50	34.98		9.52	4.57	3.42	1.06	3.70	20.72	
Pastry, apple cinnamon, frosted, low fat Pop Tarts	1	Each	52.00	191.36	2.18	39.99	0.57	2.86	0.57	1.46	0.83	0.00		
Pastry, blueberry Pop Tarts	1	Each	52.00	212.16	2.39	35.56	0.57	6.92	1.05	3.37	2.50	0.00		
Pastry, brown sugar cinnamon Pop Tarts	1	Each	50.00	219.00	2.70	32.20	0.75	9.20	1.04	3.57	4.57	0.00		
Pastry, brown sugar cinnamon, frosted Pop Tarts	1	Each	50.00	211.00	2.50	34.16	0.65	7.40	1.12	3.91	2.36	0.00		
Pastry, brown sugar cinnamon, frosted, low fat Pop Tarts	1	Each	50.00	188.00	2.35	39.15	0.60	2.75	0.60	1.45	0.65	0.00		
Pastry, cherry Pop Tarts	1	Each	52.00	204.36	2.39	37.02	0.57	5.41	0.87	2.98	1.56	0.00		
Pastry, cherry, low fat Pop Tarts	1	Each	52.00	191.88	2.34	39.78	0.62	2.86	0.62	1.56	0.68	0.00		
Pastry, chocolate fudge, frosted Pop Tarts	1	Each	52.00	201.24	2.65	37.34	0.57	4.84	0.99	2.70	1.14	0.00		
Pastry, s'mores	1	Each	52.00	203.84	3.22	36.19	0.73	5.46	1.46	3.07	0.94	0.00		
Pastry, strawberry, frosted Pop Tarts	1	Each	52.00	202.80	2.29	37.65	0.52	4.99	1.35	2.91	0.73	0.00		
Pastry, strawberry, low fat Pop Tarts	1	Each	52.00	191.88	2.34	39.78	0.62	2.86	0.62	1.56	0.68	0.00		
Sweet Roll, cinnamon raisin, cmrcl, 2 3/4" square	1	Each	60.00	223.20	3.72	30.54	1.44	9.84	1.85	2.88	4.48	39.60	37.20	
Sweet Roll, cinnamon, w/icing, refrig dough Pillsbury	1	Each	44.00	150.04	2.38	23.89		5.02	1.25	2.71	0.31			
Turnover, apple, fzn, rtb Pepperidge Farm	1	Each	89.00	283.91	3.74	31.24	1.60	16.02	4.03	8.55	0.79			
Pastry, Pie, Dessert Crusts, and Cones														
Cone, ice cream, sugar, rolled type	1	Each	10.00	40.20	0.79	8.41	0.17	0.38	0.06	0.15	0.15	0.00	0.00	
Cone, ice cream, wafer/cake type	1	Each	4.00	16.68	0.32	3.16	0.12	0.28	0.05	0.07	0.13	0.00	0.00	
Crust, cookie, chocolate, prep f/rec, chilled, 9" or 1/8 pce	1	Piece	28.00	141.68	1.43	15.23	0.42	8.71	1.88	4.12	2.16	0.28	59.08	
Crust, pastry, cream puff shell, prep f/recipe, 3 1/2"	1	Each	66.00	238.92	5.94	15.05	0.53	17.09	3.70	7.34	4.87	129.36	183.48	0.00
Crust, pastry, eclair shell, prep f/recipe, 5" × 2" × 1 3/4"	1	Each	48.00	173.76	4.32	10.94	0.38	12.43	2.69	5.34	3.54	94.08	133.44	0.00
Crust, pie, bkd f/fzn, 9" whl or 1/8 pce	1	Piece	16.00	82.24	0.70	7.94	0.16	5.25	1.69	2.51	0.65	0.00	0.00	
Crust, pie, prep f/recipe, bkd, 9" whl or 1/8 pce	1	Piece	23.00	121.21	1.47	10.93	0.39	7.96	1.98	3.49	2.10	0.00	0.00	
Crust, pie, chocolate, 1/8 of 9", Ready Crust Keebler Company Incorporated	1	Piece	18.00	87.12	1.08	12.24	0.54	3.96	0.86			0.18		
Crust, pie, Nilla, rtu, svg Nabisco	1	Each	28.00	143.64	0.98	17.67	0.25	7.59	1.44	5.24	0.38	2.80		
Crust, pie, rtb, enrich, fzn, 9" whl or 1/8 pce	1	Piece	18.00	82.26	0.70	7.94	0.16	5.26	0.78	2.24	1.98	0.00		
Crust, pie, single, prep f/rec, unbkd, 9" whl or 1/8 pce	1	Piece	24.25	113.73	1.38	10.26	0.82	7.47	1.86	3.27	1.97	0.00	0.00	
Pies														
Pie, apple, fzn Amy's Kitchen Inc	0.5	Each	114.00	240.00	2.00	37.00	2.00	8.00	4.50			25.00		
Pie, apple, prep f/recipe, 9" whl or 1/8 pce	1	Piece	155.00	410.75	3.72	57.50	2.17	19.37	4.73	8.36	5.17	0.00	17.05	
Pie, banana cream, fzn Pet Ritz	1	Piece	99.00	270.00	3.00	37.00	1.00	13.00	8.00			5.00	0.00	
Pie, banana cream, no bake, prep f/mix, 9" whl or 1/8 pce	1	Piece	92.00	230.92	3.13	29.07	0.55	11.87	6.35	4.19	0.70	26.68	87.40	
Pie, banana cream, prep f/recipe, 9" whl or 1/8 pce	1	Piece	144.00	387.36	6.34	47.38	1.01	19.58	5.41	8.24	4.74	73.44	87.84	
Pie, blackberry, prep f/recipe, 9" whl or 1/8 pce	1	Piece	150.00	402.27	3.80	56.15	4.71	18.81	3.70	8.26	5.85	0.00	24.33	0.00
Pie, blueberry, cmrcl prep, 8" whl or 1/6 pce	1	Piece	117.00	271.44	2.11	40.83	1.17	11.70	1.96	4.97	4.12	0.00	51.48	
Pie, blueberry, prep f/recipe, 9" whl or 1/8 pce	1	Piece	147.00	360.15	3.97	49.25	2.06	17.49	4.28	7.53	4.53	0.00	2.94	
Pie, cherry, cmrcl prep, 8" whl or 1/6 pce	1	Piece	117.00	304.20	2.34	46.57	0.94	12.87	3.00	6.83	2.40	0.00	60.84	
Pie, cherry, old fash, rtb, 10" whl or 1/10 pce Mrs. Smith's	1	Piece	133.00	370.00	3.00	55.00	1.00	16.00	3.50			0.00		

Vit E (mg)	Vit C	Vit B$_1$ Thia (mg)	Vit B$_2$ Ribo (mg)	Vit B$_3$ Nia (mg)	Fol (mcg)	Vit B$_6$ (mg)	Vita B$_{12}$ (mcg)	Sodi (mg)	Pota (mg)	Cal (mg)	Phos (mg)	Magn (mg)	Iron (mg)	Zinc (mg)	Caff (mg)	Alco (g)	Sol Fiber (g)	Insol Fiber (g)
0.44	0.90	0.12	0.13	1.22	44.12	0.06	0.11	192.97	50.50	49.97	58.48	17.01	0.96	0.46	0.00	0.00		
0.48	5.54	0.37	0.31	2.83	66.74	0.06	0.13	502.68	117.86	65.32	126.38	21.30	2.51	0.77	0.00	0.00		
0.24	2.77	0.19	0.16	1.41	33.37	0.03	0.06	251.34	58.93	32.66	63.19	10.65	1.26	0.38	0.00	0.00		
0.69	0.35	0.04	0.06	0.32	2.95	0.02	0.06	9.70	33.80	12.64	22.37	3.03	0.35	0.12	0.00	0.00		
	0.74	0.17	0.18	1.86	24.42	0.07	0.51	211.64	104.34	15.54	14.80	7.40	1.07	0.40	0.00	0.00		
0.00	0.00	0.16	0.16	1.98	52.00	0.21	0.00	205.92	28.08	5.72	21.32	4.68	1.82	0.16	0.00	0.00		
0.00	0.00	0.15	0.17	1.98	41.60	0.20	0.00	206.96	49.40	12.48	45.76	8.32	1.82	0.66	0.00	0.00		
0.00	0.00	0.15	0.17	2.00	40.00	0.20	0.00	214.00	67.50	15.50	31.50	8.00	1.80	0.61	0.00	0.00		
0.00	0.00	0.15	0.17	2.00	40.00	0.20	0.00	184.50	55.50	14.50	46.50	7.50	1.80	1.21	0.00	0.00		
0.00	0.00	0.15	0.15	2.00	50.00	0.20	0.00	209.50	30.50	7.00	22.50	5.00	1.80	0.15	0.00	0.00		
0.00	0.00	0.15	0.17	1.98	41.60	0.20	0.00	219.96	59.28	14.56	44.20	8.32	1.82	0.64	0.00	0.00		
0.00	0.00	0.16	0.16	1.98	52.00	0.21	0.00	221.52	29.64	5.72	22.36	4.68	1.82	0.16	0.00	0.00		
0.00	0.00	0.16	0.16	1.98	52.00	0.21	0.00	202.80	82.16	19.76	43.68	15.08	1.82	0.26		0.00		
0.00	0.00	0.16	0.16	1.98	52.00	0.21	0.00	198.64	65.00	15.08	39.00	10.92	1.82	0.21		0.00		
0.00	0.00	0.16	0.16	1.98	52.00	0.21	0.00	169.00	44.20	11.44	26.52	5.20	1.82	0.16	0.00	0.00		
0.00	0.00	0.16	0.16	1.98	52.00	0.21	0.00	221.52	29.64	5.72	22.88	4.68	1.82	0.16	0.00	0.00		
1.19	1.20	0.19	0.16	1.43	43.20	0.06	0.08	229.80	66.60	43.20	45.60	10.20	0.96	0.35	0.00	0.00	0.72	0.72
								334.40							0.00	0.00		
	0.00							176.22					1.22		0.00	0.00		
0.01	0.00	0.05	0.04	0.51	14.00	0.01	0.00	32.00	14.50	4.40	10.30	3.10	0.44	0.08	0.00	0.00		
0.03	0.00	0.01	0.01	0.18	6.92	0.00	0.00	5.72	4.48	1.00	3.88	1.04	0.14	0.03	0.00	0.00		
0.79	0.00	0.04	0.06	0.60	14.84	0.00	0.01	188.16	47.04	8.40	29.40	11.20	0.84	0.23	1.40	0.00		
1.85	0.00	0.14	0.24	1.03	34.98	0.05	0.26	367.62	64.02	23.76	78.54	7.92	1.33	0.48	0.00	0.00	0.17	0.35
1.35	0.00	0.10	0.17	0.75	25.44	0.04	0.19	267.36	46.56	17.28	57.12	5.76	0.97	0.35	0.00	0.00	0.13	0.26
0.42	0.00	0.04	0.06	0.39	8.80	0.01	0.00	103.52	17.60	3.36	9.44	2.88	0.36	0.05	0.00	0.00	0.05	0.11
0.07	0.00	0.09	0.06	0.76	15.41	0.01	0.00	124.66	15.41	2.30	15.41	3.22	0.66	0.10	0.00	0.00	0.13	0.26
	0.00							86.22		7.38			0.40			0.00		
		0.05	0.05	0.70	8.40	0.01	0.03	62.72	19.32	11.48	23.24	2.24	0.50	0.08	0.00	0.00		
0.42	0.00	0.06	0.07	0.43	12.60	0.01	0.01	103.68	17.64	3.24	9.54	2.88	0.36	0.05	0.00	0.00	0.06	0.11
0.07	0.00	0.08	0.06	0.71	17.22	0.01	0.00	116.89	14.31	2.18	14.55	2.91	0.62	0.09	0.00	0.00	0.29	0.54
	4.80							135.00		20.00			0.72		0.00	0.00		
2.94	2.63	0.23	0.17	1.91	37.20	0.05	0.00	327.05	122.45	10.85	43.40	10.85	1.74	0.29	0.00	0.00		
	0.00							250.00		20.00			0.72		0.00	0.00		
1.47	0.46	0.09	0.13	0.65	19.32	0.03	0.19	266.80	103.96	67.16	153.64	11.04	0.42	0.30	0.00	0.00		
0.58	2.30	0.20	0.30	1.52	38.88	0.19	0.36	345.60	237.60	108.00	132.48	23.04	1.50	0.69	0.00	0.00		
2.92	13.40	0.22	0.17	1.93	20.74	0.05	0.00	26.52	166.22	28.22	50.52	21.82	1.89	0.43	0.00	0.00		
1.22	3.16	0.01	0.04	0.35	31.59	0.04	0.01	380.25	58.50	9.36	26.91	5.85	0.35	0.19	0.00	0.00		
3.09	1.03	0.22	0.19	1.76	33.81	0.05	0.00	271.95	73.50	10.29	44.10	11.76	1.81	0.29	0.00	0.00		
0.89	1.05	0.03	0.03	0.23	31.59	0.05	0.01	287.82	94.77	14.04	33.93	9.36	0.56	0.21	0.00	0.00		
	0.00	0.05	0.06	0.16				260.00	159.00	0.00			0.72		0.00	0.00		

Food Name	Amount	Measure	Weight (g)	Calories	Protein (g)	Total Carb (g)	Dietary Fiber (g)	Total Fat (g)	Sat Fat (g)	Mono Fat (g)	Poly Fat (g)	Chol (mg)	Vit A (mcg RAE)	Vit D (mcg)
DESSERTS *(continued)*														
Pie, chocolate cream, gourmet, 10" whl or 1/12 pce Mrs. Smith's	1	Piece	116.00	320.00	3.00	39.00	1.00	18.00	10.00			15.00		
Pie, chocolate mousse, no bake, prep f/mix, 9"whl or 1/8 pce	1	Piece	95.00	247.00	3.32	28.12		14.63	7.79	4.83	0.77	33.25	117.80	
Pie, coconut cream, cmrcl prep, 7" whl or 1/6 pce	1	Piece	64.00	190.72	1.34	23.81	0.83	10.62	4.46	4.65	0.99	0.00	17.28	
Pie, coconut cream, gourmet, 10" whl or 1/12 pce Mrs. Smith's	1	Piece	116.00	340.00	2.00	38.00		20.00	13.00			15.00	0.00	
Pie, egg custard, cmrcl prep, 8" whl or 1/6 pce	1	Piece	105.00	220.50	5.77	21.84	1.68	12.18	2.47	5.04	3.91	34.65	59.85	
Pie, fruit, fried, 5" × 3 3/4"	1	Each	128.00	404.48	3.84	54.53	3.33	20.61	3.14	9.53	6.88	0.00	6.40	
Pie, lemon meringue, prep f/recipe, 9" whl or 1/8 pce	1	Piece	127.00	361.95	4.83	49.66	1.52	16.38	4.04	7.09	4.23	67.31	54.61	
Pie, mincemeat, prep f/recipe, 9" whl or 1/8 pce	1	Piece	165.00	476.85	4.29	79.20	4.29	17.82	4.43	7.68	4.69	0.00	1.65	
Pie, peach, 8" whl or 1/6 pce	1	Piece	117.00	260.91	2.22	38.49	0.94	11.70	1.76	4.96	4.39	0.00	11.70	
Pie, peach, old fash, 10" whl or 1/10 pce Mrs. Smith's	1	Piece	133.00	330.00	3.00	46.00	2.00	15.00	3.00			0.00		
Pie, pecan, 10" whl or 1/8 pce Mrs. Smith's	1	Piece	128.00	550.00	7.00	75.00	2.00	26.00	6.00			85.00		
Pie, pecan, cmrcl prep, 8" whl or 1/6 pce	1	Piece	113.00	452.00	4.52	64.64	3.95	20.90	4.01	12.14	3.60	36.16	57.63	
Pie, pineapple TastyKake, Inc.	1	Each	113.00	290.00	3.00	45.00	1.00	12.00	1.00			20.00	0.00	
Pie, pumpkin, 10" whl or 1/10 pce Mrs. Smith's	1	Piece	125.00	310.00	5.00	47.00	2.00	12.00	3.00			45.00		
Pie, pumpkin, cmrcl prep, 8" whl or 1/6 pce	1	Piece	109.00	228.90	4.25	29.76	2.94	10.36	1.95	4.39	3.43	21.80	488.32	
Pie, strawberry TastyKake, Inc.	1	Each	106.00	310.00	2.00	50.00	1.00	12.00	3.00			0.00	0.00	
Puddings, Custards, and Pie Fillings														
Custard, chocolate, dry mix, 2oz pkg	1	Tablespoon	9.00	32.67	0.22	8.24	0.46	0.30	0.17	0.10	0.01	0.00		
Custard, chocolate, prep f/dry mix w/whole milk	0.5	Cup	136.00	130.56	4.35	18.14	0.68	4.54	2.72	1.27	0.16	16.32	36.72	1.22
Custard, egg, prep f/dry mix w/2% milk	0.5	Cup	133.00	147.63	5.43	23.17	0.00	3.64	1.80	1.13	0.26	63.84	81.13	
Custard, flan, dry mix, 3oz pkg	1	Tablespoon	9.00	31.32	0.00	8.24	0.00	0.00	0.00	0.00	0.00	0.00	0.00	
Custard, vanilla, prep f/dry mix w/2% milk	0.5	Cup	133.00	102.41	4.07	16.41	0.00	2.35	1.41	0.64	0.09	9.31	67.83	1.22
Custard, vanilla, prep f/dry mix w/whole milk	0.5	Cup	133.00	118.37	4.03	16.24	0.00	4.08	2.46	1.12	0.15	17.29	35.91	1.22
Filling, poppy seed, Solo Sokol & Company	2	Tablespoon	36.00	119.52	1.73	20.92		3.21	0.37	0.47	2.01			
Pie Filling, apple, 21oz can	0.5	Cup	127.50	128.77	0.12	33.41	1.27	0.12	0.02	0.00	0.03	0.00	0.00	
Pie Filling, cherry, 21 oz can	0.5	Cup	132.00	151.80	0.50	36.96	0.80	0.09	0.02	0.04	0.04	0.00	13.20	
Pie Filling, pumpkin, cnd, cup	0.5	Cup	135.00	140.40	1.47	35.63	11.21	0.17	0.09	0.02	0.01	0.00	560.25	
Pudding, banana, inst, dry mix, svg, makes 1/2 cup prep	1	Each	25.00	91.75	0.00	23.18	0.00	0.15	0.02	0.04	0.09	0.00	0.00	
Pudding, chocolate, rte, 4oz snack can	1	Each	113.40	157.63	3.06	26.08	1.13	4.54	0.81	1.93	1.62	3.40	11.34	
Pudding, chocolate, sug free, rducd cal, dry mix Jell-O	1	Ounce-weight	28.35	85.05	2.84	19.85	2.84	0.00	0.00	0.00	0.00	0.00	0.00	
Pudding, coconut cream, inst, prep f/dry mix w/2% milk	0.5	Cup	147.00	157.29	4.26	28.22	0.15	3.38	2.01	0.91	0.28	8.82	66.15	
Pudding, corn, prep f/recipe	0.5	Cup	125.00	136.25	5.49	15.95	1.88	6.65	3.17	2.15	0.86	125.00	67.50	
Pudding, flan, prep f/dry mix w/2% milk Jello-O	0.5	Cup	144.00	140.00	4.00	26.00	0.00	2.50	1.50			10.00		
Pudding, lemon, rte, 5oz can	1	Each	141.75	177.19	0.14	35.44	0.14	4.25	0.64	1.84	1.62	0.00	0.00	
Pudding, pistachio, inst, prep w/2% milk Jell-O	0.5	Cup	147.00	160.00	4.00	29.00	0.00	3.00	1.50			10.00		
Pudding, rice, rte, 5oz can	1	Each	141.75	231.05	2.84	31.19	0.14	10.63	1.66	4.55	3.95	1.42	35.44	
Pudding, tapioca, fat free, rte	0.5	Cup	125.00	111.25	2.25	25.50	0.00	0.05	0.00	0.00	0.00	1.25	40.00	
Pudding, tapioca, rte, 5oz can	1	Each	141.75	168.68	2.84	27.50	0.14	5.24	0.85	2.24	1.93	1.42	0.07	
Pudding, vanilla, fat free, rte	0.5	Cup	125.00	116.25	2.75	28.35	0.00	0.08	0.03	0.03	0.01	1.25	50.00	
Pudding, vanilla, rte, 4oz snack can	1	Each	113.40	146.29	2.61	24.83	0.00	4.08	0.65	1.75	1.52	7.94	6.80	
Frosting, chocolate fudge, rte														

Vit E (mg)	Vit C	Vit B₁ Thia (mg)	Vit B₂ Ribo (mg)	Vit B₃ Nia (mg)	Fol (mcg)	Vit B₆ (mg)	Vita B₁₂ (mcg)	Sodi (mg)	Pota (mg)	Cal (mg)	Phos (mg)	Magn (mg)	Iron (mg)	Zinc (mg)	Caff (mg)	Alco (g)	Sol Fiber (g)	Insol Fiber (g)
	0.00							180.00		0.00			1.08			0.00		
1.42	0.47	0.05	0.14	0.57	24.70	0.03	0.20	437.00	270.75	73.15	219.45	30.40	1.03	0.57	0.95	0.00		
0.10	0.00	0.03	0.05	0.13	4.48	0.04	0.08	163.20	41.60	18.56	54.40	12.80	0.51	0.30	0.00	0.00		
	0.00							260.00		0.00			0.00		0.00	0.00		
0.99	0.63	0.04	0.22	0.31	21.00	0.05	0.45	252.00	111.30	84.00	117.60	11.55	0.61	0.55	0.00	0.00		
2.20	1.66	0.18	0.14	1.82	23.04	0.04	0.10	478.72	83.20	28.16	55.04	12.80	1.56	0.29	0.00	0.00		
2.29	4.19	0.15	0.20	1.20	31.75	0.03	0.15	307.34	82.55	15.24	53.34	7.62	1.27	0.36	0.00	0.00		
0.25	9.73	0.25	0.17	1.96	37.95	0.11	0.00	419.10	334.95	36.30	69.30	23.10	2.46	0.36	0.00	0.00		
1.10	1.05	0.07	0.04	0.23	33.93	0.03	0.00	315.90	146.25	9.36	25.74	7.02	0.58	0.11	0.00	0.00		
	0.00							290.00	159.00	0.00			0.00		0.00	0.00		
	0.00							510.00	90.00	0.00			0.72		0.00	0.00		
0.36	1.24	0.10	0.14	0.28	38.42	0.02	0.11	479.12	83.62	19.21	87.01	20.34	1.18	0.64	0.00	0.00		
	1.20							310.00		20.00			1.08		0.00	0.00		
	0.00	0.05	0.20	0.49				390.00	193.00	80.00			1.44		0.00	0.00		
1.12	1.09	0.06	0.17	0.20	26.16	0.06	0.28	307.38	167.86	65.40	77.39	16.35	0.86	0.49	0.00	0.00		
	9.00							300.00		20.00			1.08		0.00	0.00		
0.01	0.00	0.00	0.01	0.03	0.54	0.00	0.00	6.30	38.70	14.94	11.61	7.29	0.23	0.14	1.17	0.00		
0.13	1.09	0.05	0.21	0.14	6.80	0.06	0.44	69.36	243.44	168.64	131.92	27.20	0.41	0.68	1.36	0.00		
0.27	1.06	0.07	0.28	0.17	11.97	0.09	0.60	118.37	297.92	192.85	183.54	25.27	0.47	0.69	0.00	0.00	0.00	0.00
0.00	0.00	0.00	0.00	0.00	0.00	0.00	0.00	38.88	13.77	2.16	0.09	0.00	0.01	0.00	0.00	0.00	0.00	0.00
0.09	1.20	0.05	0.20	0.11	6.65	0.05	0.44	61.18	188.86	160.93	126.35	17.29	0.07	0.48	0.00	0.00	0.00	0.00
0.12	1.20	0.05	0.20	0.10	6.65	0.05	0.44	61.18	186.20	158.27	123.69	15.96	0.07	0.47	0.00	0.00	0.00	0.00
								26.64		115.92					0.00	0.00		
0.00	0.12	0.02	0.02	0.05	0.00	0.02	0.00	56.09	57.38	5.11	8.93	2.55	0.38	0.05	0.00	0.00	0.48	0.79
0.28	4.75	0.04	0.02	0.18	5.29	0.05	0.00	23.77	138.60	14.53	19.79	9.24	0.32	0.07	0.00	0.00		
1.08	4.73	0.02	0.16	0.51	47.25	0.22	0.00	280.80	186.30	49.95	60.75	21.60	1.44	0.37	0.00	0.00		
0.01	0.00	0.00	0.00	0.00	0.00	0.00	0.00	374.75	3.75	1.50	201.00	0.50	0.03	0.01	0.00	0.00	0.00	0.00
0.33	2.04	0.03	0.18	0.39	3.40	0.03	0.00	146.29	204.12	102.06	90.72	23.81	0.58	0.48	5.67	0.00		
	0.00							311.85	396.90	0.00			3.06			0.00		
0.06	1.18	0.05	0.20	0.13	5.88	0.06	0.44	361.62	194.04	149.94	295.47	20.58	0.22	0.49	0.00	0.00		
0.26	3.50	0.52	0.16	1.23	31.25	0.15	0.11	68.75	201.25	50.00	71.25	18.75	0.70	0.62	0.00	0.00	0.12	1.75
	0.00							65.00	200.00	150.00	100.00		0.00		0.00	0.00	0.00	0.00
0.18	0.14	0.00	0.01	0.00	0.00	0.00	0.00	198.45	1.42	2.84	7.09	1.42	0.10	0.04	0.00	0.00		
	0.00							410.00	200.00	150.00	300.00		0.00		0.00	0.00	0.00	0.00
1.96	0.71	0.03	0.10	0.23	4.25	0.04	0.30	120.49	85.05	73.71	96.39	11.34	0.43	0.69	0.00	0.00		
0.00	0.00	0.02	0.12	0.06	2.50	0.02	0.19	265.00	66.25	62.50	50.00	6.25	0.44	0.58	0.00	0.00	0.00	0.00
0.43	0.57	0.03	0.14	0.44	4.25	0.03	0.30	225.38	136.08	119.07	111.98	11.34	0.33	0.38	0.00	0.00	0.04	0.10
0.00	0.00	0.03	0.16	0.11	3.75	0.02	0.24	266.25	90.00	75.00	61.25	8.75	0.45	0.70	0.00	0.00	0.00	0.00
0.00	0.00	0.02	0.16	0.29	0.00	0.01	0.11	153.09	128.14	99.79	77.11	9.07	0.15	0.28	0.00	0.00	0.00	0.00

Food Name	Amount	Measure	Weight (g)	Calories	Protein (g)	Total Carb (g)	Dietary Fiber (g)	Total Fat (g)	Sat Fat (g)	Mono Fat (g)	Poly Fat (g)	Chol (mg)	Vit A (mcg RAE)	Vit D (mcg)
DESSERT TOPPINGS														
Creamy Supreme	2	Tablespoon	34.00	140.00	0.00	21.00	0.00	6.00	1.50			0.00	0.00	
Frosting, chocolate, creamy, dry mix, pkg	1	Ounce-weight	28.35	110.28	0.36	26.08	0.68	1.47	0.34	0.65	0.42	0.00	0.00	
Frosting, cream cheese, rte														
Creamy Supreme	2	Tablespoon	35.00	150.00	0.00	24.00	0.00	6.00	1.50			0.00	0.00	
Frosting, cream cheese, rte, 16oz can	1	Ounce-weight	28.35	117.65	0.03	19.09	0.00	4.90	1.29	1.06	1.75	0.00	0.00	
Frosting, glaze, prep f/recipe	1	Ounce-weight	28.35	101.78	0.17	20.83	0.00	2.24	0.49	0.96	0.66	0.57	24.66	
Frosting, vanilla, creamy, rte, 16oz pkg	1	Ounce-weight	28.35	119.07	0.00	19.14	0.03	4.71	0.84	1.38	2.25	0.00	0.00	
Frosting, white, fluffy, prep f/dry mix w/water	1	Ounce-weight	28.35	69.17	0.42	17.75	0.00	0.00	0.00	0.00	0.00	0.00	0.00	
Syrup, chocolate, tbsp Hershey's	2	Tablespoon	39.00	100.00	1.00	24.00		0.00	0.00	0.00	0.00	0.00	0.00	
Topping, caramel	2	Tablespoon	41.00	103.32	0.61	27.02	0.37	0.04	0.03	0.01	0.00	0.41	11.07	
Topping, hot fudge	2	Tablespoon	41.00	140.00	1.00	24.00	1.00	4.50	2.00			0.00	0.00	
Topping, marshmallow creme Jet-Puffed	2	Tablespoon	12.00	40.00	0.00	10.00	0.00	0.00	0.00	0.00	0.00	0.00	0.00	
Topping, strawberry	2	Tablespoon	42.50	107.95	0.09	28.18	0.30	0.04	0.00	0.01	0.02	0.00	0.43	
Topping, whipped, fat free, Cool Whip	2	Tablespoon	9.00	15.00	0.00	3.00	0.00	0.00	0.00	0.00	0.00	0.00	0.00	
Topping, whipped, pressurized	2	Tablespoon	8.75	23.10	0.09	1.41	0.00	1.95	1.65	0.17	0.02	0.00	0.35	
Topping, whipped, semi-solid, fzn	2	Tablespoon	9.38	29.81	0.12	2.16	0.00	2.37	2.04	0.15	0.05	0.00	0.66	
EGGS, SUBSTITUTES, AND EGG DISHES														
Egg Substitute, fzn, cup	0.25	Cup	60.00	96.00	6.77	1.92	0.00	6.67	1.16	1.46	3.74	1.20	6.60	
Egg Substitute, liquid, cup	0.25	Cup	62.75	52.71	7.53	0.40	0.00	2.08	0.41	0.56	1.01	0.63	11.29	
Egg Substitute, scrambled, prep f/fzn	0.25	Cup	35.00	57.67	3.60	1.41	0.00	4.13	0.74	1.15	2.05	0.75	33.74	0.40
Egg Whites, pwd Ener-G Foods	1	Tablespoon	15.00	56.40	12.36	0.67	0.00	0.01				0.00	0.00	0.00
Egg Whites, raw, lrg, each	1	Each	33.40	17.37	3.64	0.24	0.00	0.06	0.00	0.00	0.00	0.00	0.00	0.00
Egg Yolks, raw, lrg, each	1	Each	16.60	53.45	2.63	0.60	0.00	4.41	1.59	1.95	0.70	204.84	63.25	0.45
Eggs, deviled	1	Each	31.00	62.67	3.60	0.39	0.00	5.08	1.23	1.75	1.48	121.94	49.89	0.38
Eggs, hard bld, lrg, each	1	Each	50.00	77.50	6.29	0.56	0.00	5.30	1.63	2.04	0.71	212.00	84.50	
Eggs, poached, lrg, each	1	Each	50.00	73.50	6.26	0.38	0.00	4.95	1.54	1.90	0.68	211.00	69.50	0.43
Eggs, scrambled, fast food	1	Each	47.00	99.64	6.50	0.98	0.00	7.60	2.89	2.77	0.92	200.22	104.81	0.80
Eggs, scrambled, prep f/one lrg egg butter & milk	1	Each	61.00	101.26	6.76	1.34	0.00	7.45	2.24	2.91	1.31	214.72	87.23	0.53
Eggs, whole, lrg, fried	1	Each	46.00	92.46	6.27	0.40	0.00	7.04	1.98	2.92	1.22	210.22	91.08	0.43
Eggs, whole, raw, lrg, each	1	Each	50.00	73.50	6.29	0.38	0.00	4.97	1.55	1.90	0.68	211.50	70.00	0.43
Omelette, plain, prep w/one lrg egg margarine & salt	1	Each	61.00	93.33	6.48	0.42	0.00	7.33	2.05	3.04	1.28	217.16	94.55	0.76
ETHNIC FOODS														
Italian Foods														
Mexican Foods														
Oriental Foods														
Dish, edamame soybeans Ace Sushi Inc.	0.5	Cup	75.00	90.00	9.00	3.00		5.00	1.00			0.00	0.00	
Dish, fish curry, Thai, prep f/recipe, svg	1	Each	187.58	256.01	16.67	10.81	1.62	17.06	11.20			32.36		0.00
Dish, inari, svg Ace Sushi Inc.	3	Piece	144.00	264.00	8.40	48.00	1.20	6.00	1.20			0.00	0.00	
Dish, pad Thai, w/chicken & shrimp, prep f/recipe, svg	1	Each	317.08	590.14	30.88	41.75	4.87	35.84	6.09			161.99		1.18
Dish, spring roll, vegetable, Thai, prep f/recipe	1	Piece	63.22	158.50	4.24	19.89	0.95	6.92	0.92			2.85		0.21
Dish, sushi combo, Fujiyama Aurora Hissho Sushi	1	Each	226.00	349.00	12.00	56.00	3.00	4.00	1.00			8.00		
Dish, sushi combo, Kobe Meridian Hissho Sushi	1	Each	198.00	355.00	15.00	53.00	2.00	4.00	1.00			32.00		
Dish, sushi, California roll & inari Ace Sushi Inc.	3	Piece	117.00	200.00	6.00	36.00	1.00	4.00	1.00			3.00	0.00	
Dish, sushi, futomaki & inari Ace Sushi Inc.	3	Piece	120.00	210.00	2.00	38.00	2.00	4.00	1.00			10.00		
Dish, sushi, golden vgtrn combo Ace Sushi Inc.	4	Piece	128.00	250.00	7.00	44.00	2.00	5.00	1.00			0.00		
Dish, sweet noodles, Thai, prep f/recipe, svg	1	Each	141.75	339.25	14.47	36.92	1.69	15.46	2.44			121.49		1.27
Dish, tofu w/sour curry, Thai, prep f/recipe, svg	1	Each	297.67	421.86	25.07	15.79	4.96	31.72	4.28			0.00		0.00
Dumpling, shumai, pork, rth Ace Sushi Inc.	9	Piece	135.00	220.00	11.00	21.00	2.00	10.00	4.00			30.00	0.00	

Vit E (mg)	Vit C	Vit B₁ Thia (mg)	Vit B₂ Ribo (mg)	Vit B₃ Nia (mg)	Fol (mcg)	Vit B₆ (mg)	Vita B₁₂ (mcg)	Sodi (mg)	Pota (mg)	Cal (mg)	Phos (mg)	Magn (mg)	Iron (mg)	Zinc (mg)	Caff (mg)	Alco (g)	Sol Fiber (g)	Insol Fiber (g)
	0.00							75.00		0.00			0.72		0.00		0.00	0.00
0.28	0.00	0.00	0.01	0.04	0.85	0.02	0.00	21.55	51.03	3.12	17.58	10.77	0.34	0.23	1.70	0.00		
	0.00							70.00		0.00			0.00		0.00	0.00	0.00	0.00
1.20	0.00	0.00	0.00	0.00	0.00	0.00	0.00	54.15	9.92	0.85	0.85	0.56	0.05	0.01	0.00	0.00	0.00	0.00
0.22	0.06	0.00	0.01	0.01	0.28	0.00	0.02	26.65	8.51	6.24	5.10	0.85	0.02	0.02	0.00	0.00	0.00	0.00
0.59	0.00	0.00	0.08	0.06	2.27	0.00	0.00	52.16	9.64	0.85	5.11	0.29	0.05	0.02	0.00	0.00	0.00	0.00
0.00	0.00	0.00	0.01	0.18	0.57	0.00	0.00	44.23	21.83	1.13	1.41	0.57	0.02	0.01	0.00	0.00	0.00	0.00
	0.00							25.00		0.00			0.36		7.00	0.00		
0.00	0.12	0.00	0.04	0.02	0.82	0.01	0.04	143.09	34.44	21.73	19.27	2.87	0.08	0.08	0.00	0.00		
	0.00							100.00	85.00	40.00	60.00		0.36		0.00			
0.00	0.00							10.00	0.00	0.00			0.00		0.00	0.00	0.00	0.00
0.04	5.82	0.00	0.01	0.07	2.55	0.01	0.00	8.93	21.68	2.55	2.13	1.70	0.12	0.03	0.00	0.00		
	0.00							5.00	0.00	0.00	0.00		0.00		0.00	0.00	0.00	0.00
0.07	0.00	0.00	0.00	0.00	0.00	0.00	0.00	5.42	1.66	0.44	1.57	0.09	0.00	0.00	0.00	0.00	0.00	0.00
0.09	0.00	0.00	0.00	0.00	0.00	0.00	0.00	2.34	1.69	0.56	0.75	0.19	0.01	0.00	0.00	0.00	0.00	0.00
0.95	0.30	0.07	0.23	0.08	9.60	0.08	0.20	119.40	127.80	43.80	43.20	9.00	1.19	0.59	0.00	0.00	0.00	0.00
0.17	0.00	0.07	0.19	0.07	9.41	0.00	0.19	111.07	207.07	33.26	75.93	5.65	1.32	0.82	0.00	0.00	0.00	0.00
0.75	0.20	0.03	0.12	0.05	4.04	0.04	0.12	73.24	78.21	33.43	30.83	5.46	0.58	0.32	0.00	0.00	0.00	0.00
0.00	0.00	0.01	0.35	0.11	14.40	0.00	0.08		167.40	13.35	13.35	10.80	0.04	0.02	0.00	0.00	0.00	0.00
0.00	0.00	0.00	0.15	0.04	1.34	0.00	0.03	55.44	54.44	2.34	5.01	3.67	0.03	0.01	0.00	0.00	0.00	0.00
0.43	0.00	0.03	0.09	0.00	24.24	0.06	0.32	7.97	18.09	21.41	64.74	0.83	0.45	0.38	0.00	0.00	0.00	0.00
0.61	0.00	0.02	0.15	0.02	12.69	0.05	0.32	50.01	36.66	14.67	49.57	2.87	0.35	0.30	0.00	0.00	0.00	0.00
0.52	0.00	0.03	0.26	0.03	22.00	0.06	0.56	62.00	63.00	25.00	86.00	5.00	0.60	0.52	0.00	0.00	0.00	0.00
0.48	0.00	0.03	0.24	0.04	23.50	0.07	0.64	147.00	66.50	26.50	95.00	6.00	0.92	0.55	0.00	0.00	0.00	0.00
0.45	1.55	0.04	0.24	0.10	26.32	0.09	0.48	105.28	69.09	26.79	113.74	6.58	1.22	0.78	0.00	0.00	0.00	0.00
0.52	0.12	0.03	0.27	0.05	18.30	0.07	0.47	170.80	84.18	43.31	103.70	7.32	0.73	0.61	0.00	0.00	0.00	0.00
0.56	0.00	0.03	0.24	0.04	23.46	0.07	0.64	93.84	67.62	27.14	95.68	5.98	0.91	0.55	0.00	0.00	0.00	0.00
0.48	0.00	0.03	0.24	0.04	23.50	0.07	0.64	70.00	67.00	26.50	95.50	6.00	0.92	0.56	0.00	0.00	0.00	0.00
0.58	0.00	0.04	0.25	0.04	23.79	0.07	0.66	98.21	69.54	28.67	98.82	6.10	0.94	0.57	0.00	0.00	0.00	0.00
	2.40							0.00		40.00			1.44		0.00	0.00		
1.75	24.08	0.14	0.13	1.88	24.58	0.43	12.09	206.04	501.21	49.20	259.64	80.31	4.26	1.31	0.00	0.00		
	2.88							396.00		96.00			1.30		0.00	0.00		
2.93	10.89	0.33	0.26	4.82	119.08	0.41	0.79	2281.84	569.15	618.37	382.30	163.12	5.37	2.89	0.00	0.00		
1.30	0.95	0.18	0.14	1.89	31.74	0.03	0.01	262.83	74.59	58.25	42.36	11.89	1.79	0.39	0.00	0.00		
	5.40							1114.00		30.00			1.62		0.00	0.00		
	4.20							1046.00		20.00			1.44		0.00	0.00		
	1.20							320.00		50.00			0.72		0.00	0.00		
	1.80							280.00		50.00			0.72		0.00	0.00		
	1.20							490.00		60.00			1.44		0.00	0.00		
1.63	4.63	0.07	0.09	1.02	15.24	0.14	0.56	376.51	176.40	277.32	169.71	40.07	2.92	1.29	0.00	0.00		
4.26	19.10	0.31	0.21	1.34	61.98	0.25	0.00	409.84	625.11	1046.06	323.62	107.11	4.53	2.57	0.00	0.00		
	0.00							460.00		20.00			1.80		0.00	0.00		

Food Name	Amount	Measure	Weight (g)	Calories	Protein (g)	Total Carb (g)	Dietary Fiber (g)	Total Fat (g)	Sat Fat (g)	Mono Fat (g)	Poly Fat (g)	Chol (mg)	Vit A (mcg RAE)	Vit D (mcg)
ETHNIC FOODS *(continued)*														
Miso	1	Cup	275.00	547.25	32.15	72.79	14.85	16.53	3.13	3.42	8.81	0.00	11.00	
Sushi, California roll Ace Sushi Inc.	3	Piece	90.00	125.00	3.00	24.00	1.00	2.00	0.50			3.00		
Sushi, cucumber & imit crab Hissho Sushi	3	Ounce-weight	85.05	128.58	3.50	23.01	0.50	0.50	0.00			1.50		
Sushi, cucumber roll Ace Sushi Inc.	6	Piece	85.00	120.00	3.00	25.00	2.00	1.00	0.00			0.00		
Sushi, dynamite roll	3	Ounce-weight	85.05	141.75	5.58	20.62	0.86	2.15	0.43			6.87		
Sushi, eel roll Ace Sushi Inc.	3	Piece	85.00	130.00	4.00	24.00	2.00	2.50	0.50			20.00		
Sushi, salmon roll, spicy Hissho Sushi	3	Ounce-weight	85.05	143.03	6.01	18.47	0.43	3.01	0.43			14.61		
Sushi, shrimp roll, spicy Hissho Sushi	3	Ounce-weight	85.05	128.01	6.01	18.47	0.43	1.29	0.00			33.08		
Sushi, tuna roll Lwin Family Co.	3	Ounce-weight	85.05	148.59	8.00	21.01	0.50	1.50	0.50			9.51		
Sushi, yellowtail roll, spicy Hissho Sushi	3	Ounce-weight	85.05	135.74	6.44	18.47	0.43	2.15	0.43			13.75		
FAST FOODS/RESTAURANTS														
Generic Fast Food														
Brownie, 2" square	1	Each	60.00	243.00	2.74	38.97		10.11	3.14	3.82	2.64	9.60	3.00	
Cheeseburger, double, lrg, w/condiments & veg	1	Each	258.00	704.34	37.98	39.65		43.65	17.67	17.35	4.70	141.90	61.92	
Cheeseburger, double, plain	1	Each	155.00	457.25	27.67	22.06		28.47	13.00	11.01	1.91	110.05	99.20	
Cheeseburger, double, reg, w/condiments & veg	1	Each	166.00	416.66	21.25	35.19		21.08	8.72	7.81	2.66	59.76	71.38	
Cheeseburger, lrg, plain	1	Each	185.00	608.65	30.14	47.42		32.99	14.84	12.74	2.44	96.20	185.00	0.56
Cheeseburger, reg, plain	1	Each	102.00	319.26	14.77	31.75		15.15	6.47	5.77	1.54	49.98	45.90	0.31
Chicken, wing, pieces, hot	6	Each	134.00	450.00	24.00	23.00	1.00	29.00	6.00			145.00		
Cole Slaw, fast food	0.75	Cup	99.00	146.52	1.46	12.75		10.97	1.61	2.42	6.39	4.95	35.64	
Cornbread, hush puppies, svg	5	Piece	78.00	256.62	4.88	34.90	2.67	11.59	2.68	7.81	0.38	134.94	8.58	
Danish, cheese	1	Each	91.00	353.08	5.83	28.69		24.62	5.12	15.60	2.42	20.02	44.59	
Danish, cinnamon	1	Each	88.00	349.36	4.80	46.85	0.29	16.72	3.48	10.59	1.65	27.28	5.28	
Danish, fruit	1	Each	94.00	334.64	4.76	45.06		15.93	3.32	10.10	1.57	18.80	25.38	
Dish, corn, cob, w/butter	1	Each	146.00	154.76	4.47	31.94		3.43	1.64	1.00	0.61	5.84	33.58	
Dish, crab cake	1	Each	60.00	159.60	11.25	5.11	0.24	10.35	2.24	4.31	3.08	82.20	93.00	
Dish, mashed potatoes	0.5	Cup	121.00	100.43	2.79	19.51		1.46	0.58	0.42	0.35	2.42	13.31	
Fish, fillet, brd/batter fried	3	Ounce-weight	85.05	197.32	12.47	14.43	0.43	10.45	2.40	2.19	5.33	28.92	9.36	
French Toast, sticks	5	Piece	141.00	513.24	8.28	57.85	2.68	29.05	4.70	12.65	9.95	74.73	0.36	
Frozen Dessert, ice milk cone, vanilla, soft serve	1	Each	103.00	163.77	3.89	24.11	0.11	6.12	3.53	1.82	0.36	27.81	59.74	0.21
Hamburger, double, reg, plain	1	Each	176.00	543.84	29.92	42.93		27.90	10.38	12.11	2.34	98.56	0.00	0.70
Hamburger, double, reg, w/condiment	1	Each	215.00	576.20	31.82	38.74		32.47	12.00	14.13	2.76	103.20	2.15	
Hamburger, lrg, w/condiment	1	Each	171.50	425.32	23.03	36.72	2.06	20.94	7.90	9.28	1.59	70.32	5.15	
Hamburger, reg, plain	1	Each	90.00	274.50	12.32	30.51		11.82	4.14	5.46	0.92	35.10	0.00	0.27
Hot Dog, plain, w/bun	1	Each	98.00	242.06	10.39	18.03		14.54	5.11	6.85	1.71	44.10	0.00	
Hot Dog, w/chili & bun	1	Each	114.00	296.40	13.51	31.29		13.44	4.85	6.59	1.19	51.30	3.42	
Milk Shake, strawberry, fast food	1	Cup	283.00	319.79	9.62	53.49	1.13	7.92	4.91	2.21	0.31	31.13	73.58	0.57
Nachos, w/cheese	7	Piece	113.00	345.78	9.10	36.33		18.95	7.78	7.99	2.23	18.08	149.16	
Nachos, w/cheese & jalapeno peppers	7	Piece	204.00	607.92	16.81	60.08		34.15	14.02	14.40	4.02	83.64	573.24	
Nachos, w/cheese beans beef & peppers	7	Piece	225.00	501.75	17.46	49.25		27.09	11.02	9.69	5.02	18.00	384.75	
Onion Rings, breaded, fried, svg	8	Piece	78.11	259.33	3.48	29.47		14.60	6.54	6.26	0.62	13.28	0.78	
Oysters, brd/battered, fried	3	Ounce-weight	85.05	225.38	7.67	24.40	0.32	10.97	2.80	4.23	2.84	66.34	66.34	
Pancakes, w/butter & syrup	1	Each	116.00	259.84	4.13	45.45	0.60	6.99	2.92	2.64	0.98	29.00	40.60	
Potatoes, hash browns	0.5	Cup	72.00	151.20	1.94	16.15		9.22	4.32	3.86	0.47	9.36	1.44	
Sandwich, breakfast, egg bacon, w/biscuit	1	Each	150.00	457.50	17.00	28.59	0.75	31.10	7.95	13.44	7.47	352.50	106.50	
Sandwich, breakfast, egg cheese bacon, w/biscuit	1	Each	144.00	476.64	16.26	33.42	0.35	31.39	11.40	14.23	3.49	260.64	190.08	
Sandwich, breakfast, egg ham, w/biscuit	1	Each	192.00	441.60	20.43	30.32	0.77	27.03	5.91	10.96	7.70	299.52	236.16	
Sandwich, breakfast, egg sausage, w/biscuit	1	Each	180.00	581.40	19.15	41.15	0.90	38.70	14.98	16.40	4.45	302.40	160.20	
Sandwich, breakfast, egg steak, w/biscuit	1	Each	148.00	409.96	17.94	21.27		28.43	8.60	11.71	5.85	272.32	205.72	
Sandwich, breakfast, egg, w/biscuit	1	Each	136.00	372.64	11.60	31.91	0.82	22.07	4.73	9.07	6.40	244.80	179.52	
Sandwich, croissant, w/egg & cheese	1	Each	127.00	368.30	12.79	24.31		24.70	14.07	7.54	1.37	215.90	276.86	
Sandwich, croissant, w/egg cheese & bacon	1	Each	129.00	412.80	16.23	23.65		28.35	15.43	9.18	1.76	215.43	141.90	
Sandwich, croissant, w/egg cheese & ham	1	Each	152.00	474.24	18.92	24.20		33.58	17.48	11.39	2.36	212.80	130.72	
Sandwich, english muffin, w/cheese & sausage	1	Each	115.00	393.30	15.34	29.16	1.49	24.26	9.85	10.08	2.69	58.65	101.20	

Vit E (mg)	Vit C	Vit B₁ Thia (mg)	Vit B₂ Ribo (mg)	Vit B₃ Nia (mg)	Fol (mcg)	Vit B₆ (mg)	Vita B₁₂ (mcg)	Sodi (mg)	Pota (mg)	Cal (mg)	Phos (mg)	Magn (mg)	Iron (mg)	Zinc (mg)	Caff (mg)	Alco (g)	Sol Fiber (g)	Insol Fiber (g)
0.03	0.00	0.27	0.64	2.49	52.25	0.55	0.22	10252.00	577.50	156.75	437.25	132.00	6.85	7.04	0.00	0.00	7.12	7.73
	0.00							240.00		0.00			0.00		0.00	0.00		
	1.80							459.27		5.00			0.45		0.00	0.00		
	0.00							90.00		0.00			0.36		0.00	0.00		
	1.55							418.81		8.60			0.54		0.00	0.00		
	2.40							85.00		0.00			0.00		0.00	0.00		
	2.06							376.28		8.60			0.46		0.00	0.00		
	1.80							393.89		17.18			0.85		0.00	0.00		
	1.20							388.23		5.00			0.63		0.00	0.00		
	1.80							372.42		12.89			0.46		0.00	0.00		
	3.18	0.08	0.12	0.58	17.40	0.03	0.15	153.00	83.40	25.20	87.60	16.20	1.29	0.56	1.20	0.00		
	1.03	0.36	0.49	7.25	74.82	0.41	3.41	1148.10	595.98	239.94	394.74	51.60	5.91	6.68	0.00	0.00		
1.19	0.00	0.25	0.37	6.01	68.20	0.25	2.31	635.50	308.45	232.50	373.55	32.55	3.41	4.96	0.00	0.00		
	1.66	0.35	0.28	8.05	61.42	0.18	1.93	1050.78	335.32	170.98	242.36	29.88	3.42	3.49	0.00	0.00		
	0.00	0.48	0.57	11.17	74.00	0.28	2.53	1589.15	643.80	90.65	421.80	38.85	5.46	5.55	0.00	0.00		
0.41	0.00	0.40	0.40	3.70	54.06	0.09	0.97	499.80	164.22	140.76	195.84	21.42	2.44	2.37	0.00	0.00		
	3.60							1120.00		80.00			1.80		0.00	0.00		
3.96	8.32	0.04	0.03	0.08	38.61	0.11	0.18	267.30	177.21	33.66	35.64	8.91	0.72	0.20	0.00	0.00		
	0.00	0.00	0.03	2.03	57.72	0.10	0.17	964.86	187.98	68.64	190.32	16.38	1.43	0.43	0.00	0.00		
	2.64	0.26	0.21	2.55	54.60	0.05	0.23	319.41	116.48	70.07	80.08	15.47	1.85	0.63	0.00	0.00		
0.79	2.55	0.26	0.19	2.20	54.56	0.05	0.22	326.48	95.92	36.96	73.92	14.08	1.80	0.48	0.00	0.00		
0.85	1.60	0.29	0.21	1.80	31.02	0.06	0.23	332.76	109.98	21.62	68.62	14.10	1.40	0.48	0.00	0.00		
	6.86	0.25	0.10	2.18	43.80	0.32	0.00	29.20	359.16	4.38	108.04	40.88	0.88	0.91	0.00	0.00		
	0.18	0.06	0.08	1.17	24.60	0.15	4.40	491.40	162.00	202.20	226.80	25.20	1.12	2.12	0.00	0.00		
	0.48	0.11	0.06	1.45	9.68	0.28	0.06	274.67	355.74	25.41	66.55	21.78	0.57	0.39	0.00	0.00		
	0.00	0.09	0.09	1.79	14.46	0.09	0.94	452.47	272.16	15.31	145.44	20.41	1.79	0.37	0.00	0.00		
2.33	0.00	0.23	0.26	2.96	197.40	0.26	0.08	499.14	126.90	77.55	122.67	26.79	2.96	0.94	0.00	0.00		
0.38	1.14	0.05	0.25	0.32	12.36	0.06	0.21	91.67	168.92	153.47	139.05	15.45	0.16	0.57	0.00	0.00		
1.32	0.00	0.33	0.37	8.25	77.44	0.32	2.92	554.40	362.56	86.24	234.08	36.96	4.56	5.72	0.00	0.00		
1.61	1.08	0.34	0.41	6.73	83.85	0.37	3.33	741.75	526.75	92.45	283.80	45.15	5.55	5.81	0.00	0.00		
0.03	2.57	0.34	0.28	6.54	61.74	0.25	2.57	728.88	394.45	133.77	212.66	34.30	4.13	4.75	0.00	0.00		
0.49	0.00	0.33	0.27	3.72	53.10	0.06	0.89	387.00	144.90	63.00	102.60	18.90	2.40	2.00	0.00	0.00		
0.27	0.10	0.24	0.27	3.65	48.02	0.05	0.51	670.32	143.08	23.52	97.02	12.74	2.31	1.98	0.00	0.00		
	2.74	0.22	0.40	3.74	72.96	0.05	0.30	479.94	166.44	19.38	191.52	10.26	3.28	0.78	0.00	0.00		
0.37	2.26	0.13	0.55	0.50	8.49	0.12	0.88	234.89	515.06	319.79	283.00	36.79	0.31	1.02	0.00	0.00		
	1.24	0.19	0.37	1.54	10.17	0.20	0.82	815.86	171.76	272.33	275.72	55.37	1.28	1.79	0.00	0.00		
	1.02	0.12	0.49	2.84	18.36	0.37	1.02	1736.04	293.76	620.16	393.72	108.12	2.45	2.90	0.00	0.00		
	4.27	0.20	0.61	2.95	33.75	0.36	0.90	1588.50	398.25	339.75	342.00	85.50	2.45	3.22	0.00	0.00		
0.31	0.55	0.08	0.09	0.87	51.55	0.06	0.11	404.61	121.85	68.74	81.23	14.84	0.80	0.33	0.00	0.00		
	2.55	0.19	0.21	2.70	18.71	0.02	0.62	414.19	111.42	17.01	119.92	14.46	2.73	9.57	0.00	0.00		
0.70	1.74	0.20	0.27	1.70	25.52	0.06	0.12	552.16	125.28	63.80	237.80	24.36	1.31	0.51	0.00	0.00		
0.12	5.47	0.08	0.01	1.07	7.92	0.17	0.01	290.16	267.12	7.20	69.12	15.84	0.48	0.22	0.00	0.00		
1.96	2.70	0.14	0.22	2.40	60.00	0.14	1.03	999.00	250.50	189.00	238.50	24.00	3.74	1.64	0.00	0.00		
1.44	1.58	0.30	0.43	2.30	53.28	0.10	1.05	1260.00	230.40	164.16	459.36	20.16	2.55	1.54	0.00	0.00		
2.28	0.00	0.67	0.60	2.00	65.28	0.27	1.19	1382.40	318.72	220.80	316.80	30.72	4.55	2.23	0.00	0.00		
2.84	0.00	0.50	0.45	3.60	64.80	0.20	1.37	1141.20	320.40	154.80	489.60	25.20	3.96	2.16	0.00	0.00		
	0.15	0.36	0.52	3.06	56.24	0.18	1.41	888.00	306.36	137.64	224.96	25.16	5.30	2.80	0.00	0.00		
3.26	0.14	0.30	0.49	2.15	57.12	0.11	0.63	890.80	238.00	81.60	387.60	19.04	2.90	0.99	0.00	0.00		
	0.13	0.19	0.38	1.51	46.99	0.10	0.77	551.18	173.99	243.84	347.98	21.59	2.20	1.75	0.00	0.00		
	2.19	0.35	0.34	2.19	45.15	0.12	0.86	888.81	201.24	150.93	276.06	23.22	2.19	1.90	0.00	0.00		
	11.40	0.52	0.30	3.19	45.60	0.23	1.00	1080.72	272.08	144.40	335.92	25.84	2.13	2.17	0.00	0.00		
1.26	1.26	0.70	0.25	4.14	66.70	0.15	0.68	1036.15	215.05	167.90	186.30	24.15	2.25	1.68	0.00	0.00		

Food Name	Amount	Measure	Weight (g)	Calories	Protein (g)	Total Carb (g)	Dietary Fiber (g)	Total Fat (g)	Sat Fat (g)	Mono Fat (g)	Poly Fat (g)	Chol (mg)	Vit A (mcg RAE)	Vit D (mcg)
FAST FOODS/RESTAURANTS *(continued)*														
Sandwich, english muffin, w/egg cheese & Canadian bacon	1	Each	146.00	308.06	17.78	28.50	1.61	13.42	4.97	4.98	1.66	249.66	188.34	1.17
Shrimp, brd, fried, fast food, each	4	Each	93.70	259.55	10.79	22.85		14.22	3.07	9.93	0.36	114.31	20.61	
A&W Restaurants														
Cheeseburger, deluxe, w/bacon	1	Each	277.50	600.00	32.00	44.00	4.00	33.00	12.00			110.00		
Applebee's														
Beef, sirloin steak, house USDA SR-23	1	Each	179.00	315.04	45.88	0.00	0.00	14.66	5.81	6.70	1.03	119.93		
Chicken Fingers, kid USDA SR-23	1	Serving	109.00	288.85	20.78	17.05	1.53	15.29	2.76	3.80	7.29	46.87		
French Fries USDA SR-23	1	Serving	190.00	539.60	6.44	71.08	6.27	25.40	4.72	7.30	11.56	1.90		
Macaroni & Cheese, kid USDA SR-23	1	Serving	198.00	326.70	13.94	39.36	2.77	12.51	4.86	4.45	2.28	25.74		
Shrimp, brd, fried, double crunch USDA SR-23	1	Serving	159.00	513.57	22.55	38.03	1.91	30.21	5.77	7.68	15.46	136.74		
Sticks, mozzarella, brd, fried USDA SR-23	1	Serving	281.00	899.20	42.18	67.24	5.34	51.25	18.38	12.37	13.19	87.11		
Arby's														
Cheese, mozzarella sticks, svg	1	Each	137.00	470.00	18.00	34.00	2.00	29.00	14.00			60.00		
Sandwich, beef melt, w/cheddar	1	Each	150.00	320.00	16.00	36.00	2.00	14.00	6.00			45.00		
Sandwich, ham swiss, hot	1	Each	170.00	340.00	23.00	35.00	1.00	13.00	4.50			90.00		
Sandwich, roast beef, giant	1	Each	228.00	440.00	32.00	42.00	3.00	20.00	11.00			45.00		
Sandwich, roast beef, jr	1	Each	129.00	290.00	16.00	34.00	2.00	12.00	5.00			40.00		
Sandwich, turkey, rstd, deluxe, light	1	Each	194.00	260.00	23.00	33.00	3.00	5.00	0.50	2.20	2.30	40.00		
Baja Fresh														
Burrito, bean & cheese	1	Each	392.00	840.00	39.00	96.00	20.00	33.00	17.00			65.00		
Burrito, bean & cheese Enchilado	1	Each	812.00	1,470.00	62.00	141.00	27.00	73.00	36.00			140.00		
Burrito, bean & cheese, w/chicken	1	Each	491.00	970.00	67.00	96.00	21.00	35.00	18.00			135.00		
Burrito, bean & cheese, w/pork carnitas	1	Each	491.00	1,010.00	59.00	98.00	21.00	42.00	20.00			130.00		
Burrito, bean & cheese, w/shrimp	1	Each	505.00	950.00	61.00	96.00	20.00	34.00	17.00			310.00		
Burrito, bean & cheese, w/steak	1	Each	488.00	1,030.00	64.00	97.00	20.00	43.00	21.00			140.00		
Burrito, chicken, Baja	1	Each	440.00	790.00	52.00	65.00	8.00	38.00	15.00			120.00		
Burrito, chicken, Mexicano	1	Each	514.00	790.00	50.00	117.00	20.00	13.00	3.50			75.00		
Burrito, mahi mahi, Baja Baja	1	Each	451.00	780.00	51.00	66.00	7.00	38.00	15.00			115.00		
Burrito, pork carnitas, Baja	1	Each	440.00	830.00	45.00	67.00	8.00	45.00	18.00			115.00		
Dish, chicken, Bare Burrito Bowl	1	Each	590.00	640.00	45.00	97.00	20.00	7.00	1.00			75.00		
Dish, steak, Bare Burrito Bowl	1	Each	587.00	700.00	41.00	99.00	19.00	15.00	4.50			80.00		
Fajita, chicken, w/corn tortillas	1	Each	788.00	860.00	61.00	105.00	24.00	24.00	7.00			130.00		
Fajita, chicken, w/flour tortillas	1	Each	847.00	1,140.00	69.00	147.00	27.00	33.00	10.00			130.00		
Fajita, fish, breaded, w/mixed tortillas	1	Each	869.00	1,260.00	57.00	162.00	24.00	43.00	11.00			85.00		
Fajita, pork carnitas, w/flour tortillas	1	Each	847.00	1,190.00	58.00	150.00	26.00	43.00	14.00			120.00		
Fajita, steak, w/flour tortillas	1	Each	847.00	1,240.00	65.00	149.00	25.00	45.00	15.00			135.00		
Guacamole, 3oz	1	Side	85.00	110.00	2.00	5.00	2.00	13.00	1.00			0.00		
Guacamole, Pronto	1	Side	170.00	560.00	9.00	60.00	8.00	34.00	3.00			0.00		
Nachos, cheese	1	Entrée	782.00	1,890.00	63.00	163.00	31.00	108.00	40.00			155.00		
Nachos, chicken	1	Entrée	882.00	2,020.00	91.00	164.00	32.00	110.00	41.00			230.00		
Quesadilla, cheese	1	Each	454.00	1,200.00	47.00	84.00	8.00	78.00	37.00			140.00		
Quesadilla, chicken	1	Each	553.00	1,330.00	75.00	84.00	9.00	80.00	37.00			215.00		
Quesadilla, veggie	1	Each	565.00	1,260.00	48.00	96.00	11.00	78.00	37.00			145.00		
Salad, tostada, bean	1	Each	659.00	1,010.00	32.00	98.00	25.00	53.00	13.00			40.00		
Salad, tostada, chicken	1	Each	758.00	1,140.00	60.00	98.00	27.00	55.00	14.00			115.00		
Salsa, Baja	1	Side	227.00	70.00	2.00	7.00	4.00	2.50	0.00			0.00		
Salsa, pico de gallo	1	Side	227.00	50.00	2.00	12.00	3.00	0.50	0.00			0.00		
Taco, fish, Baja, breaded, fried	1	Each	134.00	250.00	8.00	27.00	2.00	13.00	2.00			15.00		
Taco, shrimp, Baja	1	Each	125.00	200.00	11.00	28.00	2.00	5.00	1.00			90.00		
Taco, steak, Baja	1	Each	113.00	230.00	11.00	28.00	2.00	8.00	2.00			25.00		
Baskin Robbins														
Ice Cream, chocolate	0.5	Cup	73.00	170.00	3.00	21.00	1.00	9.00	6.00			30.00		
Ice Cream, chocolate chip, 2.5 oz	1	Scoop	71.00	170.00	3.00	17.00	0.00	10.00	6.00			35.00		
Ice Cream, French vanilla, 2.5 oz	1	Scoop	71.00	180.00	3.00	16.00	0.00	11.00	7.00			75.00		
Ice Cream, fudge brownie, 2.5 oz	1	Scoop	71.00	190.00	3.00	22.00	1.00	11.00	7.00			30.00		
Ice Cream, Jamoca almond fudge, 2.5 oz	1	Scoop	71.00	170.00	3.00	19.00	1.00	9.00	4.50			25.00		
Ice Cream, mint Oreo, light, 2.5 oz	1	Scoop	71.00	150.00	3.00	25.00	1.00	4.50	2.50			15.00		
Ice Cream, Oreo cookies 'n cream, 2.5 oz	1	Scoop	71.00	170.00	3.00	20.00	0.00	9.00	5.00			30.00		
Ice Cream, vanilla, 2.5 oz	1	Scoop	71.00	170.00	3.00	17.00	0.00	10.00	6.00			40.00		

Vit E (mg)	Vit C	Vit B$_1$ Thia (mg)	Vit B$_2$ Ribo (mg)	Vit B$_3$ Nia (mg)	Fol (mcg)	Vit B$_6$ (mg)	Vita B$_{12}$ (mcg)	Sodi (mg)	Pota (mg)	Cal (mg)	Phos (mg)	Magn (mg)	Iron (mg)	Zinc (mg)	Caff (mg)	Alco (g)	Sol Fiber (g)	Insol Fiber (g)
0.60	1.90	0.53	0.48	3.55	73.00	0.16	0.72	776.72	211.70	160.60	287.62	24.82	2.60	1.66	0.00	0.00		
	0.00	0.12	0.52	0.00	57.16	0.03	0.09	826.43	104.95	47.79	196.78	22.49	1.69	0.69	0.00	0.00		
	6.00							1390.00		200.00			5.40		0.00	0.00		
		0.10	0.29	9.58		0.61	4.80	982.71	646.19	30.43	402.75	39.38	3.63	8.82	0.00	0.00	0.00	0.00
1.81		0.15	0.14	10.26		0.30	0.19	604.95	342.26	16.35	329.18	30.52	1.34	0.73	0.00	0.00		
2.62		0.19	0.03	4.38		0.43		989.90	1,029.80	39.90	256.50	57.00	1.60	0.93	0.00	0.00		
0.93		0.25	0.39	4.29		0.07	0.22	752.40	308.88	243.54	330.66	45.54	1.62	1.68	0.00	0.00		
3.83		0.05	0.02	2.18		0.09	1.00	1,135.26	198.75	46.11	518.34	33.39	1.29	1.38	0.00	0.00		
2.98		0.17	0.53	1.76		0.11	2.73	2,228.33	283.81	921.68	851.43	56.20	1.38	5.62	0.00	0.00		
	1.20							1330.00		400.00			0.72		0.00	0.00		
	0.00							850.00		80.00			2.70		0.00	0.00		
	1.20	0.83	0.37	7.80	26.00	0.31		1450.00	382.00	150.00	405.00	31.00	2.70	0.90	0.00	0.00		
	0.00	0.41	0.75	16.80				1330.00	599.00	60.00			5.40	6.00	0.00	0.00		
		0.26	0.37	9.57	10.14	0.14		700.00	291.30	60.00	86.96	11.60	2.70	2.17	0.00	0.00		
	1.20	0.08	0.41	15.32	19.90	0.52		1030.00	351.00	80.00	249.00	29.80	1.80	1.50	0.00	0.00		
								1,790.00							0.00	0.00		
								3,240.00							0.00	0.00		
								2,230.00							0.00	0.00		
								2,370.00							0.00	0.00		
								2,320.00							0.00	0.00		
								2,350.00							0.00	0.00		
								2,140.00							0.00	0.00		
								2,270.00							0.00	0.00		
								1,840.00							0.00	0.00		
								2,280.00							0.00	0.00		
								2,330.00							0.00	0.00		
								2,450.00							0.00	0.00		
								2,400.00							0.00	0.00		
								3,240.00							0.00	0.00		
								2,740.00							0.00	0.00		
								3,450.00							0.00	0.00		
								3,440.00							0.00	0.00		
								270.00							0.00	0.00		
								370.00							0.00	0.00		
								2,530.00							0.00	0.00		
								2,980.00							0.00	0.00		
								2,140.00							0.00	0.00		
								2,590.00							0.00	0.00		
								2,310.00							0.00	0.00		
								1,930.00							0.00	0.00		
								2,370.00							0.00	0.00		
								970.00							0.00	0.00		
								890.00							0.00	0.00		
								420.00							0.00	0.00		
								280.00							0.00	0.00		
								260.00							0.00	0.00		
	1.20							85.00	100.00				0.72			0.00		
	1.20							60.00	100.00				0.36			0.00	0.00	0.00
	0.00							55.00	80.00				0.00		0.00	0.00	0.00	0.00
	0.00							90.00	80.00				0.72			0.00		
	1.20							50.00	80.00				0.36					
	1.20							90.00	100.00				0.72			0.00		
	1.20							95.00	100.00				0.36			0.00	0.00	0.00
	1.20							45.00	100.00				0.00		0.00	0.00	0.00	0.00

Food Name	Amount	Measure	Weight (g)	Calories	Protein (g)	Total Carb (g)	Dietary Fiber (g)	Total Fat (g)	Sat Fat (g)	Mono Fat (g)	Poly Fat (g)	Chol (mg)	Vit A (mcg RAE)	Vit D (mcg)
FAST FOODS/RESTAURANTS *(continued)*														
Burger King														
Cheeseburger, Whopper, double	1	Each	378.00	1020.00	53.00	55.00	4.00	65.00	25.00			170.00		
Chicken, Tenders, 6 pce svg	6	Piece	92.00	250.00	16.00	15.00	1.00	14.00	4.00			35.00	0.00	
Dish, Jalapeno Poppers, 4 pce svg	4	Piece	77.00	230.00	7.00	22.00	2.00	13.00	5.00			20.00		
French Fries, lrg USDA SR-23	1	Serving	160.00	529.60	5.60	64.13	4.64	27.84						
French Fries, med USDA SR-23	1	Serving	117.00	387.27	4.09	46.89	3.39	20.36						
French Fries, sml USDA SR-23	1	Serving	74.00	244.94	2.59	29.66	2.15	12.88						
Hamburger, Whopper Jr	1	Each	167.00	410.00	18.00	32.00	2.00	23.00	7.00			50.00		
Onion Rings Burger King	1	Small	51.00	176.42	2.57	22.45	1.60	8.66	2.25			0.00	0.00	
Sandwich, breakfast, bacon egg cheese, w/biscuit	1	Each	189.00	692.11	26.62	50.58	1.33	61.23	18.63			252.89		
Milk Shake, vanilla, med	1	Each	397.00	440.00	12.00	79.00	2.00	8.00	5.00			25.00		
Sandwich, chicken tenders	1	Each	148.00	450.00	14.00	37.00	2.00	27.00	5.00			30.00		
Sandwich, chicken, club	1	Each	256.00	740.00	30.00	55.00	4.00	44.00	10.00			85.00		
Carl's Junior														
Bacon, ckd, 2 strip svg	2	Each	9.00	50.00	3.00	0.00	0.00	4.00	1.50			10.00	0.00	
Cheeseburger, double, Western Bacon	1	Each	308.00	900.00	51.00	64.00	2.00	49.00	21.00			155.00		
Hamburger, Carl's Famous Star CKE Restaurants	1	Each	254.00	580.00	25.00	49.00	2.00	32.00	9.00			70.00		
Sandwich, chicken, bbq flvr, charbroiled CKE Restaurants	1	Each	199.00	280.00	25.00	37.00	2.00	3.00	1.00			60.00		
Sandwich, chicken, club, charbroiled CKE Restaurants	1	Each	239.00	460.00	32.00	33.00	2.00	22.00	7.00			90.00		
Sandwich, chicken, crispy, bacon Swiss CKE Restaurants	1	Each	291.00	720.00	32.00	66.00	3.00	36.00	10.00			75.00		
Sandwich, chicken, crispy, ranch CKE Restaurants	1	Each	266.00	729.73	29.42	76.50	3.53	34.13	7.06			58.85		
Sandwich, chicken, Santa Fe, charbroiled CKE Restaurants	1	Each	220.00	510.00	28.00	32.00	2.00	31.00	7.00			95.00		
Chick-Fil-A														
Chicken, strips, Chick-N-Strips, 4 pce svg	4	Piece	108.00	250.00	25.00	12.00	0.00	11.00	2.50			70.00	0.00	
French Fries, waffle style, unsalted, sml	1	Serving	85.00	280.00	3.00	36.00	4.00	14.00	5.00			15.00	0.00	
Salad Dressing, ranch, w/buttermilk, pkt	1	Ind. Pkt.	35.00	190.00	1.00	2.00	0.00	20.00	3.00			10.00	0.00	
Salad, Chick-N-Strips	1	Serving	315.00	340.00	30.00	19.00	3.00	16.00	5.00			85.00		
Chipotle														
Burrito Topping, beans, black	1	Serving	113.40	120.00	7.00	23.00	11.00	1.00	0.00			0.00		
Burrito Topping, beans, pinto	1	Serving	113.40	120.00	7.00	22.00	10.00	1.00	0.00			5.00		
Burrito Topping, beef, steak	1	Serving	113.40	190.00	30.00	2.00	0.00	6.50	2.00			65.00		
Burrito Topping, cheese	1	Serving	28.35	100.00	8.00	0.00	0.00	8.50	5.00			30.00		
Burrito Topping, chicken	1	Serving	113.40	190.00	32.00	1.00	0.00	6.50	2.00			115.00		
Chips	4	Ounce-weight	113.40	570.00	8.00	73.00	8.00	27.00	3.50			0.00	0.00	
Guacamole	1	Serving	99.23	150.00	2.00	8.00	6.00	13.00	2.00			0.00		
Salad Topping, beans, black	1	Serving	113.40	120.00	7.00	23.00	11.00	1.00	0.00			0.00		
Salad Topping, beans, pinto	1	Serving	113.40	120.00	7.00	22.00	10.00	1.00	0.00			5.00		
Salad Topping, beef, steak	1	Serving	113.40	190.00	30.00	2.00	0.00	6.50	2.00			65.00		
Salad Topping, cheese	1	Serving	28.35	100.00	8.00	0.00	0.00	8.50	5.00			30.00		
Salad Topping, chicken	1	Serving	113.40	190.00	32.00	1.00	0.00	6.50	2.00			115.00		
Sour Cream	2	Tablespoon	56.70	120.00	2.00	2.00	0.00	10.00	7.00			40.00		
Tortilla, flour, burrito	1	Each	93.56	290.00	7.00	44.00	2.00	9.00	3.00			0.00	0.00	
Tortilla, flour, taco	1	Each	28.35	90.00	2.00	13.00	1.00	2.50	2.50			0.00	0.00	
Dairy Queen														
Frozen Dessert Bar, Starkiss, non dairy	1	Each	85.00	80.00	0.00	21.00	0.00	0.00	0.00	0.00	0.00	0.00	0.00	
Frozen Dessert, banana split, Royal Treats	1	Each	369.00	510.00	8.00	96.00	3.00	12.00	8.00			30.00		
Frozen Dessert, chocolate chip cookie dough, med	1	Each	439.00	950.00	17.00	143.00	2.00	36.00	19.00			75.00		
Frozen Dessert, Lemon Freez'r	0.5	Cup	92.00	80.00	0.00	20.00	0.00	0.00	0.00	0.00	0.00	0.00	0.00	
Frozen Dessert, Misty Slush, med	1	Each	595.00	290.00	0.00	74.00	0.00	0.00	0.00	0.00	0.00	0.00	0.00	
Frozen Dessert, parfait, Peanut Buster, Royal Treats	1	Each	305.00	730.00	16.00	99.00	2.00	31.00	17.00			35.00		
Hot Dog	1	Each	99.00	240.00	9.00	19.00	1.00	14.00	5.00			25.00		

Vit E (mg)	Vit C	Vit B₁ Thia (mg)	Vit B₂ Ribo (mg)	Vit B₃ Nia (mg)	Fol (mcg)	Vit B₆ (mg)	Vita B₁₂ (mcg)	Sodi (mg)	Pota (mg)	Cal (mg)	Phos (mg)	Magn (mg)	Iron (mg)	Zinc (mg)	Caff (mg)	Alco (g)	Sol Fiber (g)	Insol Fiber (g)
	9.00							1460.00		300.00			7.20		0.00	0.00		
	0.00							630.00		0.00			0.72		0.00	0.00		
	0.00							790.00		150.00			0.72		0.00	0.00		
1.22	1.12	0.28	0.05	3.75		0.28		728.00	756.80	14.40	228.80	48.00	2.06	1.76	0.00	0.00		
0.89	0.82	0.20	0.04	2.74		0.20		532.35	553.41	10.53	167.31	35.10	1.51	1.29	0.00	0.00		
0.56	0.52	0.13	0.02	1.73		0.13		336.70	350.02	6.66	105.82	22.20	0.95	0.81	0.00	0.00		
	4.80							520.00		80.00			3.60		0.00	0.00		
	0.00							256.60		64.15			0.00		0.00	0.00		
	0.00							2,129.58		199.65			3.59		0.00	0.00		
	6.00							340.00		400.00			0.00		0.00	0.00		
	3.60							680.00		60.00			1.80		0.00	0.00		
	6.00							1530.00		80.00			3.60		0.00	0.00		
	0.00							140.00		0.00			0.00		0.00	0.00	0.00	0.00
	1.20							1770.00		300.00			6.30		0.00	0.00		
	6.00							910.00		100.00			4.50		0.00	0.00		
	4.80							830.00		80.00			2.70		0.00	0.00		
	6.00							1,110.00		200.00			2.70		0.00	0.00		
	6.00							1,610.00		250.00			3.60		0.00	0.00		
	5.65							1,435.93		176.55			4.24		0.00	0.00		
	9.00							1,240.00		150.00			2.70		0.00	0.00		
	0.00							570.00		40.00			1.08		0.00	0.00	0.00	0.00
	21.00							40.00		20.00			0.00		0.00	0.00		
	0.00							330.00		20.00			0.00		0.00	0.00	0.00	0.00
	6.00							680.00		150.00			1.08		0.00	0.00		
	1.20							250.00		40.00			1.80		0.00	0.00		
	1.20							330.00		40.00			1.80		0.00	0.00		
	0.00							320.00		20.00			2.70		0.00	0.00	0.00	0.00
	0.00							180.00		200.00			0.00		0.00	0.00	0.00	0.00
	1.20							370.00		20.00			1.44		0.00	0.00	0.00	0.00
	1.20							420.00		40.00			1.08		0.00	0.00		
	12.00							190.00		20.00			0.36		0.00	0.00		
	1.20							250.00		40.00			1.80		0.00	0.00		
	1.20							330.00		40.00			1.80		0.00	0.00		
	0.00							320.00		20.00			2.70		0.00	0.00	0.00	0.00
	0.00							180.00		200.00			0.00		0.00	0.00	0.00	0.00
	1.20							370.00		20.00			1.44		0.00	0.00	0.00	0.00
	0.00							30.00		40.00			0.00		0.00	0.00	0.00	0.00
	0.00							670.00		200.00			2.70		0.00	0.00		
	0.00							200.00		60.00			0.72		0.00	0.00		
	0.00							10.00		0.00			0.00			0.00	0.00	0.00
	15.00							180.00		250.00			1.80			0.00		
	1.20							660.00		450.00			2.70			0.00		
	0.00							10.00		0.00			0.00		0.00	0.00	0.00	0.00
	0.00							30.00		0.00			0.00		0.00	0.00	0.00	0.00
	1.20							400.00		300.00			1.80			0.00		
	3.60							730.00		60.00			1.80		0.00	0.00		

Food Name	Amount	Measure	Weight (g)	Calories	Protein (g)	Total Carb (g)	Dietary Fiber (g)	Total Fat (g)	Sat Fat (g)	Mono Fat (g)	Poly Fat (g)	Chol (mg)	Vit A (mcg RAE)	Vit D (mcg)
FAST FOODS/RESTAURANTS (*continued*)														
Ice Cream Bar, Buster Bar	1	Each	149.00	450.00	10.00	41.00	2.00	28.00	12.00			15.00		
Ice Cream Bar, Dilly, chocolate	1	Each	85.00	210.00	3.00	21.00	0.00	13.00	7.00			10.00		
Ice Cream Cone, chocolate, med	1	Each	198.00	340.00	8.00	53.00	0.00	11.00	7.00			30.00		
Ice Cream Cone, chocolate, sml	1	Each	142.00	240.00	6.00	37.00	0.00	8.00	5.00			20.00		
Ice Cream Cone, dipped, med	1	Each	220.00	490.00	8.00	59.00	1.00	24.00	13.00			30.00		
Ice Cream Cone, dipped, sml	1	Each	156.00	340.00	6.00	42.00	1.00	17.00	9.00			20.00		
Ice Cream Sandwich	1	Each	85.00	200.00	4.00	31.00	1.00	6.00	3.00			10.00		
Milk Shake, chocolate malt, med	1	Each	567.00	880.00	19.00	153.00	0.00	22.00	14.00			70.00		
Potatoes, french fries, sml, svg	1	Each	113.00	350.00	4.00	42.00	3.00	18.00	3.50			0.00	0.00	
Dennys														
Chicken Strips, brd, fried, sr	1	Serving	141.75	285.00	19.00	31.00	0.00	10.00	0.00			37.00		
Dish, mini burgers, w/onion ring	1	Each	652.05	2,044.00	61.00	179.00	10.00	122.00	38.00			145.00		
Dish, nachos	1	Each	652.05	1,278.00	54.00	117.00	11.00	64.00	31.00			181.00		
Dish, steak, country fried, sr	1	Each	141.75	341.00	14.00	18.00	6.00	23.00	5.00			44.00		
French Toast, peach, w/o topping & margarine, svg	1	Serving	453.60	1,370.00	53.00	96.00	4.00	85.00	34.00			863.00		
Fried Chicken, chicken fried	1	Each	311.85	550.00	41.00	32.00	2.00	29.00	6.00			102.00		
Hamburger, classic	1	Each	311.85	694.00	40.00	56.00	4.00	35.00	12.00			100.00		
Meal, buttermilk pancake platter, w/o toppings	1	Each	311.85	660.00	23.00	83.00	3.00	25.00	8.00			50.00		
Meal, Grand Slam Slugger, w/o bread	1	Each	765.45	1,190.00	40.00	124.00	5.00	57.00	16.00			480.00		
Meal, Meat Lover's Breakfast	1	Each	595.35	1,027.00	44.00	72.00	3.00	60.00	18.00			497.00		
Meal, scramble, pepper jack & smoked sausage	1	Each	765.45	1,430.00	54.00	118.00	7.00	92.00	33.00			605.00		
Meal, Two Eggs & More Breakfast, w/o bread	1	Each	311.85	678.00	26.00	20.00	2.00	55.00	17.00			506.00		
Omelette, ham & cheddar	1	Each	283.50	595.00	41.00	5.00	0.00	47.00	16.00			783.00		
Omelette, veggie-cheese	1	Each	340.20	494.00	30.00	11.00	2.00	39.00	12.00			747.00		
Quesadilla, chicken	1	Each	454.00	827.00	50.00	43.00	2.00	55.00	23.00			181.00		
Sandwich, club	1	Each	312.00	718.00	32.00	62.00	3.00	38.00	7.00			75.00		
Salad, grilled chicken breast, w/o bread & dressing	1	Each	368.55	259.00	32.00	10.00	4.00	11.00	5.00			90.00		
Sandwich, grilled chicken, w/o dressing	1	Each	283.50	476.00	36.00	56.00	4.00	14.00	3.00			77.00		
Sandwich, Philly melt	1	Each	510.30	874.00	47.00	58.00	5.00	50.00	16.00			114.00		
Sauce, barbecue, svg	1	Each	46.00	47.00	0.00	11.00	0.00	1.00	0.00			0.00		
Shrimp, golden fried USDA SR-23	1	Serving	100.00	277.00	11.51	20.21	1.00	16.67	2.94	4.10	8.38	81.00	0.00	
Dominos Pizza														
Chicken, buffalo wings, hot	1	Each	24.90	44.92	5.46	0.50	0.19	2.39	0.65			25.58		
Pizza, deep dish, ultimate, cheese, 14" USDA SR-23	1	Piece	121.00	331.54	13.75	41.06	2.78	12.51	4.87	3.55	2.32	16.94	94.38	
Pizza, hand tossed, cheese, 14" USDA SR-23	1	Piece	106.00	272.42	11.64	36.52	1.48	8.89	3.76	2.09	1.68	13.78	64.66	0.00
Pizza, hand tossed, Hawaiian feast, 12"	2	Piece	203.74	450.26	21.18	58.28	3.30	15.64	7.20			40.78		
Pizza, hand tossed, veggie feast, 12"	2	Piece	203.16	439.30	19.16	57.28	3.74	15.82	7.10			33.82		
Dunkin' Donuts														
Bagel, poppy seed	1	Each	125.00	340.00	12.00	68.00	3.00	2.50	0.00			0.00	0.00	
Bagel, whole wheat	1	Each	125.00	320.00	12.00	63.00	5.00	1.50	0.00			0.00	0.00	
Doughnut, cake, chocolate	1	Each	59.00	210.00	3.00	19.00	1.00	14.00	3.00			0.00	0.00	
Doughnut, cake, cinnamon	1	Each	66.00	300.00	3.00	29.00	1.00	19.00	4.00			0.00	0.00	
Doughnut, cake, old fash	1	Each	60.00	280.00	3.00	24.00	1.00	19.00	4.00			0.00	0.00	
Doughnut, raised, glazed	1	Each	46.00	160.00	3.00	23.00	1.00	7.00	2.00			0.00	0.00	
Muffin, bran, low fat	1	Each	95.00	260.00	4.00	59.00	4.00	1.50	0.00			0.00	0.00	
Muffin, corn, low fat	1	Each	95.00	250.00	4.00	55.00	1.00	2.00	0.00			0.00	0.00	
El Pollo Loco														
Salad, garden, reg	1	Each	113.00	104.63	4.98	6.98	1.00	6.98	2.99			14.95		
Hardees														
Biscuit, Made from Scratch	1	Each	83.00	390.00	6.00	44.00		21.00	6.00			0.00		
Cheeseburger	1	Each	124.00	313.00	16.00	26.00	1.00	14.00	7.00			40.00		
Hamburger, Six Dollar	1	Each	353.00	911.00	41.00	50.00	2.00	61.00	27.00			137.00		
Milk Shake, chocolate	12.3	Fluid ounce	349.00	370.00	13.00	67.00	0.00	5.00	3.00			30.00		
Potatoes, french fries, Crispy Curls, reg svg	1	Each	96.00	340.00	5.00	41.00	0.00	18.00	4.00			0.00		

Vit E (mg)	Vit C	Vit B1 Thia (mg)	Vit B2 Ribo (mg)	Vit B3 Nia (mg)	Fol (mcg)	Vit B6 (mg)	Vita B12 (mcg)	Sodi (mg)	Pota (mg)	Cal (mg)	Phos (mg)	Magn (mg)	Iron (mg)	Zinc (mg)	Caff (mg)	Alco (g)	Sol Fiber (g)	Insol Fiber (g)
	0.00							280.00		150.00			1.08			0.00		
	0.00							75.00		100.00			0.36			0.00	0.00	0.00
	1.20							160.00		250.00			1.80			0.00	0.00	0.00
	0.00							115.00		150.00			1.08			0.00	0.00	0.00
	2.40							190.00		250.00			1.80			0.00		
	1.20							130.00		200.00			1.08			0.00		
	0.00							140.00		80.00			1.08			0.00		
	2.40							500.00		600.00			2.70			0.00	0.00	0.00
	3.60							880.00		20.00			1.08		0.00	0.00		
								969.00									0.00	0.00
								3,834.00										
								1,654.00										
								1,464.00										
								2,385.00										
								2,621.00										
								785.00										
								2,530.00										
								3,250.00										
								3,462.00										
								4,270.00										
								898.00										
								1,200.00									0.00	0.00
								719.00										
	54.00							1982.00		640.00			1.80		0.00	0.00		
	13.20							1666.00		120.00			4.32		0.00	0.00		
								724.00										
								1,494.00										
								2,444.00										
	2.40							595.00		10.00			0.18		0.00	0.00	0.00	0.00
		0.19	0.10	3.47		0.09	0.43	877.00	100.00	42.00	288.00	17.00	1.38	0.71	0.00	0.00		
	1.13							354.40		5.44			0.30		0.00	0.00		
1.08	0.00	0.28	0.30	5.14			0.57	678.81	198.44	179.08	244.42	30.25	3.58	1.66	0.00	0.00		
1.05	0.00	0.18	0.23	3.45		0.12	0.45	506.68	161.12	142.04	198.22	25.44	2.44	1.22	0.00	0.00		
	1.86							1,102.26		274.28			3.30		0.00	0.00		
	1.32							987.04		278.92			3.44		0.00	0.00		
	3.60							680.00		80.00			4.50		0.00	0.00		
	6.00							630.00		40.00			3.60		0.00	0.00		
	3.60							270.00		0.00			1.44			0.00		
	1.20							350.00		0.00			1.08		0.00	0.00		
	1.20							350.00		0.00			1.08		0.00	0.00		
	1.20							200.00		0.00			0.36		0.00	0.00		
	0.00							440.00		60.00			2.70		0.00	0.00		
	0.00							460.00		0.00			1.08		0.00	0.00		
	6.58							98.65		109.61			0.36		0.00	0.00		
								1000.00							0.00	0.00		
								895.00							0.00	0.00		
								1584.00							0.00	0.00		
								270.00									0.00	0.00
								950.00							0.00	0.00	0.00	0.00

Food Name	Amount	Measure	Weight (g)	Calories	Protein (g)	Total Carb (g)	Dietary Fiber (g)	Total Fat (g)	Sat Fat (g)	Mono Fat (g)	Poly Fat (g)	Chol (mg)	Vit A (mcg RAE)	Vit D (mcg)
FAST FOODS/RESTAURANTS *(continued)*														
Potatoes, french fries, reg svg	1	Each	113.00	340.00	4.00	45.00	0.00	16.00	2.00			0.00		
Sandwich, roast beef, big	1	Each	165.00	411.46	24.02	27.15	2.09	22.97	9.40			67.88		
In-N-Out Burgers														
Cheeseburger, Double Double, w/lettuce bun	1	Each	362.00	520.00	33.00	11.00	3.00	39.00	17.00			120.00		
Cheeseburger, Double Double, w/mustard & ketchup	1	Each	330.00	590.00	37.00	41.00	3.00	32.00	17.00			115.00		
Cheeseburger, Double Double, w/spread	1	Each	330.00	670.00	37.00	39.00	3.00	41.00	18.00			120.00		
Cheeseburger, protein style, wrapped w/lettuce, no bun	1	Each	300.00	330.00	18.00	11.00	2.00	25.00	9.00			60.00		
Cheeseburger, w/lettuce bun	1	Each	300.00	330.00	18.00	11.00	3.00	25.00	9.00			60.00		
Cheeseburger, w/mustard & ketchup	1	Each	268.00	400.00	22.00	41.00	3.00	18.00	9.00			60.00		
Cheeseburger, w/spread	1	Each	268.00	480.00	22.00	39.00	3.00	27.00	10.00			60.00		
Coffee	10	Fluid ounce	296.00	5.00	0.00	1.00	0.00	0.00	0.00	0.00	0.00	0.00	0.00	
Drink, lemonade	16	Fluid ounce	472.80	180.00	0.00	40.00	0.00	0.00	0.00	0.00	0.00	0.00	0.00	
Drink, lemonade, Minute Maid, light	16	Fluid ounce	472.80	8.00	0.00	1.00	0.00	0.00	0.00	0.00	0.00	0.00	0.00	
French Fries	1	Serving	125.00	400.00	7.00	54.00	2.00	18.00	5.00			0.00	0.00	
Hamburger, w/lettuce bun	1	Each	275.00	240.00	13.00	11.00	3.00	17.00	4.00			40.00		
Hamburger, w/mustard & ketchup	1	Each	243.00	310.00	16.00	41.00	3.00	10.00	4.00			35.00		
Hamburger, w/spread	1	Each	243.00	390.00	16.00	39.00	3.00	19.00	5.00			40.00		
Milk	10	Fluid ounce	305.00	180.00	12.00	18.00	0.00	6.00	4.00			30.00		
Milk Shake, chocolate	15	Fluid ounce	352.50	690.00	9.00	83.00	0.00	36.00	24.00			95.00		
Milk Shake, strawberry	15	Fluid ounce	352.50	690.00	9.00	91.00	0.00	33.00	22.00			85.00		
Milk Shake, vanilla	15	Fluid ounce	312.00	680.00	9.00	78.00	0.00	37.00	25.00			90.00		
Soda, 7 Up	16	Fluid ounce	480.00	200.00	0.00	54.00	0.00	0.00	0.00	0.00	0.00	0.00	0.00	
Soda, Coca-Cola, classic	16	Fluid ounce	497.80	198.00	0.00	54.00	0.00	0.00	0.00	0.00	0.00	0.00	0.00	
Soda, Coca-Cola, diet	16	Fluid ounce	479.00	0.00	0.00	0.00	0.00	0.00	0.00	0.00	0.00	0.00	0.00	
Soda, Dr. Pepper	16	Fluid ounce	492.00	180.00	0.00	52.00	0.00	0.00	0.00	0.00	0.00	0.00	0.00	
Soda, root beer	16	Fluid ounce	501.20	222.00	0.00	60.00	0.00	0.00	0.00	0.00	0.00	0.00	0.00	
Tea, iced	16	Fluid ounce	490.00	0.00	0.00	0.00	0.00	0.00	0.00	0.00	0.00	0.00	0.00	
Jack in the Box														
Cheeseburger	1	Each	131.00	350.00	18.00	31.00	1.00	17.00	8.00			50.00		
Cheeseburger, w/bacon, ultimate	1	Each	302.00	1020.00	58.00	37.00	1.00	71.00	26.00			210.00		
Chicken Strips, breast, brd, fried, 4 pce svg	4	Piece	201.00	500.00	35.00	36.00	3.00	25.00	6.00			80.00		
Dish, fish & chips	1	Each	281.00	780.00	19.00	86.00	6.00	39.00	9.00			45.00		
French Fries, curly, large	1	Serving	170.00	550.00	8.00	60.00	6.00	31.00	6.00			0.00		
French Fries, curly, medium	1	Serving	125.00	404.41	5.88	44.12	4.41	22.79	4.41			0.00		
French Fries, curly, sml	1	Serving	84.00	271.76	3.95	29.65	2.96	15.32	2.96			0.00		
French Fries, natural cut, large	1	Serving	196.00	530.00	8.00	69.00	5.00	25.00	6.00			0.00		
French Fries, natural cut, medium	1	Serving	133.00	359.64	5.43	46.82	3.39	16.96	4.07			0.00		
French Toast, sticks, original, svg	1	Serving	121.00	470.00	7.00	58.00	4.00	23.00	5.00			25.00		
Hamburger, deluxe	1	Each	169.00	370.00	17.00	31.00	2.00	21.00	7.00			45.00		
Milk Shake, chocolate, large	1	Each	630.00	1,310.00	23.00	178.00	2.00	57.00	36.00			225.00		
Milk Shake, Oreo cookie, large	1	Each	601.00	1,350.00	22.00	161.00	2.00	66.00	37.00			225.00		
Milk Shake, vanilla, large	1	Each	570.00	1,140.00	22.00	128.00	1.00	58.00	36.00			230.00		
Onion Rings, svg	1	Serving	119.00	500.00	6.00	51.00	3.00	30.00	6.00			0.00		
Sandwich, chicken	1	Each	145.00	400.00	15.00	38.00	2.00	21.00	4.50			35.00		
Sandwich, chicken, classic, w/ciabatta	1	Each	300.00	510.00	36.00	69.00	4.00	13.00	2.50			65.00		
Sandwich, Jack's Spicy Chicken	1	Each	270.00	620.00	25.00	61.00	4.00	31.00	6.00			50.00		
Sandwich, Jack's Spicy Chicken, w/cheese	1	Each	294.00	700.00	29.00	62.00	4.00	37.00	10.00			70.00		
Sandwich, sausage, w/croissant	1	Each	181.00	660.00	20.00	37.00	0.00	48.00	15.00			240.00		
Sauce, barbecue, dipping, svg	1	Serving	28.00	45.00	0.00	11.00	0.00	0.00	0.00	0.00	0.00	0.00		
Sauce, buttermilk house, dipping, svg	1	Serving	25.00	130.00	0.00	3.00	0.00	13.00	2.00			10.00		
Taco, monster	1	Each	138.00	270.00	12.00	19.00	4.00	17.00	6.00			30.00		
Jamba Juice														
Juice Drink, lemonade, w/grape, sml	1	Small	483.00	300.00	1.00	75.00	0.00	0.00	0.00	0.00	0.00	0.00		
Juice, carrot, sml	1	Small	472.00	100.00	3.00	23.00		0.50	0.00	0.00	0.00	0.00		
Juice, orange banana, sml	1	Small	427.00	220.00	3.00	52.00	2.00	1.00	0.00			0.00		
Juice, orange, sml	1	Small	496.00	220.00	3.00	52.00	1.00	1.00	0.00			0.00		
Juice, pineapple orange banana blend, Vibrant C, sml	1	Small	468.00	210.00	2.00	50.00	2.00	0.50	0.00			0.00		
Juice, wheatgrass, 1oz	1	Ounce-weight	28.35	4.72	0.94	0.94	0.00	0.00	0.00	0.00	0.00	0.00	0.00	

Vit E (mg)	Vit C	Vit B₁ Thia (mg)	Vit B₂ Ribo (mg)	Vit B₃ Nia (mg)	Fol (mcg)	Vit B₆ (mg)	Vita B₁₂ (mcg)	Sodi (mg)	Pota (mg)	Cal (mg)	Phos (mg)	Magn (mg)	Iron (mg)	Zinc (mg)	Caff (mg)	Alco (g)	Sol Fiber (g)	Insol Fiber (g)
								390.00							0.00	0.00	0.00	0.00
								1127.85							0.00	0.00		
	12.00							1,160.00	350.00				4.50		0.00	0.00		
	12.00							1,520.00	350.00				5.40		0.00	0.00		
	9.00							1,440.00	350.00				5.40		0.00	0.00		
	18.00							720.00	200.00				1.08		0.00	0.00		
	12.00							720.00	200.00				2.70		0.00	0.00		
	12.00							1,080.00	200.00				3.60		0.00	0.00		
	9.00							1,000.00	200.00				3.60		0.00	0.00		
	0.00							3.00	0.00				0.00		0.00	0.00	0.00	0.00
	4.80							20.00	0.00				0.00		0.00	0.00	0.00	0.00
	8.40							7.00	10.00				0.00		0.00	0.00	0.00	0.00
	0.00							245.00	20.00				1.80		0.00	0.00		
	12.00							370.00	40.00				2.70		0.00	0.00		
	12.00							730.00	40.00				3.60		0.00	0.00		
	9.00							650.00	40.00				3.60		0.00	0.00		
	3.60							190.00	450.00				0.00		0.00	0.00	0.00	0.00
	9.00							350.00	300.00				0.72			0.00	0.00	0.00
	12.00							280.00	300.00				0.00		0.00	0.00	0.00	0.00
	12.00							390.00	300.00				0.00		0.00	0.00	0.00	0.00
	0.00							60.00	0.00				0.00		0.00	0.00	0.00	0.00
	0.00							12.00	0.00				0.00		0.00	0.00	0.00	0.00
	0.00							20.00	0.00				0.00		0.00	0.00	0.00	0.00
	0.00							60.00	0.00				0.00		0.00	0.00	0.00	0.00
	0.00							48.00	0.00				0.00		0.00	0.00	0.00	0.00
	0.00							0.00	0.00				0.00		0.00	0.00	0.00	0.00
								790.00	270.00						0.00	0.00		
	0.60							1740.00	630.00	300.00			7.20		0.00	0.00		
								1,260.00	530.00						0.00	0.00		
	15.00							1740.00	1060.00	20.00			2.70		0.00	0.00		
								1,200.00	790.00						0.00	0.00		
								882.35	580.88						0.00	0.00		
								592.94	390.35						0.00	0.00		
								870.00	1,240.00						0.00	0.00		
								590.36	841.43						0.00	0.00		
								450.00	120.00						0.00	0.00		
								560.00	330.00						0.00	0.00		
								540.00	1,440.00							0.00		
								700.00	1,310.00							0.00		
								440.00	1,260.00						0.00	0.00		
								420.00	140.00						0.00	0.00		
								730.00	240.00						0.00	0.00		
								1,700.00	540.00						0.00	0.00		
								1,100.00	450.00						0.00	0.00		
								1,410.00	480.00						0.00	0.00		
	0.00							860.00	160.00	100.00			1.80		0.00	0.00	0.00	0.00
								330.00	65.00						0.00	0.00	0.00	0.00
								210.00	15.00						0.00	0.00	0.00	0.00
	2.40							630.00	365.00	200.00	217.00	49.30	1.44	1.80	0.00	0.00		
	36.00							10.00	20.00				0.00		0.00	0.00	0.00	0.00
	18.00							250.00	150.00						0.00	0.00		
	192.00							0.00	40.00				0.72		0.00	0.00		
	246.00							0.00	60.00				1.08		0.00	0.00		
	696.00							15.00	40.00				1.08		0.00	0.00		
	3.40							0.00	0.00				1.70		0.00	0.00	0.00	0.00

Food Name	Amount	Measure	Weight (g)	Calories	Protein (g)	Total Carb (g)	Dietary Fiber (g)	Total Fat (g)	Sat Fat (g)	Mono Fat (g)	Poly Fat (g)	Chol (mg)	Vit A (mcg RAE)	Vit D (mcg)
FAST FOODS/RESTAURANTS *(continued)*														
Smoothie, Aloha Pineapple, 16 fl oz	16	Fluid ounce	545.00	320.00	6.00	75.00	3.00	1.00	0.00			5.00		0.00
Smoothie, Banana Berry, 16 fl oz	16	Fluid ounce	475.00	270.00	2.00	66.00	3.00	1.50	0.00			0.00		0.00
Smoothie, Berry Lime Sublime, 16 fl oz	16	Fluid ounce	470.00	270.00	2.00	63.00	5.00	1.00	0.00			0.00		0.00
Smoothie, Berry Pizzazz, w/prot, 24 fl oz	24	Fluid ounce	710.00	440.00	20.00	92.00	6.00	1.50	0.00			0.00		9.00
Smoothie, Caribbean Passion, 16 fl oz	16	Fluid ounce	480.00	270.00	2.00	62.00	3.00	1.00	0.00			0.00		0.00
Smoothie, Chocolate Moo'd, 16 fl oz	16	Fluid ounce	451.00	540.00	12.00	112.00	2.00	6.00	3.50			20.00		3.00
Smoothie, Citrus Squeeze, 16 fl oz	16	Fluid ounce	479.00	280.00	3.00	66.00	3.00	1.50	0.00			0.00		0.00
Smoothie, Coldbuster, 16 fl oz	16	Fluid ounce	476.00	280.00	3.00	65.00	3.00	1.50	0.00			5.00		0.00
Smoothie, Cranberry Craze, 16 fl oz	16	Fluid ounce	543.00	290.00	5.00	66.00	3.00	1.00	0.50			5.00		0.00
Smoothie, Kiwi Berry Burner, 16 fl oz	16	Fluid ounce	484.00	280.00	1.00	69.00	3.00	0.00	0.00	0.00	0.00	0.00		0.00
Smoothie, Mango-A-Go-Go, 16 fl oz	16	Fluid ounce	487.00	300.00	2.00	71.00	2.00	1.00	0.50			0.00		0.00
Smoothie, Orange Berry Blitz, 16 fl oz	16	Fluid ounce	479.00	240.00	3.00	55.00	3.00	1.50	0.50			0.00		0.00
Smoothie, Orange Dream Machine, 16 fl oz	16	Fluid ounce	504.00	410.00	15.00	84.00	1.00	2.00	1.00			5.00		2.50
Smoothie, Orange-A-Peel, 16 fl oz	16	Fluid ounce	477.00	270.00	5.00	64.00	3.00	1.00	0.00			0.00		0.80
Smoothie, Peach Pleasure, 16 fl oz	16	Fluid ounce	474.00	290.00	2.00	68.00	3.00	1.00	0.00			0.00		0.00
Smoothie, Peanut Butter Moo'd, 24 fl oz	24	Fluid ounce	638.00	860.00	23.00	145.00	5.00	21.00	5.00			15.00		6.00
Smoothie, Peenya Kowlada, 16 fl oz	16	Fluid ounce	480.00	380.00	5.00	82.00	3.00	4.00	3.50			5.00		0.80
Smoothie, PowerBoost, 16 fl oz	16	Fluid ounce	519.00	280.00	4.00	67.00	6.00	1.00	0.00			0.00		6.00
Smoothie, Razzmatazz, 16 fl oz	16	Fluid ounce	490.00	300.00	2.00	72.00	3.00	1.00	0.00			0.00		0.00
Smoothie, Strawberries Wild, 16 fl oz	16	Fluid ounce	487.00	280.00	3.00	67.00	3.00	0.00	0.00	0.00	0.00	0.00		0.80
Kentucky Fried Chicken														
Baked Beans, svg Yum! Brands	0.5	Cup	166.67	281.87	9.80	56.37	8.58	1.23	1.23			0.00		0.00
Beans, green, svg	4	Ounce-weight	113.40	50.18	5.02	5.02	2.01	1.51	0.50			5.02		
Biscuit USDA SR-23	1	Each	52.00	185.12	3.77	22.11	0.78	9.07	2.18	6.08	0.60	0.52		0.03
Chicken, breast, extra crispy	1	Each	162.00	460.00	34.00	19.00	0.00	28.00	8.00			135.00	0.00	
Chicken, breast, hot & spicy	1	Each	179.00	460.00	33.00	20.00	0.00	27.00	8.00			130.00		
Chicken, breast, original rec	1	Each	161.00	380.00	40.00	11.00	0.00	19.00	6.00			145.00	0.00	
Chicken, drumstick, extra crispy	1	Each	60.00	160.00	12.00	5.00	0.00	10.00	2.50			70.00	0.00	
Chicken, drumstick, original rec	1	Each	59.00	140.00	14.00	4.00	0.00	8.00	2.00			75.00	0.00	
Chicken, thigh, extra crispy	1	Each	114.00	370.00	21.00	12.00	0.00	26.00	7.00			120.00	0.00	
Chicken, thigh, original rec	1	Each	126.00	360.00	22.00	12.00	0.00	25.00	7.00			165.00	0.00	
Chicken, wing, extra crispy	1	Each	52.00	190.00	10.00	10.00	0.00	12.00	4.00			55.00	0.00	
Chicken, wing, original rec	1	Each	47.00	150.00	11.00	5.00	0.00	9.00	2.50			60.00	0.00	
Cole Slaw, svg USDA SR-23	0.5	Cup	95.50	137.52	0.87	14.95	1.91	8.25	1.24	1.87	4.67	1.91	0.95	0.01
Corn, cob, sml Yum! Brands	1	Each	82.00	75.93	2.53	13.16	3.54	1.52	0.51			0.00	0.00	
Sandwich, chicken, honey bbq flvr, w/sauce Yum! Brands	1	Each	147.00	300.00	21.00	41.00	4.00	6.00	1.50			50.00		0.37
Sandwich, chicken, original recipe, w/o sauce Yum! Brands	1	Each	187.00	320.00	29.00	21.00	0.00	13.00	4.00			60.00		
Sandwich, chicken, tender rstd, w/o sauce Yum! Brands	1	Each	177.00	260.00	31.00	23.00	1.00	5.00	1.50			65.00	0.00	
Long John Silvers														
Cheese, cheesesticks, brd, fried	3	Each	45.00	140.00	4.00	12.00	1.00	8.00	2.00			10.00		
Chicken, strips, plank, battered	1	Piece	52.50	140.00	8.00	9.00	0.00	8.00	2.50			20.00	0.00	
Fish, batter dipped, reg	1	Piece	92.00	230.00	11.00	16.00	0.00	13.00	4.00			30.00	0.00	
McDonalds														
Cheeseburger, Big Mac	1	Each	219.00	571.59	26.15	47.15	3.07	30.88	10.95	11.30	8.50	78.84		
Cheeseburger, Quarter Pounder USDA SR-23	1	Each	199.00	513.42	29.03	39.70	2.79	28.30	11.23	9.17	0.86	93.53		
Chicken, nuggets, McNuggets, 4 pce svg	4	Piece	72.00	190.00	10.00	13.00	1.00	11.00	2.50			35.00	0.00	
Cookie, chocolate chip, pkg	1	Each	56.00	280.00	3.00	37.00	1.00	14.00	8.00			40.00		
Cookie, McDonaldland, pkg	1	Each	57.00	230.00	3.00	38.00	1.00	8.00	2.00			0.00	0.00	
Danish, apple	1	Each	105.00	340.00	5.00	47.00	2.00	15.00	3.00			20.00		
French Fries, large USDA SR-23	1	Serving	154.00	486.64	5.87	60.09	6.47	24.82	3.21	12.02	7.18	0.00	0.00	
French Fries, medium USDA SR-23	1	Serving	117.00	369.72	4.46	45.65	4.91	18.86	2.44	9.13	5.46	0.00	0.00	
French Fries, sml USDA SR-23	1	Serving	71.00	224.36	2.71	27.70	2.98	11.45	1.48	5.54	3.31	0.00	0.00	
Frozen Dessert, McFlurry, Nestle Crunch, svg	1	Each	348.00	630.00	16.00	89.00	1.00	24.00	16.00			75.00		
Hamburger	1	Each	105.00	269.85	13.03	32.34	1.68	9.76	3.64	4.06	1.27	27.30		
Milk Shake, strawberry, sml	1	Each	294.00	360.00	11.00	60.00	0.00	9.00	6.00			40.00		
Milk Shake, vanilla, sml	1	Each	293.40	360.00	11.00	59.00	0.00	9.00	6.00			40.00		
Nuggets, chicken, McNuggets, 20 pce svg USDA SR-23	20	Piece	320.00	931.20	47.90	55.10	2.56	57.82	10.03	26.17	18.87	140.80	0.00	

Vit E (mg)	Vit C	Vit B₁ Thia (mg)	Vit B₂ Ribo (mg)	Vit B₃ Nia (mg)	Fol (mcg)	Vit B₆ (mg)	Vita B₁₂ (mcg)	Sodi (mg)	Pota (mg)	Cal (mg)	Phos (mg)	Magn (mg)	Iron (mg)	Zinc (mg)	Caff (mg)	Alco (g)	Sol Fiber (g)	Insol Fiber (g)
0.00	54.00	0.15	0.14	1.20	40.00	0.40	0.12	80.00	810.00	200.00	60.00	40.00	1.44	0.30	0.00	0.00		
0.40	9.00	0.06	0.10	0.80	16.00	0.60	0.12	35.00	540.00	80.00	40.00	24.00	0.72	0.30	0.00	0.00		
0.40	42.00	0.06	0.17	4.00	100.00	0.50	0.12	45.00	420.00	80.00	60.00	24.00	1.08	0.60	0.00	0.00		
0.40	60.00	0.09	0.14	1.60	60.00	0.40	0.00	240.00	650.00	1,100.00	700.00	40.00	2.70	0.60	0.00	0.00		
0.40	42.00	0.06	0.14	3.00	60.00	0.30	0.12	40.00	530.00	80.00	60.00	24.00	1.08	0.30	0.00	0.00		
0.00	3.60	0.15	0.51	0.40	16.00	0.12	1.20	270.00	570.00	400.00	300.00	40.00	0.72	1.20	0.00	0.00		
0.40	108.00	0.23	0.17	1.20	80.00	0.30	0.12	35.00	790.00	80.00	80.00	40.00	1.08	0.30	0.00	0.00		
10.07	684.00	0.23	0.14	2.00	100.00	0.30	0.00	15.00	800.00	60.00	60.00	40.00	0.72	7.50	0.00	0.00		
0.81	30.00	0.30	0.14	4.00	80.00	0.40	0.12	80.00	390.00	200.00	60.00	16.00	1.08	0.30	0.00	0.00		
0.40	84.00	0.03	0.07	0.80	8.00	0.08	0.00	35.00	460.00	60.00	40.00	16.00	1.44	0.30	0.00	0.00		
1.21	48.00	0.12	0.17	3.00	80.00	0.50	0.12	40.00	520.00	80.00	60.00	24.00	0.72	0.30	0.00	0.00		
0.81	150.00	0.30	0.17	1.60	80.00	0.16	0.12	25.00	650.00	80.00	80.00	40.00	1.08	0.30	0.00	0.00		
0.00	78.00	0.23	0.26	0.80	60.00	0.12	0.48	230.00	540.00	400.00	300.00	32.00	0.72	0.60	0.00	0.00		
0.40	156.00	0.30	0.26	1.60	100.00	0.30	0.24	85.00	900.00	100.00	150.00	60.00	1.08	0.60	0.00	0.00		
0.40	12.00	0.03	0.14	3.00	60.00	0.50	0.12	40.00	500.00	60.00	60.00	24.00	0.36	0.30	0.00	0.00		
1.61	12.00	0.23	0.68	4.00	40.00	0.30	1.50	550.00	1,000.00	800.00	600.00	80.00	1.44	1.50	0.00	0.00		
0.00	30.00	0.15	0.26	0.80	40.00	0.30	0.36	115.00	770.00	150.00	150.00	40.00	1.08	0.60	0.00	0.00		
12.08	198.00	2.70	2.89	34.00	360.00	3.60	4.80	30.00	810.00	600.00	80.00	240.00	1.44	7.50	0.00	0.00		
0.00	36.00	0.06	0.17	4.00	100.00	0.70	0.12	45.00	570.00	80.00	60.00	24.00	1.08	0.30	0.00	0.00		
0.00	36.00	0.06	0.17	0.80	24.00	0.20	0.24	95.00	700.00	150.00	80.00	32.00	1.08	0.60	0.00	0.00		
1.45	4.41	0.14	0.08	0.59	71.39	0.18	0.00	882.37	637.23	183.83	125.23	62.80	6.62	1.38	0.00	0.00		
	1.20							461.63		0.00			0.72		0.00	0.00		
0.71	0.16	0.24	0.11	1.66	50.18	0.02	0.08	547.56	59.80	31.20	304.72	7.80	1.47	0.26	0.00	0.00		
	0.00							1230.00		0.00			1.44		0.00	0.00	0.00	0.00
	0.00							1450.00		0.00			1.14		0.00	0.00	0.00	0.00
	0.00							1150.00		0.00			1.80		0.00	0.00	0.00	0.00
	0.00							420.00		0.00			0.72		0.00	0.00	0.00	0.00
	0.00							440.00		0.00			0.72		0.00	0.00	0.00	0.00
	0.00							710.00		0.00			1.14		0.00	0.00	0.00	0.00
	0.00							1060.00		0.00			1.14		0.00	0.00	0.00	0.00
	0.00							390.00		0.00			0.38		0.00	0.00	0.00	0.00
	0.00							370.00		0.00			0.38		0.00	0.00	0.00	0.00
0.52	13.94	0.04	0.01	0.20	19.93	0.12	0.03	180.49	133.70	26.74	19.10	8.59	0.20	0.14	0.00	0.00		
	3.04							5.06		30.37			0.55		0.00	0.00		
0.36	2.40	0.48	0.37	7.55	106.92	0.32	0.31	640.00	248.77	60.00	179.98	27.79	2.70	1.60	0.00	0.00		
	0.00							890.00		40.00			1.80		0.00	0.00	0.00	0.00
	0.00							690.00		40.00			1.80		0.00	0.00		
	0.00							320.00		100.00			0.72		0.00	0.00		
	2.40							400.00		0.00			0.36		0.00	0.00	0.00	0.00
	4.80							700.00		20.00			1.80		0.00	0.00	0.00	0.00
0.13	0.66	0.40	0.44	7.95	59.13	0.37	2.78	1062.15	398.58	278.13	297.84	54.75	3.07	4.73	0.00	0.00		
	1.59	0.33	0.70	7.66	101.49		2.51	1,152.21	435.81	286.56	320.39	43.78	4.18	5.23	0.00	0.00		
0.94	0.00			4.94			0.20	360.00	201.60	9.10	191.10	16.38	0.71	0.66	0.00	0.00		
0.92	0.00	0.14	0.16	1.48				170.00	142.20	20.00	83.44	23.80	1.44	0.40	3.00	0.00		
1.00	0.00			2.04				250.00	62.70	20.00	71.25	11.34	1.80	0.39	0.00	0.00		
	15.00	0.30	0.17	2.00				340.00	113.40	60.00	0.00		1.44		0.00	0.00		
	11.24	0.51	0.06	4.25	92.40	0.80		349.58	862.40	26.18	203.28	49.28	1.32	0.68	0.00	0.00		
	8.54	0.38	0.04	3.23	70.20	0.61		265.59	655.20	19.89	154.44	37.44	1.01	0.51	0.00	0.00		
	5.18	0.23	0.03	1.96	42.60	0.37		161.17	397.60	12.07	93.72	22.72	0.61	0.31	0.00	0.00		
	2.40							230.00		500.00			0.36			0.00		
0.10	0.31	0.31	0.07	4.56	29.40	0.10	1.18	501.90	203.70	130.20	112.35	25.20	1.78	2.03	0.00	0.00		
	6.00							180.00	542.00	350.00	328.60		0.72		0.00	0.00	0.00	0.00
	1.20							250.00	533.70	350.00	326.70		0.36		0.00	0.00	0.00	0.00
	3.84	0.51	0.35	23.68	89.60	1.27	1.06	2,022.40	803.20	44.80	1,062.40	70.40	2.91	1.89	0.00	0.00		

Food Name	Amount	Measure	Weight (g)	Calories	Protein (g)	Total Carb (g)	Dietary Fiber (g)	Total Fat (g)	Sat Fat (g)	Mono Fat (g)	Poly Fat (g)	Chol (mg)	Vit A (mcg RAE)	Vit D (mcg)
FAST FOODS/RESTAURANTS *(continued)*														
Parfait, fruit & yogurt w/granola USDA SR-23	1	Each	149.00	156.45	4.07	30.87	1.49	1.94	0.06	0.16	0.14	7.45		
Parfait, fruit n' yogurt, w/o granola USDA SR-23	1	Each	142.00	127.80	3.51	25.09	1.28	1.60	0.01	0.01	0.05	7.10		
Pie, snack, apple USDA SR-23	1	Each	77.00	248.71	2.36	33.59	1.54	12.06	3.08	7.07	0.80			
Potatoes, french fries, lrg svg	1	Each	171.00	617.31	6.67	73.29	6.50	32.95	7.40	17.34	6.65		0.00	
Salad Dressing, Newman's Own, ranch, pkg USDA SR-23	2	Fluid ounce	56.00	175.28	1.47	9.38	0.17	14.88	2.44	8.60	3.56	17.92		
Salad, bacon ranch, w/crispy chicken USDA SR-23	1	Each	342.00	376.20	30.16	20.79	3.42	21.55	5.55	8.44	5.54	75.24		
Salad, bacon ranch, w/grilled chicken USDA SR-23	1	Each	321.00	260.01	33.00	11.68	3.21	10.08	3.96	3.25	1.38	89.88		
Sandwich, breakfast, bacon egg cheese, w/biscuit USDA SR-23	1	Each	142.00	431.68	19.10	31.61	1.28	26.65	11.73	7.88	3.73	237.14		
Sandwich, breakfast, McMuffin, egg cheese USDA SR-23	1	Each	139.00	298.85	17.58	28.55	1.53	12.66	4.48	3.78	2.52	229.35		
Sandwich, Filet O Fish USDA SR-23	1	Each	142.00	390.50	15.61	38.98	1.42	19.13	3.69	5.47	8.00	39.76		
Sandwich, ham egg cheese, w/bagel	1	Each	218.00	550.00	26.00	58.00	2.00	23.00	8.00			255.00		
Panda Express														
Dish, beef, w/broccoli	1	Serving	153.09	150.00	11.00	12.00	3.00	6.00	1.50			25.00		
Dish, chicken, orange, spicy	1	Serving	153.09	400.00	15.00	42.00	0.00	20.00	3.50			90.00		
Dish, chicken, sweet & sour	1	Serving	155.93	400.00	15.00	46.00	1.00	17.00	3.00			40.00		
Dish, chicken, w/broccoli	1	Serving	155.93	180.00	13.00	11.00	3.00	9.00	2.00			65.00		
Dish, eggplant & tofu, spicy	1	Serving	172.94	310.00	7.00	19.00	3.00	24.00	3.00			0.00		
Dish, fried rice	1	Serving	283.50	570.00	16.00	85.00	8.00	18.00	4.00			130.00		
Egg Roll, chicken	1	Each	85.05	200.00	8.00	16.00	2.00	12.00	4.00			20.00		
Potsticker, chicken	3	Each	93.56	220.00	7.00	23.00	1.00	11.00	2.50			20.00		
Soup, egg flower	1	Serving	289.49	90.00	3.00	15.00	1.00	2.00	0.00			60.00		
Soup, hot & sour, spicy	1	Serving	313.12	90.00	4.00	12.00	1.00	3.50	0.50			65.00		
Spring Roll, fried, veggie	2	Each	96.39	160.00	4.00	22.00	4.00	7.00	1.00			0.00		
Pizza Hut														
Pizza, cheese, 6"	1	Piece	63.00	160.00	7.00	18.00	1.00	7.00	3.00			15.00		
Pizza, cheese, med, 12"	1	Piece	79.00	200.00	10.00	21.00	1.00	8.00	4.50			25.00		
Pizza, Pepperoni Lover's, med, 12"	1	Piece	92.00	260.00	13.00	21.00	2.00	14.00	7.00			40.00		
Pizza, Pepperoni Lover's, pan, med, 12"	1	Piece	118.00	340.00	15.00	29.00	2.00	19.00	7.00			40.00		
Pizza, pepperoni, 6"	1	Piece	61.00	170.00	7.00	18.00	1.00	8.00	3.00			15.00		
Pizza, supreme, 6"	1	Piece	77.00	190.00	8.00	19.00	1.00	9.00	3.50			20.00		
Pizza, supreme, med, 12"	1	Piece	106.00	240.00	11.00	22.00	2.00	11.00	5.00			25.00		
Pizza, supreme, pan, med, 12"	1	Piece	127.00	320.00	13.00	30.00	2.00	16.00	6.00			25.00		
Pizza, supreme, super, med, 12"	1	Piece	119.00	260.00	13.00	23.00	2.00	13.00	6.00			35.00		
Pizza, supreme, super, pan, med, 12"	1	Piece	139.00	340.00	14.00	30.00	2.00	18.00	6.00			35.00		
Starbucks														
Blended Coffee, Frappuccino, caffe vanilla, light, tall	1	Each	333.00	140.00	4.00	30.00	2.00	0.50	0.00			0.00	0.00	
Blended Coffee, Frappuccino, caramel, light, tall	1	Each	328.00	130.00	4.00	25.00	2.00	1.00	0.00			6.00	0.00	
Blended Coffee, Frappuccino, caramel, w/soy milk, tall	1	Each	339.00	190.00	2.00	42.00	0.00	1.50	0.00			0.00		
Blended Coffee, Frappuccino, java chip, w/soy milk, tall	1	Each	330.00	230.00	3.00	47.00	1.00	4.00	2.00			0.00		
Blended Coffee, Frappuccino, light, tall	1	Each	340.00	90.00	4.00	18.00	2.00	0.50	0.00			0.00	0.00	
Blended Coffee, Frappuccino, mocha, light, tall	1	Each	333.00	100.00	3.00	23.00	1.00	0.50	0.00			0.00		
Blended Coffee, Frappuccino, mocha, w/soy milk, tall	1	Each	346.00	190.00	3.00	40.00	0.00	1.50	0.00			0.00		
Blended Coffee, Frappuccino, w/nonfat milk, tall	1	Each	331.00	160.00	3.00	36.00	0.00	0.00	0.00	0.00	0.00	0.00		
Blended Coffee, Frappuccino, w/soy milk, tall	1	Each	331.00	170.00	2.00	37.00	0.00	1.50	0.00			0.00		
Coffee, Americano, Caffe, tall	1	Each	315.00	10.00	1.00	2.00	0.00	0.00	0.00	0.00	0.00	0.00	0.00	
Coffee, brewed, tall	1	Each	355.20	5.00	0.00	0.00	0.00	0.00	0.00	0.00	0.00	0.00	0.00	
Coffee, Caffe Misto, w/2% milk, steamed, tall	1	Each	349.00	80.00	5.00	7.00	0.00	3.00	2.00			15.00		
Coffee, Caffe Misto, w/soy milk, steamed, tall	1	Each	351.00	70.00	4.00	10.00	1.00	2.00	0.00			0.00		

Vit E (mg)	Vit C	Vit B₁ Thia (mg)	Vit B₂ Ribo (mg)	Vit B₃ Nia (mg)	Fol (mcg)	Vit B₆ (mg)	Vita B₁₂ (mcg)	Sodi (mg)	Pota (mg)	Cal (mg)	Phos (mg)	Magn (mg)	Iron (mg)	Zinc (mg)	Caff (mg)	Alco (g)	Sol Fiber (g)	Insol Fiber (g)
	20.71	0.07	0.17	0.35	19.37		0.28	86.42	248.83	128.14	125.16	20.86	0.67	0.54	0.00	0.00		
	20.59	0.05	0.17	0.27	15.62		0.28	53.96	234.30	123.54	100.82	17.04	0.51	0.43	0.00	0.00		
1.49	24.87	0.23	0.16	2.03	87.01	0.04		153.23	48.51	14.63	27.72	5.39	1.53	0.18	0.00	0.00		
1.33	3.59	0.30	0.18	4.56	13.68	0.98		292.41	1031.13	29.07	227.43	63.27	1.50	0.94	0.00	0.00		
	0.45	0.01	0.08	0.01	0.56	0.02	0.00	534.24	67.20	43.12	42.56	1.68	0.14	0.03	0.00	0.00		
	33.17	0.21	0.24	10.35				1,008.90		157.32			2.09		0.00	0.00		
	32.74	0.18	0.27	11.89				1,004.73		154.08			2.09		0.00	0.00		
	2.98	0.37	0.59	2.78		0.13		1,225.46	171.82	154.78	475.70	17.04	3.02	1.28	0.00	0.00		
0.82	1.67	0.36	0.51	4.31	109.81	0.20	0.92	860.41	218.23	275.22	269.66	26.41	2.99	1.60	0.00	0.00		
	0.14	0.36	0.26	3.41	69.58		1.05	688.70	248.50	163.30	167.56	28.40	2.10	0.71	0.00	0.00		
	0.00							1490.00		200.00			4.50		0.00	0.00		
								720.00							0.00	0.00		
								640.00							0.00	0.00	0.00	0.00
								370.00							0.00	0.00		
								630.00							0.00	0.00		
								680.00							0.00	0.00		
								900.00							0.00	0.00		
								390.00							0.00	0.00		
								280.00							0.00	0.00		
								810.00							0.00	0.00		
								970.00							0.00	0.00		
								540.00							0.00	0.00		
	0.00							310.00		100.00			1.44		0.00	0.00		
	1.20							490.00		200.00			1.08		0.00	0.00		
	2.40							690.00		200.00			1.44		0.00	0.00		
	2.40							700.00		200.00			2.70		0.00	0.00		
	1.20							340.00		80.00			1.44		0.00	0.00		
	3.60							420.00		80.00			1.80		0.00	0.00		
	9.00							640.00		150.00			1.80		0.00	0.00		
	6.00							650.00		150.00			2.70		0.00	0.00		
	12.00							760.00		150.00			1.80		0.00	0.00		
	9.00							760.00		150.00			2.70		0.00	0.00		
	0.00							180.00		100.00			0.00		75.00	0.00		
	0.00							180.00		100.00			0.00		70.00	0.00		
	0.00							150.00		100.00			0.36		65.00	0.00	0.00	0.00
	0.00							170.00		100.00			2.70		70.00	0.00		
	0.00							160.00		100.00			0.00		70.00	0.00		
	0.00							135.00		80.00			0.72		60.00	0.00		
	0.00							150.00		80.00			0.72		70.00	0.00	0.00	0.00
	0.00							160.00		100.00			0.00		70.00	0.00	0.00	0.00
	0.00							150.00		100.00			0.36		70.00	0.00	0.00	0.00
	0.00							5.00		0.00			0.00		150.00	0.00	0.00	0.00
	0.00							10.00		0.00			0.00		260.00	0.00	0.00	0.00
	0.00							70.00		200.00			0.00		115.00	0.00	0.00	0.00
	0.00							60.00		200.00			0.72		115.00	0.00		

Food Name	Amount	Measure	Weight (g)	Calories	Protein (g)	Total Carb (g)	Dietary Fiber (g)	Total Fat (g)	Sat Fat (g)	Mono Fat (g)	Poly Fat (g)	Chol (mg)	Vit A (mcg RAE)	Vit D (mcg)
FAST FOODS/RESTAURANTS *(continued)*														
Coffee, cappuccino, w/2% milk, tall	1	Each	169.00	90.00	6.00	9.00	0.00	3.50	2.00			15.00		
Coffee, cappuccino, w/nonfat milk, tall	1	Each	170.00	60.00	6.00	9.00	0.00	0.00	0.00	0.00	0.00	6.00		
Coffee, espresso macchiato, w/2% milk, solo	1	Each	9.30	10.00	1.00	0.00	0.00	0.00	0.00	0.00	0.00	0.00	0.00	
Coffee, iced, Americano, tall	1	Each	211.00	10.00	1.00	2.00	0.00	0.00	0.00	0.00	0.00	0.00	0.00	
Coffee, iced, latte, Caffe, w/2% milk, tall	1	Each	289.00	100.00	6.00	10.00	0.00	3.50	2.50			15.00		
Coffee, iced, latte, Caffe, w/nonfat milk, tall	1	Each	289.00	70.00	6.00	10.00	0.00	0.00	0.00	0.00	0.00	6.00		
Coffee, iced, latte, caffe, w/soy milk, tall	1	Each	292.00	90.00	5.00	13.00	1.00	2.50	0.00			0.00		
Coffee, iced, latte, Caffe, w/whole milk, tall	1	Each	289.00	110.00	6.00	9.00	0.00	6.00	3.50			20.00		
Coffee, iced, latte, flvrd, skinny, w/2% milk, tall	1	Each	289.00	90.00	6.00	9.00	0.00	3.00	2.00			15.00		
Coffee, iced, latte, flvrd, w/2% milk, tall	1	Each	391.00	190.00	9.00	27.00	0.00	5.00	3.50			20.00		
Coffee, iced, latte, flvrd, w/soy milk, tall	1	Each	391.00	180.00	6.00	31.00	1.00	3.50	0.50			0.00		
Coffee, iced, latte, flvrd, w/whole milk, venti	1	Each	718.00	320.00	10.00	50.00	0.00	9.00	5.00			25.00		
Coffee, iced, w/2% milk, tall	1	Each	316.00	90.00	2.00	18.00	0.00	1.00	0.50			6.00		
Coffee, iced, w/nonfat milk, tall	1	Each	316.00	80.00	2.00	18.00	0.00	0.00	0.00	0.00	0.00	0.00		
Coffee, iced, w/soy milk, tall	1	Each	316.00	90.00	1.00	19.00	0.00	1.00	0.00			0.00		
Coffee, iced, w/whole milk, tall	1	Each	316.00	100.00	2.00	18.00	0.00	1.50	1.00			6.00		
Coffee, latte, Caffe, w/ soy milk, tall	1	Each	357.00	130.00	7.00	18.00	1.00	4.00	0.50			0.00		
Coffee, latte, Caffe, w/2% milk, tall	1	Each	352.00	150.00	10.00	14.00	0.00	6.00	3.50			25.00		
Coffee, latte, Caffe, w/nonfat milk, tall	1	Each	353.00	100.00	10.00	15.00	0.00	0.00	0.00	0.00	0.00	6.00		
Coffee, latte, Caffe, w/whole milk, tall	1	Each	352.00	180.00	10.00	14.00	0.00	9.00	5.00			30.00		
Coffee, latte, flvrd, skinny, w/2% milk, tall	1	Each	353.00	140.00	9.00	14.00	0.00	5.00	3.50			20.00		
Coffee, latte, flvrd, skinny, w/nonfat milk, tall	1	Each	353.00	90.00	9.00	14.00	0.00	0.00	0.00	0.00	0.00	6.00		
Coffee, latte, flvrd, w/2% milk, tall	1	Each	352.00	190.00	9.00	27.00	0.00	5.00	3.50			20.00		
Coffee, latte, flvrd, w/nonfat milk, tall	1	Each	353.00	150.00	9.00	28.00	0.00	0.00	0.00	0.00	0.00	6.00		
Coffee, latte, flvrd, w/soy milk, tall	1	Each	357.00	180.00	6.00	31.00	1.00	3.50	0.50			0.00		
Coffee, latte, flvrd, w/whole milk, tall	1	Each	352.00	220.00	9.00	27.00	0.00	9.00	5.00			25.00		
Hot Cocoa, w/2% milk & whip, tall	1	Each	371.00	290.00	11.00	39.00	1.00	13.00	7.00			45.00		
Hot Cocoa, w/nonfat milk, tall	1	Each	342.00	190.00	11.00	37.00	1.00	2.00	0.00			6.00		
Hot Cocoa, w/soy milk, tall	1	Each	346.00	220.00	8.00	40.00	2.00	5.00	1.00			0.00		
Hot Cocoa, w/whole milk, tall	1	Each	341.00	260.00	10.00	36.00	1.00	10.00	5.00			25.00		
Juice, apple, tall	1	Each	372.00	180.00	0.00	45.00	0.00	0.00	0.00	0.00	0.00	0.00	0.00	
Parfait, yogurt, dark cherry, w/granola	1	Each	230.00	310.00	10.00	61.00	3.00	4.00	0.50			6.00	0.00	
Parfait, yogurt, Greek, w/ honey & granola	1	Each	172.00	290.00	8.00	43.00	1.00	12.00	6.00			30.00		
Sandwich, breakfast, sausage egg & cheese, w/English muffin	1	Each	179.00	500.00	20.00	42.00	2.00	29.00	9.00			190.00		
Sandwich, breakfast, turkey bacon & egg white, w/muffin	1	Each	149.00	340.00	22.00	47.00	3.00	10.00	3.00			20.00		
Sandwich, tarragon chicken salad, w/whole wheat	1	Each	224.00	480.00	35.00	62.00	3.00	11.00	2.00			75.00		
Scone, vanilla bean, petite	1	Each	33.00	140.00	0.00	21.00	0.00	5.00	2.50			15.00		
Tea, latte, chai, w/2% milk, tall	1	Each	372.00	180.00	6.00	33.00	0.00	3.00	2.00			15.00		
Tea, latte, chai, w/nonfat milk, tall	1	Each	373.00	150.00	6.00	33.00	0.00	0.00	0.00	0.00	0.00	6.00		
Tea, latte, chai, w/soy milk, tall	1	Each	377.00	170.00	4.00	35.00	1.00	2.00	0.00			0.00		
Tea, latte, chai, w/whole milk, tall	1	Each	372.00	200.00	6.00	33.00	0.00	5.00	3.00			15.00		
Wrap, breakfast, egg white spinach & feta, w/wheat tortilla	1	Each	158.00	280.00	18.00	33.00	6.00	10.00	3.50			20.00		
Wrap, breakfast, huevos rancheros, w/wheat tortilla	1	Each	158.00	330.00	16.00	35.00	8.00	15.00	5.00			165.00		
Wrap, chicken & vegetable, w/wheat tortilla	1	Each	164.00	290.00	19.00	36.00	4.00	9.00	0.50			30.00		
Subway														
Sandwich, club, w/white, 6"	1	Each	255.00	320.00	24.00	46.00	4.00	6.00	2.00			35.00		
Sandwich, ham, w/white, 6"	1	Each	232.00	290.00	18.00	46.00	4.00	5.00	1.50			25.00		
Sandwich, turkey bacon, Southwest, w/white, 6"	1	Each	240.00	410.00	21.00	48.00	4.00	17.00	4.50			35.00		
Sandwich, turkey, deli style	1	Each	151.00	220.00	13.00	36.00	3.00	3.50	1.50			15.00		
Taco Bell														
Burrito, bean	1	Each	198.00	370.00	14.00	55.00	8.00	10.00	3.50			10.00		
Burrito, beef, grilled, Stuft	1	Each	325.00	730.00	28.00	79.00	10.00	33.00	11.00			55.00		
Burrito, beef, supreme	1	Each	248.00	440.00	18.00	51.00	7.00	18.00	8.00			40.00		
Burrito, chicken, fiesta	1	Each	184.00	370.00	18.00	48.00	3.00	12.00	3.50			30.00		

Vit E (mg)	Vit C	Vit B₁ Thia (mg)	Vit B₂ Ribo (mg)	Vit B₃ Nia (mg)	Fol (mcg)	Vit B₆ (mg)	Vita B₁₂ (mcg)	Sodi (mg)	Pota (mg)	Cal (mg)	Phos (mg)	Magn (mg)	Iron (mg)	Zinc (mg)	Caff (mg)	Alco (g)	Sol Fiber (g)	Insol Fiber (g)
	0.00							70.00	200.00				0.00		75.00	0.00	0.00	0.00
	0.00							70.00	200.00				0.00		75.00	0.00	0.00	0.00
	0.00							0.00	0.00				0.00		75.00	0.00	0.00	0.00
	0.00							5.00	0.00				0.00		150.00	0.00	0.00	0.00
	0.00							80.00	200.00				0.00		75.00	0.00	0.00	0.00
	0.00							80.00	250.00				0.00		75.00	0.00	0.00	0.00
	0.00							70.00	200.00				0.72		75.00	0.00		
	0.00							75.00	200.00				0.00		75.00	0.00	0.00	0.00
	0.00							85.00	200.00				0.00		75.00	0.00	0.00	0.00
	0.00							110.00	300.00				0.00		75.00	0.00	0.00	0.00
	0.00							95.00	300.00				1.08		75.00	0.00		
	0.00							115.00	300.00				0.00		225.00	0.00	0.00	0.00
	0.00							25.00	60.00				0.00		90.00	0.00	0.00	0.00
	0.00							25.00	60.00				0.00		90.00	0.00	0.00	0.00
	0.00							20.00	60.00				0.36		90.00	0.00	0.00	0.00
	0.00							25.00	60.00				0.00		90.00	0.00	0.00	0.00
	0.00							100.00	300.00				1.08		75.00	0.00		
	0.00							115.00	350.00				0.00		75.00	0.00	0.00	0.00
	0.00							120.00	350.00				0.00		75.00	0.00	0.00	0.00
	0.00							115.00	300.00				0.00		75.00	0.00	0.00	0.00
	0.00							125.00	300.00				0.00		75.00	0.00	0.00	0.00
	0.00							125.00	300.00				0.00		75.00	0.00	0.00	0.00
	0.00							110.00	300.00				0.00		75.00	0.00	0.00	0.00
	0.00							115.00	350.00				0.00		75.00	0.00	0.00	0.00
	0.00							95.00	300.00				1.08		75.00	0.00		
	0.00							105.00	300.00				0.00		75.00	0.00	0.00	0.00
	0.00							115.00	350.00				2.70		20.00	0.00		
	0.00							110.00	350.00				2.70		20.00	0.00		
	0.00							95.00	300.00				3.60		20.00	0.00		
	0.00							105.00	300.00				2.70		20.00	0.00		
	0.00							17.50	0.00				0.00		0.00	0.00	0.00	0.00
	3.60							150.00	250.00				1.08		0.00	0.00		
	1.20							100.00	200.00				1.08		0.00	0.00		
	0.00							980.00	350.00				3.60		0.00	0.00		
	0.00							750.00	350.00				2.70		0.00	0.00		
	3.60							121.00	150.00				3.60		0.00	0.00		
	0.00							90.00	20.00				0.72		0.00	0.00	0.00	0.00
	0.00							75.00	200.00				0.36		75.00	0.00	0.00	0.00
	0.00							75.00	200.00				0.36		75.00	0.00	0.00	0.00
	0.00							65.00	200.00				0.72		75.00	0.00		
	0.00							70.00	200.00				0.36		75.00	0.00	0.00	0.00
	9.00							900.00	250.00				2.70		0.00	0.00		
	12.00							610.00	200.00				2.70		0.00	0.00		
	36.00							530.00	350.00				3.60		0.00	0.00		
	21.00							1,300.00	60.00				5.40		0.00	0.00		
	21.00							1,270.00	60.00				3.60		0.00	0.00		
	24.00							1,230.00	60.00				3.60		0.00	0.00		
	12.00							730.00	60.00				3.60		0.00	0.00		
	4.80							1200.00	200.00				2.70		0.00	0.00		
	6.00							2080.00	350.00				4.50		0.00	0.00		
	9.00							1330.00	200.00				2.70		0.00	0.00		
	3.60							1090.00	200.00				2.70		0.00	0.00		

Food Name	Amount	Measure	Weight (g)	Calories	Protein (g)	Total Carb (g)	Dietary Fiber (g)	Total Fat (g)	Sat Fat (g)	Mono Fat (g)	Poly Fat (g)	Chol (mg)	Vit A (mcg RAE)	Vit D (mcg)
FAST FOODS/RESTAURANTS *(continued)*														
Burrito, chicken, supreme	1	Each	248.00	410.00	21.00	50.00	5.00	14.00	6.00			45.00		
Burrito, seven layer	1	Each	283.00	530.00	18.00	67.00	10.00	22.00	8.00			25.00		
Chalupa, beef, supreme	1	Each	153.00	390.00	14.00	31.00	3.00	24.00	10.00			40.00		
Dessert, cinnamon twists, svg Yum! Brands	1	Serving	35.00	160.00	1.00	28.00	0.00	5.00	1.00			0.00	0.00	
Dish, chicken, Border Bowl, zesty Yum! Brands	1	Each	417.00	730.00	23.00	65.00	12.00	42.00	9.00			45.00		
Gordita, beef, Baja Yum! Brands	1	Each	153.00	350.00	14.00	31.00	4.00	19.00	5.00			30.00		
Gordita, chicken, Baja	1	Each	153.00	320.00	17.00	29.00	2.00	15.00	3.50			40.00		
Nachos, BellGrande, svg Yum! Brands	1	Serving	308.00	780.00	20.00	80.00	12.00	43.00	13.00			35.00		
Nachos, supreme, svg USDA SR-23	1	Serving	195.00	479.70	14.80	45.03	8.00	26.62	7.77	13.69	2.79	37.05	6.83	
Pizza, Mexican Yum! Brands	1	Each	216.00	550.00	21.00	46.00	7.00	31.00	11.00			45.00		
Quesadilla, cheese	1	Each	142.00	490.00	19.00	39.00	3.00	28.00	13.00			55.00		
Salad, taco, w/salsa, w/o shell	1	Each	462.00	420.00	24.00	33.00	11.00	21.00	11.00			65.00		
Taco	1	Each	78.00	170.00	8.00	13.00	3.00	10.00	4.00			25.00		
Taco, soft, beef USDA SR-23	1	Each	99.00	216.81	11.68	19.54	2.57	10.25	4.16	4.32	1.00	27.72	3.91	
Taco, soft, chicken USDA SR-23	1	Each	99.00	199.98	14.19	19.38	1.78	7.25	2.59	2.80	1.04	36.63	1.24	
Taco, soft, chicken, supreme Yum! Brands	1	Each	134.00	230.00	15.00	21.00	1.00	10.00	5.00			45.00		
Taco, soft, steak USDA SR-23	1	Each	127.00	285.75	15.00	21.87	2.03	15.37	4.28	5.00	4.43	39.37	1.46	
Taco Johns														
Burrito, bean	1	Each	170.10	340.00	14.80	45.20		11.10	3.00			15.00		
Burrito, beef	1	Each	170.10	415.00	22.40	39.40		18.90	6.41			43.10		
Taco Time														
Burrito, veggie	1	Each	321.40	491.00	21.00	70.00	10.00	16.00	6.00			24.00		
Wendy's														
Cheeseburger, deluxe, jr	1	Each	179.00	350.00	17.00	37.00	2.00	15.00	6.00			45.00		
Cheeseburger, jr	1	Each	129.00	310.00	17.00	34.00	2.00	12.00	6.00			45.00		
Cheeseburger, w/bacon, jr	1	Each	165.00	380.00	20.00	34.00	2.00	19.00	7.00			55.00		
Frozen Dessert, Frosty, dairy, jr	1	Each	113.00	170.00	4.00	28.00	0.00	4.00	2.50			20.00		
Hamburger, Big Bacon Classic	1	Each	282.00	570.00	34.00	46.00	3.00	29.00	12.00			100.00		
Hamburger, jr	1	Each	117.00	270.00	14.00	34.00	2.00	9.00	3.00			30.00		
Hamburger, single, w/everything	1	Each	218.00	410.00	24.00	37.00	2.00	19.00	7.00			70.00		
FATS, OILS, MARGARINES, SHORTENINGS, AND SUBSTITUTES														
Fat Substitutes														
Butter Substitute, Butterlike, dried Mrs. Bateman's	0.5	Teaspoon	5.00	20.60	0.02	4.10	0.00	0.50	0.30			1.27		0.00
Butter Substitute, plain, soy, vegetarian Veggie	1	Tablespoon	14.00	40.00	1.00	2.00		3.00	0.00			0.00		
Fats and Oils, Animal														
Butter, salted, pat, 1" square × 1/3" high	1	Each	5.00	35.85	0.04	0.00	0.00	4.06	2.57	1.05	0.15	10.75	34.20	0.07
Butter, salted, whipped, pat, 1" square × 1/3" high	1	Each	3.80	27.25	0.03	0.00	0.00	3.08	1.92	0.89	0.11	8.32	25.99	
Butter, unsalted, pat, 1" square × 1/3" high	1	Each	5.00	35.85	0.04	0.00	0.00	4.06	2.57	1.05	0.15	10.75	34.20	
Fat, lard	1	Tablespoon	12.80	115.46	0.00	0.00	0.00	12.80	5.02	5.77	1.43	12.16	0.00	
Oil, fish, herring	1	Tablespoon	13.60	122.67	0.00	0.00	0.00	13.60	2.90	7.69	2.12	104.18	0.00	20.40
Fats and Oils, Vegetable														
Cooking Spray, butter flavor ConAgra Foods Pam	0.25	Second Spray	0.27	0.00	0.00	0.00	0.00	0.00	0.00	0.00	0.00	0.00	0.00	
Oil, canola, pure Crisco	1	Tablespoon	14.00	120.00	0.00	0.00	0.00	14.00	1.00	8.00	4.00	0.00	0.00	
Oil, cocoa butter	1	Tablespoon	13.60	120.22	0.00	0.00	0.00	13.60	8.12	4.47	0.41	0.00	0.00	
Oil, coconut	1	Tablespoon	13.60	117.23	0.00	0.00	0.00	13.60	11.76	0.79	0.24	0.00	0.00	
Oil, cooking spray, 0.33 second spray, svg Crisco	1	Each	0.25	2.25	0.00	0.00	0.00	0.25	0.00			0.00	0.00	
Oil, corn & canola	1	Tablespoon	14.00	123.76	0.00	0.00	0.00	14.00	1.30	5.85	6.24	0.00	0.00	
Oil, grapeseed	1	Tablespoon	13.60	120.22	0.00	0.00	0.00	13.60	1.31	2.19	9.51	0.00	0.00	
Oil, oat	1	Tablespoon	13.60	120.22	0.00	0.00	0.00	13.60	2.67	4.77	5.56	0.00	0.00	0.00
Oil, olive, extra virgin Natural Oils International	1	Tablespoon	14.00	126.00	0.00	0.00	0.00	14.00	1.96	10.78	1.26	0.00		
Oil, palm kernel	1	Tablespoon	13.60	117.23	0.00	0.00	0.00	13.60	11.08	1.55	0.22	0.00	0.00	
Oil, peanut, salad or cooking	1	Tablespoon	13.50	119.34	0.00	0.00	0.00	13.50	2.28	6.24	4.32	0.00	0.00	

Vit E (mg)	Vit C	Vit B₁ Thia (mg)	Vit B₂ Ribo (mg)	Vit B₃ Nia (mg)	Fol (mcg)	Vit B₆ (mg)	Vita B₁₂ (mcg)	Sodi (mg)	Pota (mg)	Cal (mg)	Phos (mg)	Magn (mg)	Iron (mg)	Zinc (mg)	Caff (mg)	Alco (g)	Sol Fiber (g)	Insol Fiber (g)
	9.00							1270.00		200.00			2.70		0.00	0.00		
	4.80							1360.00		300.00			3.60		0.00	0.00		
	4.80							600.00		150.00			1.80		0.00	0.00		
	0.00							150.00		0.00			0.36		0.00	0.00	0.00	0.00
	9.00							1,640.00		150.00			3.60		0.00	0.00		
	4.80							750.00		150.00			2.70		0.00	0.00		
	3.60							690.00		100.00			1.80		0.00	0.00		
	6.00							1,300.00		200.00			2.70		0.00	0.00		
1.42		0.20	0.28	1.92	56.55	0.34	0.76	838.50	471.90	142.35	384.15	89.70	4.17	2.65	0.00	0.00		
	6.00							1,030.00		350.00			3.60		0.00	0.00		
	0.00							1150.00		500.00			1.44		0.00	0.00		
	21.00							1400.00		250.00			3.60		0.00	0.00		
	2.40							350.00		60.00			1.08		0.00	0.00		
0.40		0.15	0.21	2.57	51.48	0.09	0.77	625.68	179.19	114.84	161.37	19.80	2.41	1.62	0.00	0.00		
0.35		0.21	0.16	6.30	47.52	0.15	0.37	599.94	234.63	103.95	221.76	21.78	1.70	0.78	0.00	0.00		
	4.80							570.00		150.00			1.08		0.00	0.00		
0.55		0.39	0.25	3.78	46.99	0.11	1.22	699.77	232.41	148.59	196.85	26.67	2.82	2.73	0.00	0.00		
	0.69							654.00		260.00			6.29		0.00	0.00		
	0.86							703.00		250.00			5.98		0.00	0.00		
								643.00							0.00	0.00		
	9.00							890.00	320.00	150.00			3.60		0.00	0.00		
	3.60							820.00	230.00	150.00			3.60		0.00	0.00		
	9.00							890.00	320.00	150.00			3.60		0.00	0.00		
	0.00							100.00	290.00	150.00			0.72			0.00	0.00	0.00
	15.00							1460.00	580.00	200.00			5.40		0.00	0.00		
	3.60							600.00	220.00	100.00			3.60		0.00	0.00		
	9.00							890.00	440.00	100.00			5.40		0.00	0.00		
0.00	0.02	0.00	0.00	0.00	0.02	0.00	0.00	15.85	1.02	0.85	0.57	0.22	0.02	0.00	0.00	0.00	0.00	0.00
								120.00	5.00	60.00	90.00				0.00	0.00		
0.12	0.00	0.00	0.00	0.00	0.15	0.00	0.01	28.80	1.20	1.20	1.20	0.10	0.00	0.00	0.00	0.00	0.00	0.00
0.09	0.00	0.00	0.00	0.00	0.11	0.00	0.00	31.43	0.99	0.91	0.87	0.08	0.01	0.00	0.00	0.00	0.00	0.00
0.12	0.00	0.00	0.00	0.00	0.15	0.00	0.01	0.55	1.20	1.20	1.20	0.10	0.00	0.00	0.00	0.00	0.00	0.00
0.08	0.00	0.00	0.00	0.00	0.00	0.00	0.00	0.00	0.00	0.00	0.00	0.00	0.00	0.01	0.00	0.00	0.00	0.00
1.25	0.00	0.00	0.00	0.00	0.00	0.00	0.00	0.00	0.00	0.00	0.00	0.00	0.00	0.00	0.00	0.00	0.00	0.00
	0.00							0.00		0.00			0.00		0.00		0.00	0.00
4.03	0.00							0.00		0.00			0.00		0.00	0.00	0.00	0.00
0.24	0.00	0.00	0.00	0.00	0.00	0.00	0.00	0.00	0.00	0.00	0.00	0.00	0.00	0.00	0.00	0.00	0.00	0.00
0.01	0.00	0.00	0.00	0.00	0.00	0.00	0.00	0.00	0.00	0.00	0.00	0.00	0.01	0.00	0.00	0.00	0.00	0.00
	0.00							0.00		0.00			0.00		0.00		0.00	0.00
2.83	0.00	0.00	0.00	0.00	0.00	0.00	0.00	0.00	0.00	0.00	0.00	0.00	0.00	0.00	0.00	0.00	0.00	0.00
3.92	0.00	0.00	0.00	0.00	0.00	0.00	0.00	0.00	0.00	0.00	0.00	0.00	3.60	0.00	0.00	0.00	0.00	0.00
1.96	0.00	0.00	0.00	0.00	0.00	0.00	0.00	0.00	0.00	0.00	0.00	0.00	0.00	0.00	0.00	0.00	0.00	0.00
1.74															0.00	0.00	0.00	0.00
0.52	0.00	0.00	0.00	0.00	0.00	0.00	0.00	0.00	0.00	0.00	0.00	0.00	0.00	0.00	0.00	0.00	0.00	0.00
2.12	0.00	0.00	0.00	0.00	0.00	0.00	0.00	0.00	0.00	0.00	0.00	0.00	0.00	0.00	0.00	0.00	0.00	0.00

Food Name	Amount	Measure	Weight (g)	Calories	Protein (g)	Total Carb (g)	Dietary Fiber (g)	Total Fat (g)	Sat Fat (g)	Mono Fat (g)	Poly Fat (g)	Chol (mg)	Vit A (mcg RAE)	Vit D (mcg)
FATS, OILS, MARGARINES, SHORTENINGS, AND SUBSTITUTES *(continued)*														
Oil, rice bran	1	Tablespoon	13.60	120.22	0.00	0.00	0.00	13.60	2.68	5.34	4.76	0.00	0.00	0.00
Oil, safflower Saffola	1	Tablespoon	14.00	120.00	0.00	0.00	0.00	14.00	1.00	11.00	2.00	0.00	0.00	
Oil, sesame Eden Foods, Inc.	1	Tablespoon	14.00	130.00	0.00	0.00	0.00	14.00	2.00	6.00	6.00	0.00	0.00	0.00
Oil, soybean lecithin	1	Tablespoon	13.60	103.77	0.00	0.00	0.00	13.60	2.04	1.49	6.16	0.00	0.00	
Oil, soybean, partially hydrog, winterized Archer Daniels Midland Company	1	Tablespoon	13.75	121.83	0.00	0.00	0.00	13.75	2.20	4.26	6.12	0.00	0.00	
Oil, soybean, salad or cooking	1	Tablespoon	13.60	120.22	0.00	0.00	0.00	13.60	1.96	3.17	7.87	0.00	0.00	
Oil, sunflower, greater than 60% linoleic	1	Tablespoon	13.60	120.22	0.00	0.00	0.00	13.60	1.40	2.65	8.94	0.00	0.00	
Oil, sunflower, less than 60% linoleic	1	Tablespoon	13.60	120.22	0.00	0.00	0.00	13.60	1.37	6.17	5.45	0.00	0.00	
Oil, sunflower, mid oleic, transfree, NuSun	1	Tablespoon	13.60	122.40	0.00	0.00	0.00	13.60	1.50	7.07	4.76	0.00	0.00	0.00
Oil, veg, pure Crisco	1	Tablespoon	14.00	120.00	0.00	0.00	0.00	14.00	1.50	6.00	6.00	0.00	0.00	

Margarines and Spreads

Food Name	Amount	Measure	Weight (g)	Calories	Protein (g)	Total Carb (g)	Dietary Fiber (g)	Total Fat (g)	Sat Fat (g)	Mono Fat (g)	Poly Fat (g)	Chol (mg)	Vit A (mcg RAE)	Vit D (mcg)
Margarine & Butter, blend, w/60% corn oil & 40% butter	1	Tablespoon	14.20	101.96	0.12	0.09	0.00	11.46	4.04	4.65	2.26	12.50	116.30	
Margarine, 80% fat	1	Tablespoon	14.10	99.41	0.03	0.27	0.00	11.11	2.08	5.25	3.26	0.00	115.48	
Margarine, 80% fat, unsalted	1	Tablespoon	14.20	102.10	0.13	0.13	0.00	11.43	2.20	5.54	3.17	0.00	116.30	
Margarine, hard, corn cottonseed & hydrog soybean oil, stick	1	Tablespoon	14.10	101.38	0.13	0.13	0.00	11.35	2.12	5.19	3.54	0.00	115.48	
Margarine, hard, corn hydrog soybean & cttnsd oil, stick	1	Tablespoon	14.10	101.38	0.13	0.13	0.00	11.35	2.79	4.51	3.54	0.00	115.48	
Margarine, hard, hydrog & reg soybean & palm oil, stick	1	Tablespoon	14.10	101.38	0.13	0.13	0.00	11.35	2.47	4.40	3.98	0.00	115.48	
Margarine, hard, hydrog & reg soybean oil, stick	1	Tablespoon	14.10	101.38	0.13	0.13	0.00	11.35	1.85	5.30	3.69	0.00	115.48	
Margarine, hard, hydrog corn oil, stick	1	Tablespoon	14.10	101.38	0.13	0.13	0.00	11.35	1.86	6.46	2.54	0.00	115.48	
Margarine, hard, hydrog soybean & cottonseed oil, stick	1	Tablespoon	14.10	101.38	0.13	0.13	0.00	11.35	2.13	6.67	2.06	0.00	115.48	
Margarine, hard, hydrog soybean & palm oil, stick	1	Tablespoon	14.10	101.38	0.13	0.13	0.00	11.35	2.13	4.51	4.20	0.00	115.48	
Margarine, hard, safflower hydrog&reg soy & cttnsd oil stick	1	Tablespoon	14.10	101.38	0.13	0.13	0.00	11.35	2.03	4.27	4.55	0.00	115.48	
Margarine, hard, soy hydrog corn & cttnsd oil unsalted stick	1	Tablespoon	14.10	100.67	0.07	0.07	0.00	11.32	2.12	5.17	3.53	0.00	115.48	
Margarine, hard, soybean hydrog soybean & cttnsd oil, stick	1	Tablespoon	14.10	101.38	0.13	0.13	0.00	11.35	2.20	5.09	3.57	0.00	115.48	
Margarine, hard, sunflower hydrog soybean & cttnsd oil stick	1	Tablespoon	14.10	101.38	0.13	0.13	0.00	11.35	1.68	4.02	5.16	0.00	115.48	
Margarine, hard, unspecified oil, unsalted, stick	1	Tablespoon	14.10	100.67	0.07	0.07	0.00	11.32	2.12	5.17	3.53	0.00	115.48	0.00
Margarine, liquid, cttnsd hydrog & reg soy oil	1	Tablespoon	14.20	102.38	0.27	0.00	0.00	11.45	1.87	3.99	5.08	0.00	116.30	
Margarine, unspecified oil, stick	1	Tablespoon	14.10	101.38	0.13	0.13	0.00	11.35	2.23	5.05	3.58	0.00	115.48	
Spread, 40% fat, rducd cal, stick	1	Tablespoon	14.00	49.84	0.08	0.00	0.00	5.60	0.85	2.64	1.86	0.00	114.66	
Spread, 48% fat, tub	1	Tablespoon	14.00	59.36	0.03	0.12	0.00	6.65	1.23	2.30	2.83	0.14		
Spread, rducd cal	1	Tablespoon	14.20	49.02	0.07	0.06	0.00	5.51	1.09	2.23	1.96	0.00	147.18	0.00
Spread, rducd cal, cottonseed & soybean oil, 40% fat	1	Tablespoon	14.40	49.68	0.06	0.06	0.00	5.58	1.20	2.04	2.10	0.00	117.93	
Spread, rducd cal, hydrog soy & cttnsd oil, 60% fat	1	Tablespoon	14.40	77.76	0.09	0.00	0.00	8.76	1.74	5.61	1.02	0.00	117.93	
Spread, rducd cal, hydrog soybean oil, 40%fat	1	Tablespoon	14.40	49.68	0.06	0.06	0.00	5.58	0.93	2.40	1.98	0.00	117.93	1.53
Spread, rducd cal, unspecified oil, 40%fat	1	Tablespoon	14.40	49.68	0.06	0.06	0.00	5.58	1.11	2.25	1.98	0.00	117.93	
Spread, vegetable oil butter	1	Tablespoon	14.20	77.38	0.09	0.00	0.00	8.72	1.98	4.44	1.91	0.93	103.65	0.00
Spread, vegetable oil, tub	1	Tablespoon	14.00	50.68	0.14	0.14	0.00	5.60	1.01	2.58	1.76	0.00	114.66	

Shortenings

Food Name	Amount	Measure	Weight (g)	Calories	Protein (g)	Total Carb (g)	Dietary Fiber (g)	Total Fat (g)	Sat Fat (g)	Mono Fat (g)	Poly Fat (g)	Chol (mg)	Vit A (mcg RAE)	Vit D (mcg)
Shortening, bread, hydrog soy & ctnsd oil	1	Tablespoon	12.80	113.15	0.00	0.00	0.00	12.80	2.82	4.22	5.20	0.00	0.00	
Shortening, frying, heavy duty, hydrog palm oil	1	Tablespoon	12.80	113.15	0.00	0.00	0.00	12.80	6.08	5.20	0.96	0.00	0.00	

Vit E (mg)	Vit C	Vit B₁ Thia (mg)	Vit B₂ Ribo (mg)	Vit B₃ Nia (mg)	Fol (mcg)	Vit B₆ (mg)	Vita B₁₂ (mcg)	Sodi (mg)	Pota (mg)	Cal (mg)	Phos (mg)	Magn (mg)	Iron (mg)	Zinc (mg)	Caff (mg)	Alco (g)	Sol Fiber (g)	Insol Fiber (g)
4.39	0.00	0.00	0.00	0.00	0.00	0.00	0.00	0.00	0.00	0.00	0.00	0.00	0.01	0.00	0.00	0.00	0.00	0.00
	0.00							0.00		0.00			0.00		0.00	0.00	0.00	0.00
0.57	0.00	0.00	0.00	0.00	0.00	0.00	0.00	0.00	0.00	0.00	0.00	0.00	0.00	0.00	0.00	0.57	0.00	0.00
1.25	0.00	0.00	0.00	0.00	0.00	0.00	0.00	0.00	0.00	0.00	0.00	0.00	0.00	0.00	0.00	0.00	0.00	0.00
	0.00	0.00	0.00	0.00				0.00	0.00	0.00			0.00		0.00	0.00	0.00	0.00
1.25	0.00	0.00	0.00	0.00	0.00	0.00	0.00	0.00	0.00	0.00	0.00	0.00	0.00	0.00	0.00	0.00	0.00	0.00
5.59	0.00	0.00	0.00	0.00	0.00	0.00	0.00	0.00	0.00	0.00	0.00	0.00	0.00	0.00	0.00	0.00	0.00	0.00
5.59	0.00	0.00	0.00	0.00	0.00	0.00	0.00	0.00	0.00	0.00	0.00	0.00	0.00	0.00	0.00	0.00	0.00	0.00
0.00	0.00							0.00	0.00	0.00			0.00		0.00	0.00	0.00	0.00
3.02	0.00							0.00		0.00			0.00		0.00	0.00	0.00	0.00
0.56	0.01	0.00	0.00	0.00	0.28	0.00	0.01	127.37	5.11	3.98	3.27	0.28	0.01	0.00	0.00	0.00	0.00	0.00
0.88	0.00	0.00	0.00	0.00	0.14	0.00	0.01	92.21	2.54	0.42	0.71	0.14	0.02	0.02	0.00	0.00	0.00	0.00
0.71	0.01	0.00	0.00	0.00	0.14	0.00	0.01	0.28	3.55	2.41	1.85	0.28	0.00	0.00	0.00	0.00	0.00	0.00
1.55	0.03	0.00	0.01	0.00	0.14	0.00	0.01	132.96	5.92	4.23	3.24	0.42	0.00	0.00	0.00	0.00	0.00	0.00
0.44	0.03	0.00	0.01	0.00	0.14	0.00	0.01	132.96	5.92	4.23	3.24	0.42	0.00	0.00	0.00	0.00	0.00	0.00
0.44	0.03	0.00	0.01	0.00	0.14	0.00	0.01	132.96	5.92	4.23	3.24	0.42	0.00	0.00	0.00	0.00	0.00	0.00
0.44	0.03	0.00	0.01	0.00	0.14	0.00	0.01	132.96	5.92	4.23	3.24	0.42	0.00		0.00	0.00	0.00	0.00
1.64	0.03	0.00	0.01	0.00	0.14	0.00	0.01	132.96	5.92	4.23	3.24	0.42	0.00	0.00	0.00	0.00	0.00	0.00
1.10	0.03	0.00	0.01	0.00	0.14	0.00	0.01	132.96	5.92	4.23	3.24	0.42	0.00	0.00	0.00	0.00	0.00	0.00
0.44	0.03	0.00	0.01	0.00	0.14	0.00	0.01	132.96	5.92	4.23	3.24	0.42	0.00	0.00	0.00	0.00	0.00	0.00
2.31	0.03	0.00	0.01	0.00	0.14	0.00	0.01	132.96	5.92	4.23	3.24	0.42	0.00	0.00	0.00	0.00	0.00	0.00
1.64	0.01	0.00	0.00	0.00	0.14	0.00	0.01	0.28	3.53	2.40	1.83	0.28	0.00	0.00	0.00	0.00	0.00	0.00
1.75	0.03	0.00	0.01	0.00	0.14	0.00	0.01	132.96	5.92	4.23	3.24	0.42	0.00	0.00	0.00	0.00	0.00	0.00
1.55	0.03	0.00	0.01	0.00	0.14	0.00	0.01	132.96	5.92	4.23	3.24	0.42	0.00	0.00	0.00	0.00	0.00	0.00
1.80	0.01	0.00	0.00	0.00	0.14	0.00	0.01	0.28	3.53	2.40	1.83	0.28	0.00	0.00	0.00	0.00	0.00	0.00
0.65	0.06	0.00	0.01	0.01	0.43	0.00	0.03	110.90	13.35	9.37	7.24	0.85	0.00	0.00	0.00	0.00	0.00	0.00
1.27	0.03	0.00	0.01	0.00	0.14	0.00	0.01	132.96	5.92	4.23	3.24	0.42	0.01	0.00	0.00	0.00	0.00	0.00
0.70	0.01	0.00	0.00	0.00	0.14	0.00	0.01	139.16	4.20	2.94	2.24	0.28	0.00	0.00	0.00	0.00	0.00	0.00
0.55	0.00	0.00	0.00	0.00	0.28	0.00		90.44	5.04	0.56	0.56	0.14	0.03	0.01	0.00	0.00	0.00	0.00
0.33	0.01	0.00	0.00	0.00	0.10	0.00	0.01	136.26	3.59	2.53	1.95	0.22	0.00	0.00	0.00	0.00	0.00	0.00
0.39	0.00	0.00	0.00	0.00	0.15	0.00	0.00	138.24	3.60	2.58	2.01	0.30	0.00	0.00	0.00	0.00	0.00	0.00
0.72	0.00	0.00	0.00	0.00	0.15	0.00	0.00	143.13	4.32	3.03	2.31	0.30	0.00	0.00	0.00	0.00	0.00	0.00
0.12	0.00	0.00	0.00	0.00	0.15	0.00	0.00	138.24	3.60	2.58	2.01	0.30	0.00	0.00	0.00	0.00	0.00	0.00
0.57	0.00	0.00	0.00	0.00	0.15	0.00	0.00	138.24	3.60	2.58	2.01	0.30	0.00	0.00	0.00	0.00	0.00	0.00
1.25	0.02	0.00	0.00	0.00	0.13	0.00	0.01	140.42	4.22	2.98	2.32	0.26	0.00	0.00	0.00	0.00	0.00	0.00
0.63	0.01	0.00	0.00	0.00	0.14	0.00	0.01	110.04	5.04	3.36	2.80	0.28	0.01	0.00	0.00	0.00	0.00	0.00
1.02	0.00	0.00	0.00	0.00	0.00	0.00	0.00	0.00	0.00	0.00	0.00	0.00	0.00	0.00	0.00	0.00	0.00	0.00
2.43	0.00	0.00	0.00	0.00	0.00	0.00	0.00	0.00	0.00	0.00	0.00	0.00	0.00	0.00	0.00	0.00	0.00	0.00

Food Name	Amount	Measure	Weight (g)	Calories	Protein (g)	Total Carb (g)	Dietary Fiber (g)	Total Fat (g)	Sat Fat (g)	Mono Fat (g)	Poly Fat (g)	Chol (mg)	Vit A (mcg RAE)	Vit D (mcg)
FISH, SEAFOOD, AND SHELLFISH														
Abalone, raw, mixed species	4	Ounce-weight	113.40	119.07	19.39	6.82	0.00	0.86	0.17	0.12	0.12	96.39	2.27	
Calamari, mixed species, fried USDA SR-23	3	Ounce-weight	85.05	148.84	15.26	6.63	0.00	6.36	1.60	2.34	1.82	221.13	9.36	
Clams, brd, fried	3	Ounce-weight	85.05	333.40	9.48	28.70		19.53	4.88	8.46	5.01	64.64	27.22	
Clams, brd, fried, mixed species, sml	3	Ounce-weight	85.05	171.80	12.11	8.79	0.14	9.48	2.28	3.87	2.44	51.88	77.40	
Clams, cnd, mixed species, drained	3	Ounce-weight	85.05	125.87	21.73	4.36	0.00	1.66	0.16	0.15	0.47	56.98	153.94	
Clams, minced, cnd S & W	3	Ounce-weight	85.05	30.93	6.19	1.55	0.00	0.00	0.00	0.00	0.00	15.46	0.00	
Clams, raw, mixed species, cup	4	Ounce-weight	113.40	83.92	14.48	2.91	0.00	1.10	0.11	0.09	0.32	38.56	102.06	0.11
Crab, Alaska king, imit f/surimi	3	Ounce-weight	85.05	86.75	10.22	8.69	0.00	1.11	0.22	0.17	0.57	17.01	17.01	
Crab, Alaska king, leg, raw	4	Ounce-weight	113.40	95.26	20.74	0.00	0.00	0.68	0.10	0.09	0.15	47.63	7.94	
Crab, bkd/brld	3	Ounce-weight	85.05	117.46	16.22	0.05	0.00	5.42	0.96	2.17	1.66	80.07	37.97	0.09
Crab, blue, raw	4	Ounce-weight	113.40	98.66	20.48	0.05	0.00	1.22	0.25	0.22	0.44	88.45	2.27	
Crab, dungeoness, raw	4	Ounce-weight	113.40	97.52	19.74	0.84	0.00	1.10	0.15	0.19	0.36	66.91	30.62	
Crab, soft shell, brd/floured, fried	1	Each	65.00	217.18	13.30	11.17	0.38	12.99	2.65	5.42	3.95	80.11	14.82	0.13
Eel, fillet, mixed species, raw	4	Ounce-weight	113.40	208.66	20.91	0.00	0.00	13.22	2.67	8.15	1.07	142.88	1182.76	
Eel, fillet, sashimi, mixed species	4	Ounce-weight	113.40	208.66	20.91	0.00	0.00	13.22	2.67	8.15	1.07	142.88	1182.76	
Escargot, stmd/poached	2	Each	10.00	27.40	4.77	1.55	0.00	0.08	0.01	0.01	0.00	13.00	4.68	
Fish Cake, brd, fried, heated f/fzn Universal Labs	1	Each	85.00	231.29	7.88	14.73		15.33	6.00	3.43	3.43	22.27		
Fish Cake, fried	1	Each	69.00	149.03	13.27	5.82	0.19	7.75	1.62	3.24	2.37	54.35	18.79	
Fish Paste, Japanese	1	Tablespoon	16.00	18.56	2.15	2.01	0.02	0.11	0.02	0.01	0.05	7.83	1.09	
Fish Sticks, brd, Healthy Treasures Mrs. Paul's	4	Piece	85.00	170.00	10.00	20.00	2.00	3.00	1.50			20.00	0.00	
Fish Sticks, oven breaded, fzn Van de Kamp's	6	Piece	114.00	290.00	13.00	23.00	0.00	17.00				35.00		
Fish, bass, freshwater, fillet, bkd/brld, mixed species	3	Ounce-weight	85.05	124.17	20.57	0.00	0.00	4.02	0.85	1.56	1.16	73.99	29.77	
Fish, bass, sea, fillet, bkd/brld, mixed species	3	Ounce-weight	85.05	105.46	20.10	0.00	0.00	2.18	0.56	0.46	0.81	45.08	54.43	
Fish, bass, striped, fillet, bkd/brld	3	Ounce-weight	85.05	105.46	19.33	0.00	0.00	2.54	0.55	0.72	0.85	87.60	26.37	
Fish, bluefish, fillet, bkd/brld	3	Ounce-weight	85.05	135.23	21.85	0.00	0.00	4.63	1.00	1.95	1.15	64.64	117.37	
Fish, carp, fillet, bkd/brld	3	Ounce-weight	85.05	137.78	19.44	0.00	0.00	6.10	1.18	2.54	1.56	71.44	8.51	
Fish, catfish, channel, fillet, bkd/brld, farmed	3	Ounce-weight	85.05	129.28	15.92	0.00	0.00	6.82	1.52	3.53	1.18	54.43	12.76	
Fish, catfish, channel, fillet, bkd/brld, wild	3	Ounce-weight	85.05	89.30	15.71	0.00	0.00	2.42	0.63	0.93	0.54	61.24	12.76	
Fish, cod, Atlantic, dried & salted, 5.5" × 1.5" × .5" pce	1	Piece	80.00	232.00	50.26	0.00	0.00	1.90	0.37	0.27	0.64	121.60	33.60	
Fish, cod, Atlantic, fillet, bkd/brld	3	Ounce-weight	85.05	89.30	19.42	0.00	0.00	0.73	0.14	0.11	0.25	46.78	11.91	
Fish, cod, Pacific, fillet, bkd/brld	3	Ounce-weight	85.05	89.30	19.52	0.00	0.00	0.69	0.09	0.09	0.27	39.97	8.51	
Fish, grouper, fillet, mixed species, bkd/brld	3	Ounce-weight	85.05	100.36	21.13	0.00	0.00	1.11	0.25	0.23	0.34	39.97	42.53	
Fish, haddock, fillet, bkd/brld	3	Ounce-weight	85.05	95.26	20.62	0.00	0.00	0.79	0.14	0.13	0.26	62.94	16.16	
Fish, haddock, smkd, 1" cube	3	Ounce-weight	85.05	98.66	21.46	0.00	0.00	0.80	0.15	0.15	0.25	65.49	18.71	
Fish, halibut, Atlantic/Pacific, fillet, bkd/brld	3	Ounce-weight	85.05	119.07	22.70	0.00	0.00	2.50	0.35	0.82	0.80	34.87	45.93	
Fish, halibut, Greenland, fillet, bkd/brld	3	Ounce-weight	85.05	203.27	15.67	0.00	0.00	15.09	2.64	9.14	1.49	50.18	15.31	12.76
Fish, herring, Atlantic, fillet, bkd/brld	3	Ounce-weight	85.05	172.65	19.59	0.00	0.00	9.86	2.22	4.07	2.33	65.49	30.62	
Fish, herring, Atlantic, pickled, pce, 1 3/4" × 7/8" × 1/2"	1	Piece	15.00	39.30	2.13	1.45	0.00	2.70	0.36	1.79	0.25	1.95	38.70	2.55
Fish, herring, Atlantic, smkd, kippered fillet 5" × 1.75" × .25"	1	Piece	40.00	86.80	9.83	0.00	0.00	4.95	1.12	2.04	1.17	32.80	16.00	1.20
Fish, mackerel, Atlantic, fillet, bkd/brld	3	Ounce-weight	85.05	222.83	20.28	0.00	0.00	15.15	3.55	5.96	3.66	63.79	45.93	
Fish, mackerel, king, fillet, bkd/brld	3	Ounce-weight	85.05	113.97	22.11	0.00	0.00	2.18	0.40	0.83	0.50	57.83	214.33	
Fish, mahi mahi, fillet, bkd/brld USDA SR-23	3	Ounce-weight	85.05	92.70	20.17	0.00	0.00	0.77	0.20	0.13	0.18	79.95	52.73	
Fish, monkfish, bkd/brld	3	Ounce-weight	85.05	82.50	15.79	0.00	0.00	1.66	0.46	0.32	0.82	27.22	11.91	
Fish, orange roughy, fillet, bkd/brld	3	Ounce-weight	85.05	75.69	16.03	0.00	0.00	0.77	0.02	0.52	0.01	22.11	20.41	
Fish, perch, fillet, bkd/brld, mixed species	3	Ounce-weight	85.05	99.51	21.14	0.00	0.00	1.00	0.20	0.17	0.40	97.81	8.51	
Fish, perch, ocean, Atlantic, fillet, bkd/brld	3	Ounce-weight	85.05	102.91	20.31	0.00	0.00	1.78	0.27	0.68	0.47	45.93	11.91	
Fish, pike, northen, fillet, bkd/brld	3	Ounce-weight	85.05	96.11	21.00	0.00	0.00	0.75	0.13	0.17	0.22	42.53	20.41	
Fish, pike, walleye, fillet, bkd/brld	3	Ounce-weight	85.05	101.21	20.87	0.00	0.00	1.33	0.27	0.32	0.49	93.56	20.41	
Fish, pollock, Atlantic, fillet, bkd/brld	3	Ounce-weight	85.05	100.36	21.19	0.00	0.00	1.07	0.14	0.12	0.53	77.40	10.21	
Fish, pollock, walleye, fillet, bkd/brld	3	Ounce-weight	85.05	96.11	20.00	0.00	0.00	0.95	0.20	0.15	0.45	81.65	21.26	

Vit E (mg)	Vit C	Vit B₁ Thia (mg)	Vit B₂ Ribo (mg)	Vit B₃ Nia (mg)	Fol (mcg)	Vit B₆ (mg)	Vita B₁₂ (mcg)	Sodi (mg)	Pota (mg)	Cal (mg)	Phos (mg)	Magn (mg)	Iron (mg)	Zinc (mg)	Caff (mg)	Alco (g)	Sol Fiber (g)	Insol Fiber (g)
4.54	2.27	0.22	0.11	1.70	5.67	0.17	0.83	341.33	283.50	35.15	215.46	54.43	3.62	0.93	0.00	0.00	0.00	0.00
	3.57	0.05	0.39	2.21	11.91	0.05	1.05	260.25	237.29	33.17	213.48	32.32	0.86	1.48	0.00	0.00	0.00	0.00
	0.00	0.15	0.20	2.12	31.47	0.03	0.82	616.61	196.47	15.31	176.05	22.96	2.25	1.21	0.00	0.00		
2.13	8.51	0.09	0.21	1.76	30.62	0.05	34.25	309.58	277.26	53.58	159.89	11.91	11.83	1.24	0.00	0.00	0.06	0.08
0.53	18.80	0.13	0.36	2.85	24.66	0.09	84.11	95.26	534.11	78.25	287.47	15.31	23.78	2.32	0.00	0.00	0.00	0.00
	0.00							556.69	0.00	0.00			1.11		0.00	0.00	0.00	0.00
0.35	14.74	0.09	0.24	2.00	18.14	0.07	56.06	63.50	356.08	52.16	191.65	10.21	15.85	1.55	0.00	0.00	0.00	0.00
0.09	0.00	0.03	0.02	0.15	1.70	0.03	1.36	715.27	76.55	11.06	239.84	36.57	0.33	0.28	0.00	0.00	0.00	0.00
1.02	7.94	0.05	0.05	1.25	49.90	0.17	10.21	948.02	231.34	52.16	248.35	55.57	0.67	6.75	0.00	0.00	0.00	0.00
1.40	2.65	0.08	0.04	2.64	40.73	0.14	5.85	270.34	261.52	84.77	166.09	26.57	0.73	3.38	0.00	0.00	0.00	0.00
1.13	3.40	0.09	0.05	3.06	49.90	0.17	10.21	332.26	373.09	100.93	259.69	38.56	0.84	4.01	0.00	0.00	0.00	0.00
1.02	3.97	0.05	0.19	3.56	49.90	0.17	10.21	334.53	401.44	52.16	206.39	51.03	0.42	4.84	0.00	0.00	0.00	0.00
2.07	1.43	0.15	0.13	2.55	27.10	0.11	3.36	216.59	208.97	79.51	142.67	23.50	1.36	2.46	0.00	0.00	0.19	0.19
4.54	2.04	0.17	0.05	3.97	17.01	0.08	3.40	57.83	308.45	22.68	244.94	22.68	0.57	1.84	0.00	0.00	0.00	0.00
4.54	2.04	0.17	0.05	3.97	17.01	0.08	3.40	57.83	308.45	22.68	244.94	22.68	0.57	1.84	0.00	0.00	0.00	0.00
0.03	0.60	0.00	0.02	0.16	0.95	0.06	1.09	35.02	48.58	10.83	19.74	14.62	0.91	0.33	0.00	0.00	0.00	0.00
0.51	0.00	0.03	0.06	1.37	10.54	0.04	0.86		298.11	9.42	143.06	15.42	0.34	0.34	0.00	0.00		
1.29	0.27	0.09	0.09	1.72	6.10	0.10	1.33	127.32	256.65	29.51	206.97	32.49	0.74	0.45	0.00	0.00	0.09	0.09
0.03	0.00	0.00	0.02	0.36	0.31	0.03	0.33	9.77	39.35	6.72	24.67	7.49	0.06	0.05	0.00	0.00		
	1.20							350.00		40.00			1.08		0.00	0.00		
									110.00		100.00				0.00	0.00	0.00	0.00
0.63	1.79	0.07	0.08	1.29	14.46	0.12	1.96	76.55	387.83	87.60	217.73	32.32	1.62	0.71	0.00	0.00	0.00	0.00
0.54	0.00	0.11	0.13	1.62	5.10	0.39	0.26	73.99	278.96	11.06	210.92	45.08	0.31	0.44	0.00	0.54	0.00	0.00
0.52	0.00	0.10	0.03	2.18	8.51	0.29	3.75	74.84	278.96	16.16	216.03	43.38	0.92	0.43	0.00	0.00	0.00	0.00
0.54	0.00	0.06	0.08	6.16	1.70	0.39	5.29	65.49	405.69	7.65	247.50	35.72	0.53	0.88	0.00	0.00	0.00	0.00
0.91	1.36	0.12	0.06	1.79	14.46	0.19	1.25	53.58	363.16	44.23	451.62	32.32	1.35	1.62	0.00	0.00	0.00	0.00
1.12	0.68	0.36	0.06	2.14	5.95	0.14	2.38	68.04	273.01	7.65	208.37	22.11	0.70	0.89	0.00	0.00	0.00	0.00
	0.68	0.19	0.06	2.03	8.51	0.09	2.47	42.53	356.36	9.36	258.55	23.81	0.30	0.52	0.00	0.00	0.00	0.00
2.27	2.80	0.21	0.19	6.00	20.00	0.69	8.00	5621.60	1166.40	128.00	760.00	106.40	2.00	1.27	0.00	0.00	0.00	0.00
0.69	0.85	0.07	0.07	2.14	6.80	0.24	0.89	66.34	207.52	11.91	117.37	35.72	0.42	0.49	0.00	0.00	0.00	0.00
0.29	2.55	0.02	0.04	2.11	6.80	0.39	0.88	77.40	439.71	7.65	189.66	26.37	0.28	0.43	0.00	0.00	0.00	0.00
0.53	0.00	0.07	0.01	0.32	8.51	0.30	0.59	45.08	403.99	17.86	121.62	31.47	0.97	0.43	0.00	0.00	0.00	0.00
0.42	0.00	0.03	0.04	3.94	11.06	0.29	1.18	73.99	339.35	35.72	204.97	42.53	1.15	0.41	0.00	0.00	0.00	0.00
0.45	0.00	0.05	0.05	4.30	12.76	0.35	1.35	648.93	352.96	41.67	213.48	45.93	1.20	0.45	0.00	0.00	0.00	0.00
0.93	0.00	0.06	0.08	6.06	11.91	0.34	1.17	58.68	489.89	51.03	242.39	91.00	0.91	0.45	0.00	0.00	0.00	0.00
1.05	0.00	0.06	0.09	1.64	0.85	0.41	0.82	87.60	292.57	3.40	178.61	28.07	0.72	0.43	0.00	0.00	0.00	0.00
1.17	0.60	0.10	0.25	3.51	10.21	0.30	11.18	97.81	356.36	62.94	257.70	34.87	1.20	1.08	0.00	0.00	0.00	0.00
0.26	0.00	0.01	0.02	0.50	0.30	0.03	0.64	130.50	10.35	11.55	13.35	1.20	0.18	0.08	0.00	0.00	0.00	0.00
0.62	0.40	0.05	0.13	1.76	5.60	0.17	7.48	367.20	178.80	33.60	130.00	18.40	0.60	0.54	0.00	0.00	0.00	0.00
1.57	0.34	0.14	0.35	5.83	1.70	0.39	16.16	70.59	341.05	12.76	236.44	82.50	1.34	0.80	0.00	0.00	0.00	0.00
1.47	1.36	0.10	0.49	8.90	7.65	0.43	15.31	172.65	474.58	34.02	270.46	34.87	1.94	0.61	0.00	0.00	0.00	0.00
	0.00	0.02	0.07	6.32	5.10	0.39	0.59	96.11	453.32	16.16	155.64	32.32	1.23	0.50	0.00	0.00	0.00	0.00
0.24	0.85	0.02	0.06	2.18	6.80	0.24	0.88	19.56	436.31	8.51	217.73	22.96	0.35	0.45	0.00	0.00	0.00	0.00
0.54	0.00	0.10	0.16	3.11	6.80	0.29	1.96	68.89	327.44	32.32	217.73	32.32	0.20	0.82	0.00	0.00	0.00	0.00
1.28	1.45	0.07	0.10	1.62	5.10	0.12	1.87	67.19	292.57	86.75	218.58	32.32	0.99	1.22	0.00	0.00	0.00	0.00
1.39	0.68	0.11	0.11	2.07	8.51	0.23	0.98	81.65	297.68	116.52	235.59	33.17	1.00	0.52	0.00	0.00	0.00	0.00
0.20	3.23	0.06	0.07	2.38	14.46	0.11	1.96	41.67	281.52	62.09	239.84	34.02	0.60	0.73	0.00	0.00	0.00	0.00
0.24	0.00	0.27	0.17	2.38	14.46	0.12	1.96	55.28	424.40	119.92	228.78	32.32	1.42	0.67	0.00	0.00	0.00	0.00
0.24	0.00	0.05	0.19	3.39	2.55	0.28	3.13	93.56	387.83	65.49	240.69	73.14	0.50	0.51	0.00	0.00	0.00	0.00
0.67	0.00	0.06	0.06	1.40	3.40	0.06	3.57	98.66	329.14	5.10	409.94	62.09	0.24	0.51	0.00	0.00	0.00	0.00

FISH, SEAFOOD, AND SHELLFISH (continued)

Food Name	Amount	Measure	Weight (g)	Calories	Protein (g)	Total Carb (g)	Dietary Fiber (g)	Total Fat (g)	Sat Fat (g)	Mono Fat (g)	Poly Fat (g)	Chol (mg)	Vit A (mcg RAE)	Vit D (mcg)
Fish, portions, heated f/fzn, 4" × 2" × 1/2"	1	Piece	57.00	155.04	8.92	13.54	0.80	6.97	1.79	2.89	1.80	63.84	17.67	0.10
Fish, pumpkinseed sunfish, fillet, bkd/brld	3	Ounce-weight	85.05	96.96	21.15	0.00	0.00	0.77	0.15	0.13	0.27	73.14	14.46	
Fish, salmon, Atlantic, fillet, bkd/brld, farmed	3	Ounce-weight	85.05	175.20	18.80	0.00	0.00	10.50	2.13	3.77	3.76	53.58	12.76	
Fish, salmon, Atlantic, fillet, bkd/brld, wild	3	Ounce-weight	85.05	154.79	21.64	0.00	0.00	6.91	1.07	2.29	2.77	60.39	11.06	5.95
Fish, salmon, chinook, fillet, bkd/brld	3	Ounce-weight	85.05	196.47	21.87	0.00	0.00	11.38	2.73	4.88	2.26	72.29	126.72	
Fish, salmon, chinook, smkd	3	Ounce-weight	85.05	99.51	15.55	0.00	0.00	3.67	0.79	1.72	0.85	19.56	22.11	
Fish, salmon, chum, w/bone, cnd, drained, unsalted	3	Ounce-weight	85.05	119.92	18.23	0.00	0.00	4.68	1.26	1.63	1.29	33.17	15.31	
Fish, salmon, coho, fillet, bkd/brld, f	3	Ounce-weight	85.05	151.39	20.67	0.00	0.00	7.00	1.65	3.08	1.67	53.58	50.18	
Fish, salmon, coho, fillet, bkd/brld, farmed	3	Ounce-weight	85.05	118.22	19.94	0.00	0.00	3.66	0.90	1.34	1.08	46.78	32.32	
Fish, salmon, coho, fillet, bkd/brld, wild	3	Ounce-weight	85.05	156.49	23.27	0.00	0.00	6.38	1.36	2.30	2.15	48.48	27.22	
Fish, salmon, coho, fillet, stmd/poached, wild	3	Ounce-weight	85.05	126.72	21.74	0.00	0.00	3.76	0.61	1.02	1.47	56.98	34.87	
Fish, salmon, pink, fillet, bkd/brld	3	Ounce-weight	85.05	118.22	16.82	0.00	0.00	5.15	1.31	1.54	1.74	46.78	14.46	13.27
Fish, salmon, pink, w/bone, cnd, not drained	3	Ounce-weight	85.05	176.90	20.94	0.00	0.00	9.74	1.30	3.29	4.38	120.77	27.22	5.78
Fish, sardines, Atlantic, w/bones, w/oil, drained	3	Ounce-weight	85.05	158.19	17.74	0.63	0.09	8.90	2.28	4.10	1.80	51.88	28.92	10.21
Fish, sardines, Pacific, w/bone & tomato sauce, drained	3	Ounce-weight	85.05	113.12	18.25	0.00	0.00	3.94	1.10	0.96	0.79	90.15	29.77	
Fish, sea trout, fillet, bkd/brld, mixed species	3	Ounce-weight	85.05	214.33	18.46	0.00	0.00	15.01	3.83	6.97	4.00	81.65	30.62	
Fish, shad, American, fillet, bkd/brld	3	Ounce-weight	85.05	193.91	15.84	5.43	0.00	11.75	2.73	5.05	3.15	50.18	45.93	
Fish, shark, batter dipped, fried, mixed species	4	Ounce-weight	113.40	147.42	23.79	0.00	0.00	5.11	1.05	2.05	1.36	57.83	79.38	
Fish, shark, raw, mixed species	3	Ounce-weight	85.05	108.86	22.37	0.00	0.00	1.46	0.31	0.27	0.50	39.97	29.77	
Fish, snapper, fillet, bkd/brld, mixed species	3	Ounce-weight	85.05	82.79	17.31	0.00	0.00	1.13	0.00	0.00	0.38	37.63	0.00	
Fish, sole, fillet, natural, fzn Van de Kamp's	3	Ounce-weight	85.05	131.83	21.59	0.00	0.00	4.37	1.20	1.68	1.01	42.53	34.87	
Fish, swordfish, fillet, bkd/brld	3	Ounce-weight	85.05	161.60	22.65	0.00	0.00	7.20	1.25	3.55	1.63	62.94	16.16	
Fish, trout, fillet, bkd/brld, mixed species	3	Ounce-weight	85.05	143.73	20.64	0.00	0.00	6.12	1.79	1.78	1.98	57.83	73.14	
Fish, trout, rainbow, fillet, bkd/brld, farmed	3	Ounce-weight	85.05	127.58	19.49	0.00	0.00	4.95	1.38	1.48	1.56	58.68	12.76	
Fish, trout, rainbow, fillet, bkd/brld, wild	3	Ounce-weight	85.05	156.49	25.44	0.00	0.00	5.34	1.37	1.75	1.57	41.67	643.83	
Fish, tuna, bluefin, fillet, bkd/brld	0.5	Cup	73.00	144.54	21.27	0.00	0.00	5.99	1.12	2.15	2.10	13.14	16.79	4.31
Fish, tuna, light, w/oil, drained, can	3	Ounce-weight	85.05	168.40	24.78	0.00	0.00	6.98	1.30	2.51	2.45	15.31	19.56	
Fish, tuna, light, w/oil, drained, unsalted, cnd	3	Ounce-weight	85.05	105.00	22.50	0.00	0.00	0.08	0.00			52.50	0.00	
Fish, tuna, light, w/water, chunk, cnd S & W	0.5	Cup	77.00	89.32	19.65	0.00	0.00	0.63	0.18	0.13	0.26	23.10	13.09	
Fish, tuna, light, w/water, drained, can	3	Ounce-weight	85.05	158.19	22.56	0.00	0.00	6.87	1.09	2.77	2.53	26.37	4.25	
Fish, tuna, white, w/oil, drained, cnd	3	Ounce-weight	85.05	108.86	20.09	0.00	0.00	2.53	0.67	0.67	0.94	35.72	5.10	
Fish, tuna, white, w/water, drained, cnd	3	Ounce-weight	85.05	118.22	25.49	0.00	0.00	1.04	0.26	0.17	0.31	49.33	17.01	
Fish, tuna, yellowfin, fillet, bkd/brld	3	Ounce-weight	85.05	103.76	17.50	0.00	0.00	3.21				52.73	10.21	
Fish, turbot, European, fillet, bkd/brld	3	Ounce-weight	85.05	146.29	20.81	0.00	0.00	6.39	0.99	2.18	2.34	65.49	33.17	
Fish, whitefish, fillet, bkd/brld, mixed species	3	Ounce-weight	85.05	98.66	19.97	0.00	0.00	1.44	0.34	0.38	0.50	71.44	28.92	
Fish, whiting, fillet, bkd/brld, mixed species	3	Ounce-weight	85.05	159.04	25.23	0.00	0.00	5.72				60.39	26.37	
Fish, yellowtail, fillet, bkd/brld, mixed species	1	Cup	240.00	4.80	0.96	0.24	0.00	0.05	0.00	0.00	0.01	7.20	21.60	
Juice, clam, cnd, mixed species	4	Ounce-weight	113.40	102.06	21.32	0.57	0.00	1.02	0.20	0.29	0.17	107.73	23.81	
Lobster, northern, raw	4	Ounce-weight	113.40	127.01	23.36	2.76	0.00	1.71	0.27	0.31	0.67	79.38	5.67	
Lobster, spiny, raw, mixed species	4	Ounce-weight	113.40	97.52	13.49	4.18	0.00	2.54	0.48	0.57	0.69	31.75	54.43	
Mussels, blue, raw, cup	3	Ounce-weight	85.05	67.19	5.95	6.19	0.00	1.80	0.58	0.20	0.61	32.32	16.16	
Oysters, eastern, bkd/brld, farmed, med	3	Ounce-weight	85.05	61.24	7.02	4.08	0.00	1.62	0.47	0.20	0.69	41.67	0.00	
Oysters, eastern, bkd/brld, wild, med	4	Ounce-weight	113.40	66.91	5.92	6.27	0.00	1.76	0.50	0.17	0.67	28.35	9.07	
Oysters, eastern, raw, farmed, med	3	Ounce-weight	85.05	179.46	20.15	0.00	0.00	10.33	3.83	2.82	1.24	54.43	30.62	
Pompano, Florida, fillet, bkd/brld														

Vit E (mg)	Vit C	Vit B$_1$ Thia (mg)	Vit B$_2$ Ribo (mg)	Vit B$_3$ Nia (mg)	Fol (mcg)	Vit B$_6$ (mg)	Vita B$_{12}$ (mcg)	Sodi (mg)	Pota (mg)	Cal (mg)	Phos (mg)	Magn (mg)	Iron (mg)	Zinc (mg)	Caff (mg)	Alco (g)	Sol Fiber (g)	Insol Fiber (g)
0.30	0.00	0.07	0.10	1.21	24.51	0.03	1.03	331.74	148.77	11.40	103.17	14.25	0.42	0.38	0.00	0.00		
0.22	0.85	0.08	0.07	1.24	14.46	0.12	1.96	87.60	381.87	87.60	196.47	32.32	1.31	1.69	0.00	0.00	0.00	0.00
0.75	3.15	0.29	0.11	6.84	28.92	0.55	2.38	51.88	326.59	12.76	214.33	25.52	0.29	0.37	0.00	0.00	0.00	0.00
1.07	0.00	0.23	0.41	8.57	24.66	0.80	2.59	47.63	534.11	12.76	217.73	31.47	0.88	0.70	0.00	0.00	0.00	0.00
1.45	3.49	0.04	0.13	8.54	29.77	0.39	2.44	51.03	429.50	23.81	315.54	103.76	0.77	0.48	0.00	0.00	0.00	0.00
1.15	0.00	0.02	0.09	4.01	1.70	0.24	2.77	666.79	148.84	9.36	139.48	15.31	0.72	0.26	0.00	0.00	0.00	0.00
1.36	0.00	0.02	0.14	5.95	17.01	0.32	3.74	63.79	255.15	211.77	301.08	25.52	0.60	0.85	0.00	0.00	0.00	0.00
0.48	1.28	0.09	0.10	6.29	11.91	0.48	2.70	44.23	391.23	10.21	282.37	28.92	0.33	0.40	0.00	0.00	0.00	0.00
0.69	1.19	0.06	0.12	6.76	11.06	0.48	4.25	49.33	369.12	38.27	273.86	28.07	0.52	0.48	0.00	0.00	0.00	0.00
0.69	0.85	0.10	0.14	6.62	7.65	0.47	3.81	45.08	386.98	39.12	253.45	29.77	0.60	0.44	0.00	0.00	0.00	0.00
1.07	0.00	0.17	0.06	7.25	4.25	0.20	2.94	73.14	352.11	14.46	250.90	28.07	0.84	0.60	0.00	0.00	0.00	0.00
0.54	0.00	0.02	0.16	5.56	12.76	0.26	3.74	471.18	277.26	181.16	279.81	28.92	0.71	0.78	0.00	0.00	0.00	0.00
1.74	0.00	0.07	0.19	4.46	10.21	0.14	7.60	429.50	337.65	324.89	416.75	33.17	2.48	1.11	0.00	0.00	0.00	0.00
1.22	0.85	0.04	0.20	3.57	20.41	0.10	7.65	352.11	290.02	204.12	311.28	28.92	1.96	1.19	0.00	0.00		
0.21	0.00	0.06	0.18	2.49	5.10	0.39	2.94	62.94	371.67	18.71	273.01	34.02	0.30	0.49	0.00	0.00	0.00	0.00
1.07	0.00	0.16	0.26	9.16	14.46	0.39	0.12	55.28	418.45	51.03	296.82	32.32	1.05	0.40	0.00	0.00	0.00	0.00
0.89	0.00	0.06	0.08	2.37	12.76	0.26	1.03	103.76	131.83	42.53	165.00	36.57	0.94	0.41	0.00	0.00	0.00	0.00
1.13	0.00	0.05	0.07	3.33	3.40	0.45	1.69	89.59	181.44	38.56	238.14	55.57	0.95	0.49	0.00	0.00	0.00	0.00
0.54	1.36	0.05	0.00	0.29	5.10	0.39	2.98	48.48	443.96	34.02	170.95	31.47	0.20	0.37	0.00	0.00	0.00	0.00
		0.05	0.02	1.51				94.08	376.33	15.05	150.53		0.27		0.00	0.00	0.00	0.00
0.54	0.94	0.04	0.10	10.03	1.70	0.32	1.72	97.81	313.83	5.10	286.62	28.92	0.88	1.25	0.00	0.00	0.00	0.00
0.22	0.43	0.36	0.36	4.91	12.76	0.20	6.37	56.98	393.78	46.78	267.06	23.81	1.63	0.72	0.00	0.00	0.00	0.00
0.03	2.81	0.20	0.07	7.48	20.41	0.34	4.23	35.72	375.07	73.14	226.23	27.22	0.28	0.42	0.00	0.00	0.00	0.00
0.43	1.70	0.13	0.08	4.91	16.16	0.29	5.36	47.63	381.02	73.14	228.78	26.37	0.32	0.43	0.00	0.00	0.00	0.00
1.07	0.00	0.24	0.26	8.96	1.70	0.45	9.25	42.53	274.71	8.51	277.26	54.43	1.11	0.65	0.00	0.00	0.00	0.00
0.64	0.00	0.03	0.09	9.06	3.65	0.08	1.61	258.42	151.11	9.49	227.03	22.63	1.01	0.66	0.00	0.00	0.00	0.00
1.02	0.00	0.03	0.10	10.55	4.25	0.09	1.87	42.53	176.05	11.06	264.51	26.37	1.18	0.77	0.00	0.00	0.00	0.00
	0.00							345.00	0.00	0.00			0.00		0.00	0.00	0.00	0.00
0.25	0.00	0.03	0.05	10.22	3.08	0.27	2.30	260.26	182.49	8.47	125.51	20.79	1.18	0.59	0.00	0.00	0.00	0.00
1.96	0.00	0.01	0.07	9.95	4.25	0.37	1.87	336.80	283.22	3.40	227.08	28.92	0.55	0.40	0.00	0.00	0.00	0.00
0.72	0.00	0.01	0.04	4.93	1.70	0.18	1.00	320.64	201.57	11.91	184.56	28.07	0.82	0.41	0.00	0.00	0.00	0.00
0.54	0.85	0.43	0.05	10.15	1.70	0.88	0.51	39.97	483.93	17.86	208.37	54.43	0.80	0.57	0.00	0.00	0.00	0.00
0.21	1.45	0.06	0.08	2.28	7.65	0.21	2.16	163.30	259.40	19.56	140.33	55.28	0.39	0.24	0.00	0.00	0.00	0.00
0.21	0.00	0.15	0.13	3.27	14.46	0.29	0.82	55.28	345.30	28.07	294.27	35.72	0.40	1.08	0.00	0.00	0.00	0.00
0.26	0.00	0.06	0.05	1.42	12.76	0.15	2.21	112.27	369.12	52.73	242.39	22.96	0.36	0.45	0.00	0.00	0.00	0.00
0.21	2.47	0.15	0.04	7.41	3.40	0.16	1.06	42.53	457.57	24.66	170.95	32.32	0.54	0.57	0.00	0.00	0.00	0.00
0.74	2.40	0.02	0.05	0.43	4.80	0.02	12.00	516.00	357.60	31.20	273.60	26.40	0.72	0.24	0.00	0.00	0.00	0.00
1.67	0.00	0.01	0.05	1.65	10.21	0.07	1.05	335.66	311.85	54.43	163.30	30.62	0.34	3.42	0.00	0.00	0.00	0.00
1.67	2.27	0.01	0.05	4.81	1.13	0.17	3.97	200.72	204.12	55.57	269.89	45.36	1.38	6.43	0.00	0.00	0.00	0.00
0.62	9.07	0.18	0.24	1.81	47.63	0.06	13.61	324.32	362.88	29.48	223.40	38.56	4.48	1.81	0.00	0.00	0.00	0.00
0.68	5.10	0.11	0.05	1.52	20.41	0.06	20.67	138.63	129.28	47.63	97.81	28.07	6.61	38.40	0.00	0.00	0.00	0.00
0.72	3.49	0.07	0.07	1.42	15.31	0.08	23.64	207.52	142.88	38.27	115.67	39.12	3.68	62.60	0.00	0.00	0.00	0.00
0.77	5.33	0.12	0.07	1.44	20.41	0.07	18.37	201.85	140.62	49.90	105.46	37.42	6.55	43.00	0.00	0.00	0.00	0.00
0.19	0.00	0.58	0.13	3.23	14.46	0.20	1.02	64.64	540.92	36.57	290.02	26.37	0.57	0.59	0.00	0.00	0.00	0.00

Food Name	Amount	Measure	Weight (g)	Calories	Protein (g)	Total Carb (g)	Dietary Fiber (g)	Total Fat (g)	Sat Fat (g)	Mono Fat (g)	Poly Fat (g)	Chol (mg)	Vit A (mcg RAE)	Vit D (mcg)
FISH, SEAFOOD, AND SHELLFISH *(continued)*														
Roe, black/red, granular	1	Tablespoon	16.00	40.32	3.94	0.64	0.00	2.86	0.65	0.74	1.18	94.08	89.76	0.93
Sashimi, mackerel, Pacific & jack, fillet	4	Ounce-weight	113.40	179.17	22.76	0.00	0.00	8.95	2.55	2.98	2.20	53.30	14.74	
Sashimi, salmon, chinook, fillet	4	Ounce-weight	113.40	202.99	22.60	0.00	0.00	11.83	3.52	4.99	3.17	56.70	154.22	
Sashimi, snapper, fillet, mixed species	4	Ounce-weight	113.40	113.40	23.26	0.00	0.00	1.52	0.32	0.28	0.52	41.96	34.02	
Sashimi, tuna, skipjack, fillet,	4	Ounce-weight	113.40	116.80	24.95	0.00	0.00	1.15	0.37	0.22	0.36	53.30	18.14	
Sashimi, tuna, yellowfin, fillet, w/o bone, 1" cube	4	Ounce-weight	113.40	122.47	26.51	0.00	0.00	1.08	0.27	0.17	0.32	51.03	20.41	
Sashimi, yellowtail, fillet, mixed species	4	Ounce-weight	113.40	165.56	26.24	0.00	0.00	5.94	1.45	2.26	1.61	62.37	32.89	
Scallops, raw, mixed species, lrg	4	Ounce-weight	113.40	99.79	19.03	2.68	0.00	0.86	0.09	0.04	0.30	37.42	17.01	
Shrimp, ckd, lrg, mixed species, each	3	Ounce-weight	85.05	84.20	17.78	0.00	0.00	0.92	0.25	0.17	0.37	165.85	57.83	
Shrimp, imit f/surimi, mixed species	3	Ounce-weight	85.05	85.90	10.54	7.77	0.00	1.25	0.25	0.19	0.64	30.62	17.01	
Shrimp, raw, lrg, mixed species	4	Ounce-weight	113.40	120.20	23.03	1.03	0.00	1.96	0.37	0.29	0.76	172.37	61.24	4.31
Surimi	3	Ounce-weight	85.05	84.20	12.91	5.83	0.00	0.77	0.16	0.13	0.38	25.52	17.01	
FOOD ADDITIVES														
Gums, Fibers, Starches, Pectins, Emulsifiers														
Pectin, unswtnd, dry, 1.75oz pkg	1	Each	49.61	161.24	0.00	44.65	4.47	0.00	0.00	0.00	0.00	0.00	0.00	
Starch, corn	1	Tablespoon	8.00	30.48	0.02	7.30	0.07	0.00	0.00	0.00	0.00	0.00	0.00	
Ingredient Sweeteners Nutraceuticals Nutritional Additives														
Bee Pollen	1	Teaspoon	5.00	15.70	1.21	2.18	0.39	0.25	0.17	0.02	0.03	0.00	0.00	
Multi Vitamin & Mineral, active formula, tablet Bayer Corporation	1	Each	1.75	0.00	0.00	0.00	0.00	0.00	0.00	0.00	0.00			10.00
Multi Vitamin & Mineral, Daily One Caps, w/iron, capsule Twin Laboratories	1	Each	1.75	0.00	0.00	0.03	0.00	0.00	0.00	0.00	0.00		500.00	10.00
Multi Vitamin & Mineral, Daily One Caps, w/o iron, capsule Twin Laboratories	1	Each	1.75	0.00	0.00	0.03	0.00	0.00	0.00	0.00	0.00		500.00	10.00
Multi Vitamin & Mineral, Daily One Complete, w/iron, capsule Optimum Nutrition	1	Each	1.17	0.10	0.00	0.03	0.00	0.00	0.00	0.00	0.00	0.00		10.00
Multi Vitamin & Mineral, maximum formula, tablet Bayer Corporation	1	Each	1.75	0.00	0.00	0.00	0.00	0.00	0.00	0.00	0.00	3.00		10.00
Multi Vitamin & Mineral, men's formula, tablet Bayer Corporation	1	Each	1.75	0.00	0.00	0.00	0.00	0.00	0.00	0.00	0.00			10.00
Multi Vitamin & Mineral, One A Day, women's formula, tablet Bayer Corporation	1	Each	1.75	0.00	0.00	0.00	0.00	0.00	0.00	0.00	0.00			10.00
Multi Vitamin, essential formula, tablet Bayer Corporation	1	Each	1.75	0.00	0.00	0.00	0.00	0.00	0.00	0.00	0.00			10.00
Protein, soy, conc, produced by acid wash	1	Ounce-weight	28.35	93.84	16.48	8.76	1.56	0.13	0.02	0.02	0.06	0.00	0.00	
Protein, soy, isolate	1	Ounce-weight	28.35	95.82	22.88	2.09	1.59	0.96	0.12	0.18	0.46	0.00	0.00	
Protein, soy, isolate, Supro Protein Technologies International	1	Ounce-weight	28.35	110.00	24.88	0.00	0.00	1.13	0.25	0.19	0.49	0.00	0.00	
Yeast, nutritional, flakes Now Foods	2	Tablespoon	16.00	50.00	8.00	5.00	4.00	0.65	0.00			0.00	0.00	
FRUIT, VEGETABLE, AND BLENDED JUICES														
Juice, apple, unswtnd, w/vit C, cnd/btld	1	Cup	248.00	116.56	0.15	28.97	0.25	0.27	0.05	0.01	0.08	0.00	0.12	0.00
Juice, apple, unswtnd, w/vit C, prep f/fzn conc w/water	1	Cup	239.00	112.33	0.33	27.58	0.24	0.24	0.04	0.00	0.07	0.00	0.00	0.00
Juice, apricot nectar, w/add vit C, cnd	1	Cup	251.00	140.56	0.93	36.12	1.51	0.23	0.02	0.10	0.04	0.00	165.66	
Juice, carrot	1	Cup	236.00	49.56	1.49	11.49		0.35	0.07	0.02	0.17	0.00	257.59	
Juice, cranberry cocktail, btld	1	Cup	252.80	144.10	0.00	36.40	0.25	0.25	0.02	0.04	0.11	0.00	0.51	
Juice, cranberry cocktail, prep f/fzn conc w/water	1	Cup	249.60	137.28	0.00	34.94	0.25	0.00	0.00	0.00	0.00	0.00	2.50	0.00
Juice, grape, swtnd, w/add vit C, prep f/fzn conc w/water	1	Cup	250.00	127.50	0.48	31.88	0.25	0.22	0.07	0.01	0.06	0.00	1.00	
Juice, grapefruit cocktail, ruby red, rtd Season's Best	1	Cup	247.20	130.00	1.00	33.00	0.00	0.00	0.00	0.00	0.00	0.00	0.00	
Juice, grapefruit, pink, fresh, cup	1	Cup	247.00	96.33	1.24	22.72	0.25	0.25	0.03	0.03	0.06	0.00	54.34	0.00
Juice, grapefruit, swtnd, cnd, cup	1	Cup	250.00	115.00	1.45	27.83	0.25	0.22	0.03	0.03	0.05	0.00	0.88	
Juice, grapefruit, unswtnd, cnd, cup	1	Cup	247.00	93.86	1.28	22.13	0.25	0.25	0.03	0.03	0.06	0.00	0.86	
Juice, grapefruit, unswtnd, prep f/fzn														

Vit E (mg)	Vit C	Vit B₁ Thia (mg)	Vit B₂ Ribo (mg)	Vit B₃ Nia (mg)	Fol (mcg)	Vit B₆ (mg)	Vita B₁₂ (mcg)	Sodi (mg)	Pota (mg)	Cal (mg)	Phos (mg)	Magn (mg)	Iron (mg)	Zinc (mg)	Caff (mg)	Alco (g)	Sol Fiber (g)	Insol Fiber (g)
1.12	0.00	0.03	0.10	0.02	8.00	0.05	3.20	240.00	28.96	44.00	56.96	48.00	1.90	0.15	0.00	0.00	0.00	0.00
1.13	2.27	0.13	0.48	9.43	2.27	0.37	4.99	97.52	460.40	26.08	141.75	31.75	1.32	0.76	0.00	0.00	0.00	0.00
1.38	4.54	0.06	0.13	9.55	34.02	0.45	1.47	53.30	446.80	29.48	327.73	107.73	0.28	0.50	0.00	0.00	0.00	0.00
0.57	1.81	0.05	0.00	0.32	5.67	0.45	3.40	72.58	472.88	36.29	224.53	36.29	0.20	0.41	0.00	0.00	0.00	0.00
1.13	1.13	0.04	0.11	17.46	10.21	0.96	2.15	41.96	461.54	32.89	251.75	38.56	1.42	0.93	0.00	0.00	0.00	0.00
0.57	1.13	0.49	0.05	11.11	2.27	1.02	0.59	41.96	503.50	18.14	216.59	56.70	0.83	0.59	0.00	0.00	0.00	0.00
0.20	3.18	0.16	0.05	7.71	4.54	0.18	1.47	44.23	476.28	26.08	178.04	34.02	0.56	0.59	0.00	0.00	0.00	0.00
0.00	3.40	0.01	0.07	1.30	18.14	0.17	1.74	182.57	365.15	27.22	248.35	63.50	0.33	1.08	0.00	0.00	0.00	0.00
1.17	1.87	0.03	0.03	2.20	3.40	0.11	1.27	190.51	154.79	33.17	116.52	28.92	2.63	1.33	0.00	0.00	0.00	0.00
0.09	0.00	0.02	0.03	0.14	1.70	0.03	1.36	599.60	75.69	16.16	239.84	36.57	0.51	0.28	0.00	0.00	0.00	0.00
1.25	2.27	0.03	0.04	2.89	3.40	0.12	1.32	167.83	209.79	58.97	232.47	41.96	2.73	1.26	0.00	0.00	0.00	0.00
0.54	0.00		0.02	0.19	1.70	0.03	1.36	121.62	95.26	7.65	239.84	36.57	0.22	0.28	0.00	0.00	0.00	0.00
0.00	0.00	0.00	0.00	0.00	0.50	0.00	0.00	99.22	3.47	3.47	0.99	0.50	1.49	0.00	0.00	0.00		
0.00	0.00	0.00	0.00	0.00	0.00	0.00	0.00	0.72	0.24	0.16	1.04	0.24	0.04	0.00	0.00	0.00		
0.27	2.50	0.02	0.04	0.23	0.00	0.02	0.00	0.25	11.10	4.05	4.55	2.60	0.32	0.28	0.00	0.00		
27.27	120.00	4.50	5.10	40.00	400.00	6.00	18.00		200.00	110.00	48.00	40.00	9.00	15.00	0.00	0.00	0.00	0.00
67.11	150.00	25.00	25.00	100.00	400.00	25.00	100.00		5.00	25.00		7.20	10.00	15.00	0.00	0.00	0.00	0.00
67.11	150.00	25.00	25.00	100.00	400.00	25.00	100.00		5.00	25.00		7.20		15.00	0.00	0.00	0.00	0.00
67.11	150.00	25.00	25.00	100.00	400.00	25.00	100.00		5.00	25.00		7.20	10.00	15.00	0.00	0.00	0.00	0.00
13.64	60.00	1.50	1.70	20.00	400.00	2.00	6.00		80.00	162.00	109.00	100.00	18.00	15.00	0.00	0.00	0.00	0.00
20.45	90.00	2.25	2.55	20.00	400.00	3.00	9.00		37.50			100.00		15.00	0.00	0.00	0.00	0.00
13.64	60.00	1.50	1.70	20.00	400.00	2.00	6.00			450.00			27.00	15.00	0.00	0.00	0.00	0.00
13.64	60.00	1.50	1.70	20.00	400.00	2.00	6.00								0.00	0.00	0.00	0.00
0.00	0.00	0.09	0.04	0.20	96.39	0.04	0.00	255.15	127.57	102.91	237.86	39.69	3.05	1.25	0.00	0.00	0.14	1.42
0.00	0.00	0.05	0.03	0.41	49.90	0.03	0.00	284.92	22.96	50.46	220.00	11.06	4.11	1.14	0.00	0.00		
	0.00	0.06	0.03	0.09	56.70		0.00	336.80	28.35	56.70	244.38	11.34	4.54	1.13	0.00	0.00	0.00	0.00
	0.00	9.60	9.52	56.00	240.00	9.60	7.80	5.00	320.00				0.72		0.00	0.00		
0.02	103.17	0.05	0.04	0.25	0.00	0.07	0.00	7.44	295.12	17.36	17.36	7.44	0.92	0.07	0.00	0.00	0.25	0.00
0.02	59.75	0.01	0.04	0.09	0.00	0.08	0.00	16.73	301.14	14.34	16.73	11.95	0.62	0.10	0.00	0.00	0.24	0.00
0.23	136.54	0.02	0.04	0.65	2.51	0.06	0.00	7.53	286.14	17.57	22.59	12.55	0.95	0.23	0.00	0.00	0.75	0.75
	8.92						0.00	122.72	516.84	63.72	73.16				0.00	0.00		
0.00	89.49	0.02	0.02	0.09	0.00	0.05	0.00	5.06	45.50	7.58	5.06	5.06	0.38	0.18	0.00	0.00		
0.02	24.71	0.02	0.02	0.03	0.00	0.03	0.00	7.49	34.94	12.48	2.50	4.99	0.22	0.10	0.00	0.00		
0.00	59.75	0.04	0.06	0.31	2.50	0.11	0.00	5.00	52.50	10.00	10.00	10.00	0.25	0.10	0.00	0.00	0.08	0.18
0.00	60.00	0.00		0.00	0.00	0.00		30.00	0.00	0.00			0.00		0.00	0.00	0.00	0.00
0.10	93.86	0.10	0.05	0.49	24.70	0.11	0.00	2.47	400.14	22.23	37.05	29.64	0.49	0.12	0.00	0.00		
0.10	67.25	0.10	0.06	0.80	25.00	0.05	0.00	5.00	405.00	20.00	27.50	25.00	0.90	0.15	0.00	0.00	0.08	0.18
0.10	72.12	0.10	0.05	0.57	24.70	0.05	0.00	2.47	377.91	17.29	27.17	24.70	0.49	0.22	0.00	0.00	0.07	0.17

Food Name	Amount	Measure	Weight (g)	Calories	Protein (g)	Total Carb (g)	Dietary Fiber (g)	Total Fat (g)	Sat Fat (g)	Mono Fat (g)	Poly Fat (g)	Chol (mg)	Vit A (mcg RAE)	Vit D (mcg)
FRUIT, VEGETABLE, AND BLENDED JUICES *(continued)*														
conc w/water	1	Cup	247.00	101.27	1.36	24.03	0.25	0.32	0.05	0.04	0.08	0.00	1.11	
Juice, grapefruit, white, fresh, yield per fruit	1	Each	196.00	76.44	0.98	18.03	0.20	0.20	0.03	0.03	0.05	0.00	3.92	
Juice, lemon, cnd/btld, cup	1	Cup	244.00	51.24	0.98	15.81	0.98	0.71	0.09	0.03	0.21	0.00	2.44	
Juice, lemon, fresh	1	Cup	244.00	61.00	0.93	21.06	0.98	0.00	0.00	0.00	0.00	0.00	2.44	
Juice, lime, fresh, yield per wedge	1	Each	5.00	1.25	0.02	0.42	0.02	0.00	0.00	0.00	0.00	0.00	0.10	
Juice, lime, unswtnd, cnd/btld, cup	1	Cup	246.00	51.66	0.62	16.46	0.98	0.57	0.06	0.05	0.16	0.00	2.46	
Juice, orange grapefruit, unswtnd, cnd, cup	1	Cup	247.00	106.21	1.48	25.39	0.25	0.25	0.03	0.04	0.05	0.00	14.82	
Juice, orange, fresh, yield per fruit	1	Each	86.00	38.70	0.60	8.94	0.17	0.17	0.02	0.03	0.03	0.00	8.60	
Juice, orange, unswtnd, cnd, cup	1	Cup	249.00	104.58	1.47	24.53	0.50	0.35	0.04	0.06	0.08	0.00	22.41	
Juice, orange, unswtnd, prep f/fzn conc w/water	1	Cup	249.00	112.05	1.69	26.84	0.50	0.15	0.02	0.02	0.03	0.00	12.45	
Juice, papaya nectar, cnd, cup	1	Cup	250.00	142.50	0.43	36.28	1.50	0.38	0.12	0.10	0.09	0.00	45.00	
Juice, passion fruit, purple, fresh	1	Cup	247.00	125.97	0.96	33.59	0.49	0.12	0.01	0.01	0.07	0.00	88.92	
Juice, peach nectar, w/add vit C, cnd	1	Cup	249.00	134.46	0.67	34.66	1.49	0.05	0.00	0.02	0.03	0.00	32.37	0.00
Juice, pear nectar, w/add vit C, cnd	1	Cup	250.00	150.00	0.28	39.40	1.50	0.02	0.00	0.01	0.01	0.00	0.12	0.00
Juice, pineapple, unswtnd, w/add vit C, cnd	1	Cup	250.00	140.00	0.80	34.45	0.50	0.20	0.01	0.02	0.07	0.00	0.62	0.00
Juice, tangerine, swtnd, cnd, cup	1	Cup	249.00	124.50	1.25	29.88	0.50	0.50	0.03	0.04	0.06	0.00	32.37	
Juice, tomato, cnd	1	Cup	243.00	41.31	1.85	10.30	0.97	0.12	0.02	0.02	0.06	0.00	55.89	
Juice, tomato, unsalted, cnd	1	Cup	243.00	41.31	1.85	10.30	0.97	0.12	0.02	0.02	0.06	0.00	55.89	
Juice, vegetable cocktail, cnd	1	Cup	242.00	45.98	1.52	11.01	1.94	0.22	0.03	0.03	0.09	0.00	188.76	
FRUITS														
Apples, fresh, med, 2 3/4"	1	Each	138.00	71.76	0.36	19.06	3.31	0.23	0.04	0.01	0.07	0.00	4.14	
Apples, fresh, peeled, med, 2 3/4"	1	Each	128.00	61.44	0.35	16.33	1.66	0.17	0.03	0.01	0.05	0.00	2.56	
Apples, slices, swtnd, drained, cnd, unheated	0.5	Cup	102.00	68.34	0.18	17.03	1.73	0.50	0.08	0.02	0.15	0.00	3.06	
Apples, sulfured, dehyd, unckd, cup	0.5	Cup	30.00	103.80	0.40	28.06	3.72	0.17	0.03	0.01	0.05	0.00	1.20	0.00
Apples, unswtnd, unheated, fzn	0.5	Cup	86.50	41.52	0.24	10.65	1.64	0.28	0.04	0.01	0.08	0.00	1.73	0.00
Applesauce, swtnd, cnd	0.5	Cup	127.50	96.90	0.23	25.38	1.53	0.23	0.04	0.01	0.07	0.00	1.27	0.00
Applesauce, unswtnd, w/o add Vit C, cnd	0.5	Cup	122.00	52.46	0.21	13.78	1.46	0.06	0.01	0.00	0.02	0.00	1.22	
Apricots, dried, California Sunsweet Growers Inc.	5	Each	40.00	100.00	1.00	24.00	4.00	0.00	0.00	0.00	0.00	0.00	90.00	
Apricots, fresh, whole, each	1	Each	35.00	16.80	0.49	3.89	0.70	0.14	0.01	0.06	0.03	0.00	33.60	
Apricots, halves, w/skin, w/juice, cnd	0.5	Cup	122.00	58.56	0.77	15.06	1.95	0.05	0.00	0.02	0.01	0.00	103.70	
Apricots, halves, w/skin, w/light syrup	0.5	Cup	126.50	79.69	0.67	20.86	2.02	0.06	0.00	0.03	0.01	0.00	83.49	
Apricots, swtnd, fzn	0.5	Cup	121.00	118.58	0.85	30.37	2.66	0.12	0.01	0.05	0.03	0.00	101.64	
Apricots, w/o skin, w/water, cnd	0.5	Cup	113.50	24.97	0.79	6.22	1.25	0.03	0.00	0.02	0.01	0.00	103.29	0.00
Apricots, whole, w/o skin & pit, w/heavy syrup, cnd	0.5	Cup	129.00	107.07	0.65	27.67	2.06	0.12	0.01	0.05	0.02	0.00	79.98	0.00
Avocado, avg, fresh, each	1	Each	201.00	321.60	4.02	17.15	13.47	29.47	4.27	19.70	3.65	0.00	14.07	
Avocado, Florida, fresh, each	1	Each	304.00	364.80	6.78	23.77	16.66	30.58	5.96	16.76	5.10	0.00	21.28	
Banana, chips	1	Ounce-weight	28.35	147.14	0.65	16.56	2.18	9.53	8.21	0.56	0.18	0.00	1.13	
Banana, fresh, extra lrg, 9" or longer, each	1	Each	152.00	135.28	1.66	34.72	3.95	0.50	0.17	0.05	0.11	0.00	4.56	
Banana, fresh, mashed, cup	0.5	Cup	112.50	100.12	1.23	25.70	2.92	0.37	0.13	0.03	0.08	0.00	3.37	
Banana, fresh, slices, cup	0.5	Cup	75.00	66.75	0.82	17.13	1.95	0.25	0.09	0.02	0.05	0.00	2.25	
Banana, fresh, sml, 6" to 6 7/8" long, each	1	Each	101.00	89.89	1.10	23.07	2.63	0.33	0.11	0.03	0.07	0.00	3.03	
Banana, pwd	1	Tablespoon	6.20	21.45	0.24	5.47	0.61	0.11	0.04	0.01	0.02	0.00	0.74	
Blackberries, unswtnd, fzn, cup	0.5	Cup	75.50	48.32	0.89	11.83	3.78	0.32	0.01	0.03	0.18	0.00	4.53	
Blueberries, fresh, cup	0.5	Cup	72.50	41.32	0.54	10.50	1.74	0.24	0.02	0.04	0.10	0.00	2.17	
Blueberries, unswtnd, fzn, pkg	0.5	Cup	77.50	39.52	0.33	9.43	2.09	0.50	0.04	0.07	0.22	0.00	1.55	
Blueberries, w/heavy syrup, cnd, not drained, cup	0.5	Cup	128.00	112.64	0.83	28.23	2.05	0.42	0.04	0.06	0.18	0.00	2.56	
Boysenberries, fresh, cup	0.5	Cup	72.00	30.96	1.00	6.92	3.67	0.35	0.01	0.04	0.20	0.00	7.92	
Boysenberries, unswtnd, fzn, pkg	0.5	Cup	66.00	33.00	0.73	8.05	3.50	0.17	0.00	0.01	0.10	0.00	1.98	
Breadfruit, fresh, each	0.25	Each	96.00	98.88	1.03	26.04	4.70	0.22	0.05	0.03	0.06	0.00	0.00	
Carambola, fresh, sml, 3" long, each	1	Each	70.00	21.70	0.73	4.71	1.95	0.23	0.01	0.02	0.13	0.00	2.10	
Carissa, fresh, w/o skin & seeds, each	1	Each	20.00	12.40	0.10	2.73		0.26				0.00	0.40	
Chayote, ckd, drained, 1" pces, cup	0.5	Cup	80.00	19.20	0.50	4.08	2.24	0.39	0.07	0.03	0.16	0.00	1.60	
Cherimoya, fresh, each	0.25	Each	136.75	101.20	2.26	24.20	3.15	0.85				0.00	0.00	
Cherries, maraschino, cnd, drained	1	Each	4.00	6.60	0.01	1.68	0.13	0.01	0.00	0.00	0.00	0.00	0.08	

Vit E (mg)	Vit C	Vit B₁ Thia (mg)	Vit B₂ Ribo (mg)	Vit B₃ Nia (mg)	Fol (mcg)	Vit B₆ (mg)	Vita B₁₂ (mcg)	Sodi (mg)	Pota (mg)	Cal (mg)	Phos (mg)	Magn (mg)	Iron (mg)	Zinc (mg)	Caff (mg)	Alco (g)	Sol Fiber (g)	Insol Fiber (g)
0.10	83.24	0.10	0.05	0.54	9.88	0.11	0.00	2.47	335.92	19.76	34.58	27.17	0.35	0.12	0.00	0.00	0.07	0.17
0.43	74.48	0.08	0.04	0.39	19.60	0.09	0.00	1.96	317.52	17.64	29.40	23.52	0.39	0.10	0.00	0.00	0.06	0.14
0.37	60.51	0.10	0.02	0.48	24.40	0.10	0.00	51.24	248.88	26.84	21.96	19.52	0.32	0.15	0.00	0.00	0.46	0.51
0.37	112.24	0.07	0.02	0.24	31.72	0.12	0.00	2.44	302.56	17.08	14.64	14.64	0.07	0.12	0.00	0.00	0.46	0.51
0.01	1.50	0.00	0.00	0.01	0.50	0.00	0.00	0.10	5.85	0.70	0.70	0.40	0.00	0.00	0.00	0.00		
0.30	15.74	0.08	0.01	0.40	19.68	0.07	0.00	39.36	184.50	29.52	24.60	17.22	0.57	0.15	0.00	0.00		
0.35	71.88	0.14	0.07	0.83	34.58	0.06	0.00	7.41	390.26	19.76	34.58	24.70	1.14	0.17	0.00	0.00	0.05	0.20
0.03	43.00	0.08	0.03	0.34	25.80	0.03	0.00	0.86	172.00	9.46	14.62	9.46	0.17	0.04	0.00	0.00	0.05	0.12
0.50	85.66	0.15	0.07	0.78	44.82	0.22	0.00	4.98	435.75	19.92	34.86	27.39	1.10	0.17	0.00	0.00	0.10	0.40
0.50	96.86	0.20	0.04	0.50	109.56	0.11	0.00	2.49	473.10	22.41	39.84	24.90	0.25	0.12	0.00	0.00	0.16	0.34
0.60	7.50	0.02	0.01	0.38	5.00	0.02	0.00	12.50	77.50	25.00	0.00	7.50	0.85	0.38	0.00	0.00	0.70	0.80
0.02	73.61	0.00	0.32	3.61	17.29	0.12	0.00	14.82	686.66	9.88	32.11	41.99	0.59	0.12	0.00	0.00	0.25	0.25
0.20	66.73	0.01	0.03	0.72	2.49	0.02	0.00	17.43	99.60	12.45	14.94	9.96	0.47	0.20	0.00	0.00	1.00	0.50
0.25	67.50	0.00	0.03	0.32	2.50	0.04	0.00	10.00	32.50	12.50	7.50	7.50	0.65	0.18	0.00	0.00	0.30	1.20
0.05	60.00	0.14	0.05	0.64	57.50	0.24	0.00	2.50	335.00	42.50	20.00	32.50	0.65	0.28	0.00	0.00	0.15	0.35
0.37	54.78	0.15	0.05	0.25	12.45	0.08	0.00	2.49	443.22	44.82	34.86	19.92	0.50	0.07	0.00	0.00	0.15	0.35
0.78	44.47	0.11	0.08	1.64	48.60	0.27	0.00	653.67	556.47	24.30	43.74	26.73	1.04	0.36	0.00	0.00	0.24	0.73
0.78	44.47	0.11	0.08	1.64	48.60	0.27	0.00	24.30	556.47	24.30	43.74	26.73	1.04	0.36	0.00	0.00		
0.77	67.03	0.10	0.07	1.76	50.82	0.34	0.00	653.40	467.06	26.62	41.14	26.62	1.02	0.48	0.00	0.00		
0.25	6.35	0.02	0.04	0.13	4.14	0.06	0.00	1.38	147.66	8.28	15.18	6.90	0.17	0.06	0.00	0.00	0.33	2.98
0.06	5.12	0.02	0.04	0.12	0.00	0.05	0.00	0.00	115.20	6.40	14.08	5.12	0.09	0.06	0.00	0.00	0.22	1.45
0.21	0.41	0.01	0.01	0.07	0.00	0.04	0.00	3.06	69.36	4.08	5.10	2.04	0.23	0.03	0.00	0.00	0.51	1.22
0.22	0.66	0.02	0.04	0.20	0.30	0.08	0.00	37.20	192.00	5.70	16.50	6.60	0.60	0.09	0.00	0.00		
0.93	0.09	0.01	0.01	0.04	0.87	0.03	0.00	2.60	66.61	3.46	6.92	2.60	0.15	0.04	0.00	0.00		
0.06	2.17	0.02	0.04	0.24	1.27	0.04	0.00	35.70	77.77	5.10	8.92	3.82	0.45	0.05	0.00	0.00	0.38	1.15
0.25	1.46	0.02	0.03	0.23	1.22	0.03	0.00	2.44	91.50	3.66	8.54	3.66	0.15	0.03	0.00	0.00		
	1.20						0.00	0.00	520.00	20.00			1.08		0.00	0.00		
0.31	3.50	0.01	0.01	0.21	3.15	0.02	0.00	0.35	90.65	4.55	8.05	3.50	0.14	0.07	0.00	0.00		
0.73	5.98	0.03	0.03	0.42	2.44	0.07	0.00	4.88	201.30	14.64	24.40	12.20	0.37	0.13	0.00	0.00	0.84	1.12
0.76	3.42	0.02	0.03	0.39	2.53	0.07	0.00	5.06	174.57	13.91	16.44	10.12	0.50	0.14	0.00	0.00	0.77	1.26
1.08	10.89	0.03	0.05	0.97	2.42	0.07	0.00	4.84	277.09	12.10	22.99	10.89	1.09	0.12	0.00	0.00	0.93	1.73
1.01	2.04	0.02	0.02	0.49	2.27	0.06	0.00	12.49	174.79	9.08	18.16	10.22	0.62	0.12	0.00	0.00	0.85	0.40
1.15	3.61	0.03	0.03	0.53	2.58	0.07	0.00	14.19	172.86	11.61	16.77	10.32	0.55	0.13	0.00			
4.16	20.10	0.13	0.26	3.49	162.81	0.52	0.00	14.07	974.85	24.12	104.52	58.29	1.11	1.29				
8.09	52.90	0.06	0.16	2.04	106.40	0.24	0.00	6.08	1067.04	30.40	121.60	72.96	0.52	1.22	0.00	0.00		
0.07	1.79	0.03	0.01	0.20	3.97	0.08	0.00	1.70	151.96	5.10	15.88	21.55	0.36	0.22	0.00	0.00	0.60	1.59
0.15	13.22	0.05	0.11	1.01	30.40	0.56	0.00	1.52	544.16	7.60	33.44	41.04	0.40	0.23	0.00	0.00		
0.11	9.79	0.03	0.08	0.75	22.50	0.41	0.00	1.12	402.75	5.62	24.75	30.37	0.29	0.17	0.00	0.00		
0.07	6.52	0.02	0.05	0.50	15.00	0.27	0.00	0.75	268.50	3.75	16.50	20.25	0.19	0.11	0.00	0.00		
0.10	8.79	0.03	0.07	0.67	20.20	0.37	0.00	1.01	361.58	5.05	22.22	27.27	0.26	0.15	0.00	0.00		
0.02	0.43	0.01	0.01	0.17	0.87	0.03	0.00	0.19	92.44	1.36	4.59	6.70	0.07	0.04	0.00	0.00		
0.88	2.34	0.02	0.03	0.91	25.67	0.05	0.00	0.76	105.70	21.90	22.65	16.61	0.60	0.19	0.00	0.00	0.87	2.91
0.42	7.04	0.02	0.03	0.30	4.35	0.04	0.00	0.72	55.82	4.35	8.70	4.35	0.20	0.12	0.00	0.00	0.20	1.54
0.37	1.94	0.02	0.03	0.40	5.42	0.04	0.00	0.77	41.85	6.20	8.52	3.87	0.14	0.06	0.00	0.00	0.62	1.47
0.48	1.41	0.05	0.06	0.15	2.56	0.05	0.00	3.84	51.20	6.40	12.80	5.12	0.42	0.09	0.00	0.00		
0.84	15.12	0.02	0.02	0.46	18.00	0.02	0.00	0.72	116.64	20.88	15.84	14.40	0.45	0.38	0.00	0.00		
0.58	2.05	0.03	0.02	0.50	41.58	0.04	0.00	0.66	91.74	17.82	17.82	10.56	0.56	0.15	0.00	0.00		
0.10	27.84	0.10	0.03	0.86	13.44	0.10	0.00	1.92	470.40	16.32	28.80	24.00	0.52	0.12	0.00	0.00		
0.10	24.08	0.01	0.01	0.26	8.40	0.01	0.00	1.40	93.10	2.10	8.40	7.00	0.06	0.08	0.00	0.00	0.14	1.81
	7.60	0.01	0.01	0.04			0.00	0.60	52.00	2.20	1.40	3.20	0.26		0.00	0.00		
0.09	6.40	0.02	0.03	0.34	14.40	0.09	0.00	0.80	138.40	10.40	23.20	9.60	0.18	0.24	0.00	0.00		
	15.73	0.13	0.17	0.78	24.62	0.29	0.00	5.47	367.86	10.94	35.56	21.88	0.41	0.24	0.00	0.00		
0.00	0.00	0.00	0.00	0.00	0.00	0.00	0.00	0.16	0.84	2.16	0.12	0.16	0.02	0.01	0.00	0.00		

Food Name	Amount	Measure	Weight (g)	Calories	Protein (g)	Total Carb (g)	Dietary Fiber (g)	Total Fat (g)	Sat Fat (g)	Mono Fat (g)	Poly Fat (g)	Chol (mg)	Vit A (mcg RAE)	Vit D (mcg)
FRUITS *(continued)*														
Cherries, red, sour, fresh, cup	0.5	Cup	77.50	38.75	0.77	9.44	1.24	0.23	0.06	0.06	0.07	0.00	49.60	0.00
Cherries, red, sour, unswtnd, fzn	0.5	Cup	77.50	35.65	0.71	8.54	1.24	0.34	0.08	0.09	0.10	0.00	34.10	
Cherries, red, sour, w/light syrup, cnd, not drained	0.5	Cup	126.00	94.50	0.94	24.32	1.01	0.13	0.03	0.04	0.04	0.00	45.36	0.00
Cherries, red, sour/tart, w/water, cnd, not drained	0.5	Cup	122.00	43.92	0.94	10.91	1.34	0.12	0.03	0.03	0.03	0.00	46.36	
Cherries, sweet, fresh, cup	0.5	Cup	72.50	45.67	0.77	11.61	1.52	0.14	0.03	0.04	0.04	0.00	2.17	
Cherries, sweet, swtnd, fzn, pkg	1	Ounce-weight	28.35	25.23	0.33	6.34	0.60	0.04	0.01	0.01	0.01	0.00	2.55	
Cherries, sweet, w/light syrup, cnd, not drained	0.5	Cup	126.00	84.42	0.76	21.79	1.89	0.19	0.04	0.05	0.05	0.00	10.08	0.00
Cherries, swtnd, w/juice, cnd, not drained	0.5	Cup	125.00	67.50	1.13	17.26	1.87	0.03	0.01	0.01	0.01	0.00	7.50	0.00
Cranberries, fresh, whole, cup	0.5	Cup	47.50	21.85	0.18	5.80	2.18	0.06	0.00	0.01	0.02	0.00	1.42	
Cranberry Sauce, swtnd, cnd, slice, 1/2" thick	0.25	Cup	69.25	104.57	0.14	26.94	0.69	0.10	0.01	0.01	0.05	0.00	1.38	
Currants, black, European, fresh, cup	0.5	Cup	56.00	35.28	0.78	8.61	4.14	0.22	0.01	0.03	0.10	0.00	6.72	
Dates, Deglet Noor, whole, each	5	Each	41.50	117.03	1.02	31.14	3.32	0.17	0.01	0.01	0.01	0.00	0.21	
Figs, fresh, sml, 1 1/2" each	1	Each	40.00	29.60	0.30	7.67	1.16	0.12	0.02	0.03	0.06	0.00	2.80	
Figs, stwd f/dried, cup	0.5	Cup	129.50	138.57	1.84	35.71	5.44	0.52	0.08	0.09	0.19	0.00	0.26	0.00
Figs, w/light syrup, cnd, not drained, each or cup	0.5	Cup	126.00	86.94	0.49	22.62	2.27	0.13	0.03	0.03	0.06	0.00	2.52	0.00
Fruit Cocktail, w/extra heavy syrup, cnd, not drained, cup	0.5	Cup	130.00	114.40	0.51	29.76	1.43	0.09	0.01	0.02	0.04	0.00	13.00	0.00
Fruit Cocktail, w/extra light syrup, cnd, not drained, cup	0.5	Cup	123.00	55.35	0.49	14.30	1.35	0.09	0.01	0.02	0.04	0.00	14.76	0.00
Gooseberries, fresh, cup	0.5	Cup	75.00	33.00	0.66	7.63	3.22	0.43	0.03	0.04	0.24	0.00	11.25	
Grapefruit, pink, fresh, sections, cup	0.5	Cup	115.00	36.80	0.72	9.29	1.27	0.12	0.02	0.02	0.02	0.00	52.90	
Grapefruit, w/juice, cnd, not drained, sections, cup	0.5	Cup	124.50	46.06	0.87	11.46	0.50	0.11	0.02	0.02	0.02	0.00	0.00	0.00
Grapefruit, w/light syrup, cnd, not drained, sections, cup	0.5	Cup	127.00	76.20	0.71	19.61	0.51	0.12	0.02	0.02	0.03	0.00	0.00	
Grapes, concord, fresh, cup	0.5	Cup	46.00	30.82	0.29	7.89	0.41	0.16	0.05	0.01	0.05	0.00	2.30	
Grapes, red European type varieties, fresh, each	10	Each	50.00	34.50	0.36	9.05	0.45	0.08	0.03	0.00	0.03	0.00	1.50	
Grapes, Thompson seedless, fresh, cup	0.5	Cup	80.00	55.20	0.58	14.48	0.72	0.13	0.05	0.01	0.04	0.00	2.40	
Grapes, Thompson seedless, w/heavy syrup, cnd S & W	0.5	Cup	123.00	100.00	0.00	23.00	0.00	0.00	0.00	0.00	0.00	0.00	0.00	
Guava, fresh, cup	0.5	Cup	82.50	56.10	2.10	11.82	4.46	0.78	0.22	0.07	0.33	0.00	25.58	
Huckleberries, fresh, cup	0.5	Cup	72.50	41.32	0.54	10.51	1.74	0.24	0.02	0.04	0.10	0.00	2.17	
Kiwi, fresh, w/o skin, med	1	Each	76.00	46.36	0.87	11.14	2.28	0.40	0.02	0.04	0.22	0.00	3.04	
Kumquats, fresh, each	1	Each	19.00	13.49	0.36	3.02	1.23	0.16	0.02	0.03	0.03	0.00	2.85	
Leechees, fresh, cup	0.5	Cup	80.00	52.80	0.66	13.22	1.04	0.35	0.08	0.10	0.10	0.00	0.00	
Lemon, peeled, fresh, 2 1/8"	1	Each	58.00	16.82	0.64	5.41	1.62	0.17	0.02	0.01	0.05	0.00	0.58	
Limes, med, fresh FDA	1	Each	67.00	20.00	0.00	7.00	2.00	0.00	0.00	0.00	0.00	0.00	0.00	
Litchis, dried, each	1	Each	2.50	6.93	0.10	1.77	0.12	0.03	0.01	0.01	0.01	0.00	0.00	
Loganberries, w/heavy syrup, cnd, cup	0.5	Cup	128.00	112.64	1.27	28.55	3.33	0.16	0.01	0.02	0.09	0.00	2.56	
Mandarin Oranges, fresh, sections, cup	1	Cup	195.00	103.35	1.58	26.01	3.51	0.60	0.08	0.12	0.13	0.00	66.30	
Mango, dried Sunsweet Growers Inc.	0.33	Cup	40.00	140.00	0.00	34.00	1.00	0.00	0.00	0.00	0.00	0.00	25.00	
Mango, fresh, whole, each	0.5	Each	103.50	67.27	0.52	17.59	1.86	0.28	0.07	0.10	0.05	0.00	39.33	
Melon, balls, fzn, cup	0.5	Cup	86.50	28.55	0.73	6.87	0.61	0.22	0.06	0.01	0.09	0.00	76.99	
Melon, cantaloupe, fresh Dole	0.25	Each	134.00	50.00	1.00	12.00	1.00	0.00	0.00	0.00	0.00	0.00	250.00	
Melon, casaba, fresh, cubes, cup	0.5	Cup	85.00	23.80	0.94	5.59	0.77	0.09	0.02	0.00	0.03	0.00	0.00	
Melon, honeydew, fresh, balls, cup	0.5	Cup	88.50	31.86	0.48	8.05	0.71	0.13	0.03	0.00	0.05	0.00	2.65	
Mixed Fruit, peach pear & pine, w/heavy syrup, cnd undrained	0.5	Cup	127.50	91.80	0.47	23.92	1.27	0.13	0.02	0.03	0.05	0.00	12.75	0.00
Mixed Fruit, prunes apricots & pears, dried, pkg	1	Ounce-weight	28.35	68.89	0.70	18.16	2.21	0.14	0.01	0.07	0.03	0.00	34.59	
Nectarines, fresh, 2 1/2" each	1	Each	136.00	59.84	1.44	14.35	2.31	0.44	0.03	0.12	0.15	0.00	23.12	
Oranges, Calif, navels, fresh, 2 7/8" each	1	Each	140.00	68.60	1.27	17.56	3.08	0.21	0.02	0.04	0.04	0.00	16.80	
Oranges, Calif, valencias, fresh, 2 5/8" each	1	Each	121.00	59.29	1.26	14.39	3.03	0.36	0.04	0.07	0.07	0.00	14.52	
Papaya, fresh, cubes, cup	0.5	Cup	70.00	27.30	0.42	6.86	1.26	0.10	0.03	0.02	0.02	0.00	38.50	
Passion Fruit, purple, fresh, each	1	Each	18.00	17.46	0.40	4.21	1.87	0.13	0.01	0.02	0.07	0.00	11.52	

Vit E (mg)	Vit C	Vit B$_1$ Thia (mg)	Vit B$_2$ Ribo (mg)	Vit B$_3$ Nia (mg)	Fol (mcg)	Vit B$_6$ (mg)	Vita B$_{12}$ (mcg)	Sodi (mg)	Pota (mg)	Cal (mg)	Phos (mg)	Magn (mg)	Iron (mg)	Zinc (mg)	Caff (mg)	Alco (g)	Sol Fiber (g)	Insol Fiber (g)
0.06	7.75	0.02	0.03	0.31	6.20	0.03	0.00	2.32	134.07	12.40	11.62	6.97	0.25	0.08	0.00	0.00	0.58	0.66
0.04	1.32	0.03	0.03	0.11	3.87	0.05	0.00	0.77	96.10	10.07	12.40	6.97	0.41	0.08	0.00	0.00	0.58	0.66
0.07	2.52	0.02	0.04	0.22	10.08	0.05	0.00	8.82	119.70	12.60	12.60	7.56	1.66	0.09	0.00	0.00		
0.28	2.56	0.02	0.05	0.22	9.76	0.05	0.00	8.54	119.56	13.42	12.20	7.32	1.67	0.09	0.00	0.00	0.63	0.71
0.05	5.07	0.02	0.03	0.11	2.90	0.04	0.00	0.00	160.95	9.42	15.22	7.97	0.26	0.05	0.00	0.00		
0.02	0.28	0.01	0.01	0.05	1.13	0.01	0.00	0.28	56.42	3.40	4.54	2.84	0.10	0.01	0.00	0.00	0.45	0.15
0.29	4.66	0.03	0.05	0.50	5.04	0.04	0.00	3.78	186.48	11.34	22.68	11.34	0.45	0.13	0.00	0.00		
0.29	3.12	0.03	0.03	0.51	5.00	0.04	0.00	3.75	163.75	17.50	27.50	15.00	0.72	0.12	0.00	0.00	0.88	0.99
0.57	6.32	0.00	0.01	0.05	0.48	0.02	0.00	0.95	40.38	3.80	6.18	2.85	0.12	0.04	0.00	0.00		
0.57	1.38	0.01	0.01	0.07	0.69	0.01	0.00	20.08	18.00	2.77	4.15	2.08	0.15	0.03	0.00	0.00	0.28	0.42
0.56	101.36	0.03	0.03	0.17	1.95	0.04	0.00	1.12	180.32	30.80	33.04	13.44	0.87	0.15	0.00	0.00	0.67	3.47
0.02	0.17	0.02	0.03	0.53	7.89	0.07	0.00	0.83	272.24	16.19	25.73	17.85	0.43	0.12	0.00	0.00		
0.04	0.80	0.02	0.02	0.16	2.40	0.05	0.00	0.40	92.80	14.00	5.60	6.80	0.15	0.06	0.00	0.00		
0.19	5.70	0.02	0.14	0.83	1.30	0.18	0.00	5.18	380.73	90.65	37.56	37.56	1.14	0.31	0.00	0.00		
0.13	1.26	0.03	0.04	0.55	2.52	0.09	0.00	1.26	128.52	34.02	12.60	12.60	0.37	0.13	0.00	0.00	0.45	1.82
0.38	2.47	0.03	0.03	0.48	3.90	0.06	0.00	7.80	111.80	7.80	14.30	6.50	0.36	0.10	0.00	0.00		
0.36	3.69	0.04	0.01	0.62	3.69	0.06	0.00	4.92	127.92	9.84	14.76	7.38	0.37	0.10	0.00	0.00		
0.28	20.77	0.03	0.02	0.22	4.50	0.06	0.00	0.75	148.50	18.75	20.25	7.50	0.23	0.09	0.00	0.00	1.09	2.13
0.15	39.56	0.04	0.02	0.29	11.50	0.05	0.00	0.00	159.85	13.80	9.20	9.20	0.11	0.08	0.00	0.00	0.94	0.33
0.11	42.20	0.04	0.02	0.31	11.20	0.02	0.00	8.72	210.40	18.68	14.94	13.70	0.26	0.10	0.00	0.00	0.20	0.30
0.12	27.05	0.05	0.02	0.31	11.43	0.02	0.00	2.54	163.83	17.78	12.70	12.70	0.51	0.10	0.00	0.00	0.20	0.30
0.09	1.84	0.04	0.03	0.14	1.84	0.05	0.00	0.92	87.86	6.44	4.60	2.30	0.13	0.02	0.00	0.00		
0.10	5.40	0.04	0.04	0.09	1.00	0.04	0.00	1.00	95.50	5.00	10.00	3.50	0.18	0.04	0.00	0.00		
0.15	8.64	0.06	0.06	0.15	1.60	0.07	0.00	1.60	152.80	8.00	16.00	5.60	0.29	0.06	0.00	0.00		
	0.00						0.00	20.00	120.00	0.00			1.44		0.00	0.00	0.00	0.00
0.60	188.35	0.05	0.04	0.90	40.43	0.09	0.00	1.65	344.03	14.85	33.00	18.15	0.21	0.19	0.00	0.00	2.23	2.23
0.41	7.03	0.03	0.03	0.31	4.35	0.04	0.00	0.72	55.82	4.35	8.70	4.35	0.20	0.11	0.00	0.00	0.20	1.54
1.11	70.45	0.02	0.02	0.26	19.00	0.05	0.00	2.28	237.12	25.84	25.84	12.92	0.24	0.11	0.00	0.00		
0.03	8.34	0.01	0.02	0.08	3.23	0.01	0.00	1.90	35.34	11.78	3.61	3.80	0.16	0.03	0.00	0.00	0.07	1.16
0.06	57.20	0.01	0.05	0.48	11.20	0.08	0.00	0.80	136.80	4.00	24.80	8.00	0.25	0.06				
0.09	30.74	0.02	0.01	0.06	6.38	0.05	0.00	1.16	80.04	15.08	9.28	4.64	0.35	0.03	0.00	0.00	0.52	1.10
	21.00						0.00	0.00	75.00	0.00			0.00		0.00	0.00		
0.01	4.58	0.00	0.01	0.08	0.30	0.00	0.00	0.08	27.75	0.83	4.53	1.05	0.04	0.01	0.00	0.00		
0.91	7.94	0.04	0.04	0.29	43.52	0.05	0.00	3.84	115.20	23.04	12.80	14.08	0.55	0.25	0.00	0.00	0.38	2.94
0.39	52.07	0.11	0.07	0.73	31.20	0.15	0.00	3.90	323.70	72.15	39.00	23.40	0.29	0.14	0.00	0.00	2.11	1.40
	1.20						0.00	20.00	10.00	80.00			0.36		0.00	0.00		
1.16	28.67	0.06	0.06	0.61	14.49	0.14	0.00	2.07	161.46	10.35	11.38	9.31	0.13	0.04	0.00	0.00	1.08	0.78
0.12	5.36	0.14	0.02	0.56	22.49	0.09	0.00	26.82	242.20	8.65	10.38	12.11	0.25	0.15	0.00	0.00	0.15	0.45
	48.00				40.00		0.00	25.00		20.00			0.36		0.00	0.00		
0.04	18.53	0.01	0.02	0.19	6.80	0.14	0.00	7.65	154.70	9.35	4.25	9.35	0.29	0.06	0.00	0.00		
0.02	15.93	0.03	0.01	0.37	16.81	0.08	0.00	15.93	201.78	5.31	9.73	8.85	0.15	0.03	0.00	0.00		
0.51	87.97	0.02	0.05	0.76	3.82	0.05	0.00	5.10	107.10	1.27	12.75	6.37	0.46	0.09	0.00	0.00		
0.18	1.08	0.01	0.04	0.55	1.13	0.05	0.00	5.10	225.67	10.77	21.83	11.06	0.77	0.14	0.00	0.00		
1.05	7.34	0.05	0.04	1.53	6.80	0.03	0.00	0.00	273.36	8.16	35.36	12.24	0.38	0.23	0.00	0.00	0.76	1.55
0.21	82.74	0.10	0.07	0.59	47.60	0.11	0.00	1.40	232.40	60.20	32.20	15.40	0.18	0.11	0.00	0.00	0.56	2.52
0.36	58.69	0.11	0.05	0.33	47.19	0.08	0.00	0.00	216.59	48.40	20.57	12.10	0.11	0.07	0.00	0.00	1.75	1.27
0.51	43.26	0.02	0.02	0.24	26.60	0.02	0.00	2.10	179.90	16.80	3.50	7.00	0.07	0.05	0.00	0.00		
0.00	5.40	0.00	0.02	0.27	2.52	0.02	0.00	5.04	62.64	2.16	12.24	5.22	0.29	0.02	0.00	0.00	0.94	0.94

Food Name	Amount	Measure	Weight (g)	Calories	Protein (g)	Total Carb (g)	Dietary Fiber (g)	Total Fat (g)	Sat Fat (g)	Mono Fat (g)	Poly Fat (g)	Chol (mg)	Vit A (mcg RAE)	Vit D (mcg)
FRUITS (continued)														
Peaches, fresh, lrg, w/o skin, 2 3/4" each	1	Each	157.00	61.23	1.43	14.98	2.34	0.39	0.03	0.11	0.14	0.00	25.12	
Peaches, halves, dried, sulfured, unckd	0.5	Cup	80.00	191.20	2.88	49.06	6.56	0.60	0.06	0.22	0.30	0.00	86.40	
Peaches, halves, w/heavy syrup, cnd, not drained, each	1	Each	98.00	72.52	0.44	19.54	1.27	0.10	0.01	0.03	0.05	0.00	16.66	
Peaches, halves, w/juice, cnd, not drained	0.5	Cup	124.00	54.56	0.78	14.35	1.61	0.04	0.01	0.02	0.02	0.00	23.56	
Peaches, halves, w/light syrup, cnd, not drained	0.5	Cup	125.50	67.77	0.56	18.26	1.63	0.04	0.00	0.02	0.02	0.00	22.59	
Peaches, slices, swtnd, fzn, each	5	Each	77.50	72.85	0.49	18.58	1.39	0.10	0.01	0.04	0.05	0.00	10.85	
Pears, fresh, d'anjou, lrg, each	1	Each	209.00	121.22	0.79	32.31	6.48	0.25	0.01	0.05	0.06	0.00	2.09	
Pears, halves, w/juice, cnd, not drained	0.5	Cup	124.00	62.00	0.43	16.05	1.98	0.09	0.01	0.02	0.02	0.00	0.37	
Pears, halves, w/light syrup, not drained	0.5	Cup	125.50	71.54	0.24	19.04	2.01	0.04	0.00	0.01	0.01	0.00	0.00	
Pears, sulfured, halves, ckd f/dried	0.5	Cup	90.00	235.80	1.68	62.73	6.75	0.57	0.03	0.12	0.13	0.00	0.13	
Persimmon, native, fresh	1	Each	25.00	31.75	0.20	8.38	0.38	0.10					0.00		
Pineapple, chunks, swtnd, fzn, cup	0.5	Cup	122.50	105.35	0.49	27.20	1.35	0.12	0.01	0.02	0.04	0.00	2.45	
Pineapple, chunks, w/juice, cnd, not drained, cup	0.5	Cup	124.50	74.70	0.52	19.55	1.00	0.10	0.01	0.01	0.04	0.00	2.49	
Pineapple, chunks, w/light syrup, cnd, not drained, cup	0.5	Cup	126.00	65.52	0.45	16.95	1.01	0.15	0.01	0.02	0.05	0.00	2.52	
Pineapple, fresh, dices, cup	0.5	Cup	77.50	37.20	0.42	9.79	1.08	0.09	0.01	0.01	0.03	0.00	2.32	
Pitanga, fresh, each	1	Each	7.00	2.31	0.06	0.52		0.03				0.00	5.25	
Plantain, fresh, med, each	1	Each	179.00	218.38	2.33	57.08	4.12	0.66	0.26	0.06	0.12	0.00	100.24	
Plums, fresh, 2 1/8", each	1	Each	66.00	30.36	0.46	7.54	0.92	0.18	0.01	0.09	0.03	0.00	11.22	
Plums, purple, w/juice, cnd, not drained, cup	0.5	Cup	126.00	73.08	0.64	19.09	1.13	0.03	0.00	0.02	0.01	0.00	63.00	
Plums, purple, w/light syrup, cnd, not drained, cup	0.5	Cup	126.00	79.38	0.47	20.51	1.13	0.13	0.01	0.09	0.03	0.00	15.12	
Pomegranate, fresh, 3 3/8"	1	Each	154.00	104.72	1.46	26.44	0.92	0.46	0.06	0.07	0.10	0.00	7.70	
Prickly Pears, fresh, each	1	Each	103.00	42.23	0.75	9.86	3.71	0.53	0.07	0.08	0.22	0.00	2.06	
Prunes, dried, each	5	Each	42.00	100.80	0.91	26.83	2.98	0.16	0.04	0.02	0.02	0.00	16.38	
Prunes, stwd f/dried w/o add sug	0.5	Cup	124.00	132.68	1.19	34.82	3.84	0.19	0.02	0.13	0.04	0.00	21.08	
Quince, fresh, each	1	Each	92.00	52.44	0.37	14.08	1.75	0.09	0.01	0.03	0.05	0.00	1.84	
Raisins, golden, seedless, packed cup All American Foods	0.25	Cup	41.25	124.58	1.40	32.80	1.65	0.19	0.06	0.01	0.05	0.00	0.00	
Raisins, seedless, packed cup	0.25	Cup	41.25	123.34	1.27	32.66	1.53	0.19	0.02	0.02	0.01	0.00	0.00	
Raspberries, fzn, swtnd, 10oz pkg or cup	0.5	Cup	125.00	128.75	0.87	32.70	5.50	0.20	0.01	0.02	0.11	0.00	3.75	
Raspberries, red, fresh, cup	0.5	Cup	61.50	31.98	0.74	7.34	4.00	0.40	0.01	0.04	0.23	0.00	1.23	
Raspberries, red, w/heavy syrup, cnd, not drained	0.5	Cup	128.00	116.48	1.06	29.90	4.22	0.16	0.01	0.02	0.09	0.00	2.56	
Rhubarb, ckd f/fzn w/sugar	0.5	Cup	120.00	139.20	0.47	37.44	2.40	0.07	0.02	0.01	0.03	0.00	4.80	
Rhubarb, fresh, diced, cup	0.5	Cup	61.00	12.81	0.55	2.77	1.10	0.12	0.03	0.02	0.06	0.00	3.05	
Strawberries, fresh, halves, cup	0.5	Cup	76.00	24.32	0.51	5.84	1.52	0.23	0.01	0.03	0.12	0.00	0.76	
Strawberries, fzn, unswtnd, cup	0.5	Cup	74.50	26.08	0.32	6.80	1.56	0.08	0.01	0.01	0.04	0.00	1.49	
Strawberries, w/ heavy syrup, cnd, not drained, cup	0.5	Cup	127.00	116.84	0.71	29.88	2.16	0.33	0.02	0.05	0.16	0.00	1.27	0.00
Tamar Hindi, fresh, 3" × 1", each	1	Each	2.00	4.78	0.06	1.25	0.10	0.01	0.01	0.00	0.00	0.00	0.04	
Tangerines, fresh, med, 2 3/8", each	1	Each	84.00	44.52	0.68	11.21	1.51	0.26	0.03	0.05	0.05	0.00	28.56	
Watermelon, fresh, balls, cup	0.5	Cup	77.00	23.10	0.47	5.81	0.31	0.12	0.01	0.03	0.04	0.00	21.56	
GRAINS, FLOURS, AND FRACTIONS														
Barley, pearled, ckd	0.5	Cup	78.50	96.56	1.78	22.15	2.98	0.35	0.07	0.05	0.17	0.00	0.28	
Bran, corn, crude	1	Tablespoon	4.75	10.64	0.40	4.07	3.75	0.04	0.01	0.01	0.02	0.00	0.19	
Bran, oat, ckd	1	Tablespoon	13.69	5.48	0.44	1.57	0.36	0.12	0.02	0.04	0.05	0.00	0.00	
Bran, wheat, crude	1	Tablespoon	3.63	7.84	0.56	2.34	1.55	0.15	0.02	0.02	0.08	0.00	0.02	
Buckwheat	0.25	Cup	42.50	145.77	5.63	30.38	4.25	1.44	0.31	0.44	0.44	0.00	0.00	
Buckwheat, groats, rstd, dry	0.25	Cup	41.00	141.86	4.81	30.73	4.22	1.11	0.25	0.34	0.34	0.00	0.00	
Corn, yellow, dry	0.25	Cup	41.50	151.47	3.91	30.82	3.03	1.96	0.28	0.53	0.90	0.00	4.56	
Cornmeal, white, bolted, w/wheat flour, enrich, self rising	0.25	Cup	42.50	147.90	3.57	31.21	2.68	1.22	0.17	0.33	0.55	0.00	0.00	
Cornmeal, white, degermed, enrich, self rising	0.25	Cup	34.50	122.47	2.90	25.81	2.45	0.60	0.08	0.15	0.25	0.00	0.00	
Cornmeal, white, degermed, unenrich	0.25	Cup	34.50	126.27	2.92	26.79	2.55	0.57	0.08	0.14	0.24	0.00	0.00	

Vit E (mg)	Vit C	Vit B₁ Thia (mg)	Vit B₂ Ribo (mg)	Vit B₃ Nia (mg)	Fol (mcg)	Vit B₆ (mg)	Vita B₁₂ (mcg)	Sodi (mg)	Pota (mg)	Cal (mg)	Phos (mg)	Magn (mg)	Iron (mg)	Zinc (mg)	Caff (mg)	Alco (g)	Sol Fiber (g)	Insol Fiber (g)
1.15	10.36	0.04	0.05	1.27	6.28	0.04	0.00	0.00	298.30	9.42	31.40	14.13	0.39	0.27	0.00	0.00		
0.16	3.84	0.00	0.16	3.50	0.00	0.06	0.00	5.60	796.80	22.40	95.20	33.60	3.24	0.46	0.00	0.00	2.62	3.94
0.48	2.74	0.01	0.02	0.60	2.94	0.02	0.00	5.88	90.16	2.94	10.78	4.90	0.27	0.09	0.00	0.00	0.66	0.61
0.61	4.46	0.01	0.02	0.72	3.72	0.03	0.00	4.96	158.72	7.44	21.08	8.68	0.34	0.13	0.00	0.00	0.45	1.16
0.62	3.01	0.01	0.03	0.74	3.77	0.03	0.00	6.28	121.74	3.77	13.81	6.28	0.45	0.12	0.00	0.00	0.85	0.78
0.48	73.00	0.01	0.03	0.50	2.32	0.02	0.00	4.65	100.75	2.32	8.52	3.87	0.29	0.04	0.00	0.00	0.73	0.67
0.25	8.78	0.03	0.05	0.33	14.63	0.06	0.00	2.09	248.71	18.81	22.99	14.63	0.36	0.21	0.00	0.00	1.35	5.13
0.10	1.98	0.02	0.02	0.25	1.24	0.02	0.00	4.96	119.04	11.16	14.88	8.68	0.36	0.12	0.00	0.00	0.56	1.43
0.10	0.88	0.01	0.02	0.20	1.26	0.02	0.00	6.28	82.83	6.28	8.79	5.02	0.35	0.10	0.00	0.00	0.20	1.81
0.05	6.30	0.01	0.13	1.23	0.00	0.06	0.00	5.40	479.70	30.60	53.10	29.70	1.89	0.35	0.00	0.00	1.35	5.40
0.25	16.50				2.00		0.00	0.25	77.50	6.75	6.50		0.62		0.00	0.00	0.10	0.28
0.03	9.80	0.12	0.04	0.37	13.48	0.09	0.00	2.45	122.50	11.02	4.90	12.25	0.49	0.13	0.00	0.00	0.37	0.98
0.01	11.83	0.12	0.03	0.36	6.23	0.09	0.00	1.25	151.89	17.43	7.47	17.43	0.35	0.12	0.00	0.00	0.25	0.75
0.01	9.45	0.12	0.03	0.37	6.30	0.09	0.00	1.26	132.30	17.64	8.82	20.16	0.49	0.15	0.00	0.00	0.25	0.76
0.02	28.05	0.06	0.02	0.38	11.62	0.08	0.00	0.77	89.12	10.07	6.20	9.30	0.22	0.08	0.00	0.00		
	1.84	0.00	0.00	0.02			0.00	0.21	7.21	0.63	0.77	0.84	0.01		0.00	0.00		
0.25	32.94	0.09	0.10	1.23	39.38	0.54	0.00	7.16	893.21	5.37	60.86	66.23	1.07	0.25	0.00	0.00	1.38	2.74
0.17	6.27	0.02	0.02	0.28	3.30	0.02	0.00	0.00	103.62	3.96	10.56	4.62	0.11	0.07	0.00	0.00	0.30	0.62
0.22	3.53	0.03	0.07	0.59	3.78	0.04	0.00	1.26	194.04	12.60	18.90	10.08	0.43	0.13	0.00	0.00		
0.22	0.50	0.02	0.04	0.38	3.78	0.04	0.00	25.20	117.18	11.34	16.38	6.30	1.08	0.10	0.00	0.00		
0.92	9.39	0.05	0.05	0.46	9.24	0.16	0.00	4.62	398.86	4.62	12.32	4.62	0.46	0.18	0.00	0.00	0.18	0.74
0.01	14.42	0.01	0.06	0.47	6.18	0.06	0.00	5.15	226.60	57.68	24.72	87.55	0.31	0.12	0.00	0.00	0.11	3.59
0.18	0.25	0.02	0.07	0.79	1.68	0.08	0.00	0.84	307.44	18.06	28.98	17.22	0.39	0.19	0.00	0.00	1.25	1.73
0.24	3.60	0.03	0.12	0.89	0.00	0.27	0.00	1.24	398.04	23.56	37.20	22.32	0.50	0.24	0.00	0.00		
0.51	13.80	0.02	0.03	0.18	2.76	0.04	0.00	3.68	181.24	10.12	15.64	7.36	0.64	0.04	0.00	0.00	0.41	1.33
0.05	1.32	0.00	0.08	0.47	1.24	0.13	0.00	4.95	307.73	21.86	47.44	14.44	0.74	0.13	0.00	0.00	0.50	1.16
0.05	0.95	0.04	0.05	0.32	2.06	0.07	0.00	4.54	308.96	20.62	41.66	13.20	0.77	0.09	0.00	0.00	0.22	1.31
0.90	20.62	0.03	0.05	0.29	32.50	0.04	0.00	1.25	142.50	18.75	21.25	16.25	0.81	0.22	0.00	0.00	1.74	3.76
0.54	16.11	0.02	0.02	0.37	12.92	0.04	0.00	0.62	92.87	15.38	17.84	13.53	0.43	0.26	0.00	0.00		
0.76	11.14	0.03	0.04	0.57	14.08	0.05	0.00	3.84	120.32	14.08	11.52	15.36	0.54	0.20	0.00	0.00	0.42	3.80
0.33	3.96	0.02	0.03	0.24	6.00	0.02	0.00	1.20	115.20	174.00	9.60	14.40	0.25	0.10	0.00	0.00	0.74	1.66
0.23	4.88	0.01	0.02	0.18	4.27	0.01	0.00	2.44	175.68	52.46	8.54	7.32	0.14	0.06	0.00	0.00	0.34	0.76
0.22	44.69	0.02	0.02	0.29	18.24	0.04	0.00	0.76	116.28	12.16	18.24	9.88	0.32	0.11	0.00	0.00	0.34	1.18
0.22	30.69	0.02	0.03	0.35	12.67	0.02	0.00	1.49	110.26	11.92	9.69	8.20	0.56	0.10	0.00	0.00	0.48	1.08
0.24	40.26	0.03	0.05	0.07	35.56	0.06	0.00	5.08	109.22	16.51	15.24	10.16	0.63	0.12	0.00	0.00		
0.00	0.07	0.01	0.00	0.04	0.28	0.00	0.00	0.56	12.56	1.48	2.26	1.84	0.06	0.00	0.00	0.00		
0.17	22.43	0.05	0.03	0.32	13.44	0.07	0.00	1.68	139.44	31.08	16.80	10.08	0.13	0.06	0.00	0.00	0.91	0.60
0.04	6.24	0.02	0.02	0.14	2.31	0.04	0.00	0.77	86.24	5.39	8.47	7.70	0.18	0.08	0.00	0.00	0.08	0.23
0.00	0.00	0.07	0.05	1.62	12.56	0.09	0.00	2.36	73.01	8.64	42.39	17.27	1.05	0.65	0.00	0.00	0.84	2.15
0.02	0.00	0.00	0.01	0.13	0.19	0.01	0.00	0.33	2.09	1.99	3.42	3.04	0.13	0.07	0.00	0.00	0.04	3.71
0.01	0.00	0.02	0.01	0.02	0.82	0.00	0.00	0.14	12.59	1.37	16.29	5.48	0.12	0.07	0.00	0.00	0.18	0.17
0.05	0.00	0.02	0.02	0.49	2.87	0.05	0.00	0.07	42.91	2.65	36.77	22.18	0.38	0.26	0.00	0.00	0.11	1.44
0.43	0.00	0.05	0.18	2.98	12.75	0.08	0.00	0.42	195.50	7.65	147.47	98.17	0.93	1.02	0.00	0.00		
0.42	0.00	0.09	0.11	2.10	17.22	0.15	0.00	4.51	131.20	6.97	130.79	90.61	1.01	0.99	0.00	0.00		
0.21	0.00	0.17	0.08	1.51	7.88	0.26	0.00	14.52	119.10	2.90	87.15	52.70	1.12	0.91	0.00	0.00		
0.11	0.00	0.30	0.18	2.21	112.20	0.17	0.00	560.57	87.97	127.07	276.67	22.95	2.11	0.59	0.00	0.00		
0.06	0.00	0.23	0.14	1.58	80.38	0.14	0.00	465.06	58.65	120.75	214.93	16.90	1.63	0.34	0.00	0.00	0.64	1.82
0.11	0.00	0.05	0.02	0.34	16.56	0.09	0.00	1.03	55.89	1.72	28.98	13.80	0.38	0.25	0.00	0.00	0.64	1.92

Food Name	Amount	Measure	Weight (g)	Calories	Protein (g)	Total Carb (g)	Dietary Fiber (g)	Total Fat (g)	Sat Fat (g)	Mono Fat (g)	Poly Fat (g)	Chol (mg)	Vit A (mcg RAE)	Vit D (mcg)
GRAINS, FLOURS, AND FRACTIONS *(continued)*														
Cornmeal, yellow, bolted, w/wheat flour, enrich, self rising	0.25	Cup	42.50	147.90	3.57	31.21	2.68	1.22	0.17	0.33	0.55	0.00	5.95	
Cornmeal, yellow, degermed, enrich, self rising	0.25	Cup	34.50	122.47	2.90	25.81	2.45	0.60	0.08	0.15	0.25	0.00	7.13	
Cornmeal, yellow, whole grain	0.25	Cup	30.50	110.41	2.48	23.45	2.23	1.10	0.15	0.28	0.50	0.00	3.35	
Flour, acorn, full fat	1	Ounce-weight	28.35	142.03	2.12	15.50	0.62	8.56	1.12	5.42	1.64	0.00	0.85	
Flour, all purpose, white, bleached, enrich	0.25	Cup	31.25	113.75	3.23	23.84	0.84	0.30	0.05	0.03	0.12	0.00	0.00	
Flour, all purpose, white, self rising, enrich	0.25	Cup	31.25	110.62	3.09	23.20	0.84	0.30	0.05	0.03	0.12	0.00	0.00	
Flour, amaranth, whole grain Arrowhead Mills, Inc.	0.25	Cup	22.70	90.80	3.03	15.13	1.51	1.89	0.00			0.00	0.00	
Flour, arrowroot	0.25	Cup	32.00	114.24	0.10	28.21	1.09	0.03	0.01	0.00	0.01	0.00	0.00	
Flour, barley, cup	0.25	Cup	37.00	127.65	3.89	27.58	3.74	0.59	0.12	0.07	0.28	0.00	0.00	
Flour, barley, malt	0.25	Cup	40.50	146.21	4.16	31.71	2.88	0.74	0.16	0.11	0.39	0.00	0.41	
Flour, bread, white, enrich	0.25	Cup	34.25	123.64	4.10	24.84	0.82	0.57	0.08	0.05	0.25	0.00	0.03	
Flour, buckwheat, whole groat	0.25	Cup	30.00	100.50	3.79	21.18	3.00	0.93	0.20	0.28	0.28	0.00	0.00	
Flour, cake, white, enrich, unsifted	0.25	Cup	34.25	123.98	2.81	26.73	0.58	0.30	0.05	0.02	0.13	0.00	0.00	
Flour, corn, masa, enrich	0.25	Cup	28.50	104.02	2.66	21.74	2.74	1.07	0.15	0.28	0.49	0.00	0.05	
Flour, corn, white, whole grain	0.25	Cup	29.25	105.59	2.03	22.48	2.81	1.13	0.16	0.30	0.52	0.00	0.05	
Flour, corn, yellow, degermed, unenrich, cup	0.25	Cup	31.50	118.12	1.76	26.07	0.60	0.44	0.05	0.08	0.22	0.00	3.46	
Flour, corn, yellow, whole grain	0.25	Cup	29.25	105.59	2.03	22.48	3.92	1.13	0.16	0.30	0.52	0.00	3.22	
Flour, garbanzo, tstd Arrowhead Mills, Inc.	0.25	Cup	23.00	82.80	4.60	13.80	2.76	0.92	0.00			0.00	0.00	
Flour, millet, whole grain Arrowhead Mills, Inc.	0.25	Cup	26.50	98.43	3.03	19.69	2.27	1.14	0.00			0.00	0.00	
Flour, oat, whole grain Arrowhead Mills, Inc.	0.25	Cup	22.70	90.80	3.03	15.89	2.27	2.27	0.38			0.00	0.00	
Flour, peanut, defatted	0.25	Cup	15.00	49.05	7.83	5.20	2.37	0.08	0.01	0.04	0.02	0.00	0.00	
Flour, peanut, low fat	0.25	Cup	15.00	64.20	5.07	4.69	2.37	3.28	0.46	1.63	1.04	0.00	0.00	
Flour, potato	0.25	Cup	40.00	142.80	2.76	33.23	2.36	0.13	0.04	0.00	0.07	0.00	0.00	
Flour, rice, brown	0.25	Cup	39.50	143.39	2.86	30.20	1.82	1.09	0.22	0.40	0.40	0.00	0.00	
Flour, rice, white	0.25	Cup	39.50	144.57	2.36	31.65	0.95	0.57	0.16	0.17	0.14	0.00	0.00	
Flour, rye wheat, Bohemian style, enrich Pillsbury	0.25	Cup	30.00	100.00	3.00	22.00	2.00	0.00	0.00	0.00	0.00	0.00	0.00	
Flour, rye, dark	0.25	Cup	32.00	103.68	4.49	21.99	7.23	0.86	0.10	0.11	0.38	0.00	0.32	
Flour, rye, light	0.25	Cup	25.50	93.59	2.14	20.46	3.72	0.35	0.03	0.04	0.14	0.00	0.00	
Flour, rye, med	0.25	Cup	25.50	90.27	2.40	19.76	3.72	0.45	0.05	0.05	0.20	0.00	0.00	
Flour, semolina, enrich	0.25	Cup	41.75	150.30	5.29	30.41	1.63	0.45	0.07	0.06	0.18	0.00	0.00	
Flour, semolina, unenrich	0.25	Cup	41.75	150.30	5.29	30.41	1.63	0.45	0.07	0.06	0.18	0.00	0.00	
Flour, soy, full fat, stirred, raw	0.25	Cup	21.00	91.56	7.25	7.39	2.02	4.34	0.63	0.96	2.45	0.00	1.26	
Flour, soy, low fat, stirred	0.25	Cup	22.00	81.84	10.24	8.35	2.24	1.47	0.21	0.32	0.83	0.00	0.44	
Flour, soy, whole Arrowhead Mills, Inc.	0.25	Cup	23.00	100.00	7.00	9.00	4.00	4.50	1.00	2.50	1.00	0.00	0.00	
Flour, triticale, whole grain	0.25	Cup	32.50	109.85	4.28	23.77	4.75	0.59	0.11	0.05	0.26	0.00	0.00	
Flour, whole wheat	0.25	Cup	30.00	101.70	4.11	21.77	3.66	0.56	0.10	0.07	0.23	0.00	0.14	
Grits, corn, yellow, dry Arrowhead Mills, Inc.	0.25	Cup	39.00	130.00	3.00	30.00	1.00	0.00	0.00	0.00	0.00	0.00		
Grits, soy Heller Seasonings & Ingredients Company	0.25	Cup	39.00	109.20	20.28	11.31		0.39				0.00	0.00	
Millet, ckd	0.5	Cup	87.00	103.53	3.06	20.60	1.13	0.87	0.15	0.16	0.44	0.00	0.13	
Oats, rolled, inst, non-gmo, dry; org Grain Millers, Inc.	0.25	Cup	20.37	85.76	2.85	15.07	2.36	1.41	0.26	0.45	0.51	0.00	0.00	
Oats, Scottish, non-gmo, dry Grain Millers, Inc.	0.25	Cup	29.37	123.65	4.11	21.73	3.41	2.03	0.38	0.65	0.73	0.00	0.00	
Polenta, med American Roland Food Corp.	2	Tablespoon	30.00	80.00	2.00	18.00	2.00	0.00	0.00	0.00	0.00	0.00	0.00	
Quinoa, dry	0.25	Cup	42.50	158.95	5.56	29.28	2.50	2.46	0.25	0.65	1.00	0.00	0.00	0.00
Triticale, grain, dry	0.25	Cup	48.00	161.28	6.26	34.62	8.68	1.00	0.17	0.10	0.44	0.00	0.00	
Wheat, bulgur, dry	0.25	Cup	35.00	119.70	4.30	26.55	6.40	0.47	0.08	0.06	0.19	0.00	0.16	
Wheat, durum, grain	0.25	Cup	48.00	162.72	6.57	34.14	5.99	1.18	0.21	0.16	0.47	0.00	0.00	
Wheat, germ, honey crunch, Kretschmer Quaker Oats	2	Tablespoon	16.90	62.87	4.49	9.83	1.73	1.32	0.23	0.18	0.82	0.00	0.00	0.00

Vit E (mg)	Vit C	Vit B₁ Thia (mg)	Vit B₂ Ribo (mg)	Vit B₃ Nia (mg)	Fol (mcg)	Vit B₆ (mg)	Vita B₁₂ (mcg)	Sodi (mg)	Pota (mg)	Cal (mg)	Phos (mg)	Magn (mg)	Iron (mg)	Zinc (mg)	Caff (mg)	Alco (g)	Sol Fiber (g)	Insol Fiber (g)
0.11	0.00	0.30	0.18	2.21	112.20	0.17	0.00	560.57	87.97	127.07	276.67	22.95	2.11	0.59	0.00	0.00		
0.06	0.00	0.23	0.14	1.58	80.38	0.14	0.00	465.06	58.65	120.75	214.93	16.90	1.63	0.34	0.00	0.00	0.74	1.71
0.13	0.00	0.12	0.06	1.11	7.62	0.09	0.00	10.67	87.53	1.83	73.50	38.73	1.06	0.56	0.00	0.00	1.28	0.95
	0.00	0.04	0.04	0.68	32.32	0.19	0.00	0.00	201.85	12.19	29.20	31.18	0.34	0.19	0.00	0.00		
0.02	0.00	0.25	0.16	1.84	57.19	0.01	0.00	0.62	33.44	4.69	33.75	6.87	1.45	0.22	0.00	0.00	0.32	0.52
0.02	0.00	0.21	0.12	1.82	61.25	0.02	0.00	396.87	38.75	105.62	185.94	5.94	1.46	0.20	0.00	0.00	0.28	0.56
	0.00		0.05	0.30				0.00	83.23	30.27	45.40		2.04		0.00	0.00		
	0.00	0.00	0.00	0.00	2.24	0.00	0.00	0.64	3.52	12.80	1.60	0.96	0.11	0.02	0.00	0.00		
0.21		0.14	0.04	2.32	2.96	0.15	0.00	1.48	114.33	11.84	109.52	35.52	0.99	0.74	0.00	0.00		
0.23	0.24	0.12	0.12	2.28	15.39	0.27	0.00	4.46	90.72	14.99	122.72	39.29	1.90	0.84	0.00	0.00		
0.14	0.00	0.27	0.17	2.59	62.68	0.01	0.00	0.68	34.25	5.14	33.22	8.56	1.51	0.30	0.00	0.00		
0.10	0.00	0.13	0.06	1.85	16.20	0.17	0.00	3.30	173.10	12.30	101.10	75.30	1.22	0.94	0.00	0.00		
0.01	0.00	0.31	0.15	2.33	63.70	0.01	0.00	0.68	35.96	4.79	29.11	5.48	2.51	0.22	0.00	0.00	0.21	0.38
0.05	0.00	0.41	0.22	2.80	66.40	0.10	0.00	1.42	84.93	40.18	63.55	31.35	2.05	0.50	0.00	0.00	0.83	1.91
0.13	0.00	0.07	0.02	0.56	7.31	0.11	0.00	1.46	92.14	2.05	79.56	27.20	0.69	0.51	0.00	0.00	0.70	2.11
0.05	0.00	0.02	0.02	0.84	15.12	0.03	0.00	0.31	28.35	0.63	18.90	5.67	0.28	0.12	0.00	0.00		
0.13	0.00	0.07	0.02	0.56	7.31	0.11	0.00	1.46	92.14	2.05	79.56	27.20	0.69	0.51	0.00	0.00	0.99	2.93
	0.00	0.08	0.03	0.37			0.00	0.00	184.00	36.80	78.66		1.66		0.00	0.00		
	0.00	0.17	0.11	0.61				0.00	113.57	0.00			2.04		0.00	0.00		
	0.00	0.11						0.00	79.45	15.13			1.09		0.00	0.00		
0.01	0.00	0.10	0.07	4.05	37.20	0.08	0.00	27.00	193.50	21.00	114.00	55.50	0.32	0.76	0.00	0.00	0.07	2.30
0.30	0.00	0.07	0.02	1.72	19.95	0.04	0.00	0.15	203.70	19.50	76.20	7.20	0.71	0.90	0.00	0.00	0.07	2.30
0.11	1.52	0.09	0.03	1.40	10.00	0.31	0.00	22.00	400.40	26.00	67.20	26.00	0.55	0.21	0.00	0.00		
0.26	0.00	0.17	0.03	2.50	6.32	0.29	0.00	3.16	114.16	4.35	133.12	44.24	0.78	0.97	0.00	0.00	0.20	1.62
0.04	0.00	0.05	0.01	1.03	1.58	0.17	0.00	0.00	30.02	3.95	38.71	13.83	0.14	0.32	0.00	0.00	0.24	0.71
	0.00	0.23	0.14	1.60	40.00			0.00		0.00			1.44		0.00	0.00		
0.45	0.00	0.10	0.09	1.37	19.20	0.14	0.00	0.32	233.60	17.92	202.24	79.36	2.07	1.80	0.00	0.00	1.18	6.05
0.11	0.00	0.09	0.03	0.20	5.61	0.06	0.00	0.51	59.42	5.36	49.47	17.85	0.46	0.45	0.00	0.00	1.50	2.22
0.20	0.00	0.08	0.03	0.44	4.85	0.07	0.00	0.77	86.70	6.12	52.79	19.13	0.54	0.51	0.00	0.00	0.79	2.93
0.11	0.00	0.33	0.24	2.50	76.40	0.04	0.00	0.42	77.65	7.10	56.78	19.62	1.82	0.45	0.00	0.00	0.58	1.04
0.11	0.00	0.11	0.03	1.38	30.06	0.04	0.00	0.42	77.65	7.10	56.78	19.62	0.51	0.45	0.00	0.00	0.58	1.04
0.41	0.00	0.12	0.24	0.91	72.45	0.10	0.00	2.73	528.15	43.26	103.74	90.09	1.34	0.83	0.00	0.00	0.12	1.90
0.04	0.00	0.08	0.07	0.48	90.20	0.12	0.00	3.96	565.40	41.36	130.46	50.38	1.32	0.26	0.00	0.00	0.13	2.11
	0.00	0.15	0.22	1.60				0.00	380.00	40.00			1.80		0.00	0.00		
0.29	0.00	0.12	0.04	0.93	24.05	0.13	0.00	0.65	151.45	11.38	104.33	49.73	0.85	0.87	0.00	0.00	0.79	3.95
0.25	0.00	0.13	0.06	1.91	13.20	0.10	0.00	1.50	121.50	10.20	103.80	41.40	1.16	0.88	0.00	0.00	0.62	3.04
	0.00							0.00	30.00	0.00			0.36		0.00	0.00		
0.00	0.00	0.24	0.12	1.01	0.00	0.20	0.00	3.90	963.30	124.80	284.70	122.07	3.90	2.07	0.00	0.00		
0.02	0.00	0.09	0.07	1.16	16.53	0.10	0.00	1.74	53.94	2.61	87.00	38.28	0.55	0.79	0.00	0.00	0.61	0.52
	0.00							0.90	78.22	11.61	105.92		0.94		0.00	0.00		
	0.00							1.29	112.78	16.74	152.72		1.35		0.00	0.00		
	0.00							0.00		0.00			0.36		0.00	0.00		
2.07	0.00	0.08	0.17	1.25	20.82	0.09	0.00	8.92	314.50	25.50	174.25	89.25	3.93	1.40	0.00	0.00		
0.43	0.00	0.20	0.06	0.68	35.04	0.06	0.00	2.40	159.36	17.76	171.84	62.40	1.24	1.65	0.00	0.00	1.44	7.24
0.02	0.00	0.08	0.04	1.79	9.45	0.12	0.00	5.95	143.50	12.25	105.00	57.40	0.86	0.68	0.00	0.00	1.09	5.32
0.43	0.00	0.20	0.05	3.23	20.64	0.20	0.00	0.96	206.88	16.32	243.84	69.12	1.69	1.99	0.00	0.00	0.71	5.28
3.42	0.00	0.23	0.12	0.80	102.41	0.08	0.00	1.86	162.92	8.45	170.86	45.97	1.36	2.34	0.00	0.00	0.12	1.61

Food Name	Amount	Measure	Weight (g)	Calories	Protein (g)	Total Carb (g)	Dietary Fiber (g)	Total Fat (g)	Sat Fat (g)	Mono Fat (g)	Poly Fat (g)	Chol (mg)	Vit A (mcg RAE)	Vit D (mcg)
GRAIN PRODUCTS, PREPARED AND BAKED GOODS														
Bagels														
Bagel Chips, onion & garlic, tstd Pepperidge Farm	1	Ounce-weight	28.35	111.38	3.04	18.22	2.02	4.56	1.02	3.04	0.00	0.00	0.00	
Bagel, cinnamon raisin, 4 1/2"	1	Each	118.00	323.32	11.56	65.14	2.71	2.01	0.32	0.21	0.79	0.00	24.78	
Bagel, egg, 4 1/2"	1	Each	110.00	305.80	11.66	58.30	2.53	2.31	0.46	0.46	0.71	26.40	36.30	
Bagel, everything, NY style Thomas'	1	Each	104.00	300.00	11.00	54.00	3.00	4.00	1.00			0.00	0.00	
Bagel, oat bran, 3 1/2"	1	Each	71.00	181.05	7.60	37.84	2.56	0.85	0.14	0.18	0.35	0.00	0.71	
Bagel, oat bran, mini, 2 1/2"	1	Each	26.00	66.30	2.78	13.86	0.94	0.31	0.05	0.06	0.13	0.00	0.26	
Bagel, onion, enrich, w/calc propionate, 3 1/2"	1	Each	71.00	195.25	7.45	37.91	1.63	1.14	0.16	0.09	0.49	0.00	0.00	
Bagel, onion, enrich, w/calc propionate, 4 1/2"	1	Each	110.00	302.50	11.55	58.74	2.53	1.76	0.24	0.14	0.77	0.00	0.00	
Bagel, plain, classic Bruegger's Corporation	1	Each	112.22	296.01	10.81	60.36	3.36	1.87				0.00	0.00	0.00
Bagel, salt, classic Bruegger's Corporation	1	Each	114.69	296.01	10.81	60.36	3.36	1.87				0.00	0.00	0.00
Bagel, sesame, classic Bruegger's Corporation	1	Each	114.30	311.01	10.81	60.36	3.36	1.87				0.00	0.00	0.00
Bagel, sun dried tomato basil Natural Ovens	1	Each	85.00	170.00	6.00	38.00	6.00	2.00	0.00			0.00		
Bagel, whole grain Natural Ovens	1	Each	85.00	170.00	6.00	37.00	6.00	2.00	0.00			0.00	0.00	
Biscuits														
Biscuit, buttermilk, bkd f/refrig dough, higher fat, 2 1/2"	1	Each	27.00	93.42	1.81	12.83	0.43	3.97	1.00	2.22	0.53	0.00	0.00	
Biscuit, buttermilk, bkd f/refrig dough, lower fat, 2 1/4"	1	Each	21.00	62.79	1.64	11.63	0.40	1.09	0.27	0.59	0.16	0.00	0.00	
Biscuit, buttermilk, cmrcl bkd, 2 1/2"	1	Each	35.00	127.40	2.17	16.97	0.45	5.77	0.87	2.42	2.17	0.35		
Biscuit, buttermilk, dry mix, svg Martha White	1	Each	41.00	171.38	3.03	26.44		5.94	1.12	3.44	0.57			
Biscuit, buttermilk, prep f/dry mix	1	Ounce-weight	28.35	94.97	2.07	13.72	0.51	3.43	0.79	1.19	1.22	1.13	7.37	
Biscuit, buttermilk, prep f/recipe, 2 1/2"	1	Each	60.00	212.40	4.20	26.76	0.91	9.79	2.60	4.16	2.50	1.80	13.80	
Biscuit, buttermilk, refrig dough, svg PI Grands	1	Each	61.00	194.59	4.15	25.07		8.66	2.35	4.85	0.21			
Biscuit, plain, bkd f/refrig dough, higher fat, 2 1/2"	1	Each	27.00	93.42	1.81	12.83	0.43	3.97	1.00	2.22	0.53	0.00	0.00	
Biscuit, plain, cmrcl bkd, 2 1/2"	1	Each	35.00	127.40	2.17	16.97	0.45	5.77	0.87	2.42	2.17	0.35		
Biscuit, plain, prep f/recipe, 2 1/2"	1	Each	60.00	212.40	4.20	26.76	0.91	9.79	2.60	4.16	2.50	1.80	13.80	
Breads and Rolls														
Bread, 7 grain, slice	1	Piece	26.00	65.00	2.60	12.06	1.66	0.99	0.21	0.40	0.24	0.00	0.00	
Bread, banana, homemade w/margarine, slice	1	Piece	60.00	195.60	2.58	32.76	0.66	6.30	1.34	2.69	1.88	25.80	63.60	
Bread, Boston brown, cnd, slice	1	Piece	45.00	87.75	2.34	19.48	2.11	0.67	0.13	0.09	0.25	0.45	11.25	
Bread, cracked wheat, slice, reg	1	Piece	25.00	65.00	2.17	12.38	1.38	0.98	0.23	0.48	0.17	0.00	0.00	
Bread, cracked wheat, slice, thin	1	Piece	20.00	52.00	1.74	9.90	1.10	0.78	0.18	0.38	0.14	0.00	0.00	
Bread, egg, slice	1	Piece	40.00	114.80	3.80	19.12	0.92	2.40	0.64	0.92	0.44	20.40	25.20	
Bread, focaccia Oroweat	1	Piece	57.00	150.00	4.00	31.00	1.00	1.50	0.00			0.00	0.00	
Bread, French, slice, lrg	1	Piece	96.00	263.04	8.45	49.82	2.88	2.88	0.62	1.17	0.67	0.00	0.00	
Bread, garlic Pepperidge Farm	1	Piece	47.00	160.00	5.00	14.00	1.00	10.00	3.00	4.00	1.50	30.00	0.00	
Bread, Health Nut Oroweat	1	Piece	38.00	100.00	4.00	18.00	2.00	2.00	0.00			0.00	0.00	
Bread, Italian, slice, med	1	Piece	20.00	54.20	1.76	10.00	0.54	0.70	0.17	0.16	0.28	0.00	0.00	
Bread, mixed grain, slice, lrg	1	Piece	32.00	80.00	3.20	14.85	2.05	1.22	0.26	0.49	0.30	0.00	0.00	
Bread, multigrain, Carb Counting Oroweat	1	Piece	27.00	60.00	5.00	9.00	3.00	1.50	0.00			0.00	0.00	
Bread, naan, Tandoori style, original Garden of Eatin'	1	Each	71.00	200.00	7.00	35.00	4.00	4.00	1.00			0.00	0.00	
Bread, oat bran, rducd cal, slice	1	Piece	23.00	46.23	1.84	9.50	2.76	0.74	0.10	0.16	0.38	0.00	0.02	
Bread, oat bran, slice	1	Piece	30.00	70.80	3.12	11.94	1.35	1.32	0.21	0.48	0.51	0.00	0.60	
Bread, oatmeal, slice	1	Piece	27.00	72.63	2.27	13.10	1.08	1.19	0.19	0.43	0.46	0.00	1.35	
Bread, pita, wheat, sml, 4"	1	Each	28.00	74.48	2.74	15.40	2.07	0.73	0.11	0.10	0.30	0.00	0.00	
Bread, pita, white, enrich, sml, 4"	1	Each	28.00	77.00	2.55	15.60	0.62	0.34	0.05	0.03	0.15	0.00	0.00	
Bread, pumpernickel, slice, thin	1	Piece	20.00	50.00	1.74	9.50	1.30	0.62	0.09	0.19	0.25	0.00	0.00	
Bread, pumpkin, dry quick mix Pillsbury	1	Ounce-weight	28.35	111.68	1.72	22.34	0.64	1.29	0.00			0.00		
Bread, raisin, enrich, slice	1	Piece	26.00	71.24	2.05	13.60	1.12	1.14	0.28	0.60	0.18	0.00	0.00	
Bread, rice bran, slice	1	Piece	27.00	65.61	2.40	11.75	1.32	1.24	0.19	0.45	0.48	0.00	0.01	

Vit E (mg)	Vit C	Vit B₁ Thia (mg)	Vit B₂ Ribo (mg)	Vit B₃ Nia (mg)	Fol (mcg)	Vit B₆ (mg)	Vita B₁₂ (mcg)	Sodi (mg)	Pota (mg)	Cal (mg)	Phos (mg)	Magn (mg)	Iron (mg)	Zinc (mg)	Caff (mg)	Alco (g)	Sol Fiber (g)	Insol Fiber (g)
0.00	0.00	0.22	0.14	2.02				283.50		0.00			1.46		0.00	0.00		
0.37	0.83	0.45	0.33	3.63	130.98	0.07	0.00	379.96	174.64	22.42	118.00	33.04	4.48	1.33	0.00	0.00	0.98	1.73
0.15	0.66	0.59	0.26	3.79	96.80	0.10	0.18	555.50	74.80	14.30	92.40	27.50	4.38	0.85	0.00	0.00	0.91	1.62
	0.00							510.00		100.00			3.60		0.00	0.00		
0.23	0.14	0.24	0.24	2.10	69.58	0.03	0.00	359.97	81.65	8.52	78.10	22.01	2.19	0.64	0.00	0.00	1.20	1.36
0.09	0.05	0.09	0.09	0.77	25.48	0.01	0.00	131.82	29.90	3.12	28.60	8.06	0.80	0.23	0.00	0.00	0.44	0.50
0.21	0.00	0.38	0.22	3.24	75.26	0.04	0.00	379.14	71.71	52.54	68.16	20.59	2.53	0.62	0.00	0.00	0.57	1.06
0.32	0.00	0.59	0.35	5.02	116.60	0.06	0.00	587.40	111.10	81.40	105.60	31.90	3.92	0.97	0.00	0.00	0.88	1.65
0.00	0.14	0.48	0.31	3.96	0.13	0.00	0.00	510.00	80.18	14.35	71.02	0.40	3.33	0.01	0.00	0.00		
0.00	0.14	0.48	0.31	3.96	0.13	0.00	0.00	1471.29	80.31	21.76	71.02	0.40	3.33	0.01	0.00	0.00		
0.00	0.14	0.48	0.31	3.96	0.13	0.00	0.00	510.00	80.18	14.35	71.02	0.40	6.57	0.01	0.00	0.00		
	6.00	0.45		8.00		0.60	1.80	270.00		200.00		120.00	1.08	4.50	0.00	0.00		
	0.00	0.45	0.51	8.00		0.60	1.80	200.00		200.00		120.00	1.08	4.50	0.00	0.00		
0.02	0.00	0.09	0.06	0.83	22.41	0.01	0.00	324.54	42.39	5.40	103.95	3.78	0.70	0.10	0.00	0.00	0.26	0.17
0.01	0.00	0.09	0.05	0.72	17.43	0.01	0.00	304.71	38.85	3.99	97.65	3.57	0.65	0.10	0.00	0.00	0.24	0.16
0.46	0.00	0.15	0.10	1.17	24.50	0.02	0.05	368.20	78.40	17.15	150.50	5.95	1.15	0.17	0.00	0.00	0.28	0.18
								504.30		60.68					0.00	0.00		
0.11	0.11	0.10	0.10	0.86	14.74	0.02	0.06	270.74	53.30	52.45	133.24	7.09	0.58	0.18	0.00	0.00	0.31	0.20
0.79	0.12	0.22	0.19	1.77	36.60	0.02	0.04	348.00	72.60	141.00	98.40	10.80	1.75	0.33	0.00	0.00	0.55	0.35
									605.12					1.55		0.00	0.00	
0.02	0.00	0.09	0.06	0.83	22.41	0.01	0.00	324.54	42.39	5.40	103.95	3.78	0.70	0.10	0.00	0.00	0.26	0.17
0.46	0.00	0.15	0.10	1.17	24.50	0.02	0.05	368.20	78.40	17.15	150.50	5.95	1.15	0.17	0.00	0.00	0.28	0.18
0.79	0.12	0.22	0.19	1.77	36.60	0.02	0.04	348.00	72.60	141.00	98.40	10.80	1.75	0.33	0.00	0.00	0.55	0.35
0.09	0.08	0.11	0.09	1.13	30.68	0.09	0.02	126.62	53.04	23.66	45.76	13.78	0.90	0.33	0.00	0.00	0.23	1.43
1.07	1.02	0.10	0.12	0.87	19.80	0.09	0.06	181.20	80.40	12.60	34.80	8.40	0.84	0.21	0.00	0.00		
0.14	0.00	0.01	0.05	0.50	4.95	0.04	0.00	283.95	143.10	31.50	50.40	28.35	0.94	0.22	0.00	0.00		
0.15	0.00	0.09	0.06	0.92	15.25	0.08	0.00	134.50	44.25	10.75	38.25	13.00	0.70	0.31	0.00	0.00	0.20	1.17
0.12	0.00	0.07	0.05	0.73	12.20	0.06	0.00	107.60	35.40	8.60	30.60	10.40	0.56	0.25	0.00	0.00	0.16	0.94
0.10	0.00	0.18	0.17	1.94	42.00	0.03	0.04	196.80	46.00	37.20	42.40	7.60	1.22	0.32	0.00	0.00	0.30	0.62
	0.00	0.30	0.17	2.00	0.00			320.00		0.00			1.80		0.00	0.00		
0.29	0.00	0.50	0.32	4.56	142.08	0.04	0.00	584.64	108.48	72.00	100.80	25.92	2.43	0.84	0.00	0.00	0.92	1.96
	0.00	0.23	0.14	1.60				250.00		0.00			3.60		0.00	0.00		
	0.00	0.12	0.07	1.20	24.00			180.00		20.00			1.08		0.00	0.00		
0.06	0.00	0.09	0.06	0.88	38.20	0.01	0.00	116.80	22.00	15.60	20.60	5.40	0.59	0.17	0.00	0.00	0.17	0.37
0.11	0.10	0.13	0.11	1.40	37.76	0.11	0.02	155.84	65.28	29.12	56.32	16.96	1.11	0.41	0.00	0.00	0.29	1.76
	0.00							140.00		40.00			1.08		0.00	0.00		
	0.00							330.00		20.00			1.80		0.00	0.00		
0.06	0.00	0.08	0.05	0.87	18.63	0.02	0.00	80.73	23.46	13.11	31.97	12.65	0.72	0.24	0.00	0.00	1.71	1.05
0.13	0.00	0.15	0.10	1.45	24.30	0.02	0.00	122.10	44.10	19.50	42.30	10.50	0.94	0.27	0.00	0.00		
0.13	0.00	0.11	0.06	0.85	16.74	0.02	0.01	161.73	38.34	17.82	34.02	9.99	0.73	0.28	0.00	0.00	0.29	0.79
0.17	0.00	0.09	0.02	0.80	9.80	0.07	0.00	148.96	47.60	4.20	50.40	19.32	0.86	0.43	0.00	0.00	0.91	1.16
0.08	0.00	0.17	0.09	1.30	29.96	0.01	0.00	150.08	33.60	24.08	27.16	7.28	0.73	0.24	0.00	0.00	0.27	0.34
0.08	0.00	0.07	0.06	0.62	18.60	0.03	0.00	134.20	41.60	13.60	35.60	10.80	0.57	0.30	0.00	0.00	0.60	0.70
	0.00							163.23		17.18			0.61		0.00	0.00		
0.07	0.03	0.09	0.10	0.90	27.56	0.02	0.00	101.40	59.02	17.16	28.34	6.76	0.75	0.19	0.00	0.00	0.26	0.86
0.18	0.00	0.18	0.08	1.84	23.22	0.07	0.00	118.80	58.05	18.63	48.06	21.60	0.97	0.35	0.00	0.00		

Food Name	Amount	Measure	Weight (g)	Calories	Protein (g)	Total Carb (g)	Dietary Fiber (g)	Total Fat (g)	Sat Fat (g)	Mono Fat (g)	Poly Fat (g)	Chol (mg)	Vit A (mcg RAE)	Vit D (mcg)
GRAIN PRODUCTS, PREPARED AND BAKED GOODS *(continued)*														
Bread, rye, slice	1	Piece	32.00	82.88	2.72	15.46	1.86	1.06	0.20	0.42	0.26	0.00	0.13	
Bread, sourdough, slice, med	1	Piece	64.00	175.36	5.63	33.22	1.92	1.92	0.41	0.78	0.44	0.00	0.00	
Bread, sourdough, slice, med, tstd	1	Piece	59.00	175.82	5.66	33.28	1.95	1.95	0.41	0.78	0.44	0.00	0.00	
Bread, wheat berry, slice	1	Piece	25.00	65.00	2.28	11.80	1.08	1.02	0.22	0.43	0.23	0.00	0.00	
Bread, wheat bran, slice	1	Piece	36.00	89.28	3.17	17.21	1.44	1.22	0.28	0.58	0.23	0.00	0.00	
Bread, wheat free, enrich, Papa's, 1/12 loaf or whole Ener-G Foods	1	Piece	42.00	133.05	1.01	18.99	2.77	5.96	0.46			0.00		
Bread, wheat, rducd calorie, slice	1	Piece	23.00	45.54	2.09	10.03	2.76	0.53	0.08	0.06	0.22	0.00	0.00	
Bread, white, rducd cal, slice	1	Piece	23.00	47.61	2.00	10.19	2.23	0.58	0.13	0.25	0.13	0.00	0.03	
Bread, white, soft, enrich, slice	1	Piece	25.00	66.50	1.91	12.65	0.60	0.82	0.18	0.17	0.34	0.00	0.00	
Bread, whole wheat, slice	1	Piece	28.00	68.88	2.72	12.91	1.93	1.18	0.26	0.47	0.28	0.00	0.04	
Breadsticks, focaccia, 133920, FS Pierre Foods	1	Each	42.53	133.00	3.10	22.70		3.40	0.70			0.03		
Breadsticks, plain, 7 5/8" × 5/8"	1	Each	10.00	41.20	1.20	6.84	0.30	0.95	0.14	0.36	0.36	0.00	0.01	
Breadsticks, plain, 9 1/4" × 3/8"	1	Each	6.00	24.72	0.72	4.10	0.18	0.57	0.08	0.21	0.22	0.00	0.00	
Breadsticks, plain, sml, 4 1/4" long	1	Each	5.00	20.60	0.60	3.42	0.15	0.48	0.07	0.18	0.18	0.00	0.00	
Buns, hamburger	1	Each	43.00	119.97	4.09	21.26	0.90	1.86	0.47	0.48	0.85	0.00	0.00	
Buns, hamburger, mixed grain	1	Each	43.00	113.09	4.13	19.18	1.63	2.58	0.60	1.22	0.50	0.00	0.00	
Buns, hot dog/frankfurter	1	Each	43.00	119.97	4.09	21.26	0.90	1.86	0.47	0.48	0.85	0.00	0.00	
Buns, hot dog/frankfurter, rducd cal	1	Each	43.00	84.28	3.57	18.10	2.67	0.86	0.14	0.23	0.33	0.00	0.00	
Cornbread, 2.5 × 2.5 × 1.5 pce	1	Piece	65.00	151.85	4.03	22.66	1.93	4.93	1.57	2.39	0.54	22.08	30.20	0.39
Cornbread, prep f/dry mix, pce	1	Piece	60.00	188.40	4.32	28.86	1.44	6.00	1.64	3.08	0.73	36.60	26.40	
Croissant, butter, mini	1	Each	28.35	115.10	2.32	12.98	0.74	5.95	3.31	1.57	0.31	18.99	58.40	
Dumpling, gnocchi, potato	1	Cup	188.00	268.21	4.76	33.15	1.75	13.10	8.02	3.70	0.63	35.28	123.39	
Pretzels, soft, parmesan herb Auntie Anne's Incorporated	1	Each	120.00	390.00	11.00	74.00	4.00	5.00	2.50			10.00		
Rolls, dinner, brown & serve, browned	1	Each	28.00	84.00	2.35	14.11	0.84	2.04	0.49	1.04	0.34	0.28	0.01	
Rolls, dinner, egg, 2 1/2"	1	Each	35.00	107.45	3.32	18.20	1.29	2.24	0.55	1.03	0.39	17.50	1.75	
Rolls, dinner, prep f/recipe w/2% milk, 2 1/2"	1	Each	35.00	110.60	2.97	18.69	0.66	2.55	0.63	1.01	0.70	12.25	30.45	
Rolls, dinner, wheat, 1oz each	1	Each	28.35	77.40	2.44	13.04	1.08	1.79	0.42	0.88	0.31	0.00	0.00	
Rolls, French	1	Each	38.00	105.26	3.27	19.08	1.22	1.63	0.37	0.75	0.32	0.00	0.00	
Rolls, hard, 3 1/2"	1	Each	57.00	167.01	5.64	30.04	1.31	2.45	0.35	0.65	0.98	0.00	0.00	
Rolls, onion	1	Each	43.00	129.00	3.61	21.67	1.29	3.14	0.75	1.59	0.52	0.43	0.02	
Bread Crumbs, Croutons, Breading Mixes & Batters														
Bread Crumbs, plain, grated, dry	1	Tablespoon	6.75	26.66	0.90	4.86	0.30	0.36	0.08	0.07	0.14	0.00	0.00	
Bread Crumbs, seasoned, grated, dry	1	Tablespoon	7.50	28.72	1.06	5.14	0.37	0.41	0.10	0.09	0.17	0.08	0.75	
Cracker Meal	0.25	Cup	28.75	110.11	2.67	23.26	0.75	0.49	0.08	0.05	0.21	0.00	0.00	
Croutons, plain, dry	0.25	Cup	7.50	30.52	0.89	5.52	0.39	0.49	0.12	0.22	0.10	0.00	0.00	
Croutons, seasoned, cubes	0.25	Cup	10.00	46.50	1.09	6.36	0.50	1.83	0.53	0.94	0.24	0.70	0.70	
Crackers														
Crackers, cheese sandwich	4	Each	28.00	133.56	2.60	17.28	0.53	5.91	1.72	3.15	0.72	0.56	4.76	
Crackers, cheese, 1" square, each	30	Each	30.00	150.90	3.03	17.46	0.72	7.59	2.81	3.63	0.74	3.90	8.70	
Crackers, cheese, cheddar, pkg Frito Lay	1	Each	40.00	210.00	3.00	23.00	1.00	11.00	3.00			5.00	0.00	
Crackers, cheese, cheddar, Goldfish Pepperidge Farm	55	Piece	30.00	140.00	4.00	19.00	1.00	6.00				10.00	0.00	
Crackers, cheese, low sod, gold fish	55	Piece	33.00	165.99	3.33	19.21	0.79	8.35	3.18	3.92	0.81	4.29	5.61	
Crackers, cheese, peanut butter sandwich	4	Each	28.00	138.88	3.47	15.89	0.95	7.04	1.23	3.64	1.43	0.00	0.22	0.00
Crackers, cheese, zesty, svg Snackwell's	1	Ounce-weight	28.35	122.19	2.12	21.83	0.57	2.83	0.63	0.77	0.41	1.13		
Crackers, graham, chocolate coated, 2 1/2" square	2	Each	28.00	135.52	1.62	18.62	0.87	6.50	3.74	2.16	0.29	0.00	1.40	
Crackers, graham, cinnamon, lrg rectangle	2	Each	28.00	118.44	1.93	21.50	0.78	2.83	0.43	1.15	1.07	0.00	0.03	
Crackers, graham, svg Nabisco	1	Ounce-weight	28.35	120.20	1.98	21.60	0.96	2.83	0.44	1.02	0.13	0.00	0.00	
Crackers, matzoh, egg, svg	1	Ounce-weight	28.35	110.85	3.49	22.28	0.79	0.60	0.16	0.17	0.13	23.53	3.69	
Crackers, matzoh, whole wheat, svg	1	Ounce-weight	28.35	99.51	3.71	22.37	3.35	0.43	0.07	0.05	0.19	0.00	0.00	
Crackers, melba toast, plain, rounds	10	Each	30.00	117.00	3.63	22.98	1.89	0.96	0.13	0.23	0.38	0.00	0.00	
Crackers, melba toast, pumpernickel	6	Each	30.00	116.70	3.48	23.22	2.40	1.02	0.12	0.30	0.42	0.00	0.00	
Crackers, milk	3	Each	33.00	150.15	2.51	23.00	0.63	5.21	0.87	2.13	1.89	3.63	5.28	
Crackers, peanut butter sandwich	4	Each	28.00	138.32	3.21	16.34	0.64	6.87	1.37	3.85	1.31	0.00	0.01	
Crackers, Ritz, svg Nabisco	1	Ounce-weight	28.35	139.48	2.04	18.20	0.54	6.49	1.08	4.93	0.48	0.00	0.00	
Crackers, rusk toast	3	Each	30.00	122.10	4.05	21.69	0.60	2.16	0.41	0.83	0.69	23.40	3.60	

Vit E (mg)	Vit C	Vit B₁ Thia (mg)	Vit B₂ Ribo (mg)	Vit B₃ Nia (mg)	Fol (mcg)	Vit B₆ (mg)	Vita B₁₂ (mcg)	Sodi (mg)	Pota (mg)	Cal (mg)	Phos (mg)	Magn (mg)	Iron (mg)	Zinc (mg)	Caff (mg)	Alco (g)	Sol Fiber (g)	Insol Fiber (g)
0.11	0.13	0.14	0.11	1.22	35.20	0.02	0.00	211.20	53.12	23.36	40.00	12.80	0.91	0.36	0.00	0.00	0.84	1.02
0.19	0.00	0.33	0.21	3.04	94.72	0.03	0.00	389.76	72.32	48.00	67.20	17.28	1.62	0.56	0.00	0.00	0.61	1.31
0.19	0.00	0.27	0.19	2.74	57.23	0.02	0.00	389.99	71.98	47.79	67.26	17.70	1.62	0.56	0.00	0.00	0.63	1.32
0.07	0.00	0.10	0.07	1.03	22.75	0.02	0.00	132.50	50.25	26.25	37.50	11.50	0.83	0.26	0.00	0.00	0.16	0.92
0.12	0.00	0.14	0.10	1.58	37.80	0.06	0.00	174.96	81.72	26.64	66.60	29.16	1.11	0.49	0.00	0.00		
	0.84	0.05	0.13	0.38	24.23				54.17	58.16			3.09		0.00	0.00		
0.06	0.02	0.10	0.07	0.89	20.93	0.03	0.00	117.53	28.06	18.40	23.46	8.97	0.68	0.26	0.00	0.00	0.17	2.59
0.04	0.12	0.09	0.07	0.84	21.85	0.01	0.06	104.19	17.48	21.62	27.83	5.29	0.73	0.31	0.00	0.00	0.13	2.10
0.06	0.00	0.11	0.08	1.10	27.75	0.02	0.00	170.25	25.00	37.75	24.75	5.75	0.94	0.18	0.00	0.00		
0.09	0.00	0.10	0.06	1.07	14.00	0.05	0.00	147.56	70.56	20.16	64.12	24.08	0.92	0.54	0.00	0.00	0.43	1.51
	1.42							169.70	35.30	29.00			0.54		0.00	0.00		
0.10	0.00	0.06	0.06	0.53	16.20	0.01	0.00	65.70	12.40	2.20	12.10	3.20	0.43	0.09	0.00	0.00	0.12	0.18
0.06	0.00	0.04	0.03	0.32	9.72	0.00	0.00	39.42	7.44	1.32	7.26	1.92	0.26	0.05	0.00	0.00	0.07	0.11
0.05	0.00	0.03	0.03	0.26	8.10	0.00	0.00	32.85	6.20	1.10	6.05	1.60	0.21	0.04	0.00	0.00	0.06	0.09
0.03	0.00	0.17	0.14	1.79	47.73	0.03	0.09	205.97	40.42	59.34	26.66	9.03	1.43	0.28	0.00	0.00	0.26	0.65
0.03	0.00	0.20	0.13	1.92	47.73	0.04	0.00	196.94	68.80	40.85	52.46	18.92	1.70	0.45	0.00	0.00		
0.03	0.00	0.17	0.14	1.79	47.73	0.03	0.09	205.97	40.42	59.34	26.66	9.03	1.43	0.28	0.00	0.00	0.26	0.65
0.03	0.09	0.17	0.08	2.12	47.73	0.02	0.04	190.06	33.54	25.37	36.12	8.60	1.29	0.29	0.00	0.00		
0.64	0.26	0.12	0.16	0.93	5.54	0.05	0.12	355.80	104.75	70.54	193.21	13.17	0.82	0.38	0.00	0.00		
0.72	0.06	0.15	0.16	1.23	33.00	0.06	0.10	466.80	76.80	43.80	225.60	12.00	1.14	0.38	0.00	0.00	0.79	0.65
0.24	0.06	0.11	0.07	0.62	24.95	0.02	0.05	210.92	33.45	10.49	29.77	4.54	0.58	0.21	0.00	0.00	0.49	0.24
0.31	3.51	0.25	0.19	2.19	10.40	0.19	0.13	141.06	245.15	43.68	79.27	20.74	1.44	0.44	0.00	0.00		
	1.20							780.00		80.00			1.80		0.00	0.00		
0.09	0.03	0.14	0.09	1.13	27.44	0.02	0.02	145.88	37.24	33.32	32.48	6.44	0.88	0.22	0.00	0.00	0.31	0.53
0.13	0.00	0.18	0.18	1.15	64.40	0.02	0.08	190.75	36.40	20.65	35.35	8.75	1.23	0.39	0.00	0.00		
0.34	0.07	0.14	0.14	1.21	31.50	0.02	0.05	145.25	53.20	21.00	44.10	6.65	1.04	0.24	0.00	0.00		
0.10	0.00	0.12	0.08	1.15	17.01	0.02	0.00	96.39	32.60	49.90	29.48	10.21	1.01	0.26	0.00	0.00		
0.11	0.00	0.20	0.11	1.65	42.94	0.01	0.00	231.42	43.32	34.58	31.92	7.60	1.03	0.34	0.00	0.00	0.38	0.84
0.24	0.00	0.27	0.19	2.42	54.15	0.02	0.00	310.08	61.56	54.15	57.00	15.39	1.87	0.54	0.00	0.00	0.48	0.83
0.13	0.04	0.21	0.14	1.73	42.14	0.02	0.03	224.03	57.19	51.17	49.88	9.89	1.35	0.33	0.00	0.00	0.47	0.82
0.00	0.00	0.07	0.03	0.45	7.22	0.01	0.02	49.41	13.23	12.35	11.14	2.90	0.33	0.10	0.00	0.00		
0.02	0.20	0.07	0.03	0.46	8.93	0.01	0.00	131.93	17.32	13.65	13.28	3.45	0.37	0.11	0.00	0.00		
0.12	0.00	0.20	0.13	1.64	39.10	0.01	0.00	8.05	33.06	6.61	29.90	6.90	1.33	0.20	0.00	0.00	0.29	0.46
0.02	0.00	0.04	0.02	0.41	9.90	0.00	0.00	52.35	9.30	5.70	8.62	2.32	0.31	0.06	0.00	0.00		
0.04	0.00	0.06	0.04	0.47	10.50	0.01	0.01	123.80	18.10	9.60	14.00	4.20	0.29	0.10	0.00	0.00		
0.07	0.03	0.12	0.20	1.05	28.00	0.01	0.03	392.28	120.12	71.96	113.68	10.08	0.67	0.18	0.00	0.00	0.21	0.33
0.02	0.00	0.17	0.13	1.40	45.60	0.17	0.14	298.50	43.50	45.30	65.40	10.80	1.43	0.34	0.00	0.00	0.27	0.45
	0.00							390.00		100.00			1.08		0.00	0.00		
	0.00	0.23	0.14	1.60				200.00		20.00			1.44		0.00	0.00		
0.10	0.00	0.19	0.14	1.54	29.37	0.19	0.15	151.14	34.98	49.83	71.94	11.88	1.57	0.37	0.00	0.00		
0.66	0.00	0.16	0.08	1.63	26.32	0.05	0.07	198.80	61.04	14.00	75.04	15.68	0.77	0.29	0.00	0.00		
	0.17	0.07	0.09	1.05	16.16	0.03	0.02	297.67	44.51	12.19	56.70	9.36	0.90	0.43	0.00	0.00		
0.07	0.00	0.04	0.06	0.61	5.60	0.02	0.00	81.48	58.52	16.24	37.52	16.24	1.00	0.27	12.88	0.00		
0.09	0.00	0.07	0.08	1.16	12.88	0.02	0.00	169.40	37.80	6.72	29.12	8.40	1.05	0.22	0.00	0.00	0.23	0.55
	0.00	0.07	0.07	1.07	13.04	0.03		186.83	50.18	22.40	57.27	16.73	1.17	0.55	0.00	0.00		
0.28	0.03	0.22	0.18	1.44	6.80	0.02	0.05	5.95	42.53	11.34	41.96	6.80	0.77	0.21	0.00	0.00	0.30	0.49
	0.00	0.10	0.08	1.53	9.92	0.05	0.00	0.57	89.59	6.52	86.47	37.99	1.32	0.74	0.00	0.00	0.94	2.41
0.13	0.00	0.12	0.08	1.23	37.20	0.03	0.00	248.70	60.60	27.90	58.80	17.70	1.11	0.60	0.00	0.00	0.45	1.44
0.18	0.00	0.12	0.06	1.44	25.50	0.00	0.00	269.70	57.90	23.40	54.90	11.70	1.08	0.42	0.00	0.00	0.54	1.86
0.41	0.07	0.18	0.14	1.46	29.70	0.01	0.02	195.36	37.62	56.76	99.99	7.26	1.18	0.22	0.00	0.00	0.24	0.39
0.58	0.00	0.14	0.07	1.71	24.08	0.04	0.00	201.04	60.20	22.68	76.72	15.40	0.77	0.32	0.00	0.00		
	0.00	0.08	0.09	1.08	17.01	0.01	0.00	220.00	26.37	41.67	85.05	5.67	1.15	0.42	0.00	0.00		
0.16	0.00	0.12	0.12	1.39	26.10	0.01	0.05	75.90	73.50	8.10	45.90	10.80	0.82	0.33	0.00	0.00	0.14	0.46

Food Name	Amount	Measure	Weight (g)	Calories	Protein (g)	Total Carb (g)	Dietary Fiber (g)	Total Fat (g)	Sat Fat (g)	Mono Fat (g)	Poly Fat (g)	Chol (mg)	Vit A (mcg RAE)	Vit D (mcg)
GRAIN PRODUCTS, PREPARED AND BAKED GOODS *(continued)*														
Crackers, rye, crispbread	3	Each	30.00	109.80	2.37	24.66	4.95	0.39	0.04	0.05	0.17	0.00	0.00	
Crackers, saltines, low sod, fat free	6	Each	30.00	117.90	3.15	24.69	0.81	0.48	0.07	0.04	0.21	0.00	0.00	
Crackers, saltines, low sod, rounds, lrg	3	Each	30.00	130.20	2.76	21.45	0.90	3.54	0.88	1.93	0.50	0.00	0.00	
Crackers, saltines, original, premium, svg Nabisco	10	Each	30.00	126.00	3.27	21.33	0.78	3.06	0.56	1.76	0.52	0.00	0.00	
Crackers, saltines, unsalted tops	10	Each	30.00	130.20	2.76	21.45	0.90	3.54	0.88	1.93	0.50	0.00	0.00	
Crackers, standard, snack type, rectangle	4	Each	32.00	160.64	2.37	19.52	0.51	8.10	1.21	3.40	3.05	0.00	0.00	
Crackers, Wheat Thins, original Nabisco	16	Each	29.00	136.30	2.41	20.04	0.87	5.80	0.93	2.03	0.36	0.00	0.00	
Crackers, wheat, peanut butter sandwich	4	Each	28.00	138.60	3.78	15.06	1.23	7.48	1.29	3.29	2.48	0.00	0.00	
Crackers, whole wheat	4	Each	32.00	141.76	2.82	21.95	3.36	5.50	1.09	1.88	2.11	0.00	0.00	
Crackers, whole wheat, low sod	7	Each	28.00	124.04	2.46	19.21	2.94	4.82	0.95	1.64	1.85	0.00	0.00	
Muffins														
English Muffin, cinnamon raisin Oroweat	1	Each	69.00	170.00	5.00	36.00	4.00	1.50	0.00			0.00	0.00	
English Muffin, granola	1	Each	66.00	155.10	6.01	30.56	1.85	1.19	0.15	0.55	0.37	0.00	0.00	
English Muffin, plain Thomas'	1	Each	57.00	131.67	4.96	25.99		0.85	0.17	0.25	0.44		0.00	
English Muffin, raisin cinnamon	1	Each	57.00	138.51	4.27	27.76	1.65	1.54	0.22	0.29	0.78	0.00		
English Muffin, sourdough Oroweat	1	Each	59.00	140.00	5.00	28.00	1.00	1.00	0.00			0.00	0.00	
English Muffin, wheat	1	Each	57.00	127.11	4.96	25.54	2.62	1.14	0.16	0.16	0.48	0.00	0.09	
English Muffin, whole wheat	1	Each	66.00	133.98	5.81	26.66	4.42	1.39	0.22	0.34	0.55	0.00	0.17	
Muffin, banana walnut, fzn, 4oz Krusteaz	1	Each	114.00	430.92	7.18	53.58	1.71	20.75	3.65	6.16	10.94	83.22		
Muffin, blackberry, fzn Krusteaz	1	Each	114.00	419.52	6.84	51.30	1.82	20.75	3.76	6.38	10.49	70.68		
Muffin, blueberry, cmrcl, med, 2" × 2 3/4"	1	Each	57.00	157.89	3.13	27.36	1.48	3.70	0.80	1.12	1.42	17.10	13.11	
Muffin, blueberry, dry mix, svg Martha White	1	Each	40.00	161.60	2.04	30.44		3.52	0.86	1.72	0.42			
Muffin, blueberry, prep f/recipe w/2% milk	1	Each	57.00	162.45	3.70	23.20	1.08	6.16	1.16	1.48	3.07	21.09	21.66	
Muffin, blueberry, toaster, tstd	1	Each	31.00	103.23	1.52	17.58	0.59	3.13	0.48	0.74	1.70	1.55	31.31	
Muffin, corn, prep f/recipe w/2% milk, 2" × 2 3/4"	1	Each	57.00	180.12	4.05	25.19	1.94	7.01	1.32	1.72	3.51	23.94		
Muffin, oat bran, 2 1/4" × 2 1/2"	1	Each	57.00	153.90	3.99	27.53	2.62	4.22	0.62	0.97	2.35	0.00	0.00	
Muffin, plain, prep f/recipe w/2% milk	1	Each	57.00	168.72	3.93	23.60	1.54	6.50	1.23	1.57	3.26	22.23	22.80	
Muffin, whole wheat, low fat, prep f/dry mix, 2 oz each Krusteaz	1	Each	56.70	150.00	3.00	32.00	1.00	1.00	0.00	0.50	0.50	0.00	0.00	
Pancakes, French Toast, and Waffles														
Crepe, chocolate filled	1	Each	78.00	118.58	4.30	15.56	0.66	4.49	1.82	1.65	0.63	56.20	53.92	0.70
French Toast, prep f/recipe w/2% milk	1	Piece	65.00	148.85	5.00	16.25	0.56	7.02	1.77	2.94	1.68	75.40	80.60	
French Toast, rth, fzn	1	Piece	59.00	125.67	4.37	18.94	0.65	3.60	0.91	1.20	0.72	48.38	31.86	
Pancakes, blueberry, prep f/recipe, 6"	1	Each	77.00	170.94	4.70	22.33	0.92	7.08	1.53	1.78	3.21	43.12	38.50	
Pancakes, buttermilk Eggo	1	Each	42.53	99.08	2.55	16.20	0.47	2.84	0.61	1.25	0.91	4.68		
Pancakes, buttermilk, mini, ready to microwave, fzn, svg Krusteaz	1	Each	54.00	116.10	3.62	21.71		1.62	0.24	0.67	0.27			
Pancakes, plain, prep f/complete dry mix, 4"	1	Each	38.00	73.72	1.98	13.95	0.49	0.95	0.19	0.34	0.31	4.56	3.80	
Pancakes, plain, prep f/recipe, 4"	1	Each	38.00	86.26	2.43	10.75	0.56	3.69	0.80	0.94	1.69	22.42	20.52	
Pancakes, plain, prep f/recipe, 6"	1	Each	77.00	174.79	4.93	21.79	1.14	7.47	1.63	1.90	3.42	45.43	41.58	
Pancakes, plain, rth, fzn, 4"	1	Each	36.00	82.44	1.87	15.70	0.65	1.19	0.28	0.43	0.35	3.24	10.44	
Pancakes, potato, prep f/recipe, each	1	Each	76.00	206.72	4.69	21.76	1.52	11.58	2.32	3.52	4.97	72.96	5.32	
Pancakes, whole wheat, prep f/incomplete dry mix, 4"	1	Each	44.00	91.52	3.74	12.94	1.23	2.86	0.77	0.77	1.06	26.84	28.16	
Waffles, homestyle, low fat, fzn Eggo	1	Each	35.00	82.60	2.47	15.45	0.35	1.25	0.32	0.35	0.38	8.75		
Waffles, plain, rth, fzn, 4"	1	Each	35.00	87.85	2.06	13.51	0.77	2.73	0.45	1.10	0.97	11.20	133.70	
Waffles, wildberry, fzn Hungry Jack	1	Each	35.50	100.00	1.50	16.50	0.50	3.00	1.00			0.00		
Pasta														
Couscous, ckd	0.5	Cup	78.50	87.92	2.97	18.23	1.10	0.13	0.03	0.01	0.06	0.00	0.00	
Dish, ravioli, cheese, light, preckd Di Giorno	1	Cup	101.00	280.00	15.00	40.00	2.00	7.00	4.00			40.00		
Dish, tortellini, cheese filled	1	Cup	108.00	331.56	14.58	50.76	2.05	7.81	3.89	2.23	0.50	45.36	41.04	
Pasta, chow mein noodles, ckd Frieda's Specialty Produce	3	Ounce-weight	85.05	249.00	6.75	52.50	1.50	0.75	0.00			11.25	0.00	
Pasta, egg noodles, enrich, ckd	0.5	Cup	80.00	106.40	3.80	19.87	0.88	1.18	0.25	0.34	0.32	26.40	4.80	
Pasta, egg noodles, enrich, ckd w/salt	0.5	Cup	80.00	106.40	3.80	19.87	0.88	1.18	0.25	0.34	0.32	26.40	4.80	

Vit E (mg)	Vit C	Vit B₁ Thia (mg)	Vit B₂ Ribo (mg)	Vit B₃ Nia (mg)	Fol (mcg)	Vit B₆ (mg)	Vita B₁₂ (mcg)	Sodi (mg)	Pota (mg)	Cal (mg)	Phos (mg)	Magn (mg)	Iron (mg)	Zinc (mg)	Caff (mg)	Alco (g)	Sol Fiber (g)	Insol Fiber (g)
0.24	0.00	0.07	0.04	0.31	14.10	0.06	0.00	79.20	95.70	9.30	80.70	23.40	0.73	0.72	0.00	0.00	1.09	3.86
0.04	0.00	0.16	0.18	1.71	37.20	0.03	0.00	190.80	34.50	6.60	33.90	7.80	2.32	0.28	0.00	0.00		
0.04	0.00	0.17	0.14	1.57	37.20	0.01	0.00	190.80	217.20	35.70	31.50	8.10	1.62	0.23	0.00	0.00	0.34	0.56
	0.00	0.10	0.13	1.31	25.20	0.01		381.00	29.70	57.90	29.70	6.30	1.56		0.00	0.00		
0.47	0.00	0.17	0.14	1.57	37.20	0.01	0.00	229.80	38.40	35.70	31.50	8.10	1.62	0.23	0.00	0.00	0.35	0.55
0.65	0.00	0.13	0.11	1.29	28.80	0.02	0.00	271.04	42.56	38.40	72.96	8.64	1.15	0.21	0.00	0.00	0.19	0.32
	0.00	0.09	0.09	1.16	12.18	0.03		167.62	56.26	23.20	60.32	15.08	1.07		0.00	0.00		
0.17	0.00	0.11	0.08	1.64	19.60	0.04	0.00	225.96	83.16	47.60	97.16	10.64	0.75	0.23	0.00	0.00	0.27	0.96
0.28	0.00	0.06	0.03	1.45	8.96	0.05	0.00	210.88	95.04	16.00	94.40	31.68	0.98	0.69	0.00	0.00	0.67	2.69
0.24	0.00	0.06	0.03	1.27	7.84	0.05	0.00	69.16	83.16	14.00	82.60	27.72	0.86	0.61	0.00	0.00		
	0.00	0.12	0.07	1.20	24.00			220.00		40.00			1.80		0.00	0.00		
0.00	0.00	0.28	0.21	2.36	52.80	0.03	0.00	274.56	102.96	129.36	53.46	27.06	1.99	0.92	0.00	0.00		
0.99	0.06				82.65		0.21	210.33		76.38			1.70		0.00	0.00		
0.18	0.17	0.22	0.17	2.03	63.84	0.04	0.00	254.79	118.56	83.79	39.33	8.55	1.38	0.57	0.00	0.00		
	0.00							250.00		60.00			1.80		0.00	0.00		
0.26	0.00	0.25	0.17	1.91	36.48	0.05	0.00	217.74	106.02	101.46	60.99	21.09	1.64	0.61	0.00	0.00		
0.27	0.00	0.20	0.09	2.25	32.34	0.11	0.00	420.42	138.60	174.90	186.12	46.86	1.62	1.06	0.00	0.00	1.28	3.14
	0.00							427.50	134.52	33.52	169.86		1.48		0.00	0.00		
	0.00							427.50	123.12	33.52	159.60		1.62		0.00	0.00		
0.47	0.63	0.08	0.07	0.63	42.18	0.01	0.33	254.79	70.11	32.49	112.29	9.12	0.92	0.28	0.00	0.00	0.42	1.07
								343.20							0.00	0.00		
0.97	0.85	0.16	0.16	1.26	27.36	0.02	0.08	251.37	70.11	107.73	82.65	9.12	1.29	0.31	0.00	0.00	0.29	0.79
0.30	0.00	0.06	0.09	0.60	18.29	0.01	0.00	157.79	27.28	4.34	59.52	4.65	0.17	0.15	0.00	0.00	0.12	0.47
1.03	0.17	0.17	0.18	1.36	42.75	0.05	0.09	333.45	82.65	147.63	100.89	13.11	1.49	0.35	0.00	0.00	0.13	1.81
0.38	0.00	0.15	0.05	0.24	50.73	0.09	0.01	224.01	288.99	35.91	214.32	89.49	2.39	1.05	0.00	0.00	0.82	1.81
1.03	0.17	0.16	0.17	1.32	29.07	0.02	0.09	266.19	68.97	114.00	87.21	9.69	1.36	0.32	0.00	0.00	0.40	1.14
	0.00							380.00	70.00	70.00	150.00		0.60		0.00	0.00		
0.36	0.48	0.07	0.20	0.46	7.96	0.04	0.27	86.81	126.55	81.07	89.47	12.18	0.68	0.46		0.00		
0.71	0.19	0.13	0.21	1.06	27.95	0.05	0.20	311.35	87.10	65.00	76.05	11.05	1.09	0.44	0.00	0.00		
0.40	0.18	0.16	0.23	1.60	30.68	0.30	0.99	292.05	79.06	63.13	82.01	10.03	1.30	0.46	0.00	0.00		
	1.69	0.15	0.21	1.18	27.72	0.03	0.15	317.24	106.26	158.62	116.27	12.32	1.32	0.41	0.00	0.00	0.20	0.72
0.00	0.60	0.11	0.12	1.47	22.11	0.15	0.44	225.38	43.80	14.88	145.01	7.65	1.32	0.26	0.00	0.00		
								289.98					1.46		0.00	0.00		
0.32	0.08	0.08	0.08	0.65	14.06	0.03	0.08	238.64	66.50	47.88	126.92	7.60	0.59	0.15	0.00	0.00	0.11	0.38
0.36	0.11	0.08	0.11	0.59	14.44	0.02	0.08	166.82	50.16	83.22	60.42	6.08	0.68	0.21	0.00	0.00	0.12	0.44
0.73	0.23	0.15	0.22	1.20	29.26	0.03	0.17	338.03	101.64	168.63	122.43	12.32	1.39	0.43	0.00	0.00	0.25	0.89
0.10	0.11	0.14	0.17	1.44	16.20	0.03	0.06	183.24	26.28	22.32	133.92	5.04	1.25	0.24	0.00	0.00	0.14	0.51
1.52	16.72	0.10	0.13	1.63	17.48	0.29	0.14	386.08	597.36	18.24	84.36	25.08	1.19	0.63	0.00	0.00	0.25	1.27
0.00	0.22	0.09	0.23	1.02	12.76	0.05	0.13	251.68	122.76	110.00	164.12	20.24	1.37	0.46	0.00	0.00	0.22	1.01
	0.00	0.31	0.26	2.60	26.95	0.16	0.55	154.70	50.05	20.30	28.35	23.80	1.94		0.00	0.00		
0.22	0.00	0.16	0.18	1.64	21.35	0.33	0.83	261.80	42.70	77.35	139.65	7.35	1.49	0.19	0.00	0.00	0.17	0.60
	0.00	0.15	0.17	2.00	20.00	0.20	0.60	270.00		10.00			1.80		0.00	0.00		
0.10	0.00	0.04	0.01	0.77	11.77	0.04	0.00	3.92	45.53	6.28	17.27	6.28	0.30	0.20	0.00	0.00	0.31	0.78
	0.00	0.60	0.43	3.00	60.00			400.00	170.00	250.00	250.00		1.80		0.00	0.00		
0.17	0.00	0.34	0.33	2.91	79.92	0.05	0.17	371.52	96.12	164.16	228.96	22.68	1.62	1.10	0.00	0.00		
	0.00							351.00		15.00			2.70		0.00	0.00		
0.13	0.00	0.15	0.06	1.19	51.20	0.03	0.07	5.60	22.40	9.60	55.20	15.20	1.27	0.50	0.00	0.00	0.21	0.67
0.04	0.00	0.15	0.06	1.19	51.20	0.03	0.07	132.00	22.40	9.60	55.20	15.20	1.27	0.50	0.00	0.00	0.24	0.64

Food Name	Amount	Measure	Weight (g)	Calories	Protein (g)	Total Carb (g)	Dietary Fiber (g)	Total Fat (g)	Sat Fat (g)	Mono Fat (g)	Poly Fat (g)	Chol (mg)	Vit A (mcg RAE)	Vit D (mcg)
GRAIN PRODUCTS, PREPARED AND BAKED GOODS *(continued)*														
Pasta, egg noodles, spinach, enrich, ckd	0.5	Cup	80.00	105.60	4.03	19.40	1.84	1.25	0.29	0.40	0.28	26.40	8.00	
Pasta, fettuccine noodles, spinach, preckd Di Giorno	3	Ounce-weight	85.05	228.00	9.60	45.60	2.40	1.80	0.00			0.00		
Pasta, macaroni noodles, enrich, dry	0.25	Cup	26.25	97.39	3.36	19.61	0.63	0.42	0.06	0.05	0.17	0.00	0.00	
Pasta, macaroni noodles, unenrich, dry	0.25	Cup	26.25	97.39	3.36	19.61	0.63	0.42	0.06	0.05	0.17	0.00	0.00	
Pasta, macaroni noodles, veg, enrich, dry	0.25	Cup	21.00	77.07	2.76	15.72	0.90	0.22	0.03	0.03	0.09	0.00	1.68	
Pasta, macaroni noodles, whole wheat, dry	0.25	Cup	26.25	91.35	3.84	19.70	2.18	0.37	0.07	0.05	0.15	0.00	0.00	
Pasta, noodles, cellophane, dehyd	0.25	Cup	35.00	122.85	0.06	30.13	0.18	0.02	0.01	0.00	0.01	0.00	0.00	
Pasta, noodles, fresh refrigerated, as purchased	3	Ounce-weight	85.05	244.94	9.62	46.55	3.32	1.96	0.28	0.23	0.80	62.09	11.91	
Pasta, noodles, fresh refrigerated, ckd	3	Ounce-weight	85.05	111.42	4.38	21.20	1.49	0.89	0.13	0.10	0.36	28.07	5.10	
Pasta, prep f/recipe w/o egg, ckd	3	Ounce-weight	85.05	105.46	3.72	21.37	1.36	0.83	0.12	0.16	0.43	0.00	0.00	
Pasta, ramen noodles, ckd	0.5	Cup	113.50	76.76	1.66	10.10	0.58	3.25	0.83	0.59	1.65	0.11	1.22	0.00
Pasta, ramen noodles, dry, pkg Westbrae Natural	1	Ounce-weight	28.35	96.99	2.98	20.89	2.24	0.37	0.00			0.00	0.00	
Pasta, rice noodle, ckd, cup	0.5	Cup	88.00	95.92	0.80	21.91	0.88	0.18	0.02	0.03	0.02	0.00	0.00	
Pasta, rice noodle, dry	1	Ounce-weight	28.35	103.19	0.97	23.60	0.45	0.16	0.04	0.05	0.04	0.00	0.00	
Pasta, shells, sml, enrich, ckd	0.5	Cup	57.50	81.08	2.74	16.30	0.74	0.38	0.06	0.04	0.16	0.00	0.00	
Pasta, soba noodles, dry	1	Ounce-weight	28.35	95.26	4.08	21.15		0.20	0.04	0.05	0.06	0.00	0.00	
Pasta, somen noodles, dry	1	Ounce-weight	28.35	100.93	3.22	21.01	1.22	0.23	0.03	0.03	0.09	0.00	0.00	0.00
Pasta, spaghetti noodles, enrich, ckd	0.5	Cup	70.00	98.70	3.34	19.84	1.19	0.47	0.06	0.06	0.19	0.00		
Pasta, spaghetti noodles, enrich, ckd w/salt	0.5	Cup	70.00	98.70	3.34	19.84	1.19	0.47	0.06	0.06	0.19	0.00		
Pasta, spaghetti noodles, spinach, dry	1	Ounce-weight	28.35	105.46	3.78	21.21	3.01	0.44	0.06	0.05	0.18	0.00	6.52	
Pasta, spaghetti noodles, unenrich, ckd w/salt	0.5	Cup	70.00	98.70	3.34	19.84	1.05	0.47	0.06	0.06	0.19	0.00		
Pasta, spaghetti noodles, unenrich, dry	1	Ounce-weight	28.35	105.18	3.62	21.17	0.68	0.45	0.06	0.05	0.19	0.00	0.00	
Pasta, spaghetti noodles, whole wheat, dry	1	Ounce-weight	28.35	98.66	4.15	21.27	3.60	0.40	0.07	0.06	0.16	0.00	0.00	
Pasta, spinach noodles, fresh refrigerated, as purchased	3	Ounce-weight	85.05	245.79	9.57	47.39	2.81	1.79	0.41	0.56	0.39	62.09	21.26	
Pasta, udon noodles, ckd	3	Ounce-weight	85.05	85.90	2.13	17.27	0.09	0.43					0.00	
Rice														
Bran, rice, crude	1	Tablespoon	7.38	23.32	0.98	3.67	1.55	1.54	0.31	0.56	0.55	0.00	0.00	
Rice, basmati, white, Calif, dry Lundberg Family Foods	0.25	Cup	51.20	182.78	3.92	40.72	0.33	0.63	0.21	0.16	0.23	0.00	0.00	
Rice, brown, med grain, dry	0.25	Cup	47.50	171.95	3.56	36.18	1.62	1.28	0.25	0.46	0.45	0.00	0.00	0.00
Rice, white, long grain, enrich, inst, dry	0.25	Cup	23.75	90.01	1.82	19.86	0.38	0.07	0.02	0.02	0.02	0.00	0.00	
Rice, white, long grain, enrich, parboiled, ckd	0.5	Cup	87.50	99.75	2.00	21.64	0.35	0.24	0.06	0.08	0.06	0.00	0.00	
Rice, white, med grain, ckd	0.5	Cup	93.00	120.90	2.22	26.59	0.28	0.20	0.06	0.06	0.05	0.00	0.00	0.00
Rice, white, med grain, unenrich, dry	0.25	Cup	48.75	175.50	3.22	38.68	0.57	0.28	0.08	0.09	0.08	0.00		
Stuffing and Mixes														
Baking Mix, basic, dairy free Ener-G Foods	0.33	Cup	43.00	150.73	7.25	30.13	4.29	0.10	0.03			0.00	0.00	0.00
Baking Mix, dry, Bisquick	0.33	Cup	40.00	161.60	2.80	24.40	0.72	6.00	1.60	2.48	0.52	0.00	0.00	
Baking Mix, rducd fat, Bisquick	0.33	Cup	40.00	150.00	3.00	28.00	0.50	2.50	0.50			0.00		
Stuffing, cornbread, prep f/dry mix, 6oz pkg	0.5	Cup	100.00	179.00	2.90	21.90	2.90	8.80	1.76	3.86	2.71	0.00	78.00	
Tortillas and Taco/Tostada Shells														
Taco Shells, bkd, lrg, 6 1/2"	1	Each	21.00	98.28	1.51	13.10	1.58	4.75	0.68	1.87	1.78	0.00	0.02	
Tortilla, corn, med, 6", unsalted	1	Each	26.00	57.72	1.48	12.12	1.35	0.65	0.09	0.17	0.29	0.00	0.00	
Tortilla, flour, soft taco, Mission Foods	1	Each	51.00	146.37	4.44	25.30		3.06	0.35	1.41	0.47			
Tortilla, flour, white, enrich, dry mix	0.25	Cup	27.75	112.39	2.68	18.63	0.52	2.95	1.14	1.26	0.42	0.00	0.00	
Tortilla, whole wheat	1	Each	35.00	73.15	2.94	19.98	1.89	0.45	0.08	0.06	0.19	0.00	0.00	0.00
GRANOLA BARS, CEREAL BARS, DIET BARS, SCONES, AND TARTS														
Bar, breakfast, chocolate chip, chewy Carnation	1	Each	35.96	150.00	2.00	24.00	1.00	6.00	2.00			0.00		2.50
Bar, breakfast, peanut butter chocolate chip, chewy Carnation	1	Each	35.96	150.00	3.00	22.00	0.50	5.00	1.50			0.00		2.50
Bar, cereal, apple cinnamon Nutri Grain	1	Each	37.00	136.16	1.63	26.97	0.78	2.78	0.56	1.85	0.33	0.00	224.96	
Bar, cereal, blueberry Nutri Grain	1	Each	37.00	136.16	1.63	26.97	0.78	2.78	0.56	1.85	0.33	0.00	224.96	

Vit E (mg)	Vit C	Vit B₁ Thia (mg)	Vit B₂ Ribo (mg)	Vit B₃ Nia (mg)	Fol (mcg)	Vit B₆ (mg)	Vita B₁₂ (mcg)	Sodi (mg)	Pota (mg)	Cal (mg)	Phos (mg)	Magn (mg)	Iron (mg)	Zinc (mg)	Caff (mg)	Alco (g)	Sol Fiber (g)	Insol Fiber (g)
0.46	0.00	0.20	0.10	1.18	51.20	0.09	0.11	9.60	29.60	15.20	45.60	19.20	0.87	0.50	0.00	0.00	0.32	1.52
	0.00	0.54	0.31	4.80	72.00			192.00	264.00	48.00	120.00	48.00	2.16		0.00	0.00		
0.02	0.00	0.27	0.11	1.97	72.97	0.03	0.00	1.84	42.52	4.72	39.37	12.60	1.01	0.32	0.00	0.00	0.10	0.53
0.03	0.00	0.02	0.01	0.45	4.72	0.03	0.00	1.84	42.52	4.72	39.37	12.60	0.34	0.32	0.00	0.00	0.10	0.53
0.02	0.00	0.22	0.11	1.54	58.38	0.03	0.00	9.03	59.85	7.14	24.36	9.66	0.90	0.16	0.00	0.00	0.13	0.77
0.03	0.00	0.13	0.04	1.35	14.96	0.06	0.00	2.10	56.44	10.50	,67.72	37.54	0.95	0.62	0.00	0.00	0.50	1.68
0.04	0.00	0.05	0.00	0.07	0.70	0.02	0.00	3.50	3.50	8.75	11.20	1.05	0.76	0.15	0.00	0.00		
0.28	0.00	0.60	0.37	2.85	149.69	0.08	0.26	22.11	152.24	12.76	138.63	39.12	2.85	1.04	0.00	0.00	0.52	2.81
0.13	0.00	0.18	0.13	0.84	54.43	0.03	0.12	5.10	20.41	5.10	53.58	15.31	0.97	0.47	0.00	0.00	0.22	1.27
0.13	0.00	0.15	0.13	1.14	36.57	0.02	0.00	62.94	16.16	5.10	34.02	11.91	0.96	0.32	0.00	0.00	0.27	1.09
1.17	0.01	0.01	0.01	0.13	1.57	0.01	0.00	400.95	24.54	6.53	12.10	5.18	0.19	0.09	0.00	0.00	0.09	0.49
	0.00	0.09	0.03	0.60				119.37		0.00					0.00	0.00		
	0.00	0.02	0.01	0.06	2.64	0.01	0.00	16.72	3.52	3.52	17.60	2.64	0.13	0.22	0.00	0.00		
	0.00	0.01	0.01	0.06	0.85	0.01	0.00	51.60	8.50	5.10	43.38	3.40	0.20	0.21	0.00	0.00		
0.04	0.00	0.12	0.06	0.96	44.28	0.02	0.00	0.57	17.82	4.03	31.05	10.35	0.80	0.30	0.00	0.00	0.12	0.63
	0.00	0.13	0.04	0.91	17.01	0.07	0.00	224.53	71.44	9.92	72.01	26.93	0.77	0.48	0.00	0.00		
0.02	0.00	0.03	0.01	0.25	3.97	0.02	0.00	521.64	46.49	6.52	22.68	7.94	0.38	0.13	0.00	0.00		
0.04	0.00	0.14	0.07	1.17	53.90	0.02	0.00	0.70	21.70	4.90	37.80	12.60	0.98	0.37	0.00	0.00	0.55	0.64
0.04	0.00	0.14	0.07	1.17	53.90	0.02	0.00	70.00	21.70	4.90	37.80	12.60	0.98	0.37	0.00	0.00	0.55	0.64
0.18	0.00	0.11	0.06	1.29	13.61	0.09	0.00	10.21	106.60	16.44	94.12	49.33	0.60	0.78	0.00	0.00	0.60	2.41
0.04	0.00	0.02	0.02	0.28	4.90	0.02	0.00	70.00	21.70	4.90	37.80	12.60	0.35	0.37	0.00	0.00	0.48	0.56
0.05	0.00	0.03	0.02	0.48	5.10	0.03	0.00	1.98	45.93	5.10	42.52	13.61	0.37	0.35	0.00	0.00	0.10	0.58
0.04	0.00	0.14	0.04	1.45	16.16	0.06	0.00	2.27	60.95	11.34	73.14	40.54	1.03	0.67	0.00	0.00	0.65	2.95
0.28	0.00	0.52	0.34	2.94	150.54	0.27	0.26	22.96	231.34	36.57	125.87	53.58	2.81	1.19	0.00	0.00	0.43	2.38
	0.00	0.02	0.01	0.09				38.27	5.10	5.95	15.31		0.17		0.00	0.00		
0.36	0.00	0.20	0.02	2.51	4.65	0.30	0.00	0.37	109.59	4.21	123.76	57.64	1.37	0.45	0.00	0.00	0.10	1.45
	0.14							2.51		3.54			0.22		0.00	0.00		
0.30	0.00	0.20	0.02	2.05	9.50	0.24	0.00	1.90	127.30	15.68	125.40	67.93	0.86	0.96	0.00	0.00	0.16	1.46
0.01	0.00	0.15	0.02	1.30	65.31	0.01	0.00	1.43	4.28	4.28	16.15	2.85	1.00	0.23	0.00	0.00	0.10	0.29
0.01	0.00	0.22	0.02	1.23	66.50	0.02	0.00	2.62	32.38	16.62	36.75	10.50	0.99	0.27	0.00	0.00	0.09	0.26
0.04	0.00	0.16	0.02	1.70	53.94	0.04	0.00	0.00	26.97	2.79	34.41	12.09	1.38	0.39	0.00	0.00	0.10	0.18
0.04	0.00	0.03	0.02	0.78	4.39	0.08	0.00	0.49	41.93	4.39	52.65	17.06	0.39	0.56	0.00	0.00	0.14	0.43
0.00	0.00	0.00	0.19	0.06	7.64	0.00	0.04		119.25	59.24	11.77	12.54	1.25	0.13	0.00	0.00		
	0.00	0.20	0.15	1.68				498.80	50.00	60.00			1.40		0.00	0.00		
		0.15	0.10	1.60				460.00	30.00	40.00			1.44		0.00	0.00		
0.85	0.80	0.12	0.09	1.25	97.00	0.04	0.01	455.00	62.00	26.00	34.00	13.00	0.94	0.23	0.00	0.00		
0.35	0.00	0.05	0.01	0.28	27.51	0.06	0.00	77.07	37.59	33.60	52.08	22.05	0.53	0.29	0.00	0.00		
0.04	0.00	0.03	0.02	0.39	29.64	0.06	0.00	2.86	40.04	45.50	81.64	16.90	0.36	0.24	0.00	0.00	0.23	1.12
								248.88		97.41			1.01		0.00	0.00		
0.02	0.00	0.20	0.14	1.61	37.74	0.01	0.00	187.87	27.75	56.89	58.27	5.83	1.96	0.18	0.00	0.00	0.17	0.35
0.43	0.00	0.10	0.02	0.85	8.40	0.07	0.00	171.15	81.55	10.15	81.90	25.55	0.73	0.53	0.00	0.00	0.62	1.27
6.82	15.00	0.37	0.42	5.00	99.97	0.50	1.50	80.00	55.00	500.00	250.00	99.97	4.50	3.70		0.00		
6.82	15.00	0.37	0.42	5.00	99.97	0.50	0.15	85.00	79.80	500.00	250.00	99.97	4.50	3.70		0.00		
0.00	0.00	0.37	0.41	5.00	39.96	0.52	0.00	109.89	72.89	15.17	38.11	9.99	1.80	1.52	0.00	0.00		
0.00	0.00	0.37	0.41	5.00	39.96	0.52	0.00	109.89	72.89	15.17	38.11	9.99	1.80	1.52	0.00	0.00		

Food Name	Amount	Measure	Weight (g)	Calories	Protein (g)	Total Carb (g)	Dietary Fiber (g)	Total Fat (g)	Sat Fat (g)	Mono Fat (g)	Poly Fat (g)	Chol (mg)	Vit A (mcg RAE)	Vit D (mcg)
GRANOLA BARS, CEREAL BARS, DIET BARS, SCONES, AND TARTS *(continued)*														
Bar, cereal, blueberry fruit & oatmeal Quaker Oats	1	Each	37.00	135.37	1.56	26.29	0.99	2.90	0.35	0.97	0.22	0.07		0.00
Bar, cereal, chocolate peanut butter Kashi Company	1	Each	78.00	280.00	13.00	50.00	7.00	6.00	3.00			0.00	0.00	
Bar, cereal, honey van yogurt Kashi Company	1	Each	78.00	280.00	11.00	53.00	7.00	4.00	3.00			0.00	0.00	
Bar, chocolate chip, whole grain Kudos	1	Each	37.00	161.69	2.13	25.05	1.33	6.05	3.50	1.94	0.31	50.32	5.55	
Bar, energy, ZonePerfect Fruitified, banana nut Abbott Abbott	1	Each	50.00	200.00	14.00	24.00	3.00	6.00	1.50			5.00		
Bar, energy, ZonePerfect Fruitified, blueberry Abbott Abbott	1	Each	50.00	190.00	14.00	25.00	3.00	4.00	1.00			5.00		
Bar, granola, almond, hard	1	Each	23.60	116.82	1.82	14.63	1.13	6.02	2.95	1.83	0.89	0.00	0.47	
Bar, granola, choc chip graham & marshmallow, uncoated, soft USDA SR-23	1	Each	28.00	119.56	1.71	19.82	1.12	4.34	2.57	0.82	0.71	0.28	0.66	
Bar, granola, chocolate chip, chewy General Mills Cascadian Farm	1	Each	35.00	140.00	2.00	25.00	1.00	3.00	1.00	1.00	0.50	0.00	0.00	
Bar, granola, chocolate chip, chewy PepsiCo Quaker	1	Each	18.00	75.00	0.75	13.50	0.75	2.25	1.12			0.00	0.00	
Bar, granola, chocolate chip, chocolate coated, soft, 1.25oz	1	Each	35.44	165.14	2.06	22.61	1.20	8.82	5.04	2.75	0.64	1.77	2.48	
Bar, granola, chocolate choc chip, low fat, chewy	1	Each	35.00	127.75	2.59	26.60	1.50	2.45	0.77	1.01	0.46	0.00		
Bar, granola, cookies & cream, chewy Quaker Oats	1	Each	28.00	113.81	1.53	21.93	0.84	2.49	0.46	1.15	0.30	0.03		0.00
Bar, granola, Go Lean, asrtd flvrs, chewy USDA SR-23 Kashi	1	Each	78.00	304.20	13.00	49.47	6.01	6.00	2.52	2.00	0.96	4.68	13.26	0.16
Bar, granola, Go Lean, asrtd flvrs, crunchy USDA SR-23 Kashi	1	Each	46.00	180.78	8.22	27.41	2.71	4.25	2.16	1.15	0.58	0.00	23.33	0.00
Bar, granola, honey nut, low fat, chewy	1	Each	35.00	117.95	2.87	26.60	1.50	2.10	0.28	1.12	0.56	0.00		
Bar, granola, milk chocolate, mini M & M's Kudos	1	Each	28.35	90.00	1.00	17.00	1.00	2.50	1.00			0.00		
Bar, granola, oatmeal raisin, low fat, chewy	1	Each	35.00	117.25	2.62	26.25	1.47	2.10	0.28	1.16	0.52	0.00		
Bar, granola, oats 'n honey General Mills Nature Valley	1	Each	21.00	90.00	2.00	14.50	1.00	3.00	0.25			0.00	0.00	
Bar, granola, peanut butter, w/chocolate chips, chewy Quaker Oats	1	Each	28.00	121.94	2.52	18.59	1.20	4.57	1.29	2.27	0.80	0.03		0.00
Bar, granola, raisin, uncoated, soft, 1.5oz each	1	Each	42.53	190.51	3.23	28.24	1.79	7.57	4.07	1.21	1.37	0.43	0.00	
Bar, snack, soy, chocolate Genisoy Nature Grains	1	Each	66.50	230.00	11.00	41.00	4.00	3.00	0.00			0.00		
Scone USDA Survey Database	1	Each	42.00	150.18	3.87	19.22	0.61	6.34	2.02	2.57	1.26	49.17	66.25	0.17
MEALS AND DISHES														
Canned Meals and Dishes														
Beans, baked, vegetarian, cnd Bush's Best	0.5	Cup	130.00	130.00	5.00	24.00	6.00	0.00	0.00	0.00	0.00	0.00		
Beans, baked, w/franks, cnd	0.5	Cup	129.50	183.89	8.74	19.93	8.94	8.51	3.05	3.67	1.09	7.77	5.18	
Beans, baked, w/pork, cnd B & M	0.5	Cup	131.00	180.00	8.00	33.00	7.00	2.00	0.50			3.00	0.00	
Dish, beefaroni, w/tomato sauce, cnd, svg	1	Each	212.63	184.98	8.27	31.23	2.98	2.96	1.19	1.27	0.25	17.01		
Dish, chicken & dumplings, cnd, Sweet Sue, FS Bryan Foods Inc.	1	Cup	240.00	218.40	15.12	22.80	2.64	7.44	1.80	2.95	1.62	36.00	0.00	
Dish, chicken, sweet & sour, w/veg & fruit, cnd Chun King	1	Each	254.00	165.10	5.84	31.75		1.78				22.86	0.00	
Dish, pasta, SpaghettiOs w/meatballs, cnd Franco American	1	Cup	209.00	240.00	11.00	32.00	3.00	8.00	3.50			20.00		1.00
Dish, pasta, SpaghettiOs w/sliced franks Franco American	1	Cup	209.00	230.00	9.00	27.00	5.00	10.00	5.00			20.00		1.00
Dish, pasta, w/meatballs, w/tomato sauce, cnd	1	Each	141.75	146.00	6.13	17.43	3.83	5.78	2.26	2.37	0.32	11.34	26.93	
Dish, pasta, w/sliced franks, w/tomato sauce, cnd, each	1	Each	418.00	434.72	15.47	49.74	3.76	19.23	6.14	7.94	2.50	37.62	25.08	
Dish, ravioli, beef w/tomato & meat sauce, svg Nestle Foods Company	1	Each	244.00	229.36	8.37	36.89	3.66	5.39	2.49	2.00	0.22	14.64		

Vit E (mg)	Vit C	Vit B₁ Thia (mg)	Vit B₂ Ribo (mg)	Vit B₃ Nia (mg)	Fol (mcg)	Vit B₆ (mg)	Vita B₁₂ (mcg)	Sodi (mg)	Pota (mg)	Cal (mg)	Phos (mg)	Magn (mg)	Iron (mg)	Zinc (mg)	Caff (mg)	Alco (g)	Sol Fiber (g)	Insol Fiber (g)
0.04	0.31	0.23	0.51	5.96	119.27	0.60	0.01	118.00	44.15	9.88	33.73	8.41	0.43	0.23	0.00	0.00	0.44	0.55
	0.00		0.03					150.00	130.00	0.00	20.00	8.00	0.36			0.00		
	0.00		0.03	0.40				70.00	90.00	20.00			0.36	0.30	0.00	0.00		
3.99	17.24	0.06	0.07	0.57	4.81	0.04	0.05	103.60	103.23	289.71	76.59	25.90	3.39	0.52		0.00		
	60.00	0.38	0.85	10.00	80.00	1.00	2.10	230.00	85.00	200.00	200.00	40.00	1.80	3.75	0.00	0.00		
	30.00	0.38	0.85	9.00	80.00	1.00	2.10	200.00	140.00	200.00	200.00	40.00	1.80	3.75	0.00	0.00		
0.42	0.00	0.07	0.02	0.14	2.83	0.01	0.00	60.42	64.43	7.55	53.81	19.12	0.59	0.37		0.00		
	0.00	0.04	0.04	0.28	5.88	0.01	0.00	88.48	77.00	24.92	56.56	19.88	0.72	0.36		0.00		
	0.00							125.00		0.00			1.08			0.00		
	0.00							56.25		60.00			0.27			0.00		
0.35	0.00	0.03	0.09	0.26	9.21	0.04	0.20	70.88	110.92	36.50	70.52	23.39	0.83	0.46		0.00		
		0.06	0.03	0.39				81.20	86.45	18.20			0.70			0.00		
0.33	0.11	0.06	0.03	0.37	3.74	0.02	0.01	78.30	51.97	7.82	41.70	12.34	0.50	0.31		0.00	0.27	0.57
0.63	0.31	0.11	0.12	0.53	30.42	0.07	0.12	250.38	334.62	80.34	198.90	250.38	1.26	1.09	2.34	0.00		
4.72	8.88	0.12	0.08	0.87	98.90	0.49	1.48	223.56	138.00	199.64	120.98	39.56	2.39	2.22	5.06	0.00		
		0.10	0.04	0.27				84.00	66.50	12.95			0.70		0.00	0.00		
	1.20							105.00		200.00			0.36			0.00		
		0.10	0.03	0.25				77.35	83.30	13.30					0.00	0.00		
	0.00							80.00		0.00			0.54		0.00	0.00		
0.13	0.14	0.06	0.02	0.91	4.96	0.02	0.00	103.91	70.12	10.22	58.56	16.57	0.54	0.41		0.00	0.29	0.91
0.47	0.00	0.10	0.07	0.47	8.93	0.04	0.08	119.92	153.94	42.95	93.56	30.62	1.04	0.55	0.00	0.00		
	1.20							110.00	430.00	50.00			0.90			0.00		
0.66	0.06	0.15	0.16	1.21	7.93	0.03	0.10	170.62	48.61	80.23	73.56	7.11	1.32	0.29	0.00	0.00	0.20	0.41
	0.00									40.00			0.54		0.00	0.00		
0.60	2.98	0.08	0.07	1.17	38.85	0.06	0.00	556.85	304.32	62.16	134.68	36.26	2.24	2.42	0.00	0.00	5.99	2.95
	0.00							430.00		60.00			2.70		0.00	0.00		
	0.42							801.60		17.01			1.51		0.00	0.00		
								945.60					2.57		0.00	0.00		
	30.23							563.88							0.00	0.00		
	6.00	0.15	0.17	3.00	60.00			990.00		150.00			2.70		0.00	0.00		
	6.00	0.15	0.17	3.00	80.00			930.00		150.00			2.70		0.00	0.00		
0.71	4.25	0.11	0.09	1.86	35.44	0.09	0.32	592.52	233.89	15.59	65.21	19.85	1.32	1.03	0.00	0.00		
								2014.76					3.80		0.00	0.00		
	0.24							1173.64	353.80	19.52			2.42		0.00	0.00		

Food Name	Amount	Measure	Weight (g)	Calories	Protein (g)	Total Carb (g)	Dietary Fiber (g)	Total Fat (g)	Sat Fat (g)	Mono Fat (g)	Poly Fat (g)	Chol (mg)	Vit A (mcg RAE)	Vit D (mcg)
MEALS AND DISHES *(continued)*														
Dish, ravioli, beef, w/tomato sauce, mini, cnd, svg Nestle Foods Company	1	Each	252.00	239.40	8.79	40.62	3.28	4.74	1.76	2.02	0.18	17.64		
Dish, spaghetti, w/meatballs & tomato sauce, svg Nestle Foods Company	1	Each	240.00	249.60	9.07	34.06	2.16	8.64	3.86	3.67	0.38	21.60		
Hash, beef, corned, cnd Chef-Mate	1	Cup	253.00	485.76	24.24	29.07	6.07	30.33	13.41	14.67	1.11	88.55	0.00	
Hash, beef, corned, cnd, Armour	1	Cup	236.00	497.96	23.84	12.04	1.89	39.41	15.65	17.44	0.83	96.76	0.00	
Pork & Beans, w/tomato sauce, cnd	0.5	Cup	126.50	118.91	6.51	23.65	5.06	1.18	0.33	0.60	0.18	8.86	5.06	
Dry and Prepared Meat Dishes														
Dish, beef, teriyaki, freeze dried, cnd Oregon Freeze Dry, Inc	1	Cup	65.21	260.00	12.00	44.00	3.00	4.00	1.00			15.00		
Dry and Prepared Pasta and Pasta/Rice Dishes														
Dish, cheeseburger macaroni, dry mix, svg General Mills, Inc.	1.5	Ounce-weight	42.53	167.97	4.68	27.34		4.42	1.20			3.83		
Dish, egg noodles, w/creamy alfredo sauce, dry mix, cup Lipton	0.25	Cup	23.25	97.18	3.60	14.51		2.74	1.06	0.90	0.29	26.04		
Dish, macaroni & cheese, all shapes, prep f/dry mix Kraft General Foods, Inc.	1	Cup	196.00	410.00	12.00	49.00	1.00	18.00	4.50			10.00		
Dish, macaroni & cheese, original, deluxe, prep f/mix Kraft General Foods, Inc.	1	Cup	175.00	320.00	14.00	44.00	1.00	10.00	6.00			25.00		
Dish, macaroni & cheese, original, prep f/dry mix Kraft General Foods, Inc.	1	Cup	196.00	410.00	12.00	49.00	1.00	18.00	4.50			10.00		
Dish, pad Thai, w/rice noodles, vegetarian, rth Fantastic Foods Fast Naturals	1	Each	201.00	350.00	15.00	51.00	3.00	11.00	2.50			0.00		
Dish, pasta, oriental stir fry, dry Pasta Roni	2	Ounce-weight	56.70	198.22	6.98	39.59	2.08	1.87	0.31	0.77	0.67	0.05		0.00
Dish, rice & pasta, flvrd, dry	0.25	Cup	40.75	149.96	3.82	30.70	0.76	1.00	0.18	0.26	0.40	0.82	0.00	
Dish, risotto, three cheese, meal in a cup, dry The Spice Hunter, Inc. Meals In A Cup	1	Each	63.40	234.30	7.19	45.60	1.13	2.95	1.78	0.66	0.08	9.13		0.06
Dish, spaghetti, w/meat sauce, freeze dried, sml pouch Oregon Freeze Dry, Inc	1	Each	79.38	340.00	17.00	46.00	3.00	10.00	4.50			25.00		
Dish, Thai lemon grass, w/rice noodles, vegetarian, rth Fantastic Foods Fast Naturals	1	Each	201.00	300.00	7.00	48.00	3.00	10.00	3.50			0.00		
Dish, tortellini, spinach	1	Cup	122.00	232.23	11.64	25.26	1.10	8.98	3.29	3.38	1.33	158.17	138.28	
Dish, tuna noodle casserole, creamy, Tuna Helper	1	Cup	138.00	300.00	14.00	30.00	1.70	14.00				5.00		
Dry and Prepared Rice/Grain Dishes														
Dish, pilaf, black beans & rice, Mediterranean, dry Near East	2	Ounce-weight	56.70	185.79	6.30	41.62	4.47	0.73	0.13	0.21	0.35	0.00		0.00
Dish, rice pilaf, long grain & wild, dry Rice A Roni	2	Ounce-weight	56.70	190.80	4.64	43.07	1.67	0.50	0.12	0.17	0.13	0.00		0.00
Dish, rice, broccoli cheese flvr, dry Uncle Ben's Inc.	2	Ounce-weight	56.70	200.50	5.60	41.70	1.70	1.90	1.10			4.50		
Dish, rice, fried, Oriental style, dry Uncle Ben's Inc.	2	Ounce-weight	56.70	190.00	4.00	43.00	1.00	0.50	0.00			0.00		
Dish, rice, paella, dry Uncle Ben's Inc.	2	Ounce-weight	56.70	190.00	5.00	43.00	1.00	0.50	0.00			0.00		
Dish, rice, risotto mushroom herb, seasoned, dry Uncle Ben's Inc.	2	Ounce-weight	56.70	192.50	6.20	40.40	0.80	0.80	0.20			2.20	0.00	
Dry and Prepared Vegetable and Bean Dishes														
Dish, falafel, dry Fantastic Foods International Dish	0.25	Cup	35.00	120.00	7.00	21.00	6.00	2.00	0.00			0.00	0.00	
Frozen/Refrigerated Breakfasts														
Burrito, breakfast, ham & cheese flvr, fzn	1	Each	99.00	211.86	9.60	27.82	1.39	6.93	1.99	2.08	1.80	192.06	0.00	
Burrito, breakfast, original w/scrambled eggs Swanson's Great Starts	1	Each	99.00	200.00	8.00	25.00	2.00	8.00	3.00			60.00		
Frozen/Refrigerated Children's Meals **Frozen/Refrigerated Dinners**														
Dinner, beef, pot roast, yankee, ckd f/fzn Banquet	1	Each	266.50	230.00	14.00	20.00	4.00	10.00	4.00			60.00		

Vit E (mg)	Vit C	Vit B$_1$ Thia (mg)	Vit B$_2$ Ribo (mg)	Vit B$_3$ Nia (mg)	Fol (mcg)	Vit B$_6$ (mg)	Vita B$_{12}$ (mcg)	Sodi (mg)	Pota (mg)	Cal (mg)	Phos (mg)	Magn (mg)	Iron (mg)	Zinc (mg)	Caff (mg)	Alco (g)	Sol Fiber (g)	Insol Fiber (g)
	0.25							1197.00		22.68			2.42		0.00	0.00		
	0.96							940.80		16.80			1.78		0.00	0.00		
0.33	1.52	0.22	0.30	6.31		0.58	2.45	1593.90	536.36	45.54	240.35	37.95	2.99	7.51	0.00	0.00		
								854.32					2.19		0.00	0.00		
0.13	3.80	0.07	0.06	0.62	18.98	0.08	0.00	552.81	373.18	70.84	146.74	43.01	4.10	6.93	0.00	0.00	3.06	2.00
	6.00							910.00		40.00			1.44		0.00	0.00		
								863.26							0.00	0.00		
								411.52		29.53			0.70		0.00	0.00		
	0.00	0.38	0.34	3.00	60.00			750.00	340.00	100.00	300.00	40.00	2.70		0.00	0.00		
	0.00	0.38	0.26	3.00	60.00			730.00	190.00	200.00	450.00	40.00	1.80		0.00	0.00		
	0.00	0.38	0.34	3.00	60.00			750.00	340.00	100.00	300.00	40.00	2.70		0.00	0.00		
	2.40							690.00		60.00			1.80		0.00	0.00		
0.09	0.61	0.36	0.18	2.53	82.18	0.08	0.05	987.97	163.89	23.69	85.04	27.55	1.64	0.71	0.00	0.00	0.85	1.23
0.06	0.24	0.31	0.11	2.86	84.76	0.06	0.08	760.40	85.16	18.74	64.39	16.30	1.62	0.50	0.00	0.00		
0.00	0.33	0.04	0.14	1.09	0.00	0.01	0.00	521.60	82.74	89.99	6.03	1.30	0.63	0.03	0.00	0.00		
	0.00	0.15	0.26	5.00				990.00		60.00			3.60		0.00	0.00		
	4.80							690.00		40.00			1.44		0.00	0.00		
0.86	1.01	0.24	0.37	1.85	34.80	0.10	0.48	252.02	138.44	143.34	167.54	23.70	2.42	0.98	0.00	0.00		
				6.00											0.00	0.00		
0.00	0.21	0.08	0.06	0.91	7.43	0.13	0.66	659.07	321.98	45.46	62.68	13.80	1.54	0.49	0.00	0.00	1.36	3.11
0.00	1.01	0.19	0.11	1.76	66.88	0.18	0.00	837.22	230.61	23.72	88.90	25.70	1.76	0.68	0.00	0.00	0.53	1.14
	2.40							759.00		68.70			1.44		0.00	0.00		
								560.00		35.10			1.80		0.00	0.00		
								550.00		34.10			2.16		0.00	0.00		
	3.60							848.80		33.90			0.54		0.00	0.00		
	1.20							370.00		40.00			2.70		0.00	0.00		
								404.91					3.17		0.00	0.00		
	2.40							510.00		80.00			1.44		0.00	0.00		
	3.60							1130.00		40.00			1.80		0.00	0.00		

Food Name	Amount	Measure	Weight (g)	Calories	Protein (g)	Total Carb (g)	Dietary Fiber (g)	Total Fat (g)	Sat Fat (g)	Mono Fat (g)	Poly Fat (g)	Chol (mg)	Vit A (mcg RAE)	Vit D (mcg)
MEALS AND DISHES *(continued)*														
Dinner, beef, sliced, w/gravy mashed potatoes & peas, fzn Banquet	1	Each	255.00	270.30	26.39	18.79	4.08	10.05	4.33	4.95	0.76	71.40		
Dinner, cannelloni, cheese, w/tomato sauce, low cal, fzn	1	Each	259.00	298.42	21.86	24.20	1.48	12.45	7.01	3.43	1.24	41.68	143.42	
Dinner, chicken & noodles, ckd Marie Callender's (Frozen)	1	Each	368.60	520.00	21.00	42.00	5.00	30.00	11.00			80.00		
Dinner, chicken, alfredo, w/broccoli, fzn Healthy Choice	1	Each	326.00	300.00	25.00	34.00	2.00	7.00	3.00			50.00		
Dinner, chicken, fingers, ckd Banquet	1	Each	201.30	740.00	22.00	67.00	6.00	43.00	11.00			70.00	0.00	
Dinner, chicken, fried, w/mashed potatoes & corn, fzn Banquet	1	Each	228.00	469.68	21.45	35.09	2.05	27.04	9.25	15.35	2.44	88.92	0.00	
Dinner, chicken, parmigiana, ckd f/fzn Banquet	1	Each	269.00	320.00	10.00	29.00	3.00	18.00	7.00			50.00		
Dinner, chicken, teriyaki, w/oriental veg, fzn The Budget Gourmet-Light & Healthy	1	Each	311.00	317.22	18.66	52.25	4.04	3.73	0.62	0.91	1.60	24.88	43.54	
Dinner, chicken, teriyaki, w/rice medley veg & compote, fzn Healthy Choice	1	Each	312.00	268.32	17.07	37.10	2.81	5.62	3.00	2.15	0.47	43.68		
Dinner, chow mein, chicken, w/rice, low cal, fzn	1	Each	319.00	289.65	19.01	38.22	1.95	6.28	1.76	2.39	1.44	47.05	31.01	
Dinner, enchilada, beef Van de Kamp's	1	Each	340.00	400.00	16.00	54.00		14.00				40.00		
Dinner, enchilada, cheese, ckd f/fzn Banquet	1	Each	312.00	360.00	12.00	56.00	8.00	10.00	4.00			20.00		
Dinner, enchilada, cheese, fzn	1	Each	284.00	586.74	24.46	67.16	13.78	26.20	14.12	8.40	2.12	60.92	190.99	
Dinner, enchilada, chicken, w/sauce rice corn & compote, fzn Healthy Choice	1	Each	320.00	297.60	12.99	45.98	4.16	6.72	3.10	2.59	1.02	38.40		
Dinner, fettuccine, w/broccoli & chicken, ckd f/fzn Marie Callender's (Frozen)	1	Each	368.60	710.00	26.00	53.00	6.00	43.00	17.00			85.00		
Dinner, green pepper, stuffed, fzn	1	Each	397.00	410.38	18.23	38.94	5.03	21.34	6.13	8.26	4.78	49.04	161.62	
Dinner, lasagna, extra cheese, ckd f/fzn Marie Callender's (Frozen)	1	Each	425.30	590.00	27.00	61.00	7.00	27.00	13.00			50.00		
Dinner, lasagna, w/cheese & meat, low cal, fzn	1	Each	340.00	388.82	24.27	41.32		14.40	6.67	5.50	0.84	54.81	284.47	
Dinner, lasagna, w/meat sauce, ckd f/fzn Marie Callender's (Frozen)	1	Each	425.30	629.99	29.01	59.00	3.01	30.99	15.01			75.00		
Dinner, macaroni & cheese, ckd f/fzn Banquet	1	Each	340.20	420.00	15.00	57.00	5.00	14.00	8.00			20.00	0.00	
Dinner, meatballs, swedish, ckd Marie Callender's (Frozen)	1	Each	354.40	520.00	28.00	44.00	3.00	26.00	12.00			65.00		
Dinner, meatloaf, ckd f/fzn Banquet	1	Each	269.00	280.00	12.00	23.00	3.00	16.00	6.00			60.00		
Dinner, meatloaf, extra helping, w/sauce potato carrot, fzn Banquet	1	Each	453.00	611.55	29.08	33.57	6.34	40.05	15.49	17.30	7.25	113.25		
Dinner, salisbury steak, w/red potato & veg, fzn The Budget Gourmet-Light & Healthy	1	Each	311.00	261.24	18.35	33.90	7.15	5.91	2.02	1.75	0.94	43.54	71.53	
Dinner, shrimp & vegetables, fzn Healthy Choice	1	Each	335.00	270.00	15.00	39.00	6.00	6.00	3.00			50.00		
Dinner, spaghetti, w/meat sauce & garlic bread, ckd f/fzn Marie Callender's (Frozen)	1	Each	482.00	670.00	27.00	85.00	9.00	25.00	11.00			35.00		
Dinner, steak, chicken fried, ckd Banquet	1	Each	283.50	420.00	15.00	39.00	4.00	23.00	12.00			35.00		
Dinner, stir fry, chicken & veg, oriental, fzn Healthy Choice	1	Each	337.00	360.00	19.00	57.00	5.00	6.00	2.00			25.00		
Dinner, stroganoff, beef, fzn Healthy Choice	1	Each	312.00	320.00	22.00	40.00	7.00	8.00	3.00			60.00		
Dinner, tuna & noodles, homestyle, ckd Marie Callender's (Frozen)	1	Each	340.20	600.00	18.00	52.00	5.00	35.00	18.00			90.00		
Dinner, turkey, breast meat, honey rstd, ckd f/fzn Banquet	1	Each	255.20	270.00	11.00	29.00	4.00	12.00	2.50			30.00		
Dinner, turkey, breast, w/potatoes & veg, homestyle, fzn Stouffer's	1	Each	453.60	460.00	24.00	55.00	7.00	16.00	5.00			60.00		
Dinner, turkey, w/gravy & dressing, extra helping, ckd Banquet Hearty Ones	1	Each	481.95	620.00	28.00	54.00	10.00	32.00	8.00			80.00	0.00	

Vit E (mg)	Vit C	Vit B$_1$ Thia (mg)	Vit B$_2$ Ribo (mg)	Vit B$_3$ Nia (mg)	Fol (mcg)	Vit B$_6$ (mg)	Vita B$_{12}$ (mcg)	Sodi (mg)	Pota (mg)	Cal (mg)	Phos (mg)	Magn (mg)	Iron (mg)	Zinc (mg)	Caff (mg)	Alco (g)	Sol Fiber (g)	Insol Fiber (g)
	7.65							742.05		45.90			3.75		0.00	0.00		
1.26	4.08	0.16	0.29	1.67	19.27	0.13	0.42	1221.21	226.17	268.66	262.00	29.77	1.58	1.67	0.00	0.00		
	9.00							1320.00		100.00			2.70		0.00	0.00		
	12.00							530.00		100.00			1.80		0.00	0.00		
	0.00							1070.00		40.00			2.70		0.00	0.00		
	1.37							1500.24		38.76			1.37		0.00	0.00		
	30.00							900.00		60.00			1.80		0.00	0.00		
	44.47							674.87							0.00	0.00		
	12.17							602.16	424.32	37.44	224.64		1.09		0.00	0.00		
0.49	20.04	0.21	0.19	5.66	29.29	0.34	0.12	1068.62	336.03	44.44	158.58	36.60	2.55	1.83	0.00	0.00		
								1480.00	700.00						0.00	0.00		
	2.40							1500.00		200.00			1.80		0.00	0.00		
4.27	17.84	0.27	0.38	2.72	155.85	0.43	0.47	1751.57	786.54	566.69	594.95	96.07	3.46	3.06	0.00	0.00		
	18.24							563.20	384.00	134.40	236.80		0.77		0.00	0.00		
	9.00							910.00		150.00			2.70		0.00	0.00		
2.26	67.82	0.21	0.25	5.35	44.23	0.58	1.62	1216.57	811.23	149.01	203.21	65.22	7.30	3.72	0.00	0.00		
	0.00							1230.00		800.00			2.70		0.00	0.00		
3.45	12.54	0.29	0.39	5.07	28.26	0.32	0.88	839.53	758.98	264.77	306.61	64.04	3.82	3.70	0.00	0.00		
	0.00							1230.00		500.00			2.70		0.00	0.00		
	0.00							1330.00		150.00			1.44		0.00	0.00		
	0.00							1020.00		40.00			2.70		0.00	0.00		
	0.00	0.21	0.31	6.90				1020.00	900.00	40.00			1.80		0.00	0.00		
	7.70							1943.37		77.01			3.94		0.00	0.00		
	51.00							494.49					3.05		0.00	0.00		
	30.00							580.00		150.00			1.80		0.00	0.00		
	0.00							1160.00		150.00			2.70		0.00	0.00		
	0.00							1200.00		100.00			1.80		0.00	0.00		
	4.80							600.00		40.00			2.70		0.00	0.00		
	12.00							600.00		60.00			1.80		0.00	0.00		
	0.00							1570.00		100.00			2.70		0.00	0.00		
	0.00							1310.00		60.00			1.80		0.00	0.00		
	9.00							1620.00	480.00	100.00			2.70		0.00	0.00		
	0.00	0.41	0.31	4.50		0.31		2250.00	605.80	60.00	289.00		1.44		0.00	0.00		

Food Name	Amount	Measure	Weight (g)	Calories	Protein (g)	Total Carb (g)	Dietary Fiber (g)	Total Fat (g)	Sat Fat (g)	Mono Fat (g)	Poly Fat (g)	Chol (mg)	Vit A (mcg RAE)	Vit D (mcg)
MEALS AND DISHES *(continued)*														
Dinner, turkey, w/stuffing & dessert, extra lrg, fzn	1	Each	524.00	565.24	33.74	67.93	8.36	18.11	6.10	6.69	3.90	104.59	103.56	
Dinner, veal parmigiana, w/spaghetti & veg, homestyle, fzn Stouffer's	1	Each	496.10	530.00	27.00	66.00	7.00	17.00	4.50			60.00		
Dish, teriyaki stir fry, w/chicken & pasta, fzn Everyday Foods Lean Cuisine	1	Each	283.50	290.00	18.00	45.00	4.00	4.00	1.00	1.00	1.50	20.00		
Frozen/Refrigerated Dishes														
Burrito, beef bean cheese	1	Each	101.50	165.44	7.29	19.84	2.45	6.65	3.57	2.23	0.51	61.91	75.11	
Corn Dog	1	Each	175.00	460.25	16.80	55.79		18.90	5.16	9.11	3.50	78.75	59.50	
Dinner, beef, pot roast, w/whipped potatoes, homestyle, fzn Lean Cuisine	1	Each	255.00	206.55	17.34	22.44	3.57	5.35	1.31	2.28	0.81	38.25	48.45	
Dinner, cheese spinach manicotti, w/broccoli & carrots, fzn Hearty Portions Lean Cuisine	1	Each	439.40	350.00	19.00	50.00	6.00	8.00	3.00	2.50	1.50	40.00		
Dinner, chicken, piccata, w/cheese rice & peppers, fzn Cafe Classics Lean Cuisine	1	Each	255.00	300.00	14.00	41.00	2.00	9.00	2.50	2.00	1.50	30.00		
Dinner, Italian meatballs & rigatoni pasta, w/veg, fzn Hearty Portions Lean Cuisine	1	Each	435.90	440.00	25.00	64.00	7.00	9.00	3.50	4.00	1.00	35.00		
Dinner, salisbury steak, w/macaroni & cheese, fzn Cafe Classics Lean Cuisine	1	Each	272.00	386.24	22.58	26.38		21.22	8.00	7.94	1.85	62.56	0.00	
Dish, beef & broccoli, w/rice, skillet, fzn Stouffer's Skillet Sensations	0.5	Each	354.40	320.00	17.00	51.00	3.00	5.00	2.00			30.00		
Dish, beef macaroni, fzn, svg Healthy Choice	1	Each	226.80	199.58	13.36	31.62	4.31	2.11	0.63	1.13	0.32	13.61	52.16	
Dish, beef, pepper steak, oriental, fzn La Choy	1	Cup	246.00	103.81	9.99	12.47	3.69	2.36	0.59			12.30		
Dish, beef, stroganoff, skillet, fzn Stouffer's Skillet Sensations	0.25	Each	283.50	340.00	19.00	38.00	4.00	12.00	3.50			35.00		
Dish, cannelloni, cheese, fzn Everyday Foods Lean Cuisine	1	Each	258.70	220.00	21.00	27.00	3.00	3.50	2.00	1.00	0.50	15.00		
Dish, casserole, macaroni & beef, w/tomato sauce Swanson	1	Each	284.00	270.00	18.00	39.00	2.00	5.00	5.00	0.00	0.00	35.00		
Dish, cheese ravioli, fzn Everyday Foods Lean Cuisine	1	Each	241.00	260.00	12.00	38.00	4.00	7.00	3.50	1.50	0.50	35.00		1.53
Dish, chicken & noodles, escalloped, fzn Stouffer's	1	Each	283.00	418.84	16.98	31.41		25.19	5.95	6.95	12.29	76.41	0.00	
Dish, chicken & rice, stir fry, fzn, Lunch Express Lean Cuisine	1	Each	255.00	270.30	11.73	39.52	5.86	7.39	0.93	3.47	2.02	25.50	262.65	
Dish, chicken & vegetables, w/vermicelli, fzn Cafe Classics Lean Cuisine	1	Each	297.00	252.45	18.71	32.08	5.05	5.64	1.03	2.13	1.38	23.76		
Dish, chicken a l'orange, w/broccoli & rice, fzn Cafe Classics Lean Cuisine	1	Each	255.00	267.75	24.48	38.50		1.78	0.42	0.50	0.41	45.90		
Dish, chicken alfredo, fettuccine fzn, Lunch Express Lean Cuisine	1	Each	272.00	372.64	19.04	32.64	3.81	18.50	6.99	6.26	2.39	57.12		
Dish, chicken, ala king, fzn Stouffer's	1	Each	326.00	370.00	21.00	47.00	2.00	11.00	4.00			45.00		
Dish, chicken, carbonara, pasta w/cheese sauce, fzn Cafe Classics Lean Cuisine	1	Each	255.00	280.00	17.00	36.00	4.00	7.00	1.50	2.00	2.50	30.00		
Dish, chicken, marsala, w/veg, fzn Healthy Choice	1	Each	326.00	240.00	20.00	32.00	3.00	4.00	2.00			30.00		
Dish, chicken, rstd, w/garlic sauce pasta & veg, fzn, fs Tyson Food Service	1	Each	255.00	214.20	16.93	21.52	3.57	6.71	1.30	2.35	2.14	28.05		
Dish, chicken, teriyaki, w/rice, bowl, fzn Healthy Choice	1	Each	269.00	270.00	17.00	41.00	4.00	4.00	1.00			30.00		
Dish, chili, w/beans, fzn Stouffer's	1	Each	248.10	290.00	19.00	29.00	6.00	11.00	4.00			45.00		
Dish, chow mein, beef, bi-pack, fzn La Choy	1	Cup	247.00	104.98	9.24	14.87	3.46	1.73	0.82			12.35		
Dish, chow mein, chicken, fzn La Choy	1	Each	250.00	91.25	5.32	11.40	2.10	3.65	0.95			8.75		
Dish, chow mein, shrimp, bi-pack, fzn La Choy	1	Each	141.75	35.15	2.27	6.01	1.70	0.61	0.00			17.58		
Dish, enchilada, beef, fzn Ortega	1	Each	265.78	360.00	12.00	49.00	5.00	13.00	5.00			25.00		
Dish, enchilada, cheese	1	Each	163.00	319.48	9.63	28.54		18.84	10.59	6.31	0.82	44.01	99.43	

Vit E (mg)	Vit C	Vit B₁ Thia (mg)	Vit B₂ Ribo (mg)	Vit B₃ Nia (mg)	Fol (mcg)	Vit B₆ (mg)	Vita B₁₂ (mcg)	Sodi (mg)	Pota (mg)	Cal (mg)	Phos (mg)	Magn (mg)	Iron (mg)	Zinc (mg)	Caff (mg)	Alco (g)	Sol Fiber (g)	Insol Fiber (g)
2.41	21.04	0.39	0.39	8.20	69.92	0.60	0.49	1893.74	792.08	104.88	361.95	75.98	3.80	3.87	0.00	0.00		
	27.00							1130.00	1040.00	200.00			3.60		0.00	0.00		
	0.00							590.00	610.00	40.00			1.08		0.00	0.00		
0.41	2.54	0.15	0.36	1.93	37.55	0.11	0.55	495.32	205.03	64.96	70.03	25.37	1.87	1.18	0.00	0.00		
0.70	0.00	0.28	0.70	4.16	103.25	0.09	0.44	973.00	262.50	101.50	166.25	17.50	6.18	1.31	0.00	0.00		
								494.70							0.00	0.00		
	9.00							840.00	910.00	400.00			1.80		0.00	0.00		
	12.00							690.00	290.00	100.00			0.72		0.00	0.00		
	24.00							820.00	1150.00	200.00			3.60		0.00	0.00		
	1.21							1014.56	616.12	195.84			2.28		0.00	0.00		
	9.00							1250.00	637.00	60.00			1.44		0.00	0.00		
1.59	54.89	0.26	0.15	2.94	99.79	0.18	0.11	419.58	344.74	43.09	127.01	34.02	2.56	1.15	0.00	0.00		
	7.33							969.24		23.91			0.49		0.00	0.00		
	2.40							1090.00		150.00			2.70		0.00	0.00		
	6.00	0.12	0.26	1.60		0.14	0.00	550.00	440.00	350.00		36.00	0.72	1.60	0.00	0.00		
	12.00							1060.00		60.00			2.70		0.00	0.00		
	4.80	0.06	0.26	1.20	48.00	0.20	0.30	590.00	450.00	150.00	168.00	42.00	1.44	1.50	0.00	0.00		
	0.00							1211.24	329.42	116.03			1.13		0.00	0.00		
	23.71							632.40							0.00	0.00		
	14.55							582.12	647.82	103.95			1.34		0.00	0.00		
	18.10							359.55	430.00	20.00			0.36	1.00	0.00	0.00		
	24.21							587.52		146.88					0.00	0.00		
	6.00	0.12	0.12	1.81				1300.00	450.00	100.00			0.36		0.00	0.00		
	12.00							690.00	710.00	150.00			1.44		0.00	0.00		
	3.60							440.00		40.00			0.72		0.00	0.00		
								466.65					1.56		0.00	0.00		
	12.00							570.00		20.00			1.08		0.00	0.00		
	3.60	0.10	0.10	1.20				1000.00	610.00	80.00			3.60		0.00	0.00		
	11.07							755.82		29.64			0.62		0.00	0.00		
	4.15							865.00		42.75			0.68		0.00	0.00		
	13.24							547.16		1.83			2.37		0.00	0.00		
	9.00							1460.00		150.00			1.80		0.00	0.00		
1.47	0.98	0.08	0.42	1.91	65.20	0.39	0.75	784.03	239.61	324.37	133.66	50.53	1.32	2.51	0.00	0.00		

Food Name	Amount	Measure	Weight (g)	Calories	Protein (g)	Total Carb (g)	Dietary Fiber (g)	Total Fat (g)	Sat Fat (g)	Mono Fat (g)	Poly Fat (g)	Chol (mg)	Vit A (mcg RAE)	Vit D (mcg)
MEALS AND DISHES *(continued)*														
Dish, green peppers, stuffed w/beef, w/tomato sauce, fzn Stouffer's	0.5	Each	219.50	188.77	7.90	20.85	5.27	8.12	2.72	3.75	0.53	21.95	0.00	
Dish, inari, svg Hissho Sushi	1	Each	113.00	250.00	7.00	33.00	0.00	8.00	1.00			0.00	0.00	
Dish, lasagna, bake, fzn Stouffer's	1	Each	326.00	450.00	25.00	51.00	4.00	16.00	7.00			45.00		
Dish, lasagna, Italian sausage, fzn The Budget Gourmet	1	Each	298.00	455.94	20.56	39.93	2.98	23.84	8.17	9.77	2.00	47.68		
Dish, lasagna, w/meat sauce, fzn, svg Stouffer's	1	Each	215.00	277.35	18.71	26.45	3.23	10.75	4.71	3.48	0.56	40.85	0.00	
Dish, macaroni & beef, w/tomato sauce, fzn Everyday Foods Lean Cuisine	1	Each	283.00	249.04	13.87	36.51	3.40	5.38	1.64	2.06	0.70	22.64		
Dish, macaroni & beef, w/tomato sauce, fzn, Weight Watchers	1	Each	269.00	282.45	15.60	44.65	6.73	4.57	1.58	1.77	0.61	13.45		
Dish, macaroni & cheese, fzn Stouffer's Family Style Favorites	5	Ounce-weight	226.80	380.00	16.00	40.00	2.00	17.00	8.00			35.00		
Dish, manicotti, cheese, fzn Stouffer's	1	Each	255.20	360.00	19.00	34.00	4.00	16.00	9.00			40.00		
Dish, meatballs w/pasta, Swedish, fzn Everyday Foods Lean Cuisine	1	Each	258.00	276.06	21.67	31.22	2.58	7.22	2.42	2.34	1.04	46.44	0.00	0.22
Dish, meatloaf, beef, homestyle, rtb, fzn, 4 oz, FS Travis Meats	1	Each	113.40	335.90	16.54	4.08	0.62	28.15	11.48	12.14	1.05	68.89		
Dish, noodles romanoff, fzn Stouffer's	1	Each	340.20	490.00	17.00	53.00	5.00	23.00	6.00			55.00		
Dish, pasta, w/chicken wine & mushroom sauce, low fat The Budget Gourmet	1	Each	241.00	280.00	13.00	41.00	4.00	7.00	2.00			25.00		
Dish, pea & potato curry	5	Ounce-weight	141.75	201.29	3.26	17.72	4.39	15.31					0.00	
Dish, penne pasta, w/tomato basil sauce, fzn Everyday Foods Lean Cuisine	1	Each	283.50	260.00	9.00	47.00	5.00	3.50	0.50	1.50	0.50	0.00		
Dish, penne pasta, w/tomato Italian sausage & sauce, low fat The Budget Gourmet	1	Each	226.00	270.00	10.00	46.00	3.00	6.00	1.50			10.00		
Dish, pot pie, beef, fzn	1	Each	198.00	449.46	13.27	44.15	2.18	24.35	8.51	9.68	2.67	37.62	51.48	
Dish, pot pie, chicken Swanson	1	Each	198.00	410.00	10.00	43.00	2.00	22.00	9.00			25.00		
Dish, pot pie, chicken, fzn	1	Each	217.00	483.91	13.04	42.71	1.74	29.10	9.67	12.48	4.49	41.23	256.06	
Dish, pot pie, chicken, fzn Stouffer's	1	Each	283.00	571.66	23.21	36.51	3.11	37.07	10.73	12.37	10.44	76.41		
Dish, pot pie, turkey, ckd f/fzn Banquet	1	Each	198.00	370.00	10.00	38.00	3.00	20.00	8.00			45.00		
Dish, potatoes, scalloped, fzn Stouffer's Family Style Favorites	5	Ounce-weight	141.75	140.00	4.00	19.00	2.00	5.00	1.50			3.00	0.00	
Dish, rice bowl, beef & broccoli, spicy Uncle Ben's Inc.	1	Each	340.20	370.00	21.00	62.00	5.00	4.50	1.50			25.00		
Dish, rice bowl, chicken, Szechuan Uncle Ben's Inc.	1	Each	340.20	360.00	23.00	58.00	3.00	4.00	1.00			35.00		
Dish, rice bowl, southwest style black bean & veg Uncle Ben's Inc.	1	Each	340.20	360.00	11.00	68.00	10.00	4.50	1.00			0.00		
Dish, rice bowl, teriyaki stir fry veg Uncle Ben's Inc.	1	Each	340.20	360.00	8.00	74.00	4.00	3.00	0.50			0.00		
Dish, rice pilaf, wild, w/veg The Budget Gourmet	1	Each	226.00	340.00	6.00	44.00	2.00	13.00	3.00			10.00		
Dish, rice, w/broccoli, fzn Green Giant's Rice & Vegetable Combos	1	Each	283.00	320.00	8.00	44.00	2.00	12.00	3.50			15.00		
Dish, rigatoni, w/cream sauce broccoli & chicken, low fat The Budget Gourmet	1	Each	226.00	260.00	9.00	40.00	2.00	6.00	2.00			15.00		
Dish, spaghetti, w/meat sauce, fzn Everyday Foods Lean Cuisine	1	Each	326.00	312.96	14.34	50.53	5.54	5.87	1.35	2.28	1.32	13.04		
Dish, spaghetti, w/meatballs, fzn, 12.6oz Stouffer's	1	Each	357.20	390.00	19.00	49.00	5.00	13.00	4.00			30.00		
Dish, steak, salisbury The Budget Gourmet	1	Each	241.00	350.00	15.00	23.00	2.00	23.00	9.00			55.00		
Dish, stir fry, vegetable szechuan, fzn mix Green Giant's Create-A-Meal	1	Cup	114.00	85.50	3.42	11.40	2.28	2.85	0.28			0.00		
Dish, stroganoff, beef, homestyle, fzn Stouffer's	1	Each	276.40	370.00	21.00	32.00	3.00	17.00	7.00			65.00		
Dish, tuna noodle casserole, fzn Healthy Choice	1	Each	255.00	240.00	16.00	33.00	4.00	5.00	2.00			25.00	0.00	

Vit E (mg)	Vit C	Vit B₁ Thia (mg)	Vit B₂ Ribo (mg)	Vit B₃ Nia (mg)	Fol (mcg)	Vit B₆ (mg)	Vita B₁₂ (mcg)	Sodi (mg)	Pota (mg)	Cal (mg)	Phos (mg)	Magn (mg)	Iron (mg)	Zinc (mg)	Caff (mg)	Alco (g)	Sol Fiber (g)	Insol Fiber (g)
	86.48							577.28	369.66	19.98			1.08		0.00	0.00		
	0.00							703.00		120.00			1.08		0.00	0.00	0.00	0.00
	2.40							1110.00	440.00	200.00			2.70		0.00	0.00		
								902.94		315.88			2.68		0.00	0.00		
	2.60							735.30	411.59	230.05			1.17		0.00	0.00		
	157.35							563.17	638.87	39.93			2.18		0.00	0.00		
	27.44							492.27					5.68		0.00	0.00		
	0.00							1020.00	220.00	350.00			0.72		0.00	0.00		
	4.80							850.00	525.00	450.00			1.08		0.00	0.00		
0.34	0.00	0.59	0.52	4.98	31.89	0.31	1.01	562.44	598.56	206.40	206.40	43.86	2.06	3.69	0.00	0.00		
	6.00	0.11	0.15	2.82				280.60	308.10	18.00	158.30		2.52	3.07	0.00	0.00		
	0.00	0.10	0.10	0.70				1260.00	140.00	150.00			1.44		0.00	0.00		
	1.20							670.00		60.00			1.44		0.00	0.00		
	8.51	0.07	0.06	1.70	18.43		0.00	524.48	378.47	39.69		24.10	1.28	0.57	0.00	0.00		
	6.00							390.00	520.00	60.00			1.80		0.00	0.00		
	2.40							410.00		40.00			2.70		0.00	0.00		
								736.56							0.00	0.00		
	1.20							780.00		20.00			1.80		0.00	0.00		
3.84	1.52	0.25	0.36	4.13	41.23	0.20	0.15	857.15	256.06	32.55	119.35	23.87	2.06	1.02	0.00	0.00		
	0.00							942.39		101.88			3.00		0.00	0.00		
	0.00							850.00		40.00			1.08		0.00	0.00		
	0.00							560.00	231.00	100.00			0.00		0.00	0.00		
								1550.00							0.00	0.00		
								1800.00							0.00	0.00		
								1250.00							0.00	0.00		
								1360.00							0.00	0.00		
	2.40							700.00		40.00			0.36		0.00	0.00		
	18.00							1000.00		150.00			3.60		0.00	0.00		
	2.40							480.00		100.00			1.44		0.00	0.00		
	34.88	0.30	0.34	4.00				609.62	580.00	80.00			2.12		0.00	0.00		
	4.80	0.00	0.10	1.40				850.00	500.00	60.00			1.80		0.00	0.00		
	6.00							1440.00		80.00			1.80		0.00	0.00		
	13.68						0.00	763.80		22.80			0.62		0.00	0.00		
	0.00	0.00	0.10	1.10		0.14		950.00	570.00	40.00			1.44		0.00	0.00		
	0.00							580.00		150.00			1.44		0.00	0.00		

Food Name	Amount	Measure	Weight (g)	Calories	Protein (g)	Total Carb (g)	Dietary Fiber (g)	Total Fat (g)	Sat Fat (g)	Mono Fat (g)	Poly Fat (g)	Chol (mg)	Vit A (mcg RAE)	Vit D (mcg)
MEALS AND DISHES *(continued)*														
Dish, turkey, w/gravy & mashed potato, ckd Marie Callender's (Frozen)	5	Ounce-weight	141.75	167.57	12.43	9.73	1.08	8.65	3.24			37.84	0.00	
Dish, vegetable lasagna, fzn Everyday Foods Lean Cuisine	1	Each	298.00	260.00	17.00	33.00	4.00	7.00	3.50	2.00	1.00	20.00		
Frozen/Refrigerated Dinners/Dishes—Vegetarian														
Dish, lasagna, garden vegetable, fzn Amy's Kitchen Inc	1	Each	291.00	290.00	13.00	41.00	5.00	9.00	4.00			20.00		
Dish, lasagna, tofu vegetable, fzn Amy's Kitchen Inc	1	Each	269.00	300.00	13.00	41.00	6.00	10.00	1.50			0.00		
Dish, meatloaf, meatless, w/gravy, slice Gardenburger Inc.	1	Piece	142.00	130.00	12.00	12.00	4.00	3.50	1.00			0.00		
Dish, pasta primavera, fzn Amy's Kitchen Inc	1	Each	255.00	300.00	15.00	37.00	3.00	11.00	6.00			45.00		
Dish, pot pie, vegetarian	1	Each	227.00	509.75	14.49	40.72	5.23	32.45	8.56	12.40	9.62	19.54	453.50	0.20
Dish, quiche, spinach, vegetarian	5	Ounce-weight	141.75	340.16	11.16	16.36	1.22	25.89	12.00	8.81	3.43	156.84	300.14	
Dish, ravioli, cheese, w/sauce, fzn Amy's Kitchen Inc	1	Each	227.00	340.00	15.00	43.00	3.00	12.00	5.00			25.00		
Dish, tamale pie, vgtrn, Mexican, fzn Amy's Kitchen Inc	1	Each	227.00	150.00	5.00	27.00	4.00	3.00	0.00			0.00		
Homemade and Generic Meals and Dishes														
Beef, round steak, lean, fried, med	3	Ounce-weight	85.05	197.18	28.86	0.00	0.00	8.19	2.66	3.01	1.35	83.25	0.00	0.26
Burrito, bean & cheese	1	Each	93.00	188.79	7.53	27.48		5.85	3.42	1.24	0.89	13.95	49.29	
Burrito, beef	1	Each	110.00	261.80	13.30	29.26	0.79	10.41	5.23	3.70	0.43	31.90	6.60	
Burrito, beef & cheese, w/chili peppers	1	Each	152.00	316.16	20.46	31.86		12.39	5.20	4.97	1.11	85.12	98.80	
Burrito, meat & bean	1	Each	115.50	254.10	11.24	33.01	2.49	8.91	4.16	3.51	0.61	24.25	16.17	
Chimichanga, beef	1	Each	174.00	424.56	19.61	42.80	2.00	19.68	8.51	8.06	1.14	8.70	6.96	
Chimichanga, beef & cheese	1	Each	183.00	442.86	20.06	39.33		23.44	11.18	9.43	0.73	51.24	131.76	
Chow Mein, shrimp, w/noodles USDA Survey Database	1	Cup	220.00	272.07	16.59	24.27	2.80	12.75	1.87	3.10	6.94	81.87	11.99	
Dish, beef burgundy	1	Cup	244.00	291.29	35.05	8.91	1.42	11.79	3.37	4.14	2.36	94.24	2.72	0.73
Dish, beef curry	1	Cup	236.00	435.94	27.08	13.12	2.66	31.35	7.02	14.46	7.38	69.49	286.41	
Dish, chicken curry	1	Cup	236.00	293.82	27.45	10.35	2.15	16.09	3.33	7.01	4.35	84.25	157.24	
Dish, chicken, kiev	1	Each	258.00	642.55	73.33	10.02	0.34	32.62	15.83	10.51	3.71	283.15	208.26	
Dish, chicken, kung pao	1	Cup	162.00	431.21	28.81	11.39	2.23	30.61	5.19	13.94	9.69	64.39	31.44	
Dish, chicken, parmigiana	1	Piece	182.00	319.50	28.47	15.52	1.14	15.63	5.31	4.86	4.04	137.12	118.16	
Dish, chicken thigh, sweet & sour USDA Survey Database	1	Each	78.00	70.00	4.72	8.85	0.55	1.91	0.32	0.56	0.82	13.82	7.85	
Dish, chop suey, beef, w/o noodles	1	Cup	220.00	271.46	22.13	12.35	2.74	15.08	3.70	6.50	3.49	50.36	99.34	
Dish, chow mein, pork, w/noodles	1	Cup	220.00	447.94	21.96	31.03	3.73	27.02	4.85	7.72	12.80	47.76	10.07	
Dish, curried shrimp	1	Cup	236.00	297.67	27.52	13.60	0.38	14.33	3.97	5.74	3.51	176.76	168.93	
Dish, egg foo yung patty	1	Each	86.00	113.23	6.44	3.32	0.61	8.38	1.95	3.37	2.11	185.46	84.75	
Dish, egg roll, chicken	1	Each	64.00	103.31	3.93	9.39	0.62	5.51	1.23	2.67	1.18	38.01	17.32	
Dish, egg roll, meat	1	Each	64.00	113.07	4.95	9.26	0.68	6.21	1.44	2.98	1.32	37.07	14.62	
Dish, egg roll, shrimp	1	Each	64.00	104.09	3.51	9.87	0.72	5.63	1.17	2.69	1.35	39.50	16.17	
Dish, egg roll, w/o meat	1	Each	64.00	100.82	2.54	9.82	0.82	5.81	1.23	2.86	1.33	30.16	14.83	
Dish, eggplant, parmesan casserole	1	Cup	198.00	319.43	14.47	17.21	3.16	22.16	9.22	7.83	3.90	55.02	133.32	
Dish, enchilada, beef & cheese	1	Each	192.00	322.56	11.92	30.47		17.64	9.05	6.15	1.39	40.32	97.92	
Dish, enchirito, beef, bean & cheese	1	Each	193.00	343.54	17.89	33.79		16.08	7.95	6.52	0.33	50.18	88.78	
Dish, fajitas, beef	1	Each	223.00	399.44	22.62	35.67	3.21	18.15	5.53	7.57	3.47	45.08	21.55	
Dish, fajitas, chicken	1	Each	223.00	363.16	20.01	44.27	5.11	11.98	2.25	5.53	3.12	39.30	36.03	
Dish, fried rice USDA SR-23 USDA SR-23: Chinese Restaurant	0.5	Cup	70.00	114.10	3.27	21.69	0.77	1.59	0.35	0.42	0.66	16.10		
Dish, gefilte fish, w/jellied broth, w/o add sug Manischewitz	1	Serving	70.00	80.00	7.00	3.00	1.00	3.00	1.00			21.00	0.00	
Dish, goulash, beef	1	Cup	249.00	270.26	33.08	6.98	0.95	11.62	3.24	4.32	2.47	84.38	15.47	0.37
Dish, grape leaves, stuffed w/beef & rice	6	Each	126.00	301.63	10.26	14.26	4.00	23.25	5.42	13.82	2.14	30.50	404.29	
Dish, grape leaves, stuffed w/lamb & rice	6	Each	126.00	333.01	10.54	14.97	4.24	26.41	6.70	15.25	2.76	32.19	435.09	
Dish, jambalaya, shrimp	1	Cup	243.00	310.48	27.21	27.95	1.37	9.39	1.82	3.77	2.85	180.73	104.78	
Dish, knish, cheese	1	Each	60.00	208.17	6.46	18.69	0.64	11.80	2.79	5.33	2.92	55.97	118.65	
Dish, knish, meat	1	Each	50.00	175.27	6.63	12.89	0.56	10.64	2.63	4.88	2.28	52.37	83.27	
Dish, knish, potato	1	Each	61.00	215.09	4.73	20.80	0.92	12.49	2.61	5.78	3.27	59.10	120.78	

Vit E (mg)	Vit C	Vit B₁ Thia (mg)	Vit B₂ Ribo (mg)	Vit B₃ Nia (mg)	Fol (mcg)	Vit B₆ (mg)	Vita B₁₂ (mcg)	Sodi (mg)	Pota (mg)	Cal (mg)	Phos (mg)	Magn (mg)	Iron (mg)	Zinc (mg)	Caff (mg)	Alco (g)	Sol Fiber (g)	Insol Fiber (g)
	0.00							594.59		32.43			0.19		0.00	0.00		
	4.80	0.10	0.20	0.30				580.00	540.00	350.00			1.08		0.00	0.00		
	36.00							720.00		250.00			2.70		0.00	0.00		
	21.00							630.00		100.00			4.50		0.00	0.00		
	2.40							520.00		80.00			0.72		0.00	0.00		
	18.00							670.00		300.00			1.80		0.00	0.00		
4.23	9.90	0.82	0.44	5.17	57.81	0.41	1.01	486.42	377.80	68.10	262.50	32.45	2.96	1.08	0.00	0.00		
1.73	5.32	0.18	0.39	1.13	56.19	0.13	0.39	110.79	275.35	245.08	210.26	40.33	2.17	1.32	0.00	0.00		
	1.20							580.00		250.00			2.70		0.00	0.00		
	6.00							590.00		40.00			1.80		0.00	0.00		
0.12	0.00	0.10	0.26	4.22	9.93	0.48	3.01	62.63	418.34	6.50	238.99	29.02	2.96	4.60	0.00	0.00	0.00	0.00
	0.84	0.11	0.35	1.79	37.20	0.12	0.45	583.11	248.31	106.95	90.21	39.99	1.13	0.82	0.00	0.00		
0.55	0.55	0.12	0.46	3.22	64.90	0.15	0.98	745.80	369.60	41.80	86.90	40.70	3.05	2.37	0.00	0.00		
	1.82	0.30	0.62	4.16	69.92	0.18	1.03	1045.76	332.88	110.96	158.08	34.96	3.91	3.95	0.00	0.00		
0.69	0.92	0.27	0.42	2.70	57.75	0.18	0.87	667.59	328.02	53.13	70.45	41.58	2.45	1.92	0.00	0.00		
	4.70	0.49	0.64	5.78	83.52	0.28	1.51	910.02	586.38	62.64	123.54	62.64	4.54	4.96	0.00	0.00		
	2.75	0.38	0.86	4.67	91.50	0.22	1.30	957.09	203.13	237.90	186.66	60.39	3.84	3.37	0.00	0.00		
1.34	9.38	0.23	0.24	4.47	45.08	0.18	0.59	709.70	391.14	58.12	219.91	51.19	3.42	1.35	0.00	0.00		
1.06	4.29	0.19	0.49	6.73	22.67	0.45	4.11	114.34	844.29	28.83	377.18	53.47	4.89	8.01	0.00	0.55		
5.88	24.59	0.18	0.34	5.42	20.33	0.48	3.05	801.64	977.87	43.96	291.86	59.00	4.23	6.06	0.00	0.00		
3.13	18.43	0.13	0.23	10.28	20.29	0.50	0.30	629.18	625.75	43.71	251.43	51.21	2.07	2.15	0.00	0.00		
1.54	0.00	0.25	0.35	32.00	14.18	1.37	0.87	454.23	622.71	62.79	558.18	72.82	3.27	2.51	0.00	0.00		
3.90	7.51	0.15	0.15	13.23	42.56	0.59	0.26	906.76	428.26	49.47	263.04	63.13	1.96	1.50	0.00	0.20		
2.41	8.65	0.18	0.34	8.47	16.56	0.37	0.43	640.93	470.87	198.03	316.95	45.23	2.31	2.38	0.00	0.00		
0.40	7.20	0.04	0.05	1.84	3.43	0.11	0.05	301.39	110.02	9.20	44.78	12.37	0.50	0.40	0.00	0.00		
2.03	23.42	0.18	0.25	4.20	42.01	0.41	1.96	923.87	556.38	37.50	238.00	41.54	2.91	3.48	0.00	0.00		
2.68	20.23	0.78	0.43	6.24	41.75	0.42	0.42	848.19	488.91	44.86	248.95	52.85	3.30	2.56	0.00	0.00		
2.43	3.68	0.12	0.29	3.16	11.25	0.17	1.36	342.25	443.11	229.28	367.00	60.21	3.02	1.80	0.00	0.00		
1.22	4.81	0.04	0.26	0.43	29.52	0.09	0.37	317.36	117.32	31.31	93.02	11.59	1.04	0.70	0.00	0.00		
0.73	2.35	0.08	0.11	1.06	10.97	0.05	0.08	163.87	73.20	15.15	40.95	7.73	0.85	0.33	0.00	0.00		
0.80	2.14	0.16	0.12	1.28	9.92	0.10	0.12	273.51	124.24	15.15	56.83	10.03	0.83	0.46	0.00	0.00		
0.85	2.32	0.08	0.10	0.91	9.96	0.05	0.11	292.53	99.77	17.09	46.71	9.81	0.90	0.29	0.00	0.00		
0.85	2.89	0.08	0.11	0.80	13.36	0.05	0.06	274.22	96.61	14.34	38.03	9.07	0.81	0.25	0.00	0.00		
2.62	8.10	0.14	0.25	1.63	23.52	0.19	0.45	683.97	447.44	366.34	281.40	37.52	1.30	1.52	0.00	0.00		
1.54	1.34	0.10	0.40	2.52	67.20	0.27	1.02	1319.04	574.08	228.48	167.04	82.56	3.07	2.69	0.00	0.00		
1.54	4.63	0.17	0.69	2.99	94.57	0.21	1.62	1250.64	559.70	218.09	223.88	71.41	2.39	2.76	0.00	0.00		
1.74	26.81	0.39	0.30	5.40	22.99	0.38	2.06	316.35	478.71	84.22	238.25	37.58	3.76	3.52	0.00	0.00		
1.71	36.83	0.43	0.33	6.12	41.80	0.38	0.10	343.02	533.62	100.80	188.31	48.17	3.32	1.65	0.00	0.00		
0.10		0.01	0.02	0.45	4.20	0.02	0.00	277.20	61.60	9.80	38.50	7.00	0.50	0.54	0.00	0.00		
	0.00							720.00		20.00			0.72		0.00	0.00		
1.83	8.74	0.15	0.31	5.74	21.27	0.46	3.25	225.45	698.37	18.08	336.17	45.56	3.58	5.26	0.00	0.00		
2.66	10.33	0.09	0.21	2.91	29.68	0.22	0.71	87.70	279.92	120.68	107.12	45.53	2.38	2.02	0.00	0.00		
2.78	9.04	0.11	0.20	3.51	33.04	0.22	0.76	84.30	245.67	132.61	112.78	47.54	2.38	1.97	0.00	0.00		
2.34	16.87	0.29	0.10	4.77	12.15	0.22	1.18	370.06	439.32	103.94	300.25	63.59	4.39	1.73	0.00	0.00		
1.58	0.03	0.16	0.20	1.28	10.65	0.04	0.18	203.65	61.65	24.71	75.29	7.84	1.32	0.37	0.00	0.00		
1.21	0.36	0.11	0.16	1.50	8.28	0.05	0.32	106.64	88.39	12.24	61.46	8.47	1.24	1.01	0.00	0.00		
1.71	0.94	0.17	0.18	1.48	10.37	0.07	0.13	140.22	95.50	16.07	60.01	10.07	1.34	0.37	0.00	0.00		

Food Name	Amount	Measure	Weight (g)	Calories	Protein (g)	Total Carb (g)	Dietary Fiber (g)	Total Fat (g)	Sat Fat (g)	Mono Fat (g)	Poly Fat (g)	Chol (mg)	Vit A (mcg RAE)	Vit D (mcg)
MEALS AND DISHES *(continued)*														
Dish, lamb curry	1	Cup	236.00	256.44	28.33	3.36	1.02	13.87	3.94	4.93	3.36	89.07	0.88	0.24
Dish, lo Mein, veg, vegetarian	5	Ounce-weight	141.75	95.79	4.35	19.19	2.66	0.55	0.09	0.06	0.22	0.00	46.00	
Dish, lo mein, w/pork	5	Ounce-weight	141.75	200.43	13.91	14.82	1.89	9.68	1.84	2.79	4.28	29.83	4.42	
Dish, macaroni & cheese, cnd, svg	1	Each	252.00	206.64	8.52	29.03	1.26	6.20	2.22	1.51	0.76	15.12		
Dish, pot pie, greek meat, 8"	1	Each	417.00	947.13	33.95	72.63	4.84	57.39	13.49	25.62	14.23	66.11	475.69	
Dish, quiche, cheese, w/o meat	5	Ounce-weight	141.75	420.33	12.45	19.73	0.57	32.57	15.86	10.87	3.85	178.81	241.84	
Dish, quiche, lorraine	1	Piece	176.00	526.35	14.93	25.04	0.73	40.87	18.85	14.34	5.19	221.04	275.87	1.07
Dish, rice pilaf	1	Cup	206.00	260.88	4.36	44.65	1.32	6.87	1.35	3.24	1.91	0.00	58.47	
Dish, spaghetti, w/tomato sauce & cheese, prep f/recipe	1	Cup	250.00	260.00	8.75	37.00		8.75	2.00			7.50		
Dish, spring roll, fresh	1	Each	64.00	113.07	4.95	9.26	0.68	6.21	1.44	2.98	1.32	37.07	14.62	
Dish, spring roll, meat	1	Each	64.00	113.07	4.95	9.26	0.68	6.21	1.44	2.98	1.32	37.07	14.62	
Dish, sukiyaki USDA Survey Database	1	Cup	162.00	172.47	18.69	6.75	1.27	7.73	2.89	3.10	0.73	147.76	153.34	
Dish, sweet & sour pork, w/rice	1	Cup	244.00	270.40	13.13	40.18	1.45	6.30	1.63	2.39	1.72	28.36	11.79	
Dish, turkey & noodles, w/gravy	1	Cup	224.00	303.79	19.73	27.11	1.19	12.28	3.43	4.92	2.79	77.77	29.96	
Dish, turkey & stuffing	1	Cup	200.00	273.46	34.64	18.94	0.80	5.44	1.39	1.71	1.30	104.66	19.09	
Dish, vegetables, w/pasta & cream sauce	1	Cup	162.00	180.71	7.87	20.73	1.26	7.54	2.26	3.03	1.78	6.81	272.09	
Dish, vegetables, w/pasta, New England, ckd	1	Cup	190.00	195.57	6.07	28.13		7.30	1.38	3.26	2.15	0.00	421.20	
Dish, wonton, meat filled, fried	3	Each	57.00	163.90	8.70	14.38	0.68	7.63	2.49	3.56	0.84	60.30	18.22	
Dish, ziti, w/meat, prep f/recipe	5	Ounce-weight	141.75	226.81	13.33	23.07		9.00	4.64	3.00	0.49	33.70	69.85	
Meal, sushi combo, Living Color roll Hissho Sushi Nigiri Combo	1	Each	226.00	325.00	15.00	48.00	2.00	4.00	1.00			26.00		
Meal, sushi combo, LPJ combo Hissho Sushi	1	Each	198.00	340.00	15.00	47.00	2.00	6.00	1.00			38.00		
Meal, sushi combo, Rock n Roll special Hissho Sushi Nigiri Combo	1	Each	255.00	424.00	18.00	57.00	2.00	8.00	2.00			51.00		
Meal, sushi combo, United Hissho Sushi	1	Each	198.00	320.00	9.00	49.00	2.00	6.00	2.00			15.00		
Meal, sushi combo, w/inari Hissho Sushi	1	Each	198.00	358.00	10.00	54.00	2.00	7.00	1.00			2.00		
Sandwich, bacon egg	1	Each	177.00	392.87	20.53	27.02	1.13	21.82	6.75	9.16	3.55	417.88	223.26	
Sushi, California roll Hissho Sushi Pioneer Choice	1	Each	198.00	292.00	8.00	49.00	3.00	3.00	1.00			3.00		
Sushi, cucumber imit crab avocado & carrot Hissho Sushi Healthy Choice	1	Each	170.00	260.00	6.00	46.00	2.00	2.00	0.00			1.00		
Sushi, eel roll Hissho Sushi	1	Each	198.00	296.00	11.00	42.00	1.00	5.00	1.00			44.00		
Sushi, roll, Philadelphia Hissho Sushi Pioneer Choice	1	Each	198.00	372.00	9.00	48.00	2.00	12.00	6.00			30.00		
Sushi, salmon roll Hissho Sushi Nippon Favorite	1	Each	170.00	316.00	14.00	42.00	1.00	6.00	1.00			30.00		
Sushi, snow crab roll Hissho Sushi Pioneer Choice	1	Each	198.00	291.00	11.00	45.00	2.00	3.00	1.00			31.00		
Sushi, spicy mix roll Hissho Sushi Tokyo Fantasy	1	Each	198.00	313.00	14.00	43.00	1.00	5.00	1.00			44.00		
Sushi, tuna & salmon roll Hissho Sushi Nippon Favorite	1	Each	170.00	153.00	8.00	21.00	0.00	2.00	0.00			12.00		
Sushi, w/veg & fish	3	Ounce-weight	85.05	118.67	4.57	23.90	0.98	0.35	0.09	0.08	0.11	5.75	35.48	
Sushi, w/veg, rolled in seaweed	3	Ounce-weight	85.05	99.47	1.89	22.21	0.45	0.21	0.06	0.06	0.06	0.00	16.85	
Sushi, w/veg, w/o fish	3	Ounce-weight	85.05	123.03	2.63	27.33	1.14	0.24	0.06	0.06	0.08	0.00	39.05	
Taco, sml	1	Each	171.00	369.36	20.66	26.73		20.55	11.37	6.58	0.96	56.43	107.73	
Tostada, bean & cheese	1	Each	144.00	223.20	9.60	26.52		9.86	5.37	3.05	0.75	30.24	44.64	
Tostada, beef bean & cheese	1	Each	225.00	333.00	16.09	29.66		16.94	11.48	3.51	0.60	74.25	101.25	
Pizza														
Pizza, bagel, cheese & pepperoni, fzn Ore-Ida	2	Piece	22.00	52.50	2.75	6.00	0.75	2.00	0.75			3.75		
Pizza, cheese, fzn Jeno's Crisp 'n Tasty	0.5	Each	97.50	230.00	9.50	26.00	1.00	9.50	3.00			10.00	0.00	
Pizza, combination, fzn Totino's Family Size	0.25	Each	125.00	310.00	11.00	29.00	2.00	17.00	3.50			10.00	0.00	
Pizza, combination, w/sausage & pepperoni, fzn Jeno's Crisp 'n Tasty	0.5	Each	99.00	245.52	8.41	25.84	1.39	12.08	2.85	5.96	1.53	12.87	0.00	
Pizza, combination, w/sausage & pepperoni, fzn Totino's Party Pizza	0.5	Each	152.00	384.56	14.14	36.02		20.37	4.42	10.31	2.48	12.16	0.00	
Pizza, deluxe, 1/4 ea, fzn Celeste	1	Piece	158.00	378.00	15.50	29.30	3.10	22.10				20.00		

Vit E (mg)	Vit C	Vit B₁ Thia (mg)	Vit B₂ Ribo (mg)	Vit B₃ Nia (mg)	Fol (mcg)	Vit B₆ (mg)	Vita B₁₂ (mcg)	Sodi (mg)	Pota (mg)	Cal (mg)	Phos (mg)	Magn (mg)	Iron (mg)	Zinc (mg)	Caff (mg)	Alco (g)	Sol Fiber (g)	Insol Fiber (g)
1.20	1.35	0.09	0.28	8.06	27.52	0.20	2.89	323.18	496.10	36.39	283.81	40.02	2.97	6.63	0.00	0.00		
0.25	8.52	0.16	0.17	1.99	34.08	0.14	0.00	399.45	273.82	32.91	78.19	23.10	1.44	0.66	0.00	0.00		
1.46	8.06	0.29	0.19	3.55	37.54	0.25	0.18	100.55	235.12	20.68	132.68	29.96	1.47	1.30	0.00	0.14		
	0.00	0.25	0.29	2.98		0.09	0.38	1060.92	211.68	88.20	118.44	22.68	2.27	1.13	0.00	0.00		
6.53	15.04	0.67	0.60	8.82	42.42	0.49	2.38	1032.70	750.68	45.14	355.32	62.37	6.48	4.68	0.00	0.00		
1.59	0.50	0.17	0.41	1.19	16.22	0.07	0.43	146.84	171.09	249.14	235.69	20.15	1.46	1.30	0.00	0.00		
2.02	0.63	0.26	0.49	2.01	19.26	0.10	0.61	220.69	239.29	231.09	261.32	23.95	1.88	1.50	0.00	0.00		
1.07	0.94	0.26	0.03	2.49	7.66	0.12	0.01	151.07	110.94	25.47	76.04	19.08	2.34	0.77	0.00	0.00		
2.75	12.50	0.25	0.18	2.25	8.00	0.20	0.00		407.50	80.00	135.00	26.00	2.25	1.30	0.00	0.00		
0.80	2.14	0.16	0.12	1.28	9.92	0.10	0.12	273.51	124.24	15.15	56.83	10.03	0.83	0.46	0.00	0.00		
0.80	2.14	0.16	0.12	1.28	9.92	0.10	0.12	273.51	124.24	15.15	56.83	10.03	0.83	0.46	0.00	0.00		
0.75	4.53	0.13	0.41	3.11	60.78	0.36	1.52	674.65	462.87	62.00	204.38	46.66	3.23	3.60	0.00	0.00		
0.84	14.42	0.53	0.16	3.81	9.91	0.38	0.26	617.95	310.90	28.25	142.48	34.56	1.99	1.46	0.00	0.00		
0.48	0.18	0.23	0.20	5.04	11.36	0.17	0.20	590.31	144.70	25.47	155.39	31.58	2.38	1.67	0.00	0.00		
0.61	2.92	0.23	0.31	13.11	28.69	0.45	0.36	510.90	402.72	42.53	293.10	47.49	2.28	2.54	0.00	0.00		
0.33	17.95	0.17	0.23	1.35	27.91	0.14	0.25	442.65	261.18	163.36	150.07	28.70	1.21	0.81	0.00	0.00		
1.76	39.59	0.24	0.15	2.13	47.57	0.19	0.01	125.53	307.31	43.11	99.22	35.15	1.83	0.83	0.00	0.00		
0.55	0.48	0.26	0.18	1.89	8.41	0.12	0.19	29.61	152.89	13.37	89.36	11.69	1.21	0.97	0.00	0.00		
0.67	8.36	0.14	0.19	2.43	11.48	0.14	0.57	226.31	266.00	156.46	172.90	29.13	1.78	1.92	0.00	0.00		
	4.80							976.00		20.00			1.26		0.00	0.00		
	4.20							951.00		20.00			1.44		0.00	0.00		
	4.80							1,157.00		20.00			1.62		0.00	0.00		
	4.20							1,004.00		20.00			1.26		0.00	0.00		
	3.60							1,092.00		90.00			1.44		0.00	0.00		
1.72	0.23	0.38	0.71	2.93	52.07	0.20	1.11	780.94	276.70	136.82	283.36	28.60	3.08	1.85	0.00	0.00		
	4.80							952.00		20.00			1.08		0.00	0.00		
	5.40							843.00		10.00			0.90		0.00	0.00		
	4.20							775.00		20.00			1.08		0.00	0.00		
	3.60							993.00		40.00			1.44		0.00	0.00		
	4.20							786.00		10.00			0.90		0.00	0.00		
	6.00							911.00		50.00			1.26		0.00	0.00		
	4.20							878.00		30.00			1.44		0.00	0.00		
	1.80							391.00		0.00			0.54		0.00	0.00	0.00	0.00
0.32	2.04	0.14	0.04	1.52	7.85	0.08	0.17	47.60	111.83	12.87	55.84	13.70	1.19	0.43	0.00	0.04		
0.07	1.30	0.11	0.02	1.02	5.50	0.08	0.00	2.50	54.10	11.02	32.61	11.00	0.85	0.38	0.00	0.04		
0.10	2.11	0.15	0.03	1.34	8.14	0.07	0.00	45.26	86.63	12.65	43.01	12.32	1.31	0.46	0.00	0.04		
1.88	2.22	0.15	0.44	3.21	68.40	0.24	1.04	801.99	473.67	220.59	203.49	70.11	2.41	3.93	0.00	0.00		
1.15	1.30	0.10	0.33	1.32	43.20	0.16	0.69	542.88	403.20	210.24	116.64	59.04	1.89	1.90	0.00	0.00		
1.80	4.05	0.09	0.50	2.86	85.50	0.25	1.12	870.75	490.50	189.00	173.25	67.50	2.45	3.17	0.00	0.00		
	2.25							162.50	37.50	25.00			0.36		0.00	0.00		
	0.00							430.00		175.00			0.72		0.00	0.00		
	0.00							720.00		150.00			1.80		0.00	0.00		
								619.74		83.16					0.00	0.00		
	0.00							1041.20		209.76			2.66		0.00	0.00		
3.00									352.00		357.00	38.00		3.00	0.00	0.00		

Food Name	Amount	Measure	Weight (g)	Calories	Protein (g)	Total Carb (g)	Dietary Fiber (g)	Total Fat (g)	Sat Fat (g)	Mono Fat (g)	Poly Fat (g)	Chol (mg)	Vit A (mcg RAE)	Vit D (mcg)
MEALS AND DISHES *(continued)*														
Pizza, deluxe, French bread, fzn Lean Cuisine	1	Each	173.60	290.00	16.00	43.00	3.00	6.00	2.50	2.00	1.00	25.00		
Pizza, deluxe, two cheese sausage pepperoni & onion, fzn 1/5 Red Baron Pizza	1	Piece	129.00	336.69	12.00	31.99		17.80	6.27	6.90	2.27	24.51	0.00	
Pizza, deluxe, w/sausage & pepperoni, French bread, fzn, svg Stouffer's	1	Each	175.00	428.75	16.10	44.45	3.50	20.65	6.37	8.72	2.52	33.25		
Pizza, hamburger, roll, fzn Totino's Pizza Rolls	1	Each	85.00	231.20	9.35	26.44		9.78	2.98	6.80	0.00		0.00	
Pizza, pepperoni & sausage, original, fzn, 1/5 of 12" Tombstone	1	Piece	125.00	327.50	14.38	30.62	2.12	16.38	6.09	5.62	2.30	31.25		
Pizza, pepperoni & sausage, original, fzn, svg Tombstone	1	Each	118.00	317.42	13.33	27.26	1.65	17.23	6.30	5.82	2.41	31.86		
Pizza, pepperoni, deep dish, for one, fzn, Pappalo's	1	Each	199.00	525.36	22.69	64.68	3.18	19.50	7.34	7.26	1.89	37.81	0.00	
Pizza, pepperoni, deep dish, singles, premium, fzn Red Baron Pizza	1	Each	168.00	480.48	15.96	47.88		25.03	8.20	10.77	2.79	28.56	0.00	
Pizza, pepperoni, fzn Jeno's Crisp 'n Tasty	1	Each	192.00	516.48	18.62	45.89	3.07	28.80	6.47	14.53	3.90	23.04	0.00	
Pizza, pepperoni, original, fzn, 1/4 of 12" JK Original	1	Piece	122.00	323.30	15.01	29.52		16.10	6.22	5.23	2.07	40.26		
Pizza, pepperoni, original, fzn, 12" or pce Tombstone	1	Piece	113.00	311.88	14.46	28.25		15.71	6.00	5.31	2.05	31.64		
Pizza, pepperoni, roll, fzn Totino's Pizza Rolls	1	Each	141.00	384.93	14.38	39.48	2.26	18.89	4.99	9.24	2.21	31.02	0.00	
Pizza, pepperoni, w/Italian style pastry crust, fzn Tony's Pizza Service	0.25	Each	104.75	307.97	11.31	27.55		16.97	5.79	6.89	1.96	24.09	0.00	
Pizza, sausage & mushroom, original, fzn, 1/8 of 12" Tombstone	1	Piece	132.00	306.24	14.39	31.15		13.73	5.07	4.44	2.09	26.40		
Pizza, sausage & pepperoni, fzn, 12" or 1/4 pce JK Great Combinations	1	Piece	137.00	347.98	17.40	30.14		17.54	6.60	6.12	2.27	43.84		
Pizza, sausage mushroom, 1/4 ea, fzn Celeste	1	Piece	177.00	387.00	16.90	29.40	1.47	22.40				15.00		
Pizza, sausage, for one, fzn Celeste	1	Each	213.00	571.00	22.60	48.80	4.20	31.70	10.00	7.00	3.00	20.00		
Pizza, sausage, roll, fzn Totino's Pizza Rolls	1	Each	141.00	351.09	14.10	40.18	2.82	14.95	3.45	7.18	2.17	23.97	0.00	
Pizza, supreme, w/sausage mushroom & pepperoni, fzn Red Baron Pizza	0.125	Each	85.75	216.95	8.58	20.07		11.40	3.84	4.52	1.56	14.58	0.00	
Pizza, taco, w/Mexican sausage taco sauce corn crust, fzn Tony's Pizza Service	0.25	Each	116.75	331.57	10.86	32.46		17.63	5.87	6.75	2.64	21.02		
Pizza, vegetable, 1/2 less fat, for one, fzn Tombstone	1	Each	206.00	360.00	21.00	48.00	5.00	9.00	4.00			10.00		
Pizza, vegetable, rising crust, fzn, 12" or 1/6 pce Di Giorno	1	Piece	159.00	310.00	15.00	41.00	3.00	10.00	5.00			20.00		
MEATS														
Beef														
Beef, average of all cuts, ckd, 1/4" trim	3	Ounce-weight	85.05	259.40	22.06	0.00	0.00	18.32	7.26	7.84	0.66	74.84	0.00	
Beef, average of all cuts, ckd, prime, 1/2" trim	3	Ounce-weight	85.05	344.45	19.90	0.00	0.00	28.76	11.92	12.89	1.09	78.25	0.00	
Beef, average of all cuts, lean, ckd, 1/4" trim	3	Ounce-weight	85.05	183.71	25.16	0.00	0.00	8.43	3.22	3.55	0.29	73.14	0.00	
Beef, average of all cuts, lean, ckd, prime, 1/4" trim	3	Ounce-weight	85.05	204.97	24.70	0.00	0.00	11.04	4.42	4.68	0.39	69.74	0.00	
Beef, average of all cuts, lean, ckd, select, 0" trim	3	Ounce-weight	85.05	170.95	25.42	0.00	0.00	6.88	2.63	2.89	0.24	73.14	0.00	
Beef, average of all cuts, lean, raw, choice, 1/4" trim	4	Ounce-weight	113.40	170.10	23.56	0.00	0.00	7.73	2.90	3.27	0.31	66.91	0.00	
Beef, bottom round roast, lean, brsd, 0" trim	3	Ounce-weight	85.05	182.01	28.92	0.00	0.00	6.52	2.28	2.75	0.24	88.45	0.00	
Beef, brisket, corned, cured, ckd	3	Ounce-weight	85.05	213.48	15.45	0.40	0.00	16.14	5.39	7.84	0.57	83.35	0.00	
Beef, chuck arm pot roast, lean, brsd, choice, 1/8" trim	3	Ounce-weight	85.05	190.51	29.53	0.00	0.00	7.12	2.70	3.03	0.25	68.89	0.00	
Beef, chuck blade roast, brsd, 1/4" trim	3	Ounce-weight	85.05	293.42	22.60	0.00	0.00	21.85	8.70	9.44	0.78	88.45	0.00	0.26

Vit E (mg)	Vit C	Vit B₁ Thia (mg)	Vit B₂ Ribo (mg)	Vit B₃ Nia (mg)	Fol (mcg)	Vit B₆ (mg)	Vita B₁₂ (mcg)	Sodi (mg)	Pota (mg)	Cal (mg)	Phos (mg)	Magn (mg)	Iron (mg)	Zinc (mg)	Caff (mg)	Alco (g)	Sol Fiber (g)	Insol Fiber (g)
	6.00							550.00	440.00	150.00			1.80		0.00	0.00		
								704.34		147.06			2.54		0.00	0.00		
	29.93							840.00	159.64	231.00			2.71		0.00	0.00		
		0.00						417.35							0.00	0.00		
								790.00		178.75					0.00	0.00		
								728.06		184.08					0.00	0.00		
								983.06		248.75			3.60		0.00	0.00		
								888.72		152.88			3.46		0.00	0.00		
	0.00							1221.12		203.52			1.44		0.00	0.00		
								612.44		220.82					0.00	0.00		
								551.44		202.27					0.00	0.00		
								865.74		102.93					0.00	0.00		
								632.69		163.41			2.12		0.00	0.00		
								718.08		200.64					0.00	0.00		
								708.29		224.68					0.00	0.00		
3.00									361.00		407.00	45.00		3.00	0.00	0.00		
4.00	0.00	0.30	0.77	2.85	109.00	0.23	2.00	1363.00	456.00	371.00	505.00	60.00	2.28	0.00	0.00	0.00		
								631.68	101.52						0.00	0.00		
								465.62		140.63			1.44		0.00	0.00		
								573.24		142.44			1.93		0.00	0.00		
	1.20							860.00	500.00	350.00			1.80		0.00	0.00		
	3.60							830.00	290.00	250.00			1.06		0.00	0.00		
0.17	0.00	0.07	0.18	3.10	5.95	0.28	2.08	52.73	266.21	8.51	172.65	18.71	2.23	4.98	0.00	0.00	0.00	0.00
0.20	0.00	0.06	0.17	2.77	5.95	0.25	1.96	48.48	228.78	8.51	152.24	16.16	2.08	4.29	0.00	0.00	0.00	0.00
0.12	0.00	0.09	0.20	3.51	6.80	0.31	2.25	56.98	306.18	7.65	198.17	22.11	2.54	5.89	0.00	0.00	0.00	0.00
0.15	0.00	0.09	0.21	4.05	7.65	0.35	2.40	56.98	338.50	6.80	193.06	23.81	2.42	5.67	0.00	0.00	0.00	0.00
0.09	0.00	0.08	0.20	3.40	6.80	0.30	2.25	56.13	301.08	6.80	196.47	22.11	2.54	5.78	0.00	0.00	0.00	0.00
0.15	0.00	0.12	0.20	4.08	7.94	0.50	3.69	71.44	403.70	6.80	225.67	24.95	2.42	4.90	0.00	0.00	0.00	0.00
0.38	0.00	0.07	0.16	5.20	9.36	0.39	1.60	37.42	236.44	5.95	182.01	19.56	2.41	4.95	0.00	0.00	0.00	0.00
0.14	0.00	0.02	0.14	2.58	5.10	0.20	1.39	964.47	123.32	6.80	106.31	10.21	1.58	3.90	0.00	0.00	0.00	0.00
0.39	0.00	0.06	0.20	4.46	10.21	0.29	2.29	47.63	233.89	12.76	181.16	19.56	2.59	6.97	0.00	0.00	0.00	0.00
0.17	0.00	0.06	0.20	2.06	4.25	0.22	1.94	54.43	196.47	11.06	170.10	16.16	2.64	7.08	0.00	0.00	0.00	0.00

Food Name	Amount	Measure	Weight (g)	Calories	Protein (g)	Total Carb (g)	Dietary Fiber (g)	Total Fat (g)	Sat Fat (g)	Mono Fat (g)	Poly Fat (g)	Chol (mg)	Vit A (mcg RAE)	Vit D (mcg)
MEATS (continued)														
Beef, chuck clod roast, lean, rstd, choice, 1/4" trim	3	Ounce-weight	85.05	151.39	22.20	0.00	0.00	6.30	2.02	3.32	0.25	65.49	0.00	
Beef, chuck tender steak, lean, brld, choice, 0" trim	3	Ounce-weight	85.05	136.93	21.89	0.00	0.00	4.84	1.45	2.30	0.34	55.28	0.00	
Beef, chuck, ground, extra lean, raw Maverick Ranch Naturalite	4	Ounce-weight	113.40	130.00	22.00	0.00	0.00	5.00	2.00	2.00	0.50	60.00	0.00	
Beef, corned, cured, cnd, slices, 3/4oz each	3	Ounce-weight	85.05	212.63	23.05	0.00	0.00	12.70	5.26	5.07	0.54	73.14	0.00	
Beef, cube steak, homestyle, fzn, 3oz, FS Travis Meats	3	Ounce-weight	85.05	283.97	13.79	0.00	0.00	25.21	10.28	10.90	0.92	61.88	0.00	
Beef, fajita style, flame brld, fzn, 9974, FS Pierre Foods Lean Magic	3	Ounce-weight	85.05	152.29	18.46	4.15		6.92	2.77					
Beef, flank steak, london broil, lean, brld, 0" trim	3	Ounce-weight	85.05	158.19	23.72	0.00	0.00	6.29	2.61	2.48	0.25	41.67	0.00	
Beef, ground, extra lean, raw Maverick Ranch Naturalite	4	Ounce-weight	113.40	130.00	22.00	0.00	0.00	4.50	1.50	2.00	0.50	60.00	0.00	
Beef, ground, hamburger patty, brld, 10% fat	3	Ounce-weight	85.05	184.56	22.21	0.00	0.00	9.98	3.94	4.21	0.36	72.29	0.00	
Beef, ground, hamburger patty, brld, 15% fat	3	Ounce-weight	85.05	212.63	22.05	0.00	0.00	13.17	5.01	5.67	0.41	76.55	0.00	
Beef, ground, hamburger patty, brld, 20% fat	3	Ounce-weight	85.05	230.49	21.90	0.00	0.00	15.16	5.75	6.72	0.44	77.40	0.00	
Beef, ground, hamburger, bkd, 15% fat	3	Ounce-weight	85.05	204.12	22.05	0.00	0.00	12.21	4.65	5.26	0.38	77.40	0.00	
Beef, ground, hamburger, bkd, 20% fat	3	Ounce-weight	85.05	216.03	21.48	0.00	0.00	13.75	5.92	6.09	0.40	76.55	0.00	
Beef, ground, hamburger, pan browned, 10% fat	3	Ounce-weight	85.05	195.62	24.20	0.00	0.00	10.24	4.06	4.32	0.37	75.69	0.00	
Beef, ground, hamburger, pan browned, 15% fat	3	Ounce-weight	85.05	217.73	23.58	0.00	0.00	13.01	4.93	5.61	0.41	76.55	0.00	
Beef, ground, hamburger, pan browned, 20% fat	3	Ounce-weight	85.05	231.34	22.96	0.00	0.00	14.76	6.36	6.55	0.43	75.69	0.00	
Beef, ground, hamburger, pan browned, 5% fat	3	Ounce-weight	85.05	164.15	24.81	0.00	0.00	6.45	2.93	2.67	0.32	75.69	0.00	
Beef, jerky, lrg pce	1	Each	19.80	81.18	6.57	2.18	0.36	5.07	2.15	2.24	0.20	9.50	0.00	
Beef, jerky, teriyaki, California style Snackmasters	1	Ounce-weight	28.35	81.00	13.16	5.07	0.00	1.01	0.00			20.25	0.00	
Beef, patty, salisbury shape, fzn, 3oz, FS Travis Meats	1	Each	85.00	196.50	14.05	3.00	1.40	14.47	5.88	6.23	0.57	39.42		
Beef, porterhouse steak, brld, select, 1/4" trim	3	Ounce-weight	85.05	264.51	19.96	0.00	0.00	19.84	8.05	8.79	0.85	56.13	0.00	
Beef, rib pot roast, lean, brld, choice, 1/4" trim	3	Ounce-weight	85.05	204.12	21.41	0.00	0.00	12.46	5.09	5.04	0.47	64.64	0.00	
Beef, rib pot roast, rstd, select, 1/8" trim	3	Ounce-weight	85.05	283.22	19.90	0.00	0.00	21.98	8.86	9.41	0.77	71.44	0.00	
Beef, rib steak, lean, brld, select, 1/8" trim	3	Ounce-weight	85.05	159.89	26.25	0.00	0.00	5.29	2.01	2.11	0.19	49.33	0.00	
Beef, ribs, w/bbq sauce	3	Ounce-weight	85.05	147.86	17.98	2.48	0.23	6.75	2.57	2.90	0.34	51.89	8.00	
Beef, roast, lean, rstd	3	Ounce-weight	85.05	168.57	24.11	0.00	0.00	7.27	2.77	3.02	0.23	65.59	0.00	0.26
Beef, roast, rstd	3	Ounce-weight	85.05	226.97	21.91	0.00	0.00	14.81	5.85	6.30	0.53	67.50	0.00	0.26
Beef, round eye roast, lean, raw, select, 1/8" trim	4	Ounce-weight	113.40	134.95	25.30	0.00	0.00	2.97	1.02	1.25	0.13	40.82	0.00	
Beef, round eye roast, lean, rstd, 0" trim	3	Ounce-weight	85.05	137.78	24.95	0.00	0.00	3.48	1.21	1.46	0.13	46.78	0.00	
Beef, round roast, brld, choice, 1/4" trim	3	Ounce-weight	85.05	204.12	23.26	0.00	0.00	11.58	4.39	4.97	0.46	68.04	0.00	
Beef, round tip roast, lean, rstd, choice, 1/4" trim	3	Ounce-weight	85.05	159.89	24.42	0.00	0.00	6.21	2.17	2.47	0.25	68.89	0.00	
Beef, sandwich steak, formed & thinly sliced, raw, 14oz pkg	4	Ounce-weight	113.40	350.41	18.71	0.00	0.00	30.62	13.08	12.51	0.55	80.51	0.00	
Beef, sirloin strip steak, brld, 1/8" trim	3	Ounce-weight	85.05	224.53	22.49	0.00	0.00	14.27	5.62	5.95	0.53	74.84	0.00	
Beef, sirloin strip steak, lean, brld, choice, 1/8" trim	3	Ounce-weight	85.05	170.95	24.80	0.00	0.00	7.19	2.74	2.87	0.26	67.19	0.00	
Beef, snack stick, smkd	1	Each	19.80	108.90	4.26	1.07		9.82	4.12	4.05	0.88	26.33	2.57	
Beef, steak, country fried, fzn, 1965, FS Pierre Foods	3	Ounce-weight	85.05	319.50	15.00	12.15		23.25	6.60			47.46		
Beef, taco filling, fzn Ortega	0.33	Cup	55.28	100.00	7.00	4.00	1.00	6.00	2.50			20.00		
Beef, T-bone steak, brld, choice, 1/4" trim	3	Ounce-weight	85.05	273.86	19.38	0.00	0.00	21.22	8.29	9.59	0.75	57.83	0.00	
Beef, tenderloin, filet mignon, brld, choice, 1/8" trim	3	Ounce-weight	85.05	232.19	22.48	0.00	0.00	15.12	5.95	6.30	0.56	79.10	0.00	

Vit E (mg)	Vit C	Vit B$_1$ Thia (mg)	Vit B$_2$ Ribo (mg)	Vit B$_3$ Nia (mg)	Fol (mcg)	Vit B$_6$ (mg)	Vita B$_{12}$ (mcg)	Sodi (mg)	Pota (mg)	Cal (mg)	Phos (mg)	Magn (mg)	Iron (mg)	Zinc (mg)	Caff (mg)	Alco (g)	Sol Fiber (g)	Insol Fiber (g)
0.14	0.00	0.07	0.21	2.92	7.65	0.23	2.54	60.39	313.83	5.95	181.16	18.71	2.60	5.43	0.00	0.00	0.00	0.00
0.14	0.00	0.09	0.19	3.07	6.80	0.27	2.87	62.09	249.20	6.80	199.02	19.56	2.57	6.66	0.00	0.00	0.00	0.00
	0.00			5.00			2.40	65.00		0.00			1.80	4.50	0.00	0.00	0.00	0.00
0.13	0.00	0.02	0.13	2.07	7.65	0.11	1.38	855.60	115.67	10.21	94.41	11.91	1.77	3.04	0.00	0.00	0.00	0.00
	0.00	0.07	0.12	2.35				42.53	210.12	6.30	126.97		1.44	2.62	0.00	0.00	0.00	0.00
	0.23							405.18		29.53			2.49		0.00	0.00		
0.32	0.00	0.06	0.12	6.79	7.65	0.51	1.36	48.48	297.68	15.31	184.56	19.56	1.48	4.33	0.00	0.00	0.00	0.00
	0.00			5.00			2.70	65.00		0.00			1.80	4.50	0.00	0.00	0.00	0.00
0.35	0.00	0.04	0.15	4.81	6.80	0.34	2.18	57.83	283.22	11.06	171.80	18.71	2.30	5.42	0.00	0.00	0.00	0.00
0.38	0.00	0.04	0.15	4.57	7.65	0.32	2.25	61.24	270.46	15.31	168.40	17.86	2.21	5.37	0.00	0.00	0.00	0.00
0.40	0.00	0.04	0.15	4.34	8.51	0.31	2.32	63.79	258.55	20.41	165.00	17.01	2.11	5.32	0.00	0.00	0.00	0.00
0.37	0.00	0.03	0.15	4.19	5.10	0.29	2.12	54.43	243.24	15.31	158.19	17.01	2.33	5.49	0.00	0.00	0.00	0.00
0.38	0.00	0.04	0.14	3.94	5.95	0.28	2.11	56.98	230.49	19.56	152.24	16.16	2.19	5.31	0.00	0.00	0.00	0.00
0.37	0.00	0.04	0.16	5.79	6.80	0.36	2.30	73.99	368.27	13.61	212.63	22.96	2.62	5.82	0.00	0.00	0.00	0.00
0.40	0.00	0.04	0.16	5.37	8.51	0.36	2.37	75.69	346.15	18.71	202.42	21.26	2.49	5.63	0.00	0.00	0.00	0.00
0.41	0.00	0.04	0.16	4.96	9.36	0.36	2.43	77.40	323.19	23.81	192.21	19.56	2.36	5.44	0.00	0.00	0.00	0.00
0.34	0.00	0.04	0.17	6.20	5.95	0.36	2.25	72.29	390.38	7.65	223.68	23.81	2.75	6.00	0.00	0.00	0.00	0.00
0.10	0.00	0.03	0.03	0.34	26.53	0.03	0.20	438.17	118.21	3.96	80.59	10.10	1.08	1.60	0.00	0.00		
	0.00							648.00		0.00			1.82		0.00	0.00	0.00	0.00
	1.20	0.19	0.14	3.12				224.50	333.60	33.00	148.30		1.98	4.58	0.00	0.00		
0.18	0.00	0.08	0.18	3.35	5.95	0.29	1.80	53.58	221.13	6.80	153.94	17.01	2.33	3.60	0.00	0.00	0.00	0.00
0.18	0.00	0.07	0.16	2.70	5.95	0.22	2.82	61.24	316.39	7.65	184.56	19.56	2.19	5.34	0.00	0.00	0.00	0.00
0.19	0.00	0.06	0.16	3.18	6.80	0.20	2.02	55.28	254.30	7.65	149.69	17.01	2.03	5.09	0.00	0.00	0.00	0.00
0.34	0.00	0.07	0.14	7.67	8.51	0.58	1.25	56.13	347.85	18.71	215.18	22.96	1.62	4.84	0.00	0.00	0.00	0.00
0.31	1.29	0.05	0.13	2.62	5.80	0.20	2.19	204.45	295.12	11.56	149.69	19.91	2.09	4.12	0.00	0.00		
0.12	0.00	0.08	0.19	3.42	6.86	0.29	2.17	57.07	321.29	5.23	190.65	22.31	2.19	5.50	0.00	0.00	0.00	0.00
0.16	0.00	0.07	0.17	3.07	6.06	0.27	2.04	53.43	289.67	6.18	172.55	19.64	1.98	4.79	0.00	0.00	0.00	0.00
0.32	0.00	0.10	0.16	7.53	14.74	0.74	1.47	70.31	412.78	24.95	248.35	28.35	2.18	5.06	0.00	0.00	0.00	0.00
0.31	0.00	0.06	0.14	4.48	8.51	0.33	1.38	32.32	203.27	5.10	156.49	16.16	2.08	4.26	0.00	0.00	0.00	0.00
0.16	0.00	0.08	0.18	3.39	7.65	0.32	2.56	51.88	333.40	5.10	202.42	21.26	2.15	3.67	0.00	0.00	0.00	0.00
0.12	0.00	0.09	0.23	3.18	6.80	0.34	2.46	55.28	328.29	4.25	205.82	22.96	2.50	6.01	0.00	0.00	0.00	0.00
0.24	0.00	0.04	0.18	5.20	7.94	0.28	3.08	77.11	264.22	13.61	150.82	18.14	2.11	4.11	0.00	0.00	0.00	0.00
0.39	0.00	0.06	0.11	5.98	6.80	0.47	1.33	45.93	278.96	16.16	173.50	18.71	1.44	4.04	0.00	0.00	0.00	0.00
0.35	0.00	0.07	0.13	7.32	8.51	0.52	1.55	51.03	307.88	13.61	192.21	21.26	1.68	4.65	0.00	0.00	0.00	0.00
0.06	1.35	0.03	0.09	0.90	0.00	0.04	0.20	293.04	50.89	13.46	35.64	4.16	0.67	0.48	0.00	0.00		
	0.02							320.85	177.45	13.95			2.31		0.00	0.00		
	1.20							290.00		40.00			0.72		0.00	0.00		
0.19	0.00	0.08	0.18	3.29	5.95	0.28	1.79	57.83	233.89	6.80	153.94	17.86	2.56	3.56	0.00	0.00	0.00	0.00
0.40	0.00	0.06	0.10	6.10	6.80	0.45	1.48	44.23	270.46	14.46	166.70	17.86	1.50	3.97	0.00	0.00	0.00	0.00

Food Name	Amount	Measure	Weight (g)	Calories	Protein (g)	Total Carb (g)	Dietary Fiber (g)	Total Fat (g)	Sat Fat (g)	Mono Fat (g)	Poly Fat (g)	Chol (mg)	Vit A (mcg RAE)	Vit D (mcg)
MEATS *(continued)*														
Beef, tenderloin, filet mignon, lean, rstd, 1/4" trim	3	Ounce-weight	85.05	188.81	23.57	0.00	0.00	9.76	3.68	3.81	0.44	70.59	0.00	
Beef, tenderloin, filet mignon, raw, choice, 1/8" trim	4	Ounce-weight	113.40	278.96	22.48	0.00	0.00	20.28	8.18	8.68	0.77	73.71	0.00	
Beef, top round steak, brld, choice, 1/8" trim	3	Ounce-weight	85.05	190.51	26.11	0.00	0.00	8.73	3.32	3.72	0.34	56.13	0.00	
Beef, top sirloin steak, lean, brld, choice, 1/8" trim	3	Ounce-weight	85.05	159.04	25.10	0.00	0.00	5.72	2.18	2.28	0.20	53.58	0.00	
Beef, tri-tip roast, loin, lean, rstd, 0" trim	3	Ounce-weight	85.05	154.79	22.75	0.00	0.00	7.09	2.64	3.58	0.23	60.39	0.00	
Beef, whole rib, rstd, select, 1/8" trim	3	Ounce-weight	85.05	280.67	19.65	0.00	0.00	21.80	8.78	9.36	0.77	71.44	0.00	
Game Meats														
Buffalo, burger/patty, extra lean, raw Maverick Ranch	4	Ounce-weight	113.40	140.00	24.00	0.00	0.00	4.00	1.50			55.00	0.00	
Deer, ground, pan brld	3	Ounce-weight	85.05	159.04	22.50	0.00	0.00	6.99	3.40	1.65	0.38	83.35	0.00	
Deer, top round steak, lean, 1" thick, brld	3	Ounce-weight	85.05	129.28	26.77	0.00	0.00	1.63	0.88	0.35	0.10	72.29	0.00	
Elk, rstd	3	Ounce-weight	85.05	124.17	25.68	0.00	0.00	1.62	0.60	0.41	0.34	62.09	0.00	
Rabbit, stewed, domestic	3	Ounce-weight	85.05	175.20	25.84	0.00	0.00	7.15	2.13	1.93	1.39	73.14	0.00	
Venison, rstd USDA SR-23	3	Ounce-weight	85.05	134.38	25.69	0.00	0.00	2.71	1.06	0.75	0.53	95.26	0.00	
Goat														
Lamb														
Lamb, average of all cuts, lean, raw, choice, 1/4" trim	4	Ounce-weight	113.40	151.96	23.01	0.00	0.00	5.95	2.13	2.39	0.54	73.71	0.00	
Lamb, average of all cuts, raw, choice, 1/4" trim	4	Ounce-weight	113.40	302.78	19.14	0.00	0.00	24.48	10.74	10.05	1.93	81.65	0.00	
Lamb, average of all cuts, raw, choice, 1/8" trim	4	Ounce-weight	113.40	275.56	19.89	0.00	0.00	21.16	9.15	8.68	1.68	79.38	0.00	
Lunchmeats and Sausages														
Frank, beef Oscar Mayer	1	Each	45.00	147.15	5.11	1.06	0.00	13.62	5.61	6.63	0.61	25.20	0.00	0.27
Frank, beef, fat free Oscar Mayer	1	Each	50.00	39.00	6.60	2.55	0.00	0.25	0.11	0.10	0.02	15.00	0.00	
Frank, turkey & chicken Louis Rich	1	Each	45.00	84.60	5.04	2.38	0.00	6.07	1.73	2.50	1.42	41.40	0.00	
Frank, turkey chicken & cheese, svg Louis Rich	1	Each	45.00	90.45	5.71	2.29	0.00	6.52	2.34	2.80	1.34	42.30	0.00	0.00
Frankfurter, beef, 10 per lb, 5" × 3/4"	1	Each	45.00	148.50	5.06	1.83	0.00	13.31	5.26	6.44	0.53	23.85	0.00	0.40
Frankfurter, cheese, w/pork & beef, smokies	1	Each	43.00	140.61	6.06	0.65	0.00	12.47	4.52	5.89	1.30	29.24	20.21	0.12
Frankfurter, chicken	1	Each	45.00	115.65	5.82	3.06	0.00	8.77	2.49	3.82	1.82	45.45	17.55	0.00
Frankfurter, turkey	1	Each	45.00	101.70	6.43	0.67	0.00	7.96	2.65	2.51	2.25	48.15	0.00	
Hot Dog, beef, bunsize Ball Park	1	Each	56.00	180.00	6.00	3.00	0.00	16.00	7.00			35.00	0.00	
Hot Dog, fat free Oscar Mayer	1	Each	50.00	36.50	6.30	2.15	0.00	0.30	0.10	0.10	0.06	14.50	0.00	
Hot Dog, pork & turkey, Little Wieners Oscar Mayer	6	Each	54.00	167.94	5.89	1.24	0.00	15.50	6.02	7.74	1.44	29.70	0.00	0.71
Hot Dog, pork turkey beef, light Oscar Mayer	1	Each	57.00	110.58	6.90	1.60	0.00	8.49	2.96	3.85	1.17	35.34	0.00	
Lunchmeat Loaf, beef, slice, 4" × 4" × 3/32"	1	Piece	28.35	87.32	4.08	0.82	0.00	7.43	3.17	3.46	0.24	18.14	0.00	
Lunchmeat Loaf, corned beef, jellied, slice, 4" × 4" × 3/32"	1	Piece	28.35	43.38	6.49	0.00	0.00	1.73	0.74	0.76	0.09	13.32	0.00	
Lunchmeat Loaf, ham & cheese Oscar Mayer	1	Ounce-weight	28.35	66.34	3.93	1.06	0.00	5.16	1.86	2.35	0.51	17.58	0.00	0.29
Lunchmeat Loaf, ham & cheese, slice, 4" × 4" × 3/32"	1	Piece	28.35	68.32	3.86	1.14	0.00	5.30	1.98	2.44	0.57	16.44	0.00	0.31
Lunchmeat Loaf, honey, w/pork & beef, slice, 4" × 4" × 3/32"	1	Piece	28.35	35.44	4.47	1.51	0.00	1.26	0.40	0.57	0.13	9.64	0.00	0.26
Lunchmeat Loaf, luxury, w/pork, slice, 4" × 4" × 3/32"	1	Piece	28.35	39.98	5.22	1.39	0.00	1.36	0.45	0.66	0.14	10.20	0.00	0.20
Lunchmeat Loaf, olive, w/chicken pork & turkey Oscar Mayer	1	Ounce-weight	28.35	74.56	2.80	1.95	0.00	6.18	1.99	3.16	0.75	20.13	0.00	
Lunchmeat Loaf, peppered, w/pork & beef, slice, 4" × 4" × 3/32"	1	Piece	28.35	41.96	4.90	1.30	0.00	1.81	0.65	0.85	0.14	13.04	0.00	0.23
Lunchmeat Loaf, pickle pimiento, w/chicken Oscar Mayer	1	Ounce-weight	28.35	76.26	2.72	2.58	0.00	6.13	1.98	2.96	0.80	22.68	0.00	

Vit E (mg)	Vit C	Vit B$_1$ Thia (mg)	Vit B$_2$ Ribo (mg)	Vit B$_3$ Nia (mg)	Fol (mcg)	Vit B$_6$ (mg)	Vita B$_{12}$ (mcg)	Sodi (mg)	Pota (mg)	Cal (mg)	Phos (mg)	Magn (mg)	Iron (mg)	Zinc (mg)	Caff (mg)	Alco (g)	Sol Fiber (g)	Insol Fiber (g)
0.13	0.00	0.09	0.26	2.90	7.65	0.25	2.30	51.88	332.55	5.95	203.27	22.96	3.14	4.07	0.00	0.00	0.00	0.00
0.46	0.00	0.06	0.10	7.25	12.47	0.61	1.25	56.70	343.60	28.35	200.72	22.68	1.62	3.97	0.00	0.00	0.00	0.00
0.37	0.00	0.05	0.15	4.72	8.51	0.34	1.56	34.02	210.92	5.95	159.04	17.01	2.16	4.33	0.00	0.00	0.00	0.00
0.33	0.00	0.06	0.11	6.61	7.65	0.47	1.39	51.88	313.83	14.46	196.47	21.26	1.71	4.75	0.00	0.00	0.00	0.00
0.32	0.00	0.06	0.12	6.51	7.65	0.49	1.30	46.78	289.17	14.46	179.46	19.56	1.44	4.19	0.00	0.00	0.00	0.00
0.19	0.00	0.06	0.15	2.99	5.95	0.20	2.19	55.28	263.66	9.36	153.09	17.01	2.05	4.74	0.00	0.00	0.00	0.00
	0.00							50.00		0.00			2.70	3.75	0.00	0.00	0.00	0.00
0.58	0.00	0.43	0.28	7.87	6.80	0.40	1.97	66.34	309.58	11.91	193.91	20.41	2.85	4.42	0.00	0.00	0.00	0.00
0.54	0.00	0.21	0.43	7.14	8.51	0.60	1.93	38.27	320.64	3.40	231.34	25.52	3.60	3.12	0.00	0.00	0.00	0.00
0.02	0.00				7.65		5.53	51.88	278.96	4.25	153.09	20.41	3.09	2.69	0.00	0.00	0.00	0.00
0.37	0.00	0.05	0.14	6.09	7.65	0.29	5.54	31.47	255.15	17.01	192.21	17.01	2.02	2.02	0.00	0.00	0.00	0.00
	0.00	0.15	0.51	5.71				45.93	284.92	5.95	192.21	20.41	3.80	2.34	0.00	0.00	0.00	0.00
0.24	0.00	0.15	0.26	6.80	26.08	0.18	2.97	74.84	317.52	11.34	214.33	29.48	2.01	4.60	0.00	0.00	0.00	0.00
0.24	0.00	0.14	0.25	6.92	20.41	0.15	2.71	65.77	260.82	13.61	181.44	24.95	1.78	3.78	0.00	0.00	0.00	0.00
0.24	0.00	0.14	0.25	6.88	21.55	0.16	2.77	66.91	271.03	13.61	188.24	24.95	1.84	3.99	0.00	0.00	0.00	0.00
	0.00	0.02	0.04	1.03	2.70	0.03	0.73	461.25	58.50	4.50	63.00	5.85	0.60	0.99	0.00	0.00	0.00	0.00
	0.00							463.50	233.50	10.00	64.50	9.50	0.98	1.20	0.00	0.00	0.00	0.00
	0.00							511.20	72.00	58.95	66.15	10.35	0.98	0.84	0.00	0.00	0.00	0.00
	0.00							481.50	71.10	109.35	91.80	9.90	0.95	0.81	0.00	0.81	0.00	0.00
0.09	0.00	0.02	0.07	1.07	2.25	0.04	0.77	513.00	70.20	6.30	72.00	6.30	0.68	1.11	0.00	0.00	0.00	0.00
0.00	0.00	0.11	0.07	1.25	1.29	0.06	0.74	465.26	88.58	24.94	76.54	5.59	0.46	0.97	0.00	0.00	0.00	0.00
0.10	0.00	0.03	0.05	1.39	1.80	0.14	0.11	616.50	37.80	42.75	48.15	4.50	0.90	0.47	0.00	0.00	0.00	0.00
0.28	0.00	0.02	0.08	1.86	3.60	0.10	0.13	641.70	80.55	47.70	60.30	6.30	0.83	1.40	0.00	0.00	0.00	0.00
	3.60							620.00	460.00	0.00			0.72		0.00	0.00	0.00	0.00
	0.00							487.00	235.50	7.50	81.00	10.50	0.46	0.60	0.00	0.00	0.00	0.00
	0.00	0.14	0.09	1.44	1.10	0.07	0.68	561.06	85.86	7.02	52.38	7.02	0.55	0.99	0.00	0.00	0.00	0.00
	0.00							590.52	226.29	21.66	96.33	9.69	0.73	1.01	0.00	0.00	0.00	0.00
0.06	0.00	0.03	0.06	1.04	1.42	0.06	1.10	376.77	58.97	3.12	33.74	3.97	0.66	0.72	0.00	0.00	0.00	0.00
0.05	0.00	0.00	0.03	0.50	2.27	0.03	0.36	270.18	28.63	3.12	20.70	3.12	0.58	1.16	0.00	0.00	0.00	0.00
0.00	0.00	0.16	0.05	0.98	0.85	0.07	0.21	330.84	75.13	18.99	76.55	5.39	0.24	0.52	0.00	0.00	0.00	0.00
0.08	0.00	0.17	0.06	0.98	0.85	0.08	0.23	306.18	83.35	16.44	71.72	4.54	0.26	0.56	0.00	0.00	0.00	0.00
0.06	0.00	0.14	0.07	0.89	2.27	0.10	0.30	374.22	97.24	4.82	40.54	4.82	0.38	0.68	0.00	0.00	0.00	0.00
0.06	0.00	0.20	0.08	0.98	0.56	0.09	0.39	347.29	106.88	10.20	52.45	5.67	0.30	0.86	0.00	0.00	0.00	0.00
	0.00							373.65	52.73	31.47	37.42	7.65	0.50	0.29	0.00	0.00	0.00	0.00
0.06	0.00	0.11	0.09	0.87	0.57	0.08	0.56	431.77	111.70	15.31	48.20	5.67	0.30	0.92	0.00	0.00	0.00	0.00
	0.00							361.46	49.33	31.19	42.53	8.22	0.62	0.33	0.00	0.00	0.00	0.00

Food Name	Amount	Measure	Weight (g)	Calories	Protein (g)	Total Carb (g)	Dietary Fiber (g)	Total Fat (g)	Sat Fat (g)	Mono Fat (g)	Poly Fat (g)	Chol (mg)	Vit A (mcg RAE)	Vit D (mcg)
MEATS *(continued)*														
Lunchmeat Loaf, pickle pimiento, w/pork, slice, 4" × 4" × 3/32"	1	Piece	28.35	63.79	3.18	2.40	0.17	4.52	1.50	2.00	0.80	16.44	25.80	0.31
Lunchmeat Loaf, pork & beef, Dutch brand, slice, 4" × 4" × 3/32"	1	Piece	28.35	77.40	3.40	1.11	0.06	6.49	2.58	2.86	0.87	17.01	13.32	0.28
Lunchmeat Loaf, spiced Oscar Mayer	1	Ounce-weight	28.35	66.34	3.83	1.98	0.00	4.79	1.52	2.10	0.79	18.99	0.00	
Lunchmeat Loaf, turkey, light meat, slice	1	Ounce-weight	28.35	41.67	5.30	0.15	0.00	2.05	0.57	0.71	0.49	12.19	0.00	
Lunchmeat Spread, chicken salad, rts, cnd Libby's Spreadables	1	Ounce-weight	28.35	41.11	1.39	2.87		2.66	0.55	0.83	1.02	7.37	0.00	
Lunchmeat Spread, chicken, cnd	2	Tablespoon	26.00	41.08	4.68	1.05	0.08	4.57	0.84	1.25	0.61	14.56	7.80	
Lunchmeat Spread, ham & cheese	2	Tablespoon	30.00	73.50	4.85	0.68	0.00	5.56	2.59	2.12	0.41	18.30	27.30	
Lunchmeat Spread, pork & beef	2	Tablespoon	30.00	70.50	2.30	3.58	0.06	5.20	1.79	2.29	0.77	11.40	7.80	
Lunchmeat Spread, pork chicken & beef, svg Oscar Mayer	1	Ounce-weight	28.35	67.19	1.85	4.37	0.09	4.71	1.63	2.04	0.71	12.76		
Lunchmeat Spread, poultry salad	2	Tablespoon	26.00	52.00	3.03	1.93	0.00	3.52	0.90	0.85	1.62	7.80	10.92	
Lunchmeat Spread, tuna salad	0.5	Cup	127.00	237.49	20.37	11.96	0.00	11.75	1.96	3.67	5.24	16.51	30.48	
Lunchmeat, beef, thin slice	1	Ounce-weight	28.35	42.24	5.42	0.25	0.00	2.02	0.83	0.88	0.10	19.84	0.00	
Lunchmeat, bologna, beef & pork, 4" × 1/8" slice	1	Piece	23.00	70.84	3.50	1.26	0.00	5.65	2.14	2.42	0.26	13.80	5.75	0.18
Lunchmeat, bologna, beef, 4" × 1/8" slice	1	Piece	32.00	100.48	3.29	1.27	0.00	9.02	3.56	3.91	0.25	17.92	4.16	
Lunchmeat, bologna, beef, light Oscar Mayer	1	Ounce-weight	28.35	56.70	3.33	1.59	0.00	4.11	1.65	2.03	0.13	12.47	0.00	
Lunchmeat, bologna, beef Oscar Mayer	1	Ounce-weight	28.35	89.59	3.13	0.70	0.00	8.25	3.63	4.30	0.31	18.14	0.00	0.23
Lunchmeat, bologna, pork, 4" × 1/8" slice	1	Piece	23.00	56.81	3.52	0.17	0.00	4.57	1.58	2.25	0.49	13.57	0.00	0.32
Lunchmeat, bologna, ring, Wisconsin made, svg Oscar Mayer	1	Ounce-weight	28.35	88.74	3.35	0.74	0.00	8.05	3.16	3.99	0.56	17.58	0.00	0.28
Lunchmeat, bologna, turkey	1	Ounce-weight	28.35	59.25	3.24	1.32	0.14	4.55	1.24	1.94	1.10	21.26	2.55	0.00
Lunchmeat, bologna, turkey Louis Rich	1	Ounce-weight	28.35	52.16	3.21	1.38	0.00	3.74	1.07	1.51	1.02	18.99	0.00	
Lunchmeat, chicken breast, classic, bkd/grilled Louis Rich	1	Ounce-weight	28.35	27.78	5.58	1.05	0.00	0.14	0.04	0.05	0.03	14.74	0.00	
Lunchmeat, chicken breast, honey glazed, slice Oscar Mayer	1	Ounce-weight	28.35	30.90	5.63	1.11	0.00	0.43	0.11	0.16	0.06	15.03	0.00	
Lunchmeat, chicken breast, oven rstd, deluxe Louis Rich	1	Ounce-weight	28.35	28.63	5.19	0.71	0.00	0.57	0.15	0.23	0.09	13.89	0.00	
Lunchmeat, chicken breast, oven rstd, fat free, slice Oscar Mayer	1	Ounce-weight	28.35	24.10	5.19	0.48	0.00	0.17	0.05	0.04	0.02	12.47	0.00	
Lunchmeat, chicken breast, oven rstd, resealable Healthy Choice	1	Ounce-weight	28.35	35.44	5.06	1.01	0.00	1.01	0.51			15.19	0.00	
Lunchmeat, chicken, light & dark meat, smkd, sliced, pkg Carl Buddig & Company	1	Ounce-weight	28.35	46.78	5.07	0.20	0.00	2.86	0.74	1.53	0.60	15.03		
Lunchmeat, chicken, white, oven rstd Louis Rich	1	Ounce-weight	28.35	36.29	4.82	0.65	0.00	1.59	0.41	0.66	0.28	16.73	0.00	
Lunchmeat, ham, chpd, w/natural juices Oscar Mayer	1	Ounce-weight	28.35	51.03	4.62	1.04	0.00	3.16	1.15	1.65	0.36	16.73	0.00	
Lunchmeat, ham, reg, 11% fat, sliced, 6 1/4" × 4" × 1/16"	1	Piece	28.35	46.21	4.71	1.09	0.37	2.44	0.83	1.23	0.22	16.16	0.00	0.00
Lunchmeat, ham, smkd, 40% water add, fat free, slice	1	Ounce-weight	28.35	20.41	4.14	0.54	0.00	0.20	0.06	0.08	0.04	10.77	0.00	
Lunchmeat, ham, smkd, ckd, w/water add, slice Oscar Mayer	1	Ounce-weight	28.35	28.07	4.71	0.03	0.00	1.02	0.35	0.47	0.10	13.61	0.00	
Lunchmeat, olive, w/pork, slice, 4" × 4" × 3/32"	1	Piece	28.35	66.62	3.34	2.61	0.00	4.68	1.66	2.23	0.55	10.78	17.01	0.31
Lunchmeat, pork, cnd, slice, 4.25" × 4.25" × 1/16"	1	Piece	21.00	70.14	2.63	0.44	0.00	6.36	2.26	3.00	0.75	13.02	0.00	
Lunchmeat, turkey breast & white meat, oven rstd Louis Rich	1	Ounce-weight	28.35	28.07	4.85	0.92	0.00	0.57	0.13	0.16	0.12	11.62	0.00	
Lunchmeat, turkey breast, oven rstd, fat free, slice Louis Rich	1	Ounce-weight	28.35	23.81	4.25	1.28	0.00	0.20	0.06	0.06	0.04	9.07	0.00	
Lunchmeat, turkey breast, oven rstd, fat free Louis Rich	1	Ounce-weight	28.35	25.52	5.42	0.54	0.00	0.20	0.06	0.06	0.04	11.34	0.00	
Lunchmeat, turkey breast, smkd, fat free, slice Oscar Mayer	1	Ounce-weight	28.35	22.68	4.23	1.02	0.00	0.17	0.05	0.04	0.03	8.79	0.00	

Vit E (mg)	Vit C	Vit B$_1$ Thia (mg)	Vit B$_2$ Ribo (mg)	Vit B$_3$ Nia (mg)	Fol (mcg)	Vit B$_6$ (mg)	Vita B$_{12}$ (mcg)	Sodi (mg)	Pota (mg)	Cal (mg)	Phos (mg)	Magn (mg)	Iron (mg)	Zinc (mg)	Caff (mg)	Alco (g)	Sol Fiber (g)	Insol Fiber (g)
0.12	2.21	0.14	0.04	0.97	4.54	0.09	0.22	369.68	89.58	30.90	40.54	5.96	0.38	0.54	0.00	0.00		
0.01	0.43	0.06	0.04	0.91	3.40	0.09	0.45	299.09	61.24	1.98	36.85	4.54	0.05	0.58	0.00	0.00		
	0.00							347.57	76.54	30.90	55.28	6.80	0.38	0.55	0.00	0.00	0.00	0.00
0.04	0.00	0.03	0.06	1.98	1.13	0.09	0.07	138.63	71.16	11.34	51.88	4.54	0.36	0.44	0.00	0.00	0.00	0.00
								132.68							0.00	0.00		
0.09	0.00	0.00	0.03	0.71	0.78	0.04	0.03	187.72	27.56	4.16	23.14	3.12	0.23	0.30	0.00	0.00		
	0.00	0.09	0.07	0.64	0.90	0.04	0.22	359.10	48.60	65.10	148.50	5.40	0.23	0.68	0.00	0.00	0.00	0.00
0.52	0.00	0.05	0.04	0.52	0.60	0.04	0.34	303.90	33.00	3.60	17.70	2.40	0.23	0.31	0.00	0.00		
	0.00							232.75	33.45	7.65	19.56	3.40	0.23	0.25	0.00	0.00		
0.57	0.26	0.00	0.02	0.43	1.30	0.03	0.10	98.02	47.58	2.60	8.58	2.60	0.16	0.27	0.00	0.00	0.00	0.00
1.20	2.79	0.05	0.09	8.52	10.16	0.09	1.52	510.54	226.06	21.59	226.06	24.13	1.27	0.72	0.00	0.00	0.00	0.00
0.05	0.00	0.02	0.05	1.21	3.12	0.10	0.73	400.59	121.62	3.12	47.63	5.39	0.59	1.13	0.00	0.00	0.00	0.00
0.00	0.18	0.05	0.04	0.58	1.38	0.07	0.42	169.28	72.45	19.55	37.49	3.91	0.28	0.53	0.00	0.00	0.00	0.00
0.11	4.86	0.01	0.03	0.80	2.88	0.05	0.41	345.60	55.04	9.92	55.04	4.48	0.35	2.91	0.00	0.00	0.00	0.00
	0.00				3.69			326.31	44.23	3.69	50.46	3.97	0.35	0.54	0.00	0.00	0.00	0.00
	0.00	0.02	0.03	0.69	3.69	0.05	0.41	334.25	47.63	3.40	30.90	3.97	0.39	0.58	0.00	0.00	0.00	0.00
0.06	0.00	0.12	0.04	0.90	1.15	0.06	0.21	272.32	64.63	2.53	31.97	3.22	0.18	0.47	0.00	0.00	0.00	0.00
	0.00	0.08	0.04	0.75		0.04	0.36	234.45	39.41	4.25	30.05	4.25	0.33	0.53	0.00	0.00	0.00	0.00
0.13	3.77	0.02	0.02	0.74	2.55	0.07	0.06	354.94	38.28	34.87	32.32	4.54	0.85	0.37	0.00	0.00		
	0.00				1.70			305.33	43.09	35.15	55.57	6.24	0.46	0.53	0.00	0.00	0.00	0.00
	0.00							323.76	82.50	2.27	79.95	9.07	0.37	0.25	0.00	0.00	0.00	0.00
	0.00				1.13			407.67	93.27	2.83	81.93	10.21	0.32	0.20	0.00	0.00	0.00	0.00
	0.00							336.80	75.13	1.98	75.41	6.80	0.32	0.21	0.00	0.00	0.00	0.00
	0.00							352.11	89.59	3.40	72.58	10.21	0.38	0.17	0.00	0.00	0.00	0.00
	0.00							243.00		0.00			0.00		0.00	0.00	0.00	0.00
		0.02	0.07	1.91				270.46	72.58	35.15			0.44		0.00	0.00	0.00	0.00
	0.00							339.07	85.62	4.82	70.31	6.80	0.45	0.32	0.00	0.00	0.00	0.00
	0.00				0.85			354.09	73.71	2.55	62.09	6.52	0.37	0.64	0.00	0.00	0.00	0.00
0.02	1.13	0.18	0.05	0.82	1.98	0.09	0.12	369.68	81.36	6.80	43.38	6.24	0.29	0.38	0.00	0.00		
	0.00							307.31	66.34	3.12	55.85	7.65	0.26	0.44	0.00	0.00	0.00	0.00
	0.00							344.17	75.98	2.84	66.06	8.79	0.37	0.51	0.00	0.00	0.00	0.00
0.07	0.00	0.08	0.08	0.52	0.56	0.06	0.36	420.72	84.20	30.90	36.01	5.38	0.16	0.39	0.00	0.00	0.00	0.00
0.05	0.21	0.08	0.04	0.66	1.26	0.05	0.19	270.69	45.15	1.26	17.22	2.10	0.15	0.31	0.00	0.00	0.00	0.00
	0.00				1.70			273.86	62.94	1.70	71.16	6.24	0.28	0.27	0.00	0.00	0.00	0.00
	0.00							337.93	58.12	3.12	65.77	7.65	0.31	0.24	0.00	0.00	0.00	0.00
	0.00							333.68	75.98	4.82	80.80	8.22	0.31	0.27	0.00	0.00	0.00	0.00
	0.00							310.43	61.80	2.83	68.89	8.50	0.22	0.24	0.00	0.00	0.00	0.00

Food Name	Amount	Measure	Weight (g)	Calories	Protein (g)	Total Carb (g)	Dietary Fiber (g)	Total Fat (g)	Sat Fat (g)	Mono Fat (g)	Poly Fat (g)	Chol (mg)	Vit A (mcg RAE)	Vit D (mcg)
MEATS *(continued)*														
Lunchmeat, turkey ham, cured thigh meat, slice	1	Ounce-weight	28.35	35.72	4.96	0.58	0.06	1.37	0.44	0.54	0.38	20.41	1.98	
Lunchmeat, turkey, light & dark meat, smkd, sliced, pkg Carl Buddig & Company	1	Ounce-weight	28.35	45.36	4.96	0.51	0.00	2.58	0.88	0.94	0.77	16.16		
Pastrami, beef, cured, 1 oz slice	1	Ounce-weight	28.35	41.39	6.18	0.54	0.14	1.65	0.76	0.59	0.05	19.28	9.36	
Pastrami, beef, smkd, chpd, pressed, ckd, pkg Carl Buddig & Company	1	Ounce-weight	28.35	39.97	5.56	0.28	0.00	1.84	0.85	0.91	0.09	18.43		
Pastrami, turkey, slices	1	Ounce-weight	28.35	34.87	4.62	1.04	0.03	1.23	0.34	0.42	0.32	19.28	1.14	
Salami, cotto, beef, slice Oscar Mayer	1	Ounce-weight	28.35	58.40	4.02	0.54	0.00	4.45	1.91	1.96	0.22	23.53		
Salami, hard, slice Oscar Mayer	1	Ounce-weight	28.35	104.33	7.34	0.47	0.00	8.14	3.12	4.22	0.80	27.50	1.28	0.44
Sausage, beef, smokies Oscar Mayer	1	Each	43.00	127.28	5.27	0.84	0.00	11.46	4.84	5.50	0.39	26.66	0.00	
Sausage, bockwurst, pork veal milk & eggs, raw	1	Each	65.00	180.70	7.09	0.32	0.00	16.82	6.73	8.58	1.51	60.45	0.00	0.19
Sausage, Italian, pork, link, ckd, 4 per lb	1	Each	83.00	285.52	15.87	3.54	0.08	22.67	7.91	9.92	2.72	47.31	8.30	
Sausage, knockwurst/knackwurst, beef & pork, link, 4" long	1	Each	68.00	208.76	7.55	2.18	0.00	18.84	6.94	8.71	1.99	40.80		
Sausage, pepperoni, turkey, sliced, pillow pak, svg USDA SR-23 Hormel	1	Each	30.00	72.90	9.30	1.13	0.00	3.46	1.05	1.41	1.00	36.90	4.50	
Sausage, Polish, pork, each, 10" × 1 1/4"	1	Each	227.00	740.02	32.01	3.70	0.00	65.19	23.45	30.69	6.99	158.90	0.00	
Sausage, pork & beef, smkd, link, w/nonfat dry milk, lrg, 4"	1	Each	68.00	212.84	9.03	1.31	0.00	18.77	6.61	8.60	2.05	44.20	0.00	
Sausage, pork, smkd, link, lrg, 4" × 1 1/8"	1	Each	68.00	264.52	15.10	1.43	0.00	21.56	7.70	9.95	2.56	46.24	0.00	
Sausage, smokies, links Oscar Mayer	1	Each	43.00	129.86	5.33	0.73	0.00	11.74	4.03	5.66	1.20	27.09	0.00	
Sausage, thuringer cervelat, beef, summer style, slice Oscar Mayer	1	Each	23.00	71.07	3.36	0.44	0.00	6.21	2.71	2.97	0.26	18.40		0.23
Sausage, Vienna, beef & pork, drained, 4oz can	1	Piece	16.00	36.80	1.68	0.42	0.00	3.10	1.14	1.54	0.21	13.92	0.00	
Pork and Ham														
Bacon, cured, raw, med slices, 20/lb	1	Piece	22.67	103.83	2.63	0.15	0.00	10.21	3.40	4.54	1.09	15.42	2.49	
Canadian Bacon, cured, grilled f/6oz pkg	2	Piece	46.33	85.71	11.23	0.63	0.00	3.91	1.32	1.87	0.38	26.87	0.00	
Canadian Bacon, cured, unheated, 6/6oz pkg	2	Piece	56.70	89.02	11.70	0.95	0.00	3.95	1.26	1.79	0.36	28.35	0.00	
Pork, avg of retail cuts, leg shoulder & loin, lean, ckd	3	Ounce-weight	85.05	180.31	24.89	0.00	0.00	8.22	2.90	3.70	0.64	73.14	1.70	
Pork, chop, center loin, lean, brsd	3	Ounce-weight	85.05	171.80	25.33	0.00	0.00	7.07	2.61	3.16	0.54	72.29	1.70	
Pork, chop, center rib loin, lean, brsd	3	Ounce-weight	85.05	179.46	23.77	0.00	0.00	8.62	3.37	4.12	0.62	60.39	1.70	
Pork, chop, center rib loin, w/bone, brsd	3	Ounce-weight	85.05	212.63	22.68	0.00	0.00	12.82	4.97	5.84	1.08	62.09	1.70	
Pork, chop, sirloin, lean, brsd	3	Ounce-weight	85.05	148.84	22.96	0.00	0.00	5.61	1.99	2.47	0.48	68.89	1.70	
Pork, chop, sirloin, w/bone, brsd	3	Ounce-weight	85.05	208.37	21.57	0.00	0.00	12.85	4.73	5.58	1.19	69.74	1.70	
Pork, cured ham, ckd, w/wtr add, slice Oscar Mayer	3	Ounce-weight	85.05	88.45	14.12	1.03	0.00	3.15	1.07	1.47	0.30	39.97	0.00	
Pork, cured ham, extra lean, 4% fat, cnd, unheated, cup	3	Ounce-weight	85.05	102.06	15.73	0.00	0.00	3.88	1.28	1.88	0.33	32.32	0.00	
Pork, cured ham, reg, 13% fat, cnd, rstd, cup	3	Ounce-weight	85.05	192.21	17.46	0.36	0.00	12.93	4.29	6.01	1.51	52.73	0.00	
Pork, cured ham, whole, rstd, cup	3	Ounce-weight	85.05	206.67	18.35	0.00	0.00	14.26	5.09	6.70	1.54	52.73	0.00	
Pork, ground, ckd	3	Ounce-weight	85.05	252.60	21.85	0.00	0.00	17.66	6.57	7.87	1.59	79.95	1.70	0.26
Pork, ribs, spareribs, brsd, each	3	Ounce-weight	85.05	337.65	24.72	0.00	0.00	25.77	9.46	11.46	2.32	102.91	2.55	
Pork, roast, center loin, rstd	3	Ounce-weight	85.05	199.02	22.38	0.00	0.00	11.45	4.30	5.01	1.00	68.04	1.70	
Pork, roast, center rib loin, lean, rstd	3	Ounce-weight	85.05	182.01	24.50	0.00	0.00	8.62	3.01	3.82	0.72	70.59	1.70	
Pork, roast, sirloin, lean, w/bone, rstd	3	Ounce-weight	85.05	183.71	24.50	0.00	0.00	8.75	3.08	3.84	0.74	73.14	1.70	
Pork, roast, sirloin, rstd	3	Ounce-weight	85.05	176.05	24.24	0.00	0.00	8.02	2.91	3.50	0.72	73.14	1.70	0.26
Pork, sweet & sour	3	Ounce-weight	85.05	87.00	5.65	9.44	0.59	3.11	0.80	1.19	0.85	14.50	6.03	0.26
Pork, tenderloin, lean, chop, brld	3	Ounce-weight	85.05	159.04	25.87	0.00	0.00	5.38	1.91	2.19	0.48	79.95	1.70	
Pork, tenderloin, rstd	3	Ounce-weight	85.05	147.14	23.65	0.00	0.00	5.15	1.82	2.09	0.46	67.19	1.70	0.26
Veal														
Veal, avg of all cuts, ckd	3	Ounce-weight	85.05	196.47	25.60	0.00	0.00	9.69	3.64	3.74	0.68	96.96	0.00	
Veal, sirloin roast, lean, brsd	3	Ounce-weight	85.05	173.50	28.88	0.00	0.00	5.54	1.55	1.98	0.49	96.11	0.00	
Variety Meats and By-Products														
Beef, heart, ckd	3	Ounce-weight	85.05	140.33	24.22	0.13	0.00	4.02	1.19	0.86	0.84	180.31	0.00	
Beef, liver, brsd	3	Ounce-weight	85.05	162.45	24.73	4.36	0.00	4.47	1.44	0.55	0.54	336.80	8030.42	

Vit E (mg)	Vit C	Vit B_1 Thia (mg)	Vit B_2 Ribo (mg)	Vit B_3 Nia (mg)	Fol (mcg)	Vit B_6 (mg)	Vita B_{12} (mcg)	Sodi (mg)	Pota (mg)	Cal (mg)	Phos (mg)	Magn (mg)	Iron (mg)	Zinc (mg)	Caff (mg)	Alco (g)	Sol Fiber (g)	Insol Fiber (g)
0.18	0.00	0.01	0.04	0.60	1.98	0.06	0.06	315.82	81.36	2.27	83.35	6.24	0.66	0.74	0.00	0.00		
		0.05	0.09	1.66				310.72	93.27	17.01			0.52		0.00	0.00	0.00	0.00
0.14	0.37	0.02	0.05	1.21	1.98	0.08	0.52	250.90	66.62	2.84	49.61	5.39	0.63	1.39	0.00	0.00		
		0.03	0.07	1.16				299.38	103.48	4.82			0.69		0.00	0.00	0.00	0.00
0.06	4.57	0.02	0.07	1.00	1.42	0.08	0.07	278.12	97.81	3.12	56.70	3.97	1.19	0.61	0.00	0.00		
	0.00							371.10	58.68	1.98	63.50	4.82	0.77	0.59	0.00	0.00	0.00	0.00
	0.00	0.16	0.07	1.43	0.85	0.13	0.54	560.20	100.93	3.40	51.03	5.95	0.51	0.89	0.00	0.00	0.00	0.00
	0.00				4.73			415.81	74.39	4.73	98.90	6.45	0.75	1.27	0.00	0.00	0.00	0.00
0.06	0.00	0.14	0.14	2.97	4.55	0.20	0.48	323.05	148.20	26.65	105.30	11.05	0.75	1.16	0.00	0.00	0.00	0.00
0.21	0.08	0.52	0.19	3.46	4.15	0.27	1.08	1001.81	252.32	17.43	141.10	14.94	1.19	1.98	0.00	0.00		
0.39	0.00	0.23	0.10	1.86	1.36	0.12	0.80	632.40	135.32	7.48	66.64	7.48	0.45	1.13	0.00	0.00	0.00	0.00
	0.00				1.20			557.40	134.70	7.80		12.30	0.81	1.29	0.00	0.00	0.00	0.00
0.52	2.27	1.14	0.34	7.82	4.54	0.43	2.22	1988.52	537.99	27.24	308.72	31.78	3.27	4.38	0.00	0.00	0.00	0.00
	0.00	0.13	0.15	1.93	1.36	0.12	1.07	797.64	194.48	27.88	93.16	10.88	1.00	1.33	0.00	0.00	0.00	0.00
0.17	1.36	0.48	0.18	3.08	3.40	0.24	1.11	1020.00	228.48	20.40	110.16	12.92	0.79	1.92	0.00	0.00	0.00	0.00
	0.00							433.01	77.40	4.30	103.20	7.31	0.50	0.90	0.00	0.00	0.00	0.00
	0.00	0.03	0.08	0.99	1.15	0.06	1.27	327.52	53.59	1.84	27.83	3.45	0.57	0.54	0.00	0.00	0.00	0.00
0.04	0.00	0.01	0.02	0.26	0.64	0.02	0.16	155.04	16.16	1.60	7.84	1.12	0.14	0.26	0.00	0.00	0.00	0.00
0.06	0.00	0.06	0.03	0.87	0.45	0.05	0.16	188.84	47.15	1.36	42.62	2.72	0.11	0.27	0.00	0.00	0.00	0.00
0.16	0.00	0.38	0.09	3.20	1.85	0.21	0.36	716.26	180.69	4.63	137.14	9.73	0.38	0.79	0.00	0.00	0.00	0.00
0.12	0.00	0.43	0.10	3.53	2.27	0.22	0.38	798.90	195.05	4.54	137.78	9.64	0.39	0.79	0.00	0.00	0.00	0.00
0.15	0.26	0.72	0.29	4.40	0.85	0.37	0.64	50.18	318.94	17.86	201.57	22.11	0.94	2.53	0.00	0.00	0.00	0.00
0.18	0.85	0.70	0.19	4.13	2.55	0.34	0.43	52.73	312.13	19.56	153.94	17.01	0.96	1.92	0.00	0.00	0.00	0.00
0.18	0.26	0.47	0.22	3.84	3.40	0.28	0.37	34.87	344.45	4.25	147.14	16.16	0.84	1.84	0.00	0.00	0.00	0.00
0.31	0.26	0.50	0.20	4.20	1.70	0.27	0.45	34.02	329.14	21.26	150.54	15.31	0.77	1.71	0.00	0.00	0.00	0.00
0.35	0.77	0.59	0.24	3.36	2.55	0.38	0.48	39.12	302.78	11.06	154.79	18.71	0.94	2.02	0.00	0.00	0.00	0.00
0.31	0.68	0.56	0.22	3.23	2.55	0.35	0.48	43.38	276.41	15.31	147.99	16.16	1.00	2.08	0.00	0.00	0.00	0.00
	0.00							1146.47	240.69	8.51	203.27	26.37	1.26	1.58	0.00	0.00	0.00	0.00
0.14	0.00	0.71	0.20	4.51	5.10	0.38	0.70	1067.38	309.58	5.10	190.51	14.46	0.80	1.64	0.00	0.00	0.00	0.00
0.34	11.91	0.70	0.22	4.51	4.25	0.26	0.90	800.32	303.63	6.80	206.67	14.46	1.17	2.13	0.00	0.00	0.00	0.00
0.31	0.00	0.51	0.19	3.79	2.55	0.32	0.54	1009.54	243.24	5.95	182.01	16.16	0.74	1.97	0.00	0.00	0.00	0.00
0.18	0.60	0.60	0.19	3.58	5.10	0.33	0.46	62.09	307.88	18.71	192.21	20.41	1.10	2.73	0.00	0.00	0.00	0.00
0.29	0.00	0.35	0.32	4.66	3.40	0.30	0.92	79.10	272.16	39.97	221.98	20.41	1.57	3.91	0.00	0.00	0.00	0.00
0.28	0.77	0.73	0.22	4.44	3.40	0.30	0.48	53.58	299.38	22.96	182.86	17.01	0.84	1.72	0.00	0.00	0.00	0.00
0.35	0.34	0.54	0.27	4.55	7.65	0.34	0.47	42.53	308.73	5.10	188.81	20.41	0.85	2.41	0.00	0.00	0.00	0.00
0.40	0.26	0.68	0.28	4.72	5.10	0.36	0.66	53.58	311.28	17.01	193.91	21.26	0.95	2.19	0.00	0.00	0.00	0.00
0.16	0.85	0.75	0.32	4.32	4.25	0.40	0.64	47.63	341.90	13.61	214.33	22.11	1.00	2.13	0.00	0.00	0.00	0.00
0.41	7.37	0.21	0.08	1.37	3.88	0.16	0.13	315.56	145.16	10.50	55.89	12.94	0.54	0.55	0.00	0.00		
0.41	0.85	0.84	0.33	4.37	5.10	0.45	0.85	55.28	383.58	4.25	250.90	30.62	1.22	2.51	0.00	0.00	0.00	0.00
0.16	0.34	0.79	0.33	3.97	5.10	0.35	0.47	46.78	368.27	5.10	218.58	22.96	1.23	2.21	0.00	0.00	0.00	0.00
0.34	0.00	0.05	0.27	6.78	12.76	0.26	1.34	73.99	276.41	18.71	203.27	22.11	0.98	4.05	0.00	0.00	0.00	0.00
0.37	0.00	0.05	0.32	6.00	13.61	0.32	1.35	68.89	288.32	16.16	220.28	24.66	1.05	4.04	0.00	0.00	0.00	0.00
0.25	0.00	0.09	1.03	5.68	4.25	0.21	9.19	50.18	186.26	4.25	216.03	17.86	5.43	2.44	0.00	0.00	0.00	0.00
0.43	1.62	0.16	2.91	14.91	215.18	0.86	60.03	67.19	299.38	5.10	422.70	17.86	5.56	4.51	0.00	0.00	0.00	0.00

Food Name	Amount	Measure	Weight (g)	Calories	Protein (g)	Total Carb (g)	Dietary Fiber (g)	Total Fat (g)	Sat Fat (g)	Mono Fat (g)	Poly Fat (g)	Chol (mg)	Vit A (mcg RAE)	Vit D (mcg)
MEATS *(continued)*														
Beef, liver, fried	3	Ounce-weight	85.05	148.84	22.56	4.39	0.00	3.98	1.27	0.56	0.49	324.04	6586.27	
Chicken, liver, avg, simmered, chpd, cup	3	Ounce-weight	85.05	142.03	20.80	0.74	0.00	5.54	1.75	1.20	1.08	478.83	3385.84	
Goose, liver, raw	1	Each	94.00	125.02	15.39	5.94	0.00	4.02	1.49	0.76	0.24	484.10	8750.46	
Pate, liver, unspecified, cnd	1	Tablespoon	13.00	41.47	1.85	0.19	0.00	3.64	1.24	1.61	0.41	33.15	128.83	
MEAT SUBSTITUTES, SOY TOFU AND VEGETABLE														
Bacon Substitute, vegetarian, strips	3	Each	15.00	46.50	1.60	0.95	0.39	4.43	0.69	1.06	2.32	0.00	0.60	
Beef Substitute, vegetarian, ground round, Italian Yves Veggie Cuisine	0.33	Cup	55.00	60.00	10.00	4.00	3.00	0.00	0.00	0.00	0.00	0.00	0.00	
Beef Substitute, vegetarian, Burger Crumbles, svg Morningstar Farms	0.5	Cup	55.00	115.50	11.08	3.31	2.53	6.46	1.63	2.31	2.46	0.00	0.00	
Beef Substitute, vegetarian, meatballs Gardenburger Inc.	6	Piece	85.00	110.00	12.00	8.00	4.00	4.50	1.00			0.00	0.00	
Burger Substitute, vegetarian, black bean, spicy Morningstar Farms	1	Each	78.00	114.66	11.79	15.20	4.76	0.78	0.18	0.25	0.35	0.78		
Burger Substitute, vegetarian, Diner Deluxe Gardenburger Inc.	1	Each	71.00	110.00	12.00	6.00	4.00	5.00	0.50			0.00		
Burger Substitute, vegetarian, flame grilled Gardenburger Inc.	1	Each	71.00	120.00	14.00	7.00	4.00	4.00	0.00			0.00	0.00	
Burger Substitute, vegetarian, fzn Morningstar Better 'N Burger	1	Each	85.00	90.95	13.91	7.53	4.25	0.54	0.10	0.28	0.15	0.00	0.00	
Burger Substitute, vegetarian, garden vegan Gardenburger Inc.	1	Each	71.00	90.00	10.00	12.00	2.00	0.00	0.00	0.00	0.00	0.00	0.00	
Burger Substitute, vegetarian, garden veggie, fzn Morningstar Farms	1	Each	67.00	119.26	11.21	10.20	4.02	3.77	0.54	1.07	2.16	0.67	134.00	
Burger Substitute, vegetarian, Harvest Burger, original, fzn Green Giant	1	Each	90.00	137.70	18.00	7.02	5.67	4.14	1.02	2.13	0.27	0.00	0.00	
Burger Substitute, vegetarian, roasted garlic Boca Foods Company	1	Each	71.00	100.00	14.00	7.00	5.00	2.00	0.50			3.00	0.00	
Burger Substitute, vegetarian, savory portabella Gardenburger Inc.	1	Each	71.00	120.00	6.00	18.00	4.00	2.50	1.00			20.00		
Burger Substitute, vegetarian, soy	1	Each	70.00	125.30	12.54	9.38	3.22	4.18	0.50	0.77	1.65	0.00	0.00	
Burger Substitute, vegetarian, vegan, fzn Morningstar Better 'N Burger	1	Each	85.00	90.95	13.91	7.53	4.25	0.54	0.10	0.28	0.15	0.00	0.00	
Chicken Substitute, vegetarian, Chik Patties, fzn Morningstar Farms	1	Each	71.00	148.18	9.51	13.65	2.83	6.17	0.86	1.60	3.61	0.58	0.00	
Hot Dog Substitute, vegetarian Morningstar Farms	1	Each	45.00	111.60	10.39	3.70	2.74	6.16	0.89	1.95	3.31	0.45	0.00	
Hot Dog Substitute, vegetarian	1	Each	51.00	102.00	10.20	4.08	2.35	5.10	0.81	1.24	2.64	0.00	0.00	
Hot Dog Substitute, vegetarian, Big Franks, cnd Loma Linda	1	Each	51.00	118.32	12.12	1.51	1.32	7.08	0.81	1.52	3.69	0.00		
Meat Extender	1	Cup	88.00	275.44	33.54	33.72	15.40	2.61	0.37	0.57	1.46	0.00	1.76	
Meat Substitute, vegetarian, prot, pces, Quorn Myco Marlow Foods Limited	3	Ounce-weight	85.05	67.04	10.21	5.40	4.20	2.40	0.40			0.00	0.00	
Sausage Substitute, vegetarian, breakfast links, fzn Morningstar Farms	1	Each	22.50	32.11	4.48	1.22	0.72	1.03	0.18	0.27	0.53	0.67	0.00	
Sausage Substitute, vegetarian, breakfast patty, fzn Morningstar Farms	1	Each	38.00	79.42	9.92	3.72	1.98	2.77	0.51	0.69	1.32	0.76	0.00	
Tempeh	0.5	Cup	83.00	160.19	15.39	7.79		8.96	1.85	2.49	3.17	0.00	0.00	
Tofu, fermented & salted, block	3	Ounce-weight	85.05	98.66	6.93	4.38	0.23	6.80	0.98	1.50	3.84	0.00	6.80	
Tofu, firm, silken, light, slice Mori-Nu	3	Ounce-weight	85.05	31.47	5.36	0.93	0.00	0.68	0.11	0.11	0.38	0.00	0.00	
Tofu, firm, silken, slice Mori-Nu	3	Ounce-weight	85.05	52.73	5.87	2.05	0.08	2.30	0.34	0.46	1.27	0.00	0.00	
Tofu, fried, each pce	3	Ounce-weight	85.05	230.49	14.62	8.93	3.32	17.16	2.48	3.79	9.69	0.00	0.85	
Tofu, soft, silken, slice Mori-Nu	3	Ounce-weight	85.05	46.78	4.08	2.47	0.08	2.30	0.30	0.45	1.32	0.00	0.00	
Vegetarian Meat, chicken, Chik'n Buffalo wings, hot & spicy Kraft Boca Foods	3	Ounce-weight	85.00	156.32	13.68	13.68	2.93	6.84	0.49			0.00	0.00	
NUTS, SEEDS, AND PRODUCTS														
Almond Butter, unsalted	2	Tablespoon	32.00	202.56	4.83	6.79	1.18	18.91	1.79	12.28	3.97	0.00	0.00	
Cashew Butter, plain, unsalted	2	Tablespoon	32.00	187.84	5.62	8.82	0.64	15.82	3.12	9.32	2.68	0.00	0.00	
Coconut, creamed f/dry	2	Tablespoon	30.00	205.20	1.59	6.46	4.29	20.72	18.38	0.88	0.23	0.00	0.00	
Coconut, dried, flaked, swtnd, pkg	2	Tablespoon	9.25	43.85	0.30	4.40	0.40	2.97	2.64	0.13	0.03	0.00	0.00	
Coconut, dried, unswtnd	2	Tablespoon	9.25	61.05	0.64	2.19	1.51	5.97	5.29	0.25	0.07	0.00	0.00	

Vit E (mg)	Vit C	Vit B₁ Thia (mg)	Vit B₂ Ribo (mg)	Vit B₃ Nia (mg)	Fol (mcg)	Vit B₆ (mg)	Vita B₁₂ (mcg)	Sodi (mg)	Pota (mg)	Cal (mg)	Phos (mg)	Magn (mg)	Iron (mg)	Zinc (mg)	Caff (mg)	Alco (g)	Sol Fiber (g)	Insol Fiber (g)
0.39	0.60	0.15	2.91	14.86	221.13	0.87	70.70	65.49	298.53	5.10	412.49	18.71	5.25	4.45	0.00	0.00	0.00	0.00
0.70	23.73	0.25	1.70	9.39	491.59	0.64	14.33	64.64	223.68	9.36	344.45	21.26	9.89	3.38	0.00	0.00	0.00	0.00
1.35	4.23	0.53	0.84	6.11	693.72	0.71	50.76	131.60	216.20	40.42	245.34	22.56	28.70	2.89	0.00	0.00	0.00	0.00
	0.26	0.00	0.08	0.43	7.80	0.01	0.42	90.61	17.94	9.10	26.00	1.69	0.71	0.37	0.00	0.00	0.00	0.00
1.04	0.00	0.66	0.07	1.13	6.30	0.07	0.00	219.75	25.50	3.45	10.50	2.85	0.36	0.06	0.00	0.00	0.29	0.11
	0.00	0.23	0.14	3.00		0.20	1.50	270.00	240.00	40.00			2.70	3.00	0.00	0.00		
0.35	0.00	4.96	0.18	1.49		0.27	2.18	238.15	89.10	39.60	86.90	1.10	3.20	0.82	0.00	0.00		
	0.00							400.00		60.00			1.80		0.00	0.00		
0.36	0.00	8.06	0.14	0.00		0.21	0.07	499.20	269.10	56.16	149.76	43.68	1.84	0.93	0.00	0.00		
	0.00							380.00		80.00			1.44		0.00	0.00		
	0.00							300.00		0.00			0.00		0.00	0.00		
0.01	0.00	0.26	0.55	4.11	245.65	0.20	0.00	382.50	433.50	86.70	181.05	16.15	2.90	0.75	0.00	0.00		
	0.00							230.00		40.00			4.50		0.00	0.00		
0.55	0.00	6.47	0.10	0.00	58.96	0.00	0.00	381.90	179.56	48.24	123.95	29.48	1.21	0.58	0.00	0.00		
1.56	0.00	0.31	0.20	6.30	21.60	0.39	0.00	411.30	432.00	101.70	225.00	70.20	3.85	8.07	0.00	0.00		
	1.20							400.00		100.00			1.80		0.00	0.00		
	0.00							370.00		100.00			0.36		0.00	0.00	4.00	0.00
1.21	0.00	0.63	0.42	7.00	54.60	0.84	1.68	385.00	126.00	20.30	240.80	12.60	1.47	1.26	0.00	0.00		
0.01	0.00	0.26	0.55	4.11	245.65	0.20	0.00	382.50	433.50	86.70	181.05	16.15	2.90	0.75	0.00	0.00		
	0.00	1.39	0.23	2.26		0.18	2.47	513.90	173.88	23.93	124.25		2.31	0.58	0.00	0.00		
1.26	0.00	0.14	0.02	0.00		0.01	0.01	430.65	49.95	17.10	42.30	3.60	0.61	0.38	0.00	0.00		
0.98	0.00	0.56	0.61	8.16	39.78	0.50	1.22	219.30	76.50	16.83	175.44	9.18	0.92	0.61	0.00	0.00		
		0.28	0.68	5.78		0.67	2.94	223.89	60.69	10.20	84.66		0.99	1.20	0.00	0.00		
0.44	0.00	0.62	0.78	19.38	174.24	1.18	5.28	8.80	1673.76	179.52	562.32	190.08	10.55	1.94	0.00	0.00		
	0.00							170.10		3.00			1.00		0.00	0.00		
	0.00	2.72	0.08	1.25		0.19	1.16	177.68	22.95	4.52	32.40		0.89	0.17	0.00	0.00		
0.30	0.00	5.38	0.13	1.84		0.19	1.50	259.16	101.84	18.24	106.40	1.14	1.92	0.37	0.00	0.00		
0.02	0.00	0.07	0.29	2.19	19.92	0.18	0.07	7.47	341.96	92.13	220.78	67.23	2.25	0.95	0.00	0.00		
0.02	0.17	0.13	0.09	0.32	24.66	0.08	0.00	2443.49	63.79	39.12	62.09	44.23	1.68	1.33	0.00	0.00	0.11	0.12
0.05	0.00	0.03	0.02	0.09		0.00	0.00	72.29	53.58	30.62	68.89	8.51	0.64	0.28	0.00	0.00	0.00	0.00
0.16	0.00	0.08	0.03	0.21		0.01	0.00	30.62	165.00	27.22	76.55	22.96	0.88	0.52	0.00	0.00		
0.03	0.00	0.14	0.04	0.09	22.96	0.08	0.00	13.61	124.17	316.39	244.09	51.03	4.14	1.69	0.00	0.00	1.59	1.73
0.17	0.00	0.08	0.03	0.25		0.01	0.00	4.25	153.09	26.37	52.73	24.66	0.70	0.45	0.00	0.00		
	8.79							683.91		39.08			2.64		0.00	0.00		
6.50	0.22	0.04	0.20	0.92	20.80	0.02	0.00	3.52	242.56	86.40	167.36	96.96	1.18	0.98	0.00	0.00		
0.50	0.00	0.10	0.06	0.52	21.76	0.08	0.00	4.80	174.72	13.76	146.24	82.56	1.60	1.66	0.00	0.00	0.36	0.28
0.41	0.45	0.02	0.03	0.18	2.70	0.09	0.00	11.10	165.30	7.80	62.70	27.60	1.01	0.61	0.00	0.00		
0.04	0.00	0.00	0.00	0.03	0.74	0.02	0.00	23.68	29.23	1.30	9.25	4.44	0.17	0.16	0.00	0.00	0.04	0.35
0.04	0.14	0.01	0.01	0.06	0.83	0.03	0.00	3.42	50.23	2.41	19.06	8.33	0.31	0.19	0.00	0.00	0.12	1.39

Food Name	Amount	Measure	Weight (g)	Calories	Protein (g)	Total Carb (g)	Dietary Fiber (g)	Total Fat (g)	Sat Fat (g)	Mono Fat (g)	Poly Fat (g)	Chol (mg)	Vit A (mcg RAE)	Vit D (mcg)
NUTS, SEEDS, AND PRODUCTS (continued)														
Coconut, milk, cnd	2	Tablespoon	28.25	55.65	0.57	0.79	0.32	6.03	5.34	0.26	0.07	0.00	0.00	
Coconut, milk, fzn	2	Tablespoon	30.00	60.60	0.48	1.67	0.67	6.24	5.53	0.27	0.07	0.00	0.00	
Coconut, tstd f/dried	2	Tablespoon	9.25	54.76	0.49	4.11	0.59	4.35	3.86	0.18	0.05	0.00	0.00	
Nut Butter, almond Futters	2	Tablespoon	32.00	170.00	7.00	5.00	4.00	15.00	1.00			0.00		
Nuts, acorns, raw	1	Ounce-weight	28.35	109.71	1.75	11.56		6.77	0.88	4.28	1.30	0.00	0.57	
Nuts, almonds	0.25	Cup	35.50	205.19	7.55	7.01	4.19	17.97	1.37	11.42	4.33	0.00	0.09	
Nuts, almonds, dry rstd, salted, whole	22	Each	28.35	169.25	6.27	5.47	3.35	14.98	1.14	9.54	3.58	0.00	0.02	
Nuts, almonds, oil rstd, salted	22	Each	28.35	172.08	6.02	5.01	2.98	15.64	1.19	9.87	3.84	0.00	0.02	
Nuts, almonds, oil rstd, whole, blanched Blue Diamond Growers	0.25	Cup	35.50	217.61	7.35	5.08		20.41				0.00		
Nuts, Brazil, dried, lrg	6	Each	28.35	185.98	4.06	3.48	2.13	18.83	4.29	6.96	5.83	0.00	0.00	
Nuts, butternuts, dried	0.25	Cup	30.00	183.60	7.47	3.62	1.41	17.09	0.39	3.13	12.82	0.00	1.80	
Nuts, cashews, dry rstd, salted	0.25	Cup	34.25	196.59	5.24	11.20	1.03	15.88	3.14	9.36	2.68	0.00	0.00	
Nuts, cashews, dry rstd, unsalted	0.25	Cup	34.25	196.59	5.24	11.20	1.03	15.88	3.14	9.36	2.68	0.00	0.00	
Nuts, cashews, oil rstd, salted	0.25	Cup	32.50	188.83	5.47	9.80	1.07	15.52	2.75	8.43	2.77	0.00	0.00	
Nuts, cashews, oil rstd, unsalted	0.25	Cup	32.50	188.50	5.47	9.71	1.07	15.52	2.75	8.43	2.77	0.00	0.00	
Nuts, chestnuts, Chinese, dried	1	Ounce-weight	28.35	102.91	1.94	22.61	0.64	0.51	0.08	0.26	0.13	0.00	4.54	
Nuts, chestnuts, European, rstd, cup	0.25	Cup	35.75	87.59	1.13	18.94	1.82	0.79	0.14	0.27	0.31	0.00	0.36	
Nuts, chestnuts, Japanese, ckd	1	Ounce-weight	28.35	15.88	0.24	3.58	0.10	0.06	0.01	0.03	0.02	0.00	0.28	
Nuts, hazelnuts, chpd	0.25	Cup	28.75	180.55	4.30	4.80	2.79	17.47	1.28	13.13	2.28	0.00	0.29	
Nuts, macadamia, dried	11	Each	28.35	203.55	2.24	3.92	2.44	21.48	3.42	16.69	0.43	0.00	0.00	
Nuts, mixed, w/o peanuts, oil rstd, salted	0.25	Cup	36.00	221.40	5.59	8.02	1.98	20.22	3.28	11.93	4.12	0.00	0.14	
Nuts, mixed, w/o peanuts, oil rstd, unsalted	0.25	Cup	36.00	221.40	5.59	8.02	1.98	20.22	3.28	11.93	4.12	0.00	0.36	
Nuts, mixed, w/peanuts, dry rstd, salted	0.25	Cup	34.25	203.44	5.93	8.69	3.08	17.63	2.36	10.75	3.69	0.00	0.09	
Nuts, mixed, w/peanuts, dry rstd, unsalted	0.25	Cup	34.25	203.44	5.93	8.69	3.08	17.63	2.36	10.75	3.69	0.00	0.34	
Nuts, mixed, w/peanuts, oil rstd, salted	0.25	Cup	35.50	219.03	5.95	7.60	3.19	20.00	3.10	11.25	4.72	0.00	0.13	
Nuts, mixed, w/peanuts, oil rstd, unsalted	0.25	Cup	35.50	219.03	5.95	7.60	3.51	20.00	3.10	11.25	4.72	0.00	0.35	
Nuts, peanuts, dry rstd, salted, each	30	Each	30.00	175.50	7.10	6.45	2.40	14.90	2.07	7.39	4.71	0.00	0.00	
Nuts, peanuts, dry rstd, unsalted	30	Each	30.00	175.50	7.10	6.45	2.40	14.90	2.07	7.39	4.71	0.00	0.00	
Nuts, peanuts, oil rstd, salted, each	30	Each	27.00	161.73	7.57	4.12	2.54	14.17	2.34	7.00	4.12	0.00	0.00	
Nuts, peanuts, oil rstd, unsalted, each	32	Each	28.00	162.68	7.38	5.30	1.93	13.80	1.91	6.85	4.36	0.00	0.00	
Nuts, peanuts, raw	0.25	Cup	36.50	206.96	9.42	5.89	3.10	17.97	2.49	8.92	5.68	0.00	0.00	
Nuts, peanuts, Spanish, raw	0.25	Cup	36.50	208.05	9.55	5.78	3.47	18.10	2.79	8.15	6.28	0.00	0.00	
Nuts, pecans, chpd	0.25	Cup	29.75	205.57	2.73	4.13	2.86	21.41	1.83	12.14	6.43	0.00	0.89	
Nuts, pecans, dry rstd, salted	1	Ounce-weight	28.35	201.28	2.69	3.85	2.66	21.05	1.78	12.46	5.83	0.00	1.98	
Nuts, pecans, dry rstd, unsalted	1	Ounce-weight	28.35	201.28	2.69	3.85	2.66	21.05	1.78	12.46	5.83	0.00	1.98	
Nuts, pine, pinon/pinyon, dried	10	Each	1.00	6.29	0.12	0.19	0.11	0.61	0.09	0.23	0.26	0.00	0.01	
Nuts, pistachio, dry rstd, salted	0.25	Cup	32.00	181.76	6.83	8.57	3.30	14.71	1.77	7.75	4.45	0.00	4.17	
Nuts, pistachio, dry rstd, unsalted	0.25	Cup	32.00	182.72	6.83	8.85	3.30	14.71	1.77	7.75	4.45	0.00	4.17	
Nuts, walnuts, English, dried, chpd	0.25	Cup	30.00	196.20	4.57	4.11	2.01	19.56	1.84	2.68	14.15	0.00	0.30	
Peanut Butter, chunky	2	Tablespoon	32.00	188.48	7.70	6.90	2.56	15.98	2.59	7.86	4.74	0.00	0.00	0.00
Peanut Butter, chunky, unsalted	2	Tablespoon	32.00	188.48	7.70	6.90	2.56	15.98	2.59	7.86	4.74	0.00	0.00	
Peanut Butter, creamy, unsalted	2	Tablespoon	32.00	188.16	8.03	6.26	1.92	16.12	3.29	7.59	4.44	0.00	0.00	
Peanut Butter, natural, creamy, rducd fat The J.M. Smucker Co.	2	Tablespoon	35.00	200.00	9.00	12.00	2.00	12.00	2.00			0.00	0.00	
Seeds, flax/linseed, ground, Canada Flax Council of Canada	1	Tablespoon	8.00	36.00	1.68	2.72	2.24	3.36		0.94	1.01		0.08	
Seeds, sunflower, kernels, dry rstd, salted	0.25	Cup	32.00	186.24	6.19	7.70	2.88	15.94	1.67	3.04	10.53	0.00	0.15	
Seeds, sunflower, kernels, dry rstd, unsalted	0.25	Cup	32.00	186.24	6.19	7.70	3.55	15.94	1.67	3.04	10.53	0.00	0.15	
Seeds, sunflower, oil rstd, salted	0.25	Cup	33.75	199.80	6.77	7.73	3.58	17.31	2.38	2.72	11.58	0.00	0.16	
Tahini, f/raw & stone ground kernels	2	Tablespoon	30.00	171.00	5.34	7.86	2.79	14.40	2.02	5.44	6.31	0.00	0.90	
POULTRY														

Chicken—BBQ, Breaded, Fried, Glazed, Grilled, Raw

Food Name	Amount	Measure	Weight (g)	Calories	Protein (g)	Total Carb (g)	Dietary Fiber (g)	Total Fat (g)	Sat Fat (g)	Mono Fat (g)	Poly Fat (g)	Chol (mg)	Vit A (mcg RAE)	Vit D (mcg)
Chicken, breast, teriyaki	3	Ounce-weight	85.05	118.19	17.77	4.43	0.27	2.43	0.62	0.71	0.60	54.59	9.99	
Chicken, broiler/fryer, breast, w/o skin, fried	3	Ounce-weight	85.05	159.04	28.44	0.43	0.00	4.01	1.10	1.46	0.91	77.40	5.95	
Chicken, broiler/fryer, breast, w/o skin, rstd, each or cup	3	Ounce-weight	85.05	140.33	26.38	0.00	0.00	3.04	0.86	1.05	0.65	72.29	5.10	

Vit E (mg)	Vit C	Vit B₁ Thia (mg)	Vit B₂ Ribo (mg)	Vit B₃ Nia (mg)	Fol (mcg)	Vit B₆ (mg)	Vita B₁₂ (mcg)	Sodi (mg)	Pota (mg)	Cal (mg)	Phos (mg)	Magn (mg)	Iron (mg)	Zinc (mg)	Caff (mg)	Alco (g)	Sol Fiber (g)	Insol Fiber (g)
0.18	0.28	0.01	0.00	0.18	3.95	0.01	0.00	3.67	62.15	5.08	27.12	12.99	0.93	0.16	0.00	0.00		
0.20	0.33	0.01	0.00	0.20	4.20	0.01	0.00	3.60	69.60	1.20	17.70	9.60	0.24	0.18	0.00	0.00		
0.09	0.14	0.01	0.01	0.06	0.83	0.03	0.00	3.42	51.25	2.50	19.52	8.51	0.31	0.19	0.00	0.00	0.06	0.53
								0.00							0.00	0.00		
	0.00	0.03	0.04	0.52	24.66	0.15	0.00	0.00	152.81	11.62	22.40	17.58	0.23	0.14	0.00	0.00		
9.18	0.00	0.08	0.28	1.40	10.29	0.05	0.00	0.35	258.44	88.04	168.27	97.62	1.53	1.20	0.00	0.00	0.51	3.68
7.37	0.00	0.02	0.25	1.10	9.36	0.04	0.00	96.11	211.49	75.41	138.63	81.08	1.28	1.00	0.00	0.00	0.37	2.98
7.36	0.00	0.03	0.22	1.04	7.65	0.04	0.00	96.11	198.17	82.50	132.11	77.68	1.04	0.87	0.00	0.00	0.33	2.65
		0.27	0.50	1.51			0.00	0.00	205.90	81.65			1.74		0.00	0.00		
1.62	0.20	0.17	0.01	0.08	6.24	0.03	0.00	0.85	186.83	45.36	205.54	106.60	0.69	1.15	0.00	0.00		
1.05	0.96	0.11	0.04	0.31	19.80	0.17	0.00	0.30	126.30	15.90	133.80	71.10	1.21	0.94	0.00	0.00		
0.32	0.00	0.07	0.07	0.48	23.63	0.09	0.00	219.20	193.51	15.41	167.82	89.05	2.05	1.92	0.00	0.00	0.55	0.48
0.32	0.00	0.07	0.07	0.48	23.63	0.09	0.00	5.48	193.51	15.41	167.82	89.05	2.05	1.92	0.00	0.00	0.55	0.48
0.30	0.10	0.12	0.08	0.56	8.13	0.11	0.00	100.10	205.40	13.98	172.58	88.73	1.97	1.74	0.00	0.00	0.56	0.51
0.30	0.10	0.12	0.08	0.56	8.13	0.11	0.00	4.23	205.40	13.98	172.58	88.73	1.97	1.74	0.00	0.00	0.56	0.51
0.26	16.58	0.08	0.09	0.37	31.18	0.19	0.00	1.42	205.82	8.22	43.94	38.84	0.65	0.40	0.00	0.00		
0.18	9.30	0.08	0.06	0.48	25.03	0.18	0.00	0.72	211.64	10.37	38.25	11.80	0.32	0.20	0.00	0.00	0.45	1.37
0.03	2.69	0.04	0.02	0.15	4.82	0.03	0.00	1.42	33.74	3.12	7.37	5.10	0.15	0.11	0.00	0.00		
4.32	1.81	0.18	0.03	0.52	32.49	0.16	0.00	0.00	195.50	32.77	83.37	46.86	1.35	0.71	0.00	0.00	0.89	1.90
0.15	0.34	0.34	0.05	0.70	3.12	0.08	0.00	1.42	104.33	24.10	53.30	36.86	1.05	0.37	0.00	0.00	0.88	1.56
2.95	0.18	0.18	0.18	0.71	20.16	0.06	0.00	110.16	195.84	38.16	161.64	90.36	0.92	1.68	0.00	0.00		
2.16	0.18	0.18	0.18	0.71	20.16	0.06	0.00	3.96	195.84	38.16	161.64	90.36	0.92	1.68	0.00	0.00		
3.74	0.14	0.07	0.07	1.61	17.12	0.10	0.00	229.13	204.47	23.97	148.99	77.06	1.27	1.30	0.00	0.00		
2.05	0.14	0.07	0.07	1.61	17.12	0.10	0.00	4.11	204.47	23.97	148.99	77.06	1.27	1.30	0.00	0.00		
2.56	0.18	0.18	0.08	1.80	29.46	0.08	0.00	148.74	206.25	38.34	164.72	83.42	1.14	1.80	0.00	0.00		
2.13	0.18	0.18	0.08	1.80	29.46	0.08	0.00	3.90	206.25	38.34	164.72	83.42	1.14	1.80	0.00	0.00		
2.34	0.00	0.13	0.03	4.06	43.50	0.08	0.00	243.90	197.40	16.20	107.40	52.80	0.68	0.99	0.00	0.00	0.67	1.73
2.08	0.00	0.13	0.03	4.06	43.50	0.08	0.00	1.80	197.40	16.20	107.40	52.80	0.68	0.99	0.00	0.00		
1.87	0.22	0.03	0.03	3.73	32.40	0.13	0.00	86.40	196.02	16.47	107.19	47.52	0.41	0.88	0.00	0.00	0.07	2.47
1.93	0.00	0.07	0.03	3.99	35.28	0.07	0.00	1.68	190.96	24.64	144.76	51.80	0.51	1.86	0.00	0.00	0.53	1.40
3.04	0.00	0.23	0.05	4.40	87.60	0.12	0.00	6.57	257.33	33.58	137.24	61.32	1.67	1.19	0.00	0.00	0.86	2.24
2.70	0.00	0.24	0.05	5.82	87.60	0.12	0.00	8.03	271.56	38.69	141.62	68.62	1.42	0.78	0.00	0.00	0.97	2.49
0.42	0.33	0.20	0.04	0.35	6.55	0.06	0.00	0.00	121.98	20.83	82.41	36.00	0.75	1.35	0.00	0.00	0.88	1.97
0.37	0.20	0.13	0.03	0.33	4.54	0.06	0.00	108.58	120.20	20.41	83.07	37.42	0.79	1.44	0.00	0.00	0.64	2.02
0.37	0.20	0.13	0.03	0.33	4.54	0.06	0.00	0.28	120.20	20.41	83.07	37.42	0.79	1.44	0.00	0.00	0.64	2.02
0.04	0.02	0.01	0.00	0.04	0.58	0.00	0.00	0.72	6.28	0.08	0.35	2.34	0.03	0.04	0.00	0.00	0.02	0.09
0.62	0.73	0.27	0.05	0.45	16.01	0.41	0.00	129.60	333.44	35.21	155.20	38.40	1.34	0.73	0.00	0.00	0.09	3.21
0.62	0.73	0.27	0.05	0.45	16.01	0.41	0.00	3.21	333.44	35.21	155.20	38.40	1.34	0.73	0.00	0.00	0.09	3.21
0.21	0.39	0.10	0.05	0.34	29.40	0.16	0.00	0.60	132.30	29.40	103.80	47.40	0.87	0.93	0.00	0.00	0.66	1.35
2.02	0.00	0.03	0.04	4.38	29.44	0.13	0.00	155.52	238.40	14.40	102.08	51.20	0.61	0.89	0.00	0.00	0.72	1.84
2.02	0.00	0.03	0.04	4.38	29.44	0.13	0.00	5.44	238.40	14.40	102.08	51.20	0.61	0.89	0.00	0.00	0.72	1.84
2.88	0.00	0.02	0.03	4.29	23.68	0.17	0.00	5.44	207.68	13.76	114.56	49.28	0.60	0.93	0.00	0.00	0.54	1.38
	0.00			5.00	24.00	0.12	0.00	120.00		0.00		60.00	0.72	0.90	0.00	0.00		
0.03		0.06	0.02	0.35		0.06	0.04	3.68	60.00	20.00	52.00	28.00	0.80	0.16	0.00	0.00	0.56	1.68
8.35	0.45	0.03	0.07	2.25	75.84	0.26	0.00	131.20	272.00	22.40	369.60	41.28	1.22	1.70	0.00	0.00	0.92	1.96
8.35	0.45	0.03	0.07	2.25	75.84	0.26	0.00	0.96	272.00	22.40	369.60	41.28	1.22	1.70	0.00	0.00	1.14	2.42
12.26	0.37	0.11	0.09	1.40	78.97	0.27	0.00	138.38	163.01	29.36	384.41	42.86	1.44	1.76	0.00	0.00	1.15	2.43
0.66	0.00	0.38	0.15	1.78	29.40	0.04	0.00	22.20	124.20	126.00	225.60	28.80	0.75	1.39	0.00	0.00		
0.23	2.11	0.05	0.13	5.82	8.06	0.31	0.19	1118.49	205.16	18.01	131.93	23.44	1.14	1.31	0.00	0.56		
0.36	0.00	0.07	0.11	12.57	3.40	0.54	0.31	67.19	234.74	13.61	209.22	26.37	0.97	0.92	0.00	0.00	0.00	0.00
0.23	0.00	0.06	0.10	11.66	3.40	0.51	0.29	62.94	217.73	12.76	193.91	24.66	0.88	0.85	0.00	0.00	0.00	0.00

Food Name	Amount	Measure	Weight (g)	Calories	Protein (g)	Total Carb (g)	Dietary Fiber (g)	Total Fat (g)	Sat Fat (g)	Mono Fat (g)	Poly Fat (g)	Chol (mg)	Vit A (mcg RAE)	Vit D (mcg)
POULTRY (continued)														
Chicken, broiler/fryer, breast, w/o skin, stwd	3	Ounce-weight	85.05	128.43	24.65	0.00	0.00	2.58	0.72	0.88	0.56	65.49	5.10	
Chicken, broiler/fryer, breast, w/skin, rstd	3	Ounce-weight	85.05	167.55	25.34	0.00	0.00	6.62	1.86	2.58	1.41	71.44	22.96	
Chicken, broiler/fryer, breast, w/skin, stwd	3	Ounce-weight	85.05	156.49	23.30	0.00	0.00	6.31	1.77	2.47	1.34	63.79	20.41	
Chicken, broiler/fryer, dark meat, w/o skin, fried, cup	3	Ounce-weight	85.05	203.27	24.66	2.20	0.00	9.88	2.65	3.67	2.36	81.65	20.41	
Chicken, broiler/fryer, dark meat, w/o skin, rstd	3	Ounce-weight	85.05	174.35	23.28	0.00	0.00	8.28	2.26	3.03	1.92	79.10	18.71	
Chicken, broiler/fryer, dark meat, w/o skin, stwd	3	Ounce-weight	85.05	163.30	22.09	0.00	0.00	7.64	2.08	2.77	1.78	74.84	17.86	
Chicken, broiler/fryer, dark meat, w/skin, rstd	3	Ounce-weight	85.05	215.18	22.09	0.00	0.00	13.42	3.72	5.26	2.97	77.40	51.03	
Chicken, broiler/fryer, dark meat, w/skin, stwd	3	Ounce-weight	85.05	198.17	19.99	0.00	0.00	12.47	3.45	4.89	2.76	69.74	47.63	
Chicken, broiler/fryer, leg, w/o skin, rstd, each or cup	3	Ounce-weight	85.05	162.45	22.99	0.00	0.00	7.17	1.95	2.59	1.68	79.95	16.16	
Chicken, broiler/fryer, leg, w/o skin, stwd, each or cup	3	Ounce-weight	85.05	157.34	22.33	0.00	0.00	6.86	1.87	2.49	1.60	75.69	15.31	
Chicken, broiler/fryer, leg, w/skin, rstd, each or cup	3	Ounce-weight	85.05	197.32	22.08	0.00	0.00	11.45	3.16	4.46	2.55	78.25	33.17	
Chicken, broiler/fryer, leg, w/skin, stwd, each or cup	3	Ounce-weight	85.05	187.11	20.56	0.00	0.00	10.99	3.04	4.29	2.44	71.44	30.62	
Chicken, broiler/fryer, light meat, w/o skin, fried, cup	3	Ounce-weight	85.05	163.30	27.91	0.36	0.00	4.71	1.29	1.68	1.07	76.55	7.65	
Chicken, broiler/fryer, light meat, w/skin, stwd	3	Ounce-weight	85.05	170.95	22.23	0.00	0.00	8.48	2.38	3.33	1.80	62.94	24.66	
Chicken, broiler/fryer, thigh, w/o skin, fried	3	Ounce-weight	85.05	185.41	23.97	1.00	0.00	8.76	2.36	3.25	2.07	86.75	17.86	
Chicken, broiler/fryer, thigh, w/o skin, rstd	3	Ounce-weight	85.05	177.75	22.06	0.00	0.00	9.25	2.58	3.53	2.11	80.80	17.01	
Chicken, broiler/fryer, thigh, w/o skin, stwd	3	Ounce-weight	85.05	165.85	21.26	0.00	0.00	8.33	2.30	3.15	1.91	76.55	16.16	
Chicken, broiler/fryer, thigh, w/skin, rstd	3	Ounce-weight	85.05	210.07	21.31	0.00	0.00	13.17	3.68	5.23	2.91	79.10	40.82	
Chicken, broiler/fryer, thigh, w/skin, stwd	3	Ounce-weight	85.05	197.32	19.78	0.00	0.00	12.54	3.50	4.97	2.76	71.44	37.42	
Chicken, broiler/fryer, whole, w/skin, rstd, each or cup	3	Ounce-weight	85.05	203.27	23.22	0.00	0.00	11.57	3.22	4.54	2.53	74.84	39.97	
Chicken, broiler/fryer, whole, w/skin, stwd, each or cup	3	Ounce-weight	85.05	186.26	20.99	0.00	0.00	10.68	2.98	4.19	2.33	66.34	35.72	
Chicken, broiler/fryer, wing, w/o skin, fried	3	Ounce-weight	85.05	179.46	25.64	0.00	0.00	7.78	2.13	2.62	1.76	71.44	15.31	
Chicken, broiler/fryer, wing, w/o skin, rstd	3	Ounce-weight	85.05	172.65	25.91	0.00	0.00	6.91	1.92	2.22	1.51	72.29	15.31	
Chicken, broiler/fryer, wing, w/o skin, stwd	3	Ounce-weight	85.05	153.94	23.12	0.00	0.00	6.11	1.70	1.96	1.34	62.94	13.61	
Chicken, broiler/fryer, wing, w/skin, rstd, each or cup	3	Ounce-weight	85.05	246.65	22.84	0.00	0.00	16.55	4.64	6.50	3.52	71.44	39.97	
Chicken, broiler/fryer, wing, w/skin, stwd	3	Ounce-weight	85.05	211.77	19.37	0.00	0.00	14.31	4.01	5.61	3.04	59.54	34.02	
Chicken, nuggets, brd, fzn, 1598, FS Pierre Foods	1	Each	17.00	50.00	3.10	2.60		3.00	0.60					
Chicken, patty, southern fried, w/o bone, ckd f/fzn Banquet	1	Each	63.79	190.00	8.00	10.00	1.00	13.00	3.00			25.00	0.00	
Chicken, w/o skin, w/broth, can	3	Ounce-weight	85.05	140.33	18.52	0.00	0.00	6.76	1.87	2.68	1.49	52.73	28.92	
Dish, chicken patty, breaded strips Swanson	1	Each	150.00	340.00	11.00	31.00	3.00	19.00	3.50			30.00		
Turkey														
Bacon, turkey, svg Louis Rich	1	Ounce-weight	28.35	70.88	4.27	0.47	0.00	5.75	1.50	2.13	1.34	25.52	0.00	
Turkey, breast, prebasted, w/skin, rstd	3	Ounce-weight	85.05	107.16	18.85	0.00	0.00	2.94	0.83	0.97	0.71	35.72	0.00	
Turkey, fryer/roaster, dark meat, w/o skin, raw	4	Ounce-weight	113.40	125.87	23.20	0.00	0.00	3.03	1.02	0.69	0.91	91.85	0.00	
Turkey, fryer/roaster, leg, w/skin, raw	4	Ounce-weight	113.40	133.81	22.83	0.00	0.00	4.05	1.25	1.22	1.10	98.66	1.13	
Turkey, fryer/roaster, light meat, w/o skin, raw	4	Ounce-weight	113.40	122.47	27.42	0.00	0.00	0.56	0.18	0.10	0.15	74.84	0.00	
Turkey, fryer/roaster, whole, w/o skin, raw	4	Ounce-weight	113.40	124.74	25.31	0.00	0.00	1.79	0.60	0.40	0.53	82.78	0.00	
Turkey, fryer/roaster, wing, w/o skin, rstd	3	Ounce-weight	85.05	138.63	26.24	0.00	0.00	2.93	0.94	0.51	0.78	86.75	0.00	
Turkey, ground, 8% fat, raw	4	Ounce-weight	113.40	168.97	19.80	0.00	0.00	9.37	2.55	3.52	2.27	89.59	2.27	
Turkey, ham, dark meat, USDA, smkd, fzn, svg	3	Ounce-weight	85.05	100.36	13.86	2.64	0.00	3.40	1.02	1.14	0.74	54.43	13.61	
Turkey, hen, back, w/skin, raw	4	Ounce-weight	113.40	247.21	19.86	0.00	0.00	18.06	5.00	6.94	4.41	77.11	2.27	

Vit E (mg)	Vit C	Vit B₁ Thia (mg)	Vit B₂ Ribo (mg)	Vit B₃ Nia (mg)	Fol (mcg)	Vit B₆ (mg)	Vita B₁₂ (mcg)	Sodi (mg)	Pota (mg)	Cal (mg)	Phos (mg)	Magn (mg)	Iron (mg)	Zinc (mg)	Caff (mg)	Alco (g)	Sol Fiber (g)	Insol Fiber (g)
0.23	0.00	0.04	0.10	7.20	2.55	0.28	0.20	53.58	159.04	11.06	140.33	20.41	0.75	0.82	0.00	0.00	0.00	0.00
0.23	0.00	0.06	0.10	10.81	3.40	0.48	0.27	60.39	208.37	11.91	182.01	22.96	0.91	0.87	0.00	0.00	0.00	0.00
0.23	0.00	0.03	0.10	6.64	2.55	0.25	0.18	52.73	151.39	11.06	132.68	18.71	0.78	0.82	0.00	0.00	0.00	0.00
0.49	0.00	0.08	0.21	6.01	7.65	0.31	0.28	82.50	215.18	15.31	159.04	21.26	1.27	2.47	0.00	0.00	0.00	0.00
0.23	0.00	0.06	0.19	5.57	6.80	0.31	0.27	79.10	204.12	12.76	152.24	19.56	1.13	2.38	0.00	0.00	0.00	0.00
0.23	0.00	0.05	0.17	4.03	5.95	0.18	0.19	62.94	153.94	11.91	121.62	17.01	1.16	2.26	0.00	0.00	0.00	0.00
0.48	0.00	0.06	0.18	5.41	5.95	0.26	0.25	73.99	187.11	12.76	142.88	18.71	1.16	2.12	0.00	0.00	0.00	0.00
0.51	0.00	0.04	0.15	3.84	5.10	0.14	0.17	59.54	141.18	11.91	113.12	15.31	1.11	1.92	0.00	0.00	0.00	0.00
0.23	0.00	0.06	0.20	5.37	6.80	0.31	0.27	77.40	205.82	10.21	155.64	20.41	1.11	2.43	0.00	0.00	0.00	0.00
0.23	0.00	0.05	0.18	4.08	6.80	0.18	0.20	66.34	161.60	9.36	126.72	17.86	1.19	2.36	0.00	0.00	0.00	0.00
0.23	0.00	0.06	0.18	5.27	5.95	0.28	0.26	73.99	191.36	10.21	147.99	19.56	1.13	2.21	0.00	0.00	0.00	0.00
0.23	0.00	0.05	0.16	3.90	5.10	0.15	0.17	62.09	149.69	9.36	118.22	17.01	1.15	2.07	0.00	0.00	0.00	0.00
0.26	0.00	0.06	0.11	11.37	3.40	0.54	0.31	68.89	223.68	13.61	196.47	24.66	0.97	1.08	0.00	0.00	0.00	0.00
0.22	0.00	0.03	0.10	5.90	2.55	0.23	0.17	53.58	142.03	11.06	124.17	17.01	0.83	0.97	0.00	0.00	0.00	0.00
0.49	0.00	0.07	0.22	6.06	7.65	0.32	0.28	80.80	220.28	11.06	169.25	22.11	1.24	2.37	0.00	0.00	0.00	0.00
0.23	0.00	0.06	0.20	5.55	6.80	0.30	0.26	74.84	202.42	10.21	155.64	20.41	1.11	2.19	0.00	0.00	0.00	0.00
0.23	0.00	0.05	0.19	4.42	5.95	0.18	0.18	63.79	155.64	9.36	126.72	17.86	1.21	2.19	0.00	0.00	0.00	0.00
0.23	0.00	0.06	0.18	5.41	5.95	0.26	0.25	71.44	188.81	10.21	147.99	18.71	1.14	2.01	0.00	0.00	0.00	0.00
0.23	0.00	0.05	0.16	4.16	5.10	0.14	0.16	60.39	144.59	9.36	118.22	16.16	1.17	1.91	0.00	0.00	0.00	0.00
0.23	0.00	0.05	0.14	7.22	4.25	0.34	0.26	69.74	189.66	12.76	154.79	19.56	1.07	1.65	0.00	0.00	0.00	0.00
0.23	0.00	0.04	0.13	4.76	4.25	0.19	0.17	56.98	141.18	11.06	118.22	16.16	0.99	1.50	0.00	0.00	0.00	0.00
0.26	0.00	0.04	0.11	6.16	3.40	0.50	0.29	77.40	176.90	12.76	139.48	17.86	0.97	1.80	0.00	0.00	0.00	0.00
0.23	0.00	0.04	0.11	6.22	3.40	0.50	0.29	78.25	178.61	13.61	141.18	17.86	0.99	1.82	0.00	0.00	0.00	0.00
0.23	0.00	0.04	0.09	4.42	2.55	0.27	0.19	62.09	130.13	11.06	113.97	15.31	0.95	1.72	0.00	0.00	0.00	0.00
0.23	0.00	0.04	0.11	5.65	2.55	0.36	0.25	69.74	156.49	12.76	128.43	16.16	1.08	1.55	0.00	0.00	Sol Fiber	Insol Fiber
0.23	0.00	0.03	0.09	3.93	2.55	0.19	0.15	56.98	118.22	10.21	102.91	13.61	0.96	1.39	0.00	0.00	0.00	0.00
	0.00							98.80		5.90			0.42		0.00	0.00		
	1.20	0.08	0.03	2.88				430.00	135.00	0.00	117.00		0.72		0.00	0.00		
0.22	1.70	0.01	0.11	5.38	3.40	0.30	0.25	427.80	117.37	11.91	94.41	10.21	1.34	1.20	0.00	0.00	0.00	0.00
	6.00							560.00		20.00			1.44		0.00	0.00		
	0.00			2.27				343.89	58.97	11.34	56.42	5.39	0.41	0.71	0.00	0.00	0.00	0.00
	0.00	0.05	0.11	7.71	4.25	0.27	0.27	337.65	210.92	7.65	182.01	17.86	0.56	1.30	0.00	0.00	0.00	0.00
0.73	0.00	0.06	0.23	3.35	12.47	0.42	0.46	78.25	276.70	14.74	193.91	24.95	1.88	3.02	0.00	0.00	0.00	0.00
0.73	0.00	0.05	0.23	2.97	11.34	0.40	0.45	78.25	278.96	12.47	190.51	23.81	1.97	3.29	0.00	0.00	0.00	0.00
0.10	0.00	0.04	0.13	6.52	9.07	0.65	0.52	58.97	312.98	11.34	222.26	29.48	1.38	1.58	0.00	0.00	0.00	0.00
0.39	0.00	0.05	0.18	4.94	10.21	0.53	0.50	69.17	294.84	13.61	208.66	27.22	1.63	2.30	0.00	0.00	0.00	0.00
0.08	0.00	0.03	0.14	3.51	5.95	0.50	0.35	66.34	173.50	22.11	147.99	18.71	1.51	3.26	0.00	0.00	0.00	0.00
0.40	0.00	0.06	0.15	3.96	7.94	0.40	0.39	106.60	264.22	14.74	176.90	21.55	1.42	2.19	0.00	0.00	0.00	0.00
	0.00	0.20	0.23	3.50		0.05	0.68	773.10	215.18	5.95	245.79	13.61	0.85	1.79	0.00	0.00	0.00	0.00
0.72	0.00	0.07	0.20	2.69	10.21	0.31	0.40	69.17	261.95	20.41	173.50	20.41	2.02	2.87	0.00	0.00	0.00	0.00

Food Name	Amount	Measure	Weight (g)	Calories	Protein (g)	Total Carb (g)	Dietary Fiber (g)	Total Fat (g)	Sat Fat (g)	Mono Fat (g)	Poly Fat (g)	Chol (mg)	Vit A (mcg RAE)	Vit D (mcg)
POULTRY *(continued)*														
Turkey, light & dark meat, diced, seasoned	3	Ounce-weight	85.05	117.37	15.90	0.85	0.00	5.10	1.49	1.68	1.30	46.78	0.00	
Turkey, nuggets, brd, svg Louis Rich	3	Piece	84.00	231.84	12.02	12.94	0.42	14.70	2.85	6.88	4.61	33.60	0.00	
Turkey, sticks, brd, batter fried, 2.25oz each	1	Each	63.79	177.97	9.06	10.84	0.34	10.78	2.79	4.41	2.80	40.83	7.65	
Turkey, thigh, prebasted, w/skin, w/o bone, rstd	3	Ounce-weight	85.05	133.53	15.99	0.00	0.00	7.26	2.25	2.15	2.00	52.73	0.00	
Duck, Emu, Ostrich and Other														
Cornish Game Hen, whole, w/o skin, rstd	3	Ounce-weight	85.05	113.97	19.82	0.00	0.00	3.29	0.84	1.05	0.80	90.15	17.01	
Cornish Game Hen, whole, w/skin, rstd	3	Ounce-weight	85.05	221.13	18.94	0.00	0.00	15.49	4.30	6.80	3.06	111.42	27.22	
Dove, whole, ckd	3	Ounce-weight	85.05	186.26	20.33	0.00	0.00	11.06	3.18	4.65	2.32	98.66	23.81	
Duck, breast, w/o skin, raw, wild	4	Ounce-weight	113.40	139.48	22.51	0.00	0.00	4.82	1.50	1.37	0.66	87.32	18.14	
Duck, domesticated, whole, rstd	3	Ounce-weight	85.05	286.62	16.15	0.00	0.00	24.11	8.22	10.97	3.10	71.44	53.63	
Duck, whole, w/o skin, rstd, domesticated	3	Ounce-weight	85.05	170.95	19.97	0.00	0.00	9.53	3.55	3.15	1.22	75.69	19.56	
Duck, whole, w/skin, rstd, domesticated	3	Ounce-weight	85.05	286.62	16.15	0.00	0.00	24.11	8.22	10.97	3.10	71.44	53.58	
Duckling, white pekin, breast, w/o skin, brld, cup	3	Ounce-weight	85.05	119.07	23.47	0.00	0.00	2.13	0.49	0.74	0.32	121.62		
Emu, ground, brld	3	Ounce-weight	85.05	138.63	24.18	0.00	0.00	3.95	1.06	1.66	0.58	73.99	0.00	
Goose, whole, w/o skin, raw	4	Ounce-weight	113.40	182.57	25.80	0.00	0.00	8.09	3.16	2.10	1.02	95.26	13.61	
Goose, whole, w/o skin, rstd	3	Ounce-weight	85.05	202.42	24.64	0.00	0.00	10.78	3.88	3.69	1.31	81.65	10.21	
Guinea Hen, whole, w/skin, raw	4	Ounce-weight	113.40	179.17	26.54	0.00	0.00	7.31	2.01	2.76	1.60	83.92	31.75	
Ostrich, ground, brld	3	Ounce-weight	85.05	148.84	22.24	0.00	0.00	6.01	1.52	1.83	0.63	70.59	0.00	
SALAD DRESSINGS, DIPS, AND MAYONNAISE														
Dips														
Dip, avocado Kraft General Foods, Inc.	2	Tablespoon	32.00	60.00	1.00	4.00	0.00	4.00	3.00			0.00	0.00	
Dip, baba ganoush, all natural, low fat, dry mix Casbah	0.5	Tablespoon	7.00	35.00	1.00	4.00	0.00	1.50	0.00			0.00	0.00	
Dip, bean, black Old El Paso	2	Tablespoon	30.00	25.00	1.00	5.00	1.00	0.00	0.00	0.00	0.00	0.00	0.00	
Dip, bean, black, mild Guiltless Gourmet	2	Tablespoon	30.00	30.00	2.00	5.00	1.00	0.00	0.00	0.00	0.00	0.00	0.00	
Dip, cheese, mild cheddar PepsiCo Fritos	2	Tablespoon	34.00	60.00	1.00	3.00	0.00	4.00	1.50			5.00	0.00	
Dip, hummus, original, dry mix Fantastic Foods International Dish	2	Tablespoon	19.00	80.00	3.00	11.00	1.00	3.00	0.50			0.00	0.00	
Dip, jalapeno Old El Paso	2	Tablespoon	29.00	30.00	1.00	4.00	2.00	1.00	0.00			3.00	0.00	
Dip, ranch Kraft General Foods, Inc.	2	Tablespoon	31.00	60.00	1.00	3.00	0.00	4.50	3.00			0.00	0.00	
Dip, ranch PepsiCo Frito Lay Ruffles	2	Tablespoon	33.00	60.00	1.00	1.00	0.25	5.00	2.50			3.00	0.00	
Guacamole, Rancho Grande, zesty, fzn JR Simplot	2	Tablespoon	30.00	40.00	0.00	3.00	1.00	3.50	0.50			0.00	5.00	
Guacamole, svg	1	Each	21.00	35.00	0.00	2.00	1.00	3.00	0.00			0.00	0.00	
Guacamole, w/tomatoes	2	Tablespoon	29.13	34.15	0.47	2.03	1.10	3.05	0.48	1.90	0.40	0.00	8.05	0.00
Mayonnaise														
Mayonnaise, light Kraft General Foods, Inc.	1	Tablespoon	15.00	50.10	0.09	1.28	0.02	4.94	0.75			5.25		
Mayonnaise, rducd fat, Just 2 Good!, jar Best Foods	1	Tablespoon	15.00	25.00	0.00	2.00	0.00	2.00	0.50			0.00	0.00	
Mayonnaise, soybean oil	1	Tablespoon	13.80	98.95	0.15	0.54	0.00	10.79	1.64	2.70	5.89	5.24	11.18	
Mayonnaise, soybean oil, unsalted	1	Tablespoon	13.80	98.95	0.15	0.37	0.00	10.96	1.63	3.13	5.12	8.14	11.59	0.04
Salad Dressings—Lower Calorie/Fat/Sodium/Cholesterol														
Dip, hummus, low fat, dry mix Casbah	2	Tablespoon	15.00	75.00	3.00	7.50	1.50	3.00	0.00			0.00	0.00	
Salad Dressing, blue cheese, low cal	2	Tablespoon	30.00	29.70	1.53	0.87	0.00	2.16	0.77	0.53	0.73	0.30	0.05	
Salad Dressing, French, diet, 5cal/tsp	2	Tablespoon	32.60	75.63	0.18	9.54	0.36	4.39	0.36	1.92	1.64	0.00	8.80	
Salad Dressing, honey dijon, fat free Kraft General Foods, Inc.	2	Tablespoon	34.00	45.00	0.00	10.00	1.00	0.00	0.00	0.00	0.00	0.00	0.00	
Salad Dressing, Italian, diet, 2cal/tsp, cmrcl	2	Tablespoon	30.00	22.50	0.14	1.37	0.00	1.91	0.14	0.66	0.51	1.80	0.30	
Salad Dressing, ranch, fat free	1	Ounce-weight	28.35	33.74	0.08	7.51	0.03	0.55	0.12	0.11	0.20	1.98	0.28	
Salad Dressing, ranch, fat free Kraft General Foods, Inc.	2	Tablespoon	35.00	48.30	0.24	10.71	0.21	0.35	0.07			0.35		
Salad Dressing, thousand island, diet, 10cal/tsp	2	Tablespoon	30.60	62.42	0.27	6.79	0.40	4.03	0.22	1.98	0.83	0.31	4.90	
Salad Dressing, vinaigrette, raspberry, fat free Seven Seas	2	Tablespoon	34.00	30.00	0.00	7.00	0.00	0.00	0.00	0.00	0.00	0.00	0.00	

Vit E (mg)	Vit C	Vit B$_1$ Thia (mg)	Vit B$_2$ Ribo (mg)	Vit B$_3$ Nia (mg)	Fol (mcg)	Vit B$_6$ (mg)	Vita B$_{12}$ (mcg)	Sodi (mg)	Pota (mg)	Cal (mg)	Phos (mg)	Magn (mg)	Iron (mg)	Zinc (mg)	Caff (mg)	Alco (g)	Sol Fiber (g)	Insol Fiber (g)
	0.00	0.03	0.09	4.08	4.25	0.24	0.20	722.93	263.66	0.85	204.12	14.46	1.53	1.72	0.00	0.00	0.00	0.00
	0.00							570.36	147.84	7.56	165.48	17.64	0.73	1.54	0.00	0.00		
1.28	0.00	0.06	0.11	1.34	18.50	0.13	0.15	534.56	165.85	8.93	149.27	9.57	1.40	0.93	0.00	0.00		
0.82	0.00	0.07	0.22	2.05	5.10	0.20	0.20	371.67	204.97	6.80	145.44	14.46	1.28	3.50	0.00	0.00	0.00	0.00
0.20	0.51	0.06	0.19	5.34	1.70	0.30	0.26	53.58	212.63	11.06	126.72	16.16	0.65	1.30	0.00	0.00	0.00	0.00
0.31	0.43	0.06	0.17	5.02	1.70	0.26	0.24	54.43	208.37	11.06	124.17	15.31	0.77	1.27	0.00	0.00	0.00	0.00
0.05	2.47	0.24	0.30	6.46	5.10	0.48	0.35	48.48	217.73	14.46	282.37	22.11	5.03	3.26	0.00	0.00	0.00	0.00
0.33	7.03	0.47	0.35	3.91	28.35	0.71	0.86	64.64	303.91	3.40	210.92	24.95	5.11	0.84	0.00	0.00	0.00	0.00
0.60	0.00	0.15	0.23	4.10	5.10	0.15	0.26	50.18	173.50	9.36	132.68	13.61	2.30	1.58	0.00	0.00	0.00	0.00
0.60	0.00	0.22	0.40	4.34	8.51	0.21	0.34	55.28	214.33	10.21	172.65	17.01	2.30	2.21	0.00	0.00	0.00	0.00
0.60	0.00	0.15	0.23	4.10	5.10	0.15	0.26	50.18	173.50	9.36	132.68	13.61	2.30	1.58	0.00	0.00	0.00	0.00
	2.72		8.80	8.80				89.30		7.65			3.82		0.00	0.00	0.00	0.00
0.20	0.00	0.27	0.46	7.59	7.65	0.71	7.25	55.28	318.94	6.80	228.78	24.66	4.26	3.88	0.00	0.00		
1.30	8.16	0.15	0.43	4.85	35.15	0.73	0.56	98.66	476.28	14.74	353.81	27.22	2.91	2.65	0.00	0.00		
1.32	0.00	0.08	0.33	3.47	10.21	0.40	0.42	64.64	329.99	11.91	262.80	21.26	2.44	2.70	0.00	0.00		
0.34	1.47	0.07	0.12	8.69	5.67	0.43	0.39	75.98	218.86	12.47	173.50	24.95	0.95	1.28	0.00	0.00	0.00	0.00
0.20	0.00	0.18	0.23	5.58	11.91	0.43	4.88	68.04	274.71	6.80	190.51	19.56	2.92	3.68	0.00	0.00	0.00	0.00
	0.00							240.00	25.00	0.00	0.00		0.00		0.00	0.00	0.00	0.00
	1.20							100.00		0.00			0.36		0.00	0.00	0.00	0.00
	0.00							280.00		0.00			0.36		0.00	0.00		
	1.20							100.00		20.00			0.36		0.00	0.00		
	0.00							330.00		60.00			0.00		0.00	0.00		0.00
	0.00							280.00		20.00			1.44		0.00	0.00		
	0.00							125.00		0.00			0.36		0.00	0.00		
	0.00							210.00	20.00	0.00			0.00		0.00	0.00	0.00	0.00
	0.00							240.00		0.00			0.00		0.00	0.00		
	3.60							110.00		0.00			0.36		0.00	0.00		
	0.00							100.00		0.00			0.00		0.00	0.00		
0.29	3.53	0.03	0.03	0.42	13.66	0.06	0.00	2.62	136.98	3.08	10.26	8.68	0.24	0.09	0.00	0.00		
0.57	0.05							119.55	7.80	0.90	8.70		0.03		0.00	0.00		
	0.00							130.00		0.00			0.00		0.00	0.00	0.00	0.00
0.72	0.00	0.00	0.00	0.00	1.10	0.08	0.04	78.38	4.69	2.48	3.86	0.14	0.07	0.02	0.00	0.00	0.00	0.00
2.87	0.00	0.00	0.00	0.00	1.06	0.08	0.04	4.14	4.69	2.48	3.86		0.07		0.00	0.00	0.00	0.00
	0.00							240.00		0.00			0.54		0.00	0.00		
0.08	0.09	0.01	0.03	0.02	0.90	0.01	0.07	360.00	1.50	26.70	24.90	2.10	0.15	0.08	0.00	0.00	0.00	0.00
0.10	0.00	0.01	0.02	0.15	0.65	0.02	0.00	262.10	34.88	3.59	5.22	2.61	0.28	0.07	0.00	0.00		
	0.00							330.00	35.00	0.00	20.00		0.00		0.00	0.00		
0.06	0.00	0.00	0.00	0.00	0.00	0.02	0.00	409.80	25.50	2.70	3.30	1.20	0.20	0.06	0.00	0.00	0.00	0.00
0.05	0.00	0.01	0.01	0.00	1.70	0.01	0.00	214.04	31.47	14.17	32.04	2.27	0.30	0.11	0.00	0.00		
	0.03							353.85	30.80	9.10	27.65		0.02		0.00	0.00		
0.31	0.00	0.01	0.01	0.13	0.00	0.00	0.00	254.29	61.81	4.90	4.28	2.14	0.29	0.06	0.00	0.00		
	0.00							320.00	15.00	0.00	0.00		0.00		0.00	0.00	0.00	0.00

Food Name	Amount	Measure	Weight (g)	Calories	Protein (g)	Total Carb (g)	Dietary Fiber (g)	Total Fat (g)	Sat Fat (g)	Mono Fat (g)	Poly Fat (g)	Chol (mg)	Vit A (mcg RAE)	Vit D (mcg)
SALAD DRESSINGS, DIPS, AND MAYONNAISE *(continued)*														
Salad Dressings—Regular														
Salad Dressing, blue cheese, cmrcl	2	Tablespoon	30.60	154.22	1.47	2.26	0.00	16.00	3.03	3.76	8.51	5.20	20.50	0.09
Salad Dressing, caesar	2	Tablespoon	29.40	155.23	0.35	0.91	0.03	16.96	2.58	3.97	9.66	0.59	0.59	
Salad Dressing, French, cmrcl	2	Tablespoon	31.20	142.58	0.24	4.86	0.00	13.98	1.76	2.63	6.56	0.00	7.18	
Salad Dressing, honey dijon Kraft General Foods, Inc.	2	Tablespoon	31.00	110.00	0.00	6.00	0.00	10.00	1.50			0.00	0.00	
Salad Dressing, Newman's Own, ranch, pkg USDA SR-23 McDonald's	2	Fluid ounce	56.00	175.28	1.47	9.38	0.17	14.88	2.44	8.60	3.56	17.92		
Salad Dressing, Italian, cmrcl	2	Tablespoon	29.40	85.55	0.11	3.07	0.00	8.34	1.31	1.85	3.80	0.00	0.59	
Salad Dressing, ranch Kraft General Foods, Inc.	2	Tablespoon	29.00	147.90	0.41	1.33	0.09	15.57	2.38			8.12		
Salad Dressing, ranch, cmrcl	1	Ounce-weight	28.35	137.21	0.29	1.90	0.20	14.57	2.28	3.23	8.03	9.36	2.83	0.02
Salad Dressing, sesame seed	2	Tablespoon	30.60	135.56	0.95	2.63	0.30	13.83	1.90	3.64	7.68	0.00	0.61	
Salad Dressing, sweet and sour	2	Tablespoon	32.00	4.80	0.03	1.18	0.00	0.00	0.00	0.00	0.00	0.00	0.00	
Salad Dressing, thousand island Kraft General Foods, Inc.	2	Tablespoon	31.00	110.00	0.00	5.00	0.00	10.00	1.50			10.00	0.00	
Salad Dressing, vinaigrette, herb Seven Seas	2	Tablespoon	30.00	140.00	0.00	1.00	0.00	15.00	2.00			0.00	0.00	
Salad Dressing, vinegar & oil, prep f/recipe	2	Tablespoon	31.20	140.09	0.00	0.78	0.00	15.63	2.84	4.62	7.52	0.00	0.00	
SALADS														
Cole Slaw, prep f/recipe	0.5	Cup	60.00	41.40	0.77	7.45	0.90	1.57	0.23	0.42	0.81	4.80	31.80	
Salad, bean, three	0.5	Cup	75.00	70.05	2.17	7.45	2.66	3.79	0.55	0.85	2.19	0.00	5.79	
Salad, fruit, w/ight syrup, cnd, not drained, cup	0.5	Cup	126.00	73.08	0.43	19.08	1.26	0.09	0.01	0.02	0.04	0.00	26.46	
Salad, fruit, w/juice, cnd, not drained, cup	0.5	Cup	124.50	62.25	0.63	16.25	1.25	0.04	0.00	0.01	0.01	0.00	37.35	
Salad, macaroni, elbow, classic, FS Orval Kent Food Company	0.5	Cup	106.00	196.86	3.03	24.99	1.51	9.09	1.51			7.57		
Salad, potato, prep f/recipe	0.5	Cup	125.00	178.75	3.35	13.96	1.62	10.25	1.79	3.10	4.67	85.00	40.00	
Salad, seafood	0.5	Cup	104.00	163.88	12.88	2.28	0.35	11.46	1.59	7.98	1.18	65.76	17.21	
Salad, tabouli/tabbouleh	0.5	Cup	80.00	99.56	1.31	8.02	1.87	7.50	1.02	5.41	0.69	0.00	17.14	
SANDWICHES														
Cheeseburger, reg, w/condiments	1	Each	113.00	294.93	15.96	26.53		14.15	6.31	5.35	1.09	37.29	85.88	
Pizza, pocket, pepperoni, fzn Chef America, Inc.	1	Each	128.00	367.36	13.57	38.66		17.66	6.63	6.35	2.00	40.96		
Sandwich, bbq beef, w/bun	1	Each	186.00	357.53	18.26	36.33	2.38	14.78	5.03	6.59	1.43	46.44	36.28	
Sandwich, bbq pork, w/bun	1	Each	186.00	321.95	22.76	34.36	2.25	9.57	2.80	4.37	1.42	50.65	35.49	
Sandwich, breakfast, egg cheese, w/biscuit, preckd, fzn Sunny Fresh	1	Each	99.23	224.26	9.89	24.64	0.00	8.89	2.36	1.14	3.68	111.14		
Sandwich, breakfast, egg ham cheese, w/biscuit, preckd, fzn Sunny Fresh	1	Each	120.40	243.21	12.24	25.21	0.12	9.70	2.63	1.23	3.77	114.38		
Sandwich, chicken, bbq	1	Each	119.00	251.42	20.53	26.85	1.32	6.19	1.58	2.40	1.40	50.10	14.22	
Sandwich, chicken, fillet, plain	1	Each	182.00	515.06	24.12	38.69		29.45	8.53	10.41	8.38	60.06	30.94	
Sandwich, egg patty cheese, vegetarian, w/English muffin Morningstar Farms	1	Each	171.00	277.88	30.01	32.71	7.01	2.99				3.69		
Sandwich, fajita beef, w/cheese, w/pita	1	Each	207.00	292.45	19.36	28.05	2.49	11.37	4.42	3.21	2.69	39.39	70.09	
Sandwich, fish, w/tartar sauce	1	Each	158.00	431.34	16.94	41.02	0.40	22.77	5.23	7.69	8.25	55.30	33.18	
Sandwich, ham cheese, grilled	1	Each	141.00	380.90	20.57	29.77	1.19	19.59	7.91	7.86	2.42	54.15	98.97	
Sandwich, ham cheese, pocket, fzn Chef America, Inc.	1	Each	128.00	340.48	14.85	38.40		14.21	5.79	4.42	1.48	49.92	0.00	
Sandwich, meatball, w/mozzarella, pocket, fzn Chef America, Inc.	1	Each	128.00	320.00	13.00	41.00	2.00	11.00	5.00			35.00	0.00	
Sandwich, meatball, w/mozzarella, pocket, fzn Chef America, Inc.	1	Each	128.00	300.00	13.00	44.00	2.00	7.00	3.50			30.00	0.00	
Sandwich, philly steak cheese, pocket, fzn Chef America, Inc.	1	Each	128.00	350.00	12.00	40.00	2.00	16.00	7.00			45.00	0.00	
Sandwich, philly steak cheese, pocket, fzn Chef America, Inc.	1	Each	128.00	290.00	12.00	43.00	2.00	7.00	3.00			30.00	0.00	
Sandwich, roast beef, plain	1	Each	139.00	346.11	21.50	33.44		13.76	3.61	6.80	1.71	51.43	11.12	
Sandwich, roast beef, w/cheese	1	Each	176.00	473.44	32.23	45.37		18.00	9.03	3.66	3.50	77.44	58.08	

Vit E (mg)	Vit C	Vit B₁ Thia (mg)	Vit B₂ Ribo (mg)	Vit B₃ Nia (mg)	Fol (mcg)	Vit B₆ (mg)	Vita B₁₂ (mcg)	Sodi (mg)	Pota (mg)	Cal (mg)	Phos (mg)	Magn (mg)	Iron (mg)	Zinc (mg)	Caff (mg)	Alco (g)	Sol Fiber (g)	Insol Fiber (g)
1.84	0.61	0.00	0.03	0.03	8.57	0.01	0.08	334.76	11.32	24.79	22.64	0.00	0.06	0.08	0.00	0.00	0.00	0.00
1.54	0.00	0.00	0.00	0.01	0.88	0.00	0.01	316.93	8.53	7.06	5.59	0.59	0.05	0.03	0.00	0.00		
1.56	0.00	0.01	0.02	0.06	0.00	0.00	0.04	260.83	20.90	7.49	5.93	1.56	0.25	0.09	0.00	0.00	0.00	0.00
	0.00							210.00	35.00	0.00	0.00		0.00		0.00	0.00	0.00	0.00
	0.45	0.01	0.08	0.01	0.56	0.02	0.00	534.24	67.20	43.12	42.56	1.68	0.14	0.03	0.00	0.00		
1.47	0.00	0.00	0.01	0.00	0.00	0.02	0.00	486.28	14.11	2.06	2.65	0.88	0.19	0.04	0.00	0.00	0.00	0.00
	0.06							287.10	14.21	8.41	26.39		0.05		0.00	0.00		
1.34	0.96	0.03	0.02	0.00	1.13	0.01	0.09	231.34	17.58	8.79	45.64	1.42	0.18	0.11	0.00	0.00		
1.53	0.00	0.00	0.00	0.00	0.00	0.00	0.00	306.00	48.04	5.81	11.32	0.00	0.18	0.03	0.00	0.00		
0.82	2.59	0.00	0.00	0.02	0.64	0.00	0.00	66.56	10.56	1.28	0.96	0.96	0.01	0.01	0.00	0.00	0.00	0.00
	0.00							310.00	40.00	0.00	0.00		0.00		0.00	0.00	0.00	0.00
	0.00							250.00	10.00	0.00	0.00		0.00		0.00	0.00	0.00	0.00
1.44	0.00	0.00	0.00	0.00	0.00	0.00	0.00	0.31	2.50	0.00	0.00	0.00	0.00	0.00	0.00	0.00	0.00	0.00
0.06	19.62	0.04	0.04	0.16	16.20	0.08	0.00	13.80	108.60	27.00	19.20	6.00	0.35	0.12	0.00	0.00		
0.87	2.02	0.04	0.05	0.22	28.00	0.02	0.01	260.09	123.26	17.64	37.82	13.74	0.74	0.29	0.00	0.00		
0.82	3.15	0.02	0.03	0.46	3.78	0.04	0.00	7.56	103.32	8.82	11.34	6.30	0.37	0.09	0.00	0.00		
0.75	4.11	0.01	0.02	0.44	3.74	0.03	0.00	6.23	144.42	13.70	17.43	9.96	0.31	0.17	0.00	0.00	0.61	0.63
								560.29							0.00	0.00		
2.32	12.50	0.10	0.07	1.12	8.75	0.18	0.00	661.25	317.50	23.75	65.00	18.75	0.81	0.38	0.00	0.00		
2.00	6.19	0.04	0.05	1.18	15.67	0.09	0.92	176.13	251.49	46.22	141.39	27.12	0.99	1.65	0.00	0.00		
1.08	14.25	0.04	0.03	0.57	15.54	0.06	0.00	399.53	122.78	14.49	31.78	17.79	0.62	0.24	0.00	0.00		
0.53	1.92	0.25	0.23	3.72	54.24	0.11	0.94	615.85	222.61	110.74	176.28	20.34	2.43	2.09	0.00	0.00		
								675.84	280.32				3.16		0.00	0.00		
1.28	5.84	0.29	0.27	5.73	21.75	0.23	1.52	1008.14	367.68	92.42	149.28	35.53	3.63	3.16	0.00	0.00		
1.25	5.70	0.76	0.37	5.65	19.71	0.34	0.45	947.67	426.09	94.40	197.79	39.16	2.89	2.21	0.00	0.00		
1.98	0.00	0.24	0.30	2.02	11.91	0.04	0.27	564.62	39.69	101.21	49.62	2.98	2.25	0.30	0.00	0.00	0.00	0.00
2.41	0.12	0.24	0.31	2.02	12.04	0.04	0.29	724.81	46.96	105.95	54.18	3.61	2.44	0.33	0.00	0.00		
0.43	0.85	0.28	0.28	7.25	21.20	0.30	0.19	422.13	217.40	65.86	159.11	28.39	2.33	1.51	0.00	0.00		
	8.92	0.33	0.24	6.81	100.10	0.20	0.38	957.32	353.08	60.06	232.96	34.58	4.68	1.87	0.00	0.00		
	0.00	5.30	1.06	7.83		0.10	1.32	1051.14	354.14	283.35	579.69		6.05	2.77	0.00	0.00		
1.46	33.41	0.34	0.30	4.16	36.85	0.42	1.66	777.86	464.05	182.39	251.77	38.55	2.54	2.72	0.00	0.00		
0.87	2.84	0.33	0.22	3.40	85.32	0.11	1.07	614.62	339.70	83.74	211.72	33.18	2.61	1.00	0.00	0.00		
1.11	0.01	0.71	0.44	5.01	16.41	0.27	0.81	1464.85	337.38	233.26	342.97	32.40	2.41	2.47	0.00	0.00		
								665.60	250.88				2.61		0.00	0.00		
	0.00							660.00	250.00				3.60		0.00	0.00		
	0.00							600.00	300.00				3.60		0.00	0.00		
	0.00							630.00	250.00				2.70		0.00	0.00		
	0.00							560.00	250.00				3.60		0.00	0.00		
0.19	2.08	0.38	0.31	5.87	56.99	0.26	1.22	792.30	315.53	54.21	239.08	30.58	4.23	3.39	0.00	0.00		
	0.00	0.39	0.46	5.90	63.36	0.33	2.06	1633.28	344.96	183.04	401.28	40.48	5.05	5.37	0.00	0.00		

Food Name	Amount	Measure	Weight (g)	Calories	Protein (g)	Total Carb (g)	Dietary Fiber (g)	Total Fat (g)	Sat Fat (g)	Mono Fat (g)	Poly Fat (g)	Chol (mg)	Vit A (mcg RAE)	Vit D (mcg)
SANDWICHES *(continued)*														
Sandwich, sausage, w/biscuit, fzn, Jimmy Dean, FS Travis Meats	1	Each	48.00	192.48	4.75	11.57	0.72	14.11	4.31			15.84		
Sandwich, steak	1	Each	204.00	459.00	30.33	51.96		14.08	3.81	5.34	3.35	73.44	20.40	
Sandwich, submarine, w/cold cuts	1	Each	228.00	456.00	21.84	51.05	1.70	18.63	6.81	8.23	2.28	36.48	70.68	
Sandwich, submarine, w/roast beef	1	Each	216.00	410.40	28.64	44.30		12.96	7.09	1.84	2.61	73.44	30.24	
Sandwich, submarine, w/tuna salad	1	Each	256.00	583.68	29.70	55.37		27.98	5.33	13.40	7.30	48.64	46.08	
SAUCES AND GRAVIES														
Gravies														
Gravy, au jus, dry mix	1	Teaspoon	3.00	9.39	0.28	1.42		0.29	0.06	0.14	0.01	0.12	0.03	
Gravy, beef, can	0.25	Cup	58.25	30.87	2.18	2.80	0.23	1.37	0.67	0.56	0.05	1.75	0.58	
Gravy, beef, hearty, jar Pepperidge Farm	0.25	Cup	60.00	25.80	1.80	3.72		0.42	0.14	0.15	0.04	3.00	0.00	
Gravy, brown, dry mix	1	Tablespoon	6.00	22.02	0.64	3.56	0.12	0.58	0.20	0.27	0.02	0.18	0.48	
Gravy, brown, dry mix, 16oz pkg Trio	1	Tablespoon	6.00	24.36	0.63	3.47	0.21	0.89	0.26	0.16	0.46	0.00		
Gravy, brown, homestyle, savory, cnd Heinz	0.25	Cup	60.00	24.60	0.90	3.41		0.78	0.32	0.28	0.04	2.40		
Gravy, chicken, can	0.25	Cup	59.50	47.01	1.15	3.22	0.24	3.40	0.84	1.52	0.89	1.19	0.60	
Gravy, chicken, dry pkt	1	Tablespoon	8.00	30.48	0.90	4.97		0.78	0.23	0.37	0.15	1.52	3.04	
Gravy, country, dry mix, 22oz pkg Trio	1	Tablespoon	8.00	34.64	0.73	5.19	0.72	1.22	0.32	0.14	0.54	0.48	0.00	
Gravy, mushroom, dry mix, svg, makes 1 cup prep	1	Each	21.30	69.86	2.13	13.77	1.02	0.85	0.50	0.28	0.03	0.64	0.01	
Gravy, pork, dry mix, svg	1	Each	6.70	24.59	0.59	4.26	0.16	0.58	0.29	0.26	0.03	0.67	2.28	
Gravy, southern, dry mix Trio	1	Tablespoon	10.00	48.10	0.25	6.05	0.00	2.55	0.56	0.30	1.19	0.20		
Gravy, turkey, dry mix, svg	1	Each	7.00	25.69	0.73	4.56		0.50	0.14	0.18	0.15	0.98	0.56	
Sauces														
Marinade, cooking sauce, teriyaki S & W	1	Tablespoon	18.00	25.00	1.00	5.00	0.00	0.00	0.00	0.00	0.00	0.00	0.00	
Sauce, alfredo Unilever Carb Options	0.25	Cup	61.00	110.00	1.00	2.00	0.00	10.00	3.50			30.00		
Sauce, alfredo, creamy garlic, dry mix McCormick & Co.	2	Tablespoon	18.00	90.00	3.00	4.00		6.00				20.00		
Sauce, alfredo, dry mix Corn Products International	2	Tablespoon	15.00	61.80	2.22	7.13		2.72	1.61	1.01	0.09	5.40		
Sauce, barbecue USDA SR-23	1	Fluid ounce	31.25	46.88	0.00	11.33	0.19	0.09	0.00	0.02	0.05	0.00	3.67	0.00
Sauce, bearnaise, dehyd, svg, makes 1 cup prep	1	Each	16.50	59.73	2.32	9.86	0.10	1.49	0.22	0.64	0.56	0.17	0.17	
Sauce, cheese, cheddar, basic, rts Chef-Mate	0.25	Cup	62.00	81.84	1.80	8.02	0.00	4.70	1.57			6.20		
Sauce, cheese, cheddar, inst, dry mix, FS Custom Food Products Superb	2	Tablespoon	14.20	60.07	1.13	8.02	0.62	2.60	1.51	0.95	0.14	3.83		
Sauce, cheese, dry mix, 2lb pkg Nestle Foods Company	2	Tablespoon	12.00	53.52	0.89	7.31	0.00	2.30	0.78	0.88	0.63	2.28		
Sauce, cheese, nacho, dry mix, 2lb pkg Nestle Foods Company	2	Tablespoon	12.00	51.36	1.07	7.57	0.07	1.86	0.80	0.54	0.42	2.04		
Sauce, cheese, nacho, rts, pkg Ortega	0.25	Cup	63.00	127.89	5.24	4.02	0.44	10.10	5.80			28.98		
Sauce, cocktail Kraft	0.25	Cup	66.00	60.00	1.00	13.00	1.00	0.50	0.00			0.00		
Sauce, creole, rts, pkg Chef-Mate	0.25	Cup	62.00	24.80	0.92	3.71	0.81	0.69	0.07	0.23	0.29	0.00		
Sauce, curry, dehyd, pkt	1	Each	35.40	151.16	3.31	17.93	0.46	8.18	1.21	3.51	3.08	0.35	1.76	
Sauce, enchilada, rts Ortega	2	Tablespoon	30.00	15.00	0.44	2.01	0.30	0.59	0.09	0.17	0.28	0.00		
Sauce, fish, rts	2	Tablespoon	36.00	12.60	1.82	1.31	0.00	0.00	0.00	0.00	0.00	0.00	1.44	
Sauce, hoisin, rts	2	Tablespoon	32.00	70.40	1.06	14.11	0.90	1.08	0.18	0.31	0.54	0.96	0.10	
Sauce, hollandaise, prep f/recipe	2	Tablespoon	20.00	85.44	1.00	0.26		9.09	5.13	2.78	0.50	89.99	96.94	
Sauce, lemon, rts, pkg Chef-Mate	2	Tablespoon	32.00	42.88	0.07	10.21	0.00	0.19	0.02	0.05	0.09	0.00		
Sauce, marinara Di Giorno	0.5	Cup	127.00	70.00	2.00	15.00	2.00	0.00	0.00	0.00	0.00	0.00	25.00	
Sauce, mole poblano, prep f/recipe	2	Tablespoon	30.30	49.69	1.07	3.92	1.27	3.32		1.46	0.86	0.28	45.45	
Sauce, mushroom, dehyd, svg, makes 1 cup prep	1	Each	22.70	79.22	3.26	12.42		2.16	0.32	0.93	0.81	0.00	0.00	
Sauce, oyster, rts	2	Tablespoon	8.00	4.08	0.11	0.87	0.02	0.02	0.00	0.01	0.01	0.00	0.00	
Sauce, pasta, fresh mushroom, jar Prego	0.5	Cup	122.80	120.00	2.00	21.00	3.00	3.50	1.50			0.00		
Sauce, pasta, marinara, jar Prego	0.5	Cup	122.80	90.00	2.00	10.00	3.00	5.00	1.50			0.00		
Sauce, pasta, pesto, dry mix Knorr	2	Teaspoon	5.00	15.00	1.00	3.00	0.00	0.00	0.00	0.00	0.00	0.00		
Sauce, pasta, smooth, traditional, jar, Old World Style Ragu	0.5	Cup	125.00	80.00	1.88	12.11	2.62	2.62	0.36	0.55	1.29	0.00	32.50	
Sauce, pepper/hot, rts	1	Teaspoon	4.70	0.52	0.02	0.08	0.01	0.02	0.00	0.00	0.01	0.00	0.38	

Vit E (mg)	Vit C	Vit B₁ Thia (mg)	Vit B₂ Ribo (mg)	Vit B₃ Nia (mg)	Fol (mcg)	Vit B₆ (mg)	Vita B₁₂ (mcg)	Sodi (mg)	Pota (mg)	Cal (mg)	Phos (mg)	Magn (mg)	Iron (mg)	Zinc (mg)	Caff (mg)	Alco (g)	Sol Fiber (g)	Insol Fiber (g)
								440.64		37.92			0.79		0.00	0.00		
	5.51	0.41	0.37	7.30	89.76	0.37	1.57	797.64	524.28	91.80	297.84	48.96	5.16	4.53	0.00	0.00		
	12.31	1.00	0.80	5.49	86.64	0.14	1.09	1650.72	394.44	189.24	287.28	68.40	2.51	2.58	0.00	0.00		
	5.62	0.41	0.41	5.96	71.28	0.32	1.81	844.56	330.48	41.04	192.24	66.96	2.81	4.38	0.00	0.00		
	3.58	0.46	0.33	11.34	102.40	0.23	1.61	1292.80	335.36	74.24	220.16	79.36	2.64	1.87	0.00	0.00		
0.01	0.03	0.01	0.01	0.12	2.43	0.01	0.01	347.64	8.37	4.20	4.59	1.68	0.28	0.02	0.00	0.00		
0.01	0.00	0.02	0.02	0.38	1.16	0.01	0.06	326.20	47.18	3.49	17.47	1.16	0.41	0.58	0.00	0.00		
								378.60							0.00	0.00		
0.02	0.02	0.01	0.02	0.22	1.86	0.01	0.04	290.58	15.72	7.92	12.18	2.04	0.10	0.07	0.00	0.00		
0.04	0.00	0.00	0.00	0.01	1.56	0.00	0.00	261.78	0.84	2.16	7.32	0.48	0.11	0.04	0.00	0.00		
								351.60							0.00	0.00		
0.08	0.00	0.01	0.03	0.26	1.19	0.01	0.06	343.32	64.86	11.90	17.26	1.19	0.28	0.48	0.00	0.00		
0.02	0.05	0.02	0.05	0.32	10.00	0.02	0.04	332.16	32.32	11.68	19.92	3.20	0.11	0.11	0.00	0.00		
0.07	0.00	0.01	0.02	0.10	0.80	0.00	0.01	204.72	11.12	5.20	8.88	1.12	0.10	0.05	0.00	0.00		
0.03	1.49	0.04	0.09	0.79	6.60	0.02	0.15	1401.54	55.81	48.99	43.24	7.24	0.21	0.33	0.00	0.00		
0.02	0.09	0.01	0.02	0.15	2.08	0.01	0.03	358.85	15.75	9.31	12.60	2.28	0.26	0.07	0.00	0.00		
0.43	0.07	0.00	0.01	0.01	0.30	0.00	0.02	290.00	13.80	7.50	6.60	1.40	0.06	0.03	0.00	0.00	0.00	0.00
0.01	0.01	0.01	0.03	0.19	5.74	0.01	0.04	307.44	29.96	10.22	17.78	3.08	0.23	0.09	0.00	0.00		
	3.00							480.00	40.00	0.00			0.00		0.00	0.00	0.00	0.00
	0.00							390.00		40.00			0.00		0.00	0.00	0.00	0.00
								860.00							0.00	0.00		
								730.20							0.00	0.00		
0.21	0.22	0.00	0.01	0.15	0.62	0.01	0.00	264.69	65.00	3.75	5.31	3.75	0.07	0.04	0.00	0.00		
0.05	0.33	0.02	0.03	0.10	2.15	0.01	0.07	559.35	48.18	27.23	24.42	4.62	0.08	0.12	0.00	0.00		
1.24	0.56	0.00	0.04	0.04	1.86	0.01	0.06	471.20	16.12	45.88	50.84	3.72	0.18	0.33	0.00	0.00	0.00	0.00
0.33	0.14	0.03	0.10	0.34	19.03	0.03	0.07	685.15	60.78	40.47	40.19	5.11	0.07	0.16	0.00	0.00		
0.28	0.00	0.03	0.08	0.29	16.08	0.02	0.06	309.60	51.36	21.96	33.96	4.32	0.09	0.13	0.00	0.00	0.00	0.00
0.28	0.29	0.03	0.08	0.29	16.08	0.02	0.06	338.40	51.36	20.04	33.96	4.32	0.09	0.13	0.00	0.00		
0.26	0.44	0.00	0.08	0.02	3.15	0.01	0.09	579.60	20.16	180.81	105.21	6.30	0.15	0.65	0.00	0.00		
	6.00							800.00					0.36		0.00	0.00		
0.61		0.03	0.02	0.53	8.68	0.07	0.00	339.14	187.24	34.72	17.36	8.68	0.31	0.10	0.00	0.00		
	0.71	0.04	0.08	0.29	3.19	0.01	0.14	1444.32	124.61	62.66	52.75	14.51	1.10	0.31	0.00	0.00		
0.00	2.13	0.02	0.01	0.32	2.40	0.04	0.00	77.40	83.40	7.20	10.50	5.10	0.31	0.06	0.00	0.00		
0.00	0.18	0.00	0.02	0.83	18.36	0.14	0.17	2779.20	103.68	15.48	2.52	63.00	0.28	0.07	0.00	0.00	0.00	0.00
0.09	0.13	0.00	0.07	0.37	7.36	0.02	0.00	516.80	38.08	10.24	12.16	7.68	0.32	0.10	0.00	0.00		
0.32	0.85	0.01	0.04	0.01	8.49	0.02	0.18	77.83	9.79	9.88	28.88	0.82	0.21	0.18	0.00	0.00		
0.01	2.75	0.00	0.00	0.01	0.32	0.00	0.00	2.56	6.40	1.28	1.28	0.64	0.12	0.01	0.00	0.00	0.00	0.00
		0.09	0.10	1.60	0.00		0.00	220.00	400.00	40.00	20.00		0.72		0.00	0.00		
0.44	0.00	0.01	0.00	0.50	8.48	0.08	0.01	40.60	98.78	7.27	24.85	9.70	0.56	0.14	0.00	0.00		
0.00	0.00	0.02	0.11	1.04	6.13	0.02	0.00	1414.21	98.29	2.04	30.19	4.09	0.23	0.20	0.00	0.00		
0.00	0.01	0.00	0.01	0.12	1.20	0.00	0.03	218.64	4.32	2.56	1.76	0.32	0.01	0.01	0.00	0.00		
	2.40							560.00		20.00			1.08		0.00	0.00		
	2.40							550.00		40.00			0.72		0.00	0.00		
	0.00							490.00		0.00			0.00		0.00	0.00	0.00	0.00
								756.25					1.02		0.00	0.00		
0.01	3.52	0.00	0.00	0.01	0.28	0.01	0.00	124.22	6.77	0.38	0.52	0.23	0.02	0.01	0.00	0.00		

Food Name	Amount	Measure	Weight (g)	Calories	Protein (g)	Total Carb (g)	Dietary Fiber (g)	Total Fat (g)	Sat Fat (g)	Mono Fat (g)	Poly Fat (g)	Chol (mg)	Vit A (mcg RAE)	Vit D (mcg)
SAUCES AND GRAVIES *(continued)*														
Sauce, pesto USDA Survey Database	2	Tablespoon	29.00	155.03	5.60	2.03	0.88	14.20	3.82	8.70	1.00	10.00	30.04	0.00
Sauce, pizza, traditional, all natural, Prince Heinz	1	Ounce-weight	28.35	12.23	0.55	2.27	0.62	0.10	0.02	0.06	0.02	0.29	10.66	
Sauce, plum, rts	2	Tablespoon	38.13	70.15	0.34	16.32	0.27	0.40	0.06	0.09	0.22	0.00	0.76	
Salsa, rts	2	Tablespoon	32.38	8.74	0.50	2.03	0.52	0.05	0.01	0.01	0.04	0.00	4.86	
Sauce, sofrito, prep f/recipe, tbsp	2	Tablespoon	29.80	70.63	3.81	1.63	0.51	5.42						
Sauce, sour cream, dehyd, svg	1	Ounce-weight	28.35	145.16	4.45	13.69		8.89	4.45	3.03	1.00	22.68	20.42	
Sauce, spaghetti, w/meat, cnd Del Monte Foods	0.5	Cup	125.00	60.00	3.00	14.00	3.00	1.00	0.00			0.00		
Sauce, spaghetti/marinara, rts	0.5	Cup	125.00	92.50	2.44	14.09	0.50	2.97	0.41	0.95	1.18	0.00	33.75	
Sauce, sweet & sour ConAgra Foods La Choy	1	Ounce-weight	28.35	48.20	0.05	11.94	0.00	0.04	0.00			0.00	0.00	
Sauce, sweet & sour, dehyd, svg	1	Ounce-weight	28.35	110.28	0.27	27.24	0.54	0.03	0.00	0.00	0.03	0.00	0.00	
Sauce, szechuan, rts Chef-Mate	2	Tablespoon	32.00	41.60	0.46	5.84	0.10	1.82	0.24	0.53	0.88			
Sauce, tartar Kraft	2	Tablespoon	31.00	70.00		4.00		6.00	1.00			5.00	0.00	
Sauce, teriyaki, rts Chef-Mate	2	Tablespoon	32.00	41.60	0.30	7.48	0.00	1.16	0.12	0.34	0.56	0.00	0.00	
Sauce, tzatziki FAGE USA FAGE Total	2	Tablespoon	28.00	30.00	1.00	2.00	0.00	2.00	1.00			5.00	0.00	
Sauce, white, thick, prep f/recipe	2	Tablespoon	31.25	58.12	1.25	3.63	0.09	4.32	1.07	1.83	1.22	1.88	36.56	
Tomato Paste, 6oz can	0.25	Cup	65.50	53.71	2.84	12.38	2.95	0.31	0.07	0.04	0.15	0.00	49.78	
Tomato Sauce, cnd	0.5	Cup	122.50	39.20	1.61	9.02	1.84	0.29	0.04	0.04	0.12	0.00	20.83	
SNACK FOODS—CHIPS, PRETZELS, POPCORN														
Cheese Puffs, white cheddar, svg Season's Enterprises, Ltd.	1	Each	30.00	180.00	3.00	13.00	2.00	13.00	3.00			5.00	0.00	
Chips, bagel	5	Piece	70.00	298.18	6.18	52.41	4.25	7.33	1.26	2.08	3.45	0.00		
Chips, corn cones, plain, extruded	1	Ounce-weight	28.35	144.58	1.64	17.83	0.31	7.63	6.45	0.48	0.22	0.00	4.54	
Chips, corn, bbq flvr, extruded, 7oz bag	1	Ounce-weight	28.35	148.27	1.98	15.93	1.47	9.27	1.27	2.68	4.58	0.00	8.79	
Chips, corn, plain, extruded, 7oz bag	1	Ounce-weight	28.35	152.81	1.87	16.13	1.39	9.47	1.29	2.74	4.67	0.00	1.42	
Chips, potato, bbq flvr, 7 oz bag	1	Ounce-weight	28.35	139.20	2.18	14.97	1.25	9.19	2.29	·1.85	4.64	0.00	3.12	
Chips, potato, bkd	1	Ounce-weight	28.35	132.96	1.42	20.25	1.37	5.15	0.76	2.81	1.20	0.00	0.00	
Chips, potato, cheese flvr, f/dried potato, can	1	Ounce-weight	28.35	156.21	1.98	14.35	0.96	10.49	2.71	2.02	5.29	1.13	0.28	
Chips, potato, fat free, Wow! Lays	1	Ounce-weight	28.35	75.00	2.00	18.00	1.00	0.00	0.00	0.00	0.00	0.00	0.00	
Chips, potato, Kettle, lightly salted Season's Enterprises, Ltd.	1	Ounce-weight	28.35	140.00	2.00	17.00	1.00	8.00	1.50			0.00	0.00	
Chips, potato, plain, bag	1	Ounce-weight	28.35	151.96	1.98	15.00	1.28	9.81	3.11	2.79	3.45	0.00	0.00	
Chips, potato, plain, unsalt, w/part hydrog soy oil, bag	1	Ounce-weight	28.35	151.96	1.98	15.00	1.36	9.81	1.54	5.10	2.60	0.00	0.00	
Chips, potato, plain, w/part hydrog soy oil, bag	1	Ounce-weight	28.35	151.96	1.98	15.00	1.36	9.81	1.54	5.10	2.60	0.00	0.00	
Chips, potato, rducd fat, unsalted	1	Ounce-weight	28.35	138.06	2.01	19.22	1.73	5.90	1.18	1.36	3.10	0.00	0.00	
Chips, potato, sour cream & onion flvr, bag	1	Ounce-weight	28.35	150.54	2.30	14.60	1.47	9.61	2.52	1.74	4.94	1.98	3.97	
Chips, sweet potato USDA SR-23	1	Serving	28.00	138.88	0.98	18.15	0.98	6.92	0.62	2.55	3.43	0.00	331.44	0.00
Chips, taro	1	Ounce-weight	28.35	141.18	0.65	19.31	2.04	7.06	1.82	1.26	3.65	0.00	1.98	
Chips, tortilla, blue corn, Blue Chips Garden of Eatin'	1	Ounce-weight	28.35	140.00	2.00	18.00	2.00	7.00	0.50			0.00	0.00	
Chips, veggie Robert's American Gourmet	1	Ounce-weight	28.35	120.00	1.00	19.00	1.00	4.00	0.50			0.00	0.00	
Chips, tortilla, nacho flvr, rducd fat, bag	1	Ounce-weight	28.35	126.16	2.47	20.30	1.36	4.31	0.82	2.54	0.60	0.85	6.80	
Chips, tortilla, nacho, made w/enrich masa flour	1	Ounce-weight	28.35	141.18	2.21	17.69	1.50	7.26	1.39	4.28	1.00	0.85	6.80	
Chips, tortilla, plain, bag	1	Ounce-weight	28.35	142.03	1.98	17.83	1.84	7.43	1.43	4.38	1.03	0.00	1.13	
Chips, tortilla, ranch flvr, bag	1	Ounce-weight	28.35	138.91	2.15	18.31	1.11	6.75	1.29	3.99	0.94	0.28	4.25	
Chips, tortilla, taco flvr, bag	1	Ounce-weight	28.35	136.08	2.24	17.89	1.50	6.86	1.31	4.05	0.95	1.42	12.76	
Chips, tortilla, w/cinnamon & sugar	1	Ounce-weight	28.35	153.94	1.87	16.49	0.86	9.36	4.73	3.08	1.08	10.21	1.42	
Corn Nuts, bbq flvr	1	Ounce-weight	28.35	123.61	2.55	20.33	2.38	4.05	0.73	2.09	0.92	0.00	4.82	
Corn Nuts, plain	1	Ounce-weight	28.35	126.44	2.41	20.37	1.96	4.43	0.69	2.68	0.87	0.00	0.00	
Fruit Leather, roll, sml	1	Each	14.00	51.94	0.01	12.00	0.46	0.42	0.09	0.21	0.08	0.00	0.84	
Popcorn, air popped	1	Cup	8.00	30.56	0.96	6.23	1.21	0.34	0.05	0.09	0.15	0.00	0.80	
Popcorn, caramel coated, w/o peanuts	1	Ounce-weight	28.35	122.19	1.08	22.42	1.47	3.63	1.02	0.81	1.27	1.42	0.57	
Popcorn, cheese flvrd	1	Cup	11.00	57.86	1.02	5.68	1.09	3.65	0.70	1.07	1.69	1.21	4.18	
Popcorn, oil popped	1	Cup	11.00	55.00	0.99	6.29	1.10	3.09	0.54	0.90	1.48	0.00	0.88	
Popcorn, white, air popped USDA SR-23	1	Cup	8.00	30.56	0.96	6.23	1.21	0.34	0.05	0.09	0.15	0.00	0.11	
Popcorn, white, oil popped	1	Cup	11.00	55.00	0.99	6.29	1.10	3.09	0.54	0.90	1.48	0.00	0.11	
Pork Skins, bbq flvr	1	Ounce-weight	28.35	152.52	16.41	0.45		9.02	3.28	4.26	0.98	32.60	18.43	

Vit E (mg)	Vit C	Vit B$_1$ Thia (mg)	Vit B$_2$ Ribo (mg)	Vit B$_3$ Nia (mg)	Fol (mcg)	Vit B$_6$ (mg)	Vita B$_{12}$ (mcg)	Sodi (mg)	Pota (mg)	Cal (mg)	Phos (mg)	Magn (mg)	Iron (mg)	Zinc (mg)	Caff (mg)	Alco (g)	Sol Fiber (g)	Insol Fiber (g)
1.42	2.27	0.01	0.06	0.20	7.25	0.04	0.18	238.01	90.81	220.29	113.45	15.77	1.06	0.54	0.00	0.00		
	1.73	0.02	0.04	0.43				134.17	113.90	3.54	14.54	5.35	0.16	0.07	0.00	0.00		
0.08	0.19	0.01	0.03	0.39	2.29	0.03	0.00	205.11	98.74	4.57	8.39	4.57	0.55	0.07	0.00	0.00		
0.38	0.62	0.01	0.01	0.02	1.29	0.06	0.00	194.25	96.15	8.74	10.04	4.86	0.15	0.12	0.00	0.00		
	6.08	0.08	0.06	0.87	12.81	0.11		341.21	119.50	5.96	41.42	7.45	0.28	0.42	0.00	0.00		
	0.13	0.03	0.13	0.13	1.13	0.03	0.10	357.21	146.00	102.90	33.44	5.96	0.19	0.52	0.00	0.00		
	9.00							720.00		40.00			1.44		0.00	0.00		
2.55	3.88	0.03	0.08	4.90	13.75	0.22	0.00	601.25	470.00	33.75	45.00	26.25	1.06	0.68	0.00	0.00		
	0.00							100.64		1.75			0.03		0.00	0.00	0.00	0.00
0.00		0.00	0.03	0.30	0.84	0.15		291.99	24.66	15.30	17.01	3.39	0.60	0.03	0.00	0.00		
0.14	0.51	0.00	0.01	0.19	1.28	0.02	0.24	436.16	25.60	3.52	11.84	3.20	0.24	0.04	0.00	0.00		
	0.00							230.00		0.00			0.00		0.00	0.00	0.00	0.00
0.05	0.00	0.00	0.01	0.19	0.96	0.01		318.72	16.00	2.56	6.72	2.56	0.18	0.03	0.00	0.00	0.00	0.00
	0.00							120.00		20.00			0.00		0.00	0.00	0.00	0.00
0.12	0.22	0.03	0.06	0.18	3.44	0.01	0.08	116.56	46.56	34.69	30.00	4.38	0.16	0.12	0.00	0.00		
2.82	14.34	0.04	0.11	2.01	7.86	0.13	0.00	517.45	664.17	23.58	54.37	27.51	1.94	0.41	0.00	0.00	0.76	2.18
2.55	8.58	0.02	0.08	1.20	11.03	0.12	0.00	641.90	405.48	15.93	31.85	19.60	1.25	0.25	0.00	0.00		
	0.00							270.00		40.00			0.36		0.00	0.00		
1.70	0.00	0.14	0.12	1.61	46.04	0.16	0.00	418.90	167.42	8.94	144.62	39.22	1.38	0.89	0.00	0.00		
0.54	0.00	0.09	0.07	0.40	0.85	0.01	0.00	289.74	22.96	0.85	12.47	3.12	0.72	0.06	0.00	0.00		
0.38	0.48	0.02	0.06	0.46	11.06	0.07	0.00	216.31	66.91	37.14	58.68	21.83	0.43	0.30	0.00	0.00		
0.39	0.00	0.01	0.04	0.33	5.67	0.07	0.00	178.60	40.26	36.00	52.45	21.55	0.38	0.36	0.00	0.00		
1.42	9.61	0.06	0.06	1.33	23.53	0.18	0.00	212.62	357.49	14.17	52.73	21.26	0.55	0.26	0.00	0.00		
0.61	0.00	0.09	0.02	1.16	0.00	0.14	0.00	259.97	204.40	35.44	77.68	12.19	0.24	0.12	0.00	0.00		
1.38	2.41	0.05	0.04	0.74	5.10	0.15	0.00	214.04	108.01	31.18	46.21	15.03	0.45	0.18	0.00	0.00		
	6.00	0.02	0.04	0.27				200.00	76.00	0.00	44.00		0.36	0.40	0.00	0.00		
	18.00							80.00		0.00			0.36		0.00	0.00		
2.58	8.82	0.05	0.06	1.09	12.76	0.19	0.00	168.40	361.46	6.80	46.78	18.99	0.46	0.31	0.00	0.00		
1.38	8.82	0.05	0.06	1.09	12.76	0.19	0.00	2.27	361.46	6.80	46.78	18.99	0.46	0.31	0.00	0.00		
1.38	8.82	0.05	0.06	1.09	12.76	0.19	0.00	168.40	361.46	6.80	46.78	18.99	0.46	0.31	0.00	0.00		
1.55	7.29	0.06	0.08	1.98	2.83	0.19	0.00	2.27	494.42	5.95	54.72	25.23	0.39	0.28	0.00	0.00		
1.38	10.57	0.06	0.06	1.14	17.58	0.19	0.28	177.19	377.34	20.41	49.90	20.98	0.45	0.27	0.00	0.00		
3.21	1.42	0.05	0.01	0.14	5.67	0.12	0.00	96.96	214.04	17.01	37.14	23.81	0.34	0.10	0.00	0.00		
2.75	0.00	0.02	0.05	0.58	10.36	0.15	0.00	9.80	259.00	19.88	40.60	18.20	0.71	0.15	0.00	0.00		
	0.00							60.00		20.00			0.36		0.00	0.00		
	0.00							250.00		0.00			0.36		0.00	0.00		
0.23	0.06	0.07	0.08	0.11	7.37	0.07	0.00	284.35	77.11	45.08	90.15	27.50	0.46		0.00	0.00		
	0.51	0.11	0.10	1.13	36.85	0.09	0.02	200.72	61.24	41.67	69.17	23.25	1.05	0.34	0.00	0.00		
1.00	0.00	0.02	0.06	0.36	2.83	0.09	0.00	149.69	55.85	43.66	58.12	24.95	0.43	0.43	0.00	0.00		
0.39	0.26	0.03	0.07	0.42	4.82	0.06	0.00	173.50	69.17	39.97	67.76	25.23	0.42	0.35	0.00	0.00		
0.39	0.26	0.07	0.06	0.57	5.95	0.09	0.00	223.11	61.52	43.94	67.76	24.95	0.58	0.36	0.00	0.00		
	2.07	0.05	0.11	1.02	1.98	0.05	0.44	114.25	20.41	22.11	8.50	5.10	0.76	0.15	0.00	0.00		
0.28	0.11	0.10	0.04	0.43	0.00	0.06	0.00	276.70	81.08	4.82	80.23	30.90	0.48	0.53	0.00	0.00		
0.56	0.00	0.01	0.04	0.48	0.00	0.07	0.00	155.64	78.81	2.55	77.96	32.04	0.47	0.50	0.00	0.00		
0.08	16.80	0.01	0.00	0.01	0.56	0.04	0.00	44.38	41.16	4.48	4.34	2.80	0.14	0.03	0.00	0.00		
0.02	0.00	0.02	0.02	0.15	1.84	0.02	0.00	0.32	24.08	0.80	24.00	10.48	0.21	0.27	0.00	0.00		
0.34	0.00	0.02	0.02	0.62	1.42	0.01	0.00	58.40	30.90	12.19	23.53	9.92	0.49	0.16	0.00	0.00		
0.01	0.06	0.01	0.03	0.16	1.21	0.03	0.06	97.79	28.71	12.43	39.71	10.01	0.25	0.22	0.00	0.00		
0.55	0.03	0.01	0.01	0.17	1.87	0.02	0.00	97.24	24.75	1.10	27.50	11.88	0.30	0.29	0.00	0.00		
	0.00	0.02	0.02	0.16	1.84	0.02	0.00	0.32	24.08	0.80	24.00	10.48	0.21	0.28	0.00	0.00		
0.03	0.03	0.01	0.01	0.17	1.87	0.02	0.00	97.24	24.75	1.10	27.50	11.88	0.30	0.29	0.00	0.00		
	0.43	0.03	0.12	0.95	8.79	0.05	0.04	756.09	51.03	12.19	62.37	0.00	0.29	0.20	0.00	0.00		

Food Name	Amount	Measure	Weight (g)	Calories	Protein (g)	Total Carb (g)	Dietary Fiber (g)	Total Fat (g)	Sat Fat (g)	Mono Fat (g)	Poly Fat (g)	Chol (mg)	Vit A (mcg RAE)	Vit D (mcg)
SNACK FOODS-CHIPS, PRETZELS, POPCORN (continued)														
Pretzels, hard	10	Each	60.00	228.60	5.46	47.52	1.92	2.10	0.46	0.82	0.74	0.00	0.00	
Pretzels, hard, unsalted, w/unenrich flour	5	Each	30.00	114.30	2.73	23.76	0.84	1.05	0.23	0.41	0.37	0.00	0.00	
Pretzels, hard, whole wheat	1	Ounce-weight	28.35	102.63	3.15	23.02	2.18	0.74	0.16	0.29	0.24	0.00	0.00	
Rice Cake, brown rice & buckwheat, salted	1	Each	9.00	34.20	0.81	7.21	0.34	0.32	0.06	0.10	0.10	0.00	0.00	
Rice Cake, brown rice & multigrain, unsalted	1	Each	9.00	34.83	0.77	7.21	0.38	0.32	0.05	0.11	0.13	0.00	0.00	
Rice Cake, brown rice, plain, unsalted	1	Each	9.00	34.83	0.74	7.34	0.38	0.25	0.05	0.09	0.09	0.00	0.00	
Rice Krispies Treats, square, single svg Kellogg's Company	1	Each	37.00	153.18	1.26	29.79	0.22	3.33	0.52	0.93	1.89	0.00	119.88	
Snack Mix, Chex, traditional Ralston Foods	0.66	Cup	30.00	130.00	3.00	22.00	1.00	3.50	1.00			0.00	0.00	
Snack Mix, oriental, rice based	1	Ounce-weight	28.35	143.45	4.90	14.64	3.74	7.25	1.08	2.80	3.01	0.00	0.00	
Trail Mix, regular	0.25	Cup	37.50	173.25	5.18	16.84	1.92	11.02	2.09	4.70	3.62	0.00	0.38	
Trail Mix, w/chocolate chips salted nuts & seeds	0.25	Cup	36.25	175.45	5.15	16.28	2.02	11.56	2.21	4.91	4.10	1.45	0.73	
SOUPS, STEWS AND CHILIS														
Canned/Frozen/Prepared Soups, Stews and Chilis														
Beans, chili style, med, cnd Bush's Best	0.5	Cup	130.00	120.00	6.00	20.00	6.00	1.00	0.50			0.00		
Bowl, enchilada, Santa Fe, fzn Amy's	1	Each	283.00	340.00	17.00	47.00	10.00	9.00	2.00			5.00		0.00
Bowl, fried rice Seapoint Farms	1	Serving	340.00	450.00	18.00	77.00	6.00	8.00	0.50			0.00		0.00
Bowl, rice, brown, w/vegetables, fzn Amy's	1	Each	283.00	240.00	9.00	36.00	5.00	8.00	1.00			0.00		0.23
Bowl, rice, white, teriyaki, w/tofu & vegetables, fzn Amy's	1	Each	283.00	300.00	10.00	59.00	3.00	2.00	0.00			0.00		
Bouillon/Broth, beef, cond, prep w/water, can	1	Cup	240.00	16.80	2.74	0.10	0.00	0.53	0.26	0.22	0.02	0.00	0.00	
Broth, chicken, prep f/cnd w/water, cmrcl	1	Cup	244.00	39.04	4.93	0.93	0.00	1.39	0.39	0.59	0.27	0.00	0.00	
Burrito, bean & rice, fzn Amy's	1	Each	177.00	270.00	9.00	48.00	5.00	6.00	0.50			0.00		0.00
Chili, con carne	1	Cup	253.00	255.53	24.62	21.94		8.27	3.43	3.41	0.53	134.09	83.49	
Chili, con carne, w/beans, cnd, svg	1	Cup	222.00	268.62	15.74	25.37	8.66	11.68	3.86	4.76	0.95	28.86		
Chili, mild vegetarian, w/soy protein, low fat, cnd Health Valley Foods	1	Cup	245.00	160.00	14.00	30.00	11.00	1.00	0.00			0.00		
Chili, vegetarian lentil, w/soy protein, low fat, cnd Health Valley Foods	1	Cup	245.00	160.00	15.00	28.00	11.00	1.00	0.00			0.00		
Chili, vegetarian, w/beans, cnd	1	Cup	247.00	205.01	11.93	38.01	9.88	0.69	0.12	0.07	0.40	0.00		
Chili, w/beans, classic, cnd	1	Cup	247.00	323.57	17.22	29.22	7.41	16.33	6.69	6.89	1.11	41.99		
Chili, w/beans, cnd	1	Cup	256.00	286.72	14.62	30.49	11.26	14.05	6.02	5.97	0.93	43.52	43.52	
Chili, w/beans, cnd Chef-Mate	1	Cup	253.00	412.39	17.74	29.04	11.13	25.02	10.93	10.75	1.40	55.66		
Chili, w/beans, dynamite, cnd Hormel Foods Corporation	1	Cup	247.00	333.45	18.28	30.73	8.15	15.36	5.66	6.79	0.91	44.46		
Chili, w/black beans, spicy, vegetarian, fat free, cnd Health Valley Foods	1	Cup	245.00	160.00	13.00	28.00	12.00	1.00	0.00			0.00		
Chowder, clam, Manhattan style, chunky, rts, can	1	Cup	240.00	134.40	7.25	18.82	2.88	3.38	2.11	0.98	0.12	14.40	168.00	
Chowder, clam, New England, prep f/cnd w/milk, cmrcl	1	Cup	248.00	163.68	9.47	16.62	1.49	6.60	2.95	2.26	1.09	22.32	57.04	
Chowder, clam, New England, prep f/cnd w/water, cmrcl	1	Cup	244.00	95.16	4.81	12.42	1.46	2.88	0.41	1.22	1.10	4.88	2.44	
Dish, beef, teriyaki, w/vegetables, fzn Birds Eye Foods Birds Eye Reduced Carb Voila	1.67	Cup	210.00	160.00	15.00	15.00	4.00	4.00	1.50			25.00		
Dish, Jaipur vegetables Preferred Brands Intl Tasty Bite	1	Serving	142.50	169.00	7.00	10.00	4.00	11.00	3.00			3.00	0.00	
Dish, Jodhpur lentils Preferred Brands Intl Tasty Bite	1	Serving	142.50	106.00	6.00	12.00	7.00	4.00	2.00			0.00	0.00	
Dish, Kashmir spinach Preferred Brands Intl Tasty Bite	1	Serving	142.50	133.00	6.00	8.00	3.00	8.00	3.00			0.00		
Dish, Kerala vegetables Preferred Brands Intl Tasty Bite	1	Serving	142.50	140.00	2.00	15.00	2.00	4.00	1.00			0.00	10.00	
Dish, red curry Preferred Brands Intl Tasty Bite	1	Serving	142.50	100.00	2.00	11.00	1.50	6.00	5.00			0.00	5.00	
Dish, rice & lentils, cnd Eden	0.5	Cup	130.00	120.00	4.00	23.00	2.00	1.00	0.00			0.00	0.00	

Vit E (mg)	Vit C	Vit B₁ Thia (mg)	Vit B₂ Ribo (mg)	Vit B₃ Nia (mg)	Fol (mcg)	Vit B₆ (mg)	Vita B₁₂ (mcg)	Sodi (mg)	Pota (mg)	Cal (mg)	Phos (mg)	Magn (mg)	Iron (mg)	Zinc (mg)	Caff (mg)	Alco (g)	Sol Fiber (g)	Insol Fiber (g)
0.22	0.00	0.28	0.38	3.16	102.60	0.06	0.00	1029.00	87.60	21.60	67.80	21.00	2.60	0.52	0.00	0.00		
0.06	0.00	0.05	0.03	0.58	24.90	0.03	0.00	86.70	43.80	10.80	33.90	10.50	0.50	0.26	0.00	0.00		
0.07	0.28	0.12	0.09	1.85	15.31	0.08	0.00	57.55	121.90	7.94	35.44	8.50	0.77	0.18	0.00	0.00		
0.01	0.00	0.01	0.01	0.73	1.89	0.01	0.00	10.44	26.91	0.99	34.20	13.59	0.10	0.23	0.00	0.00		
0.01	0.00	0.01	0.02	0.59	1.80	0.01	0.00	0.36	26.46	1.89	33.30	12.33	0.18	0.23	0.00	0.00		
0.11	0.00	0.01	0.02	0.70	1.89	0.02	0.00	2.34	26.10	0.99	32.40	11.79	0.14	0.27	0.00	0.00		
0.00	0.00	0.47	0.51	6.03	40.33	0.33	0.00	129.87	14.43	1.11	15.54	4.81	0.47	0.19	0.00	0.00		
	0.60	0.30	0.03	3.00	60.00	0.30	0.90	280.00		0.00			4.50		0.00	0.00		
1.59	0.09	0.09	0.04	0.87	10.77	0.02	0.00	117.09	92.99	15.31	74.28	33.45	0.69	0.76	0.00	0.00		
1.34	0.52	0.18	0.08	1.76	26.62	0.11	0.00	85.88	256.88	29.25	129.38	59.25	1.15	1.21	0.00	0.00		
3.88	0.47	0.15	0.08	1.60	23.56	0.10	0.00	43.86	234.90	39.51	140.29	58.36	1.23	1.14	2.18	0.00		
	1.20							480.00		20.00			1.44		0.00	0.00		
1.75	24.00	0.27	0.18	1.73	159.47	0.41	0.14	780.00	649.94	100.00	334.39	82.84	3.60	2.10	0.00	0.00		
0.65	3.60	0.59	0.22	5.87	222.57	0.55	0.00	1,090.00	480.78	150.00	282.90	75.12	6.30	1.61	0.00	0.00		
1.46	21.00	0.22	0.25	4.19	89.71	0.38	0.00	510.00	486.76	80.00	223.30	78.09	1.80	1.69	0.00	0.00		
	30.00							780.00		20.00			2.70		0.00	0.00		
0.00	0.00	0.00	0.05	1.87	4.80	0.02	0.17	782.40	129.60	14.40	31.20	4.80	0.41	0.00	0.00	0.00	0.00	0.00
0.05	0.00	0.01	0.07	3.35	4.88	0.02	0.24	775.92	209.84	9.76	73.20	2.44	0.51	0.24	0.00	0.00	0.00	0.00
2.15	6.00	0.22	0.09	2.35	65.91	0.23	0.00	550.00	320.82	40.00	173.52	63.65	2.70	1.30	0.00	0.00		
1.62	1.52	0.13	1.14	2.48	45.54	0.33	1.14	1006.94	690.69	68.31	197.34	45.54	5.19	3.57	0.00	0.00		
0.29	3.11	0.12	0.22	2.16	57.72	0.28	1.44	941.28	608.28	84.36	215.34	64.38	5.79	2.31	0.00	0.00		
	12.00							390.00		40.00			5.40		0.00	0.00		
	9.00							390.00		40.00			3.60		0.00	0.00		
	1.24							778.05	802.75	96.33		81.51	3.46	1.73	0.00	0.00		
	2.47							824.98	785.46	91.39		64.22	3.95	2.72	0.00	0.00		
1.46	4.35	0.12	0.27	0.92	58.88	0.34	0.00	1336.32	934.40	120.32	394.24	115.20	8.78	5.12	0.00	0.00		
1.21	0.76	0.11	0.20	3.48		0.23	1.44	1171.39	511.06	88.55	166.98	45.54	4.83	3.87	0.00	0.00		
	2.96							862.03	778.05	103.74		69.16	4.45	2.72	0.00	0.00		
	12.00							320.00		40.00			3.60		0.00	0.00		
1.61	12.24	0.06	0.06	1.85	9.60	0.26	7.92	1000.80	384.00	67.20	84.00	19.20	2.64	1.68	0.00	0.00		
0.45	3.47	0.07	0.24	1.03	9.92	0.13	10.24	992.00	300.08	186.00	156.24	22.32	1.49	0.79	0.00	0.00		
0.24	1.95	0.02	0.04	0.96	4.88	0.08	8.00	915.00	146.40	43.92	53.68	7.32	1.49	0.76	0.00	0.00		
	12.00							950.00		20.00			0.72		0.00	0.00		
	3.00							372.00		90.00			2.16		0.00	0.00		
	3.00							664.00		30.00			1.08		0.00	0.00		
	3.00							693.00		150.00			2.88		0.00	0.00		
	1.20							430.00		40.00			1.08		0.00	0.00		
	2.40							305.00		20.00			1.08		0.00	0.00		
	0.00	0.12	0.06	1.06	30.00			120.00	190.00	26.00	110.00	45.50	1.27	1.90	0.00	0.00	1.00	1.00

Food Name	Amount	Measure	Weight (g)	Calories	Protein (g)	Total Carb (g)	Dietary Fiber (g)	Total Fat (g)	Sat Fat (g)	Mono Fat (g)	Poly Fat (g)	Chol (mg)	Vit A (mcg RAE)	Vit D (mcg)
SOUPS, STEWS AND CHILIS *(continued)*														
Dish, rice bowl, cheddar broccoli, microwv General Mills Betty Crocker Bowl Appetit	1	Bowl	74.00	290.00	8.00	51.00	2.00	7.00	2.50			10.00	0.00	
Dish, rice bowl, kung pao vegetables Seapoint Farms	1	Serving	340.00	450.00	17.00	75.00	6.00	8.00	0.50			0.00		0.00
Dish, rice bowl, sweet & sour vegetables Seapoint Farms	1	Serving	340.00	430.00	14.00	82.00	6.00	4.50	0.00			0.00		0.00
Dish, rice bowl, Szechuan vegetables Seapoint Farms	1	Serving	340.00	410.00	15.00	77.00	6.00	4.00	0.00			0.00		0.00
Dish, rice bowl, teriyaki, microwv General Mills Betty Crocker Bowl Appetit	1	Bowl	71.00	260.00	7.00	54.00	2.00	3.00	0.50			0.00		
Dish, rice bowl, teriyaki vegetables Seapoint Farms	1	Serving	340.00	450.00	15.00	86.00	6.00	4.50	0.00			0.00		0.00
Dish, satay vegetables Preferred Brands Intl Tasty Bite	1	Serving	142.50	200.00	4.00	31.00	3.00	11.00	1.50			0.00	15.00	
Dish, spinach dal Preferred Brands Intl Tasty Bite	1	Serving	142.00	115.00	5.00	13.00	4.00	5.00	0.70			0.00	22.50	
Dish, vegetables, Asian, w/sesame ginger sauce, fzn Birds Eye Foods	1	Cup	116.00	60.00	2.00	12.00	2.00	1.00	0.00			0.00		
Dish, vegetables, sweet, Chinese, preserved USDA Survey Database	0.5	Cup	81.50	301.82	0.30	77.73	0.31	0.04	0.01	0.00	0.02	0.00	4.00	
Dish, vegetables, Szechuan, w/sesame sauce, fzn Birds Eye Foods	1	Cup	110.00	60.00	1.00	9.00	2.00	2.00	0.00			0.00		
Egg Roll, chicken, mini, ckd ConAgra Foods Chun King	6	Each	205.50	210.00	6.00	25.00	2.00	9.00	2.50			15.00		
Egg Roll, pork & shrimp, bite size, ckd ConAgra Foods La Choy	12	Each	212.60	210.00	6.00	25.00	2.00	10.00	2.50			10.00		
Egg Roll, shrimp, mini, ckd ConAgra Foods Chun King	6	Each	205.50	190.00	5.00	28.00	2.00	6.00	1.50			10.00		
Egg Roll, sweet & sour, restaurant style, ckd, svg ConAgra Foods La Choy	1	Each	170.10	220.00	6.00	29.00	2.00	9.00	2.00			15.00		
Fettuccini, alfredo, fzn Nestle Stouffer's Lean Cuisine	1	Each	262.24	280.00	14.00	42.00	1.00	6.00	3.00	1.50	1.00	15.00	0.00	1.29
Meal, Asian pot stickers, chicken, w/rice & veg, fzn Nestle Stouffer's Lean Cuisine	1	Each	255.15	260.00	9.00	47.00	3.00	4.00	1.00	1.50	1.00	15.00		
Meal, chicken, sweet & sour, ckd ConAgra Foods Marie Callender's (Frozen)	1	Each	396.90	570.00	23.00	86.00	7.00	15.00	2.50			40.00		
Meal, enchilada, beef, w/beans & rice Don Miguel El Charrito	1	Each	311.85	420.00	13.00	63.00	10.00	14.00	6.00			15.00		
Refried Beans, spicy pinto, cnd Eden	0.5	Cup	130.00	90.00	6.00	19.00	7.00	1.00	0.00			0.00	0.00	
Soup, beef barley, 99% fat free, rts, cnd Progresso Healthy Classics	8	Ounce-weight	226.80	129.28	11.57	16.10	3.41	1.54	0.66	0.68	0.21	18.14	95.26	
Soup, beef mushroom, cond, cmrcl, can	1	Cup	251.00	153.11	11.55	13.05	0.50	6.02	3.01	2.51	0.25	12.55	0.00	
Soup, beef noodle, cond, cmrcl, can	1	Cup	251.00	168.17	9.66	17.97	1.51	6.17	2.28	2.48	0.98	10.04	27.61	
Soup, beef, w/country veg, chunky, rts, cnd	8	Ounce-weight	226.80	142.88	11.56	14.97		4.08	1.22	1.01	1.16	22.68	204.12	
Soup, black bean, cond, cnd, cmrcl	0.5	Cup	128.50	116.93	6.21	19.81	8.74	1.70	0.44	0.62	0.53	0.00	28.27	
Soup, broccoli cheese, cond, cmrcl, can	4	Ounce-weight	113.40	98.66	2.38	8.73	2.04	6.01	1.81	2.27	1.93	4.54	74.84	
Soup, chicken gumbo, cond, cmrcl, can	0.5	Cup	125.50	56.47	2.64	8.37	2.01	1.43	0.33	0.65	0.35	3.76	6.27	
Soup, chicken mushroom, prep f/cnd w/water, cmrcl	1	Cup	244.00	131.76	4.39	9.27	0.24	9.15	2.39	4.03	2.32	9.76	56.12	
Soup, chicken noodle, chunky, rts, can	8	Ounce-weight	226.80	106.60	7.26	12.93		2.95	0.73	1.13	0.59	22.68	122.47	
Soup, chicken rice, chunky, rts, cnd	1	Cup	240.00	127.20	12.26	12.98	0.96	3.19	0.96	1.44	0.67	12.00	292.80	
Soup, chicken vegetable, cond, cnd, cmrcl	0.5	Cup	123.00	75.03	3.62	8.62	0.86	2.85	0.85	1.28	0.60	8.61	134.07	
Soup, crab, rts, can	1	Cup	244.00	75.64	5.49	10.30	0.73	1.51	0.39	0.68	0.39	9.76	24.40	
Soup, cream of asparagus, cond, cnd, cmrcl	0.5	Cup	125.50	86.59	2.28	10.69	0.50	4.09	1.03	0.94	1.83	5.02	32.63	
Soup, cream of asparagus, prep f/cnd w/water, cmrcl	1	Cup	244.00	85.40	2.29	10.69	0.49	4.10	1.05	0.95	1.85	4.88	36.60	
Soup, cream of celery, prep f/cnd w/milk, cmrcl	1	Cup	248.00	163.68	5.68	14.53	0.74	9.70	3.94	2.46	2.65	32.24	114.08	
Soup, cream of celery, prep f/cnd w/water, cmrcl	1	Cup	244.00	90.28	1.66	8.83	0.73	5.59	1.42	1.29	2.51	14.64	56.12	
Soup, cream of chicken, prep f/cnd w/milk, cmrcl	1	Cup	248.00	190.96	7.46	14.98	0.25	11.46	4.64	4.46	1.64	27.28	178.56	

Vit E (mg)	Vit C	Vit B₁ Thia (mg)	Vit B₂ Ribo (mg)	Vit B₃ Nia (mg)	Fol (mcg)	Vit B₆ (mg)	Vita B₁₂ (mcg)	Sodi (mg)	Pota (mg)	Cal (mg)	Phos (mg)	Magn (mg)	Iron (mg)	Zinc (mg)	Caff (mg)	Alco (g)	Sol Fiber (g)	Insol Fiber (g)
	0.00	0.23	0.26	1.60	60.00			950.00	350.00	150.00			1.44		0.00	0.00		
1.33	9.00	0.55	0.21	6.19	190.70	0.59	0.00	730.00	565.98	100.00	270.53	74.98	6.30	1.76	0.00	0.00		
0.59	15.00	0.55	0.18	5.58	204.98	0.50	0.00	200.00	426.46	100.00	226.26	59.49	6.30	1.33	0.00	0.00		
0.49	18.00	0.61	0.18	6.40	232.95	0.53	0.00	310.00	395.12	100.00	242.46	59.46	6.30	1.45	0.00	0.00		
	0.00	0.15		1.60	60.00			1,160.00	190.00	20.00			1.80		0.00	0.00		
0.47	9.00	0.46	0.21	5.34	169.80	0.47	0.00	810.00	467.72	100.00	244.01	66.41	6.30	1.34	0.00	0.00		
	2.40							450.00		40.00			1.44		0.00	0.00		
	3.60							534.00		100.00			2.34		0.00	0.00		
	9.00							630.00		20.00			0.36		0.00	0.00		
0.03	1.76	0.02	0.02	0.10	4.62	0.02	0.00	1.55	66.31	4.69	9.90	5.75	0.16	0.07	0.00	0.00		
	15.00							460.00		20.00			0.36		0.00	0.00		
	0.00	0.19	0.12	1.36				650.00	232.60	20.00	174.50		1.08		0.00	0.00		
	0.00							540.00		20.00			0.72		0.00	0.00		
	0.00	0.17	0.06	0.78				730.00	155.10	20.00	96.90		1.08		0.00	0.00		
	2.40							550.00		20.00			1.08		0.00	0.00		
0.22	0.00	0.77	0.80	4.43	93.66	0.53	0.99	690.00	270.00	200.00	246.75	35.17	1.52	1.27	0.00	0.00		
	2.40							530.00	190.00	40.00					0.00	0.00		
	0.00							700.00		40.00			1.80		0.00	0.00		
	4.80							1,160.00		100.00			4.50		0.00	0.00		
	0.00	0.10	0.09	0.63	0.00			180.00	420.00	46.80	117.00	50.00	1.37	1.26	0.00	0.00		
								496.69					1.48		0.00	0.00		
	0.00	0.05	0.15	2.26	17.57	0.10	0.40	1940.23	316.26	10.04	72.79	17.57	1.76	2.76	0.00	0.00		
2.51	0.75	0.14	0.12	2.13	37.65	0.08	0.40	1905.09	198.29	30.12	92.87	12.55	2.21	3.09	0.00	0.00		
								809.68					2.02		0.00	0.00		
0.46	0.26	0.05	0.05	0.53	25.70	0.09	0.00	1246.45	321.25	44.97	96.37	42.40	1.93	1.41	0.00	0.00		
0.82	2.27	0.02	0.04	0.28	45.36	0.07	0.02	774.52	234.74	46.49	47.63	14.74	0.34	0.29	0.00	0.00		
0.45	5.02	0.25	0.38	0.67	6.27	0.06	0.03	955.05	75.30	23.84	25.10	3.76	0.89	0.38	0.00	0.00		
1.22	0.00	0.02	0.11	1.63	0.00	0.05	0.05	941.84	153.72	29.28	26.84	9.76	0.88	0.98	0.00	0.00		
								816.48					1.11		0.00	0.00		
0.58	3.84	0.02	0.10	4.10	4.80	0.05	0.31	888.00	108.00	33.60	72.00	9.60	1.87	0.96	0.00	0.00		
0.31	0.98	0.04	0.06	1.23	4.92	0.05	0.12	948.33	154.98	17.22	40.59	6.15	0.87	0.37	0.00	0.00		
0.24	0.00	0.20	0.07	1.34	14.64	0.12	0.20	1234.64	326.96	65.88	87.84	14.64	1.22	1.46	0.00	0.00		
0.61	2.76	0.05	0.08	0.78	23.84	0.01	0.05	981.41	173.19	28.86	38.90	3.76	0.80	0.88	0.00	0.00		
0.66	2.68	0.05	0.08	0.78	21.96	0.01	0.05	980.88	173.24	29.28	39.04	4.88	0.81	0.88	0.00	0.00		
0.97	1.49	0.07	0.25	0.44	7.44	0.06	0.50	1009.36	310.00	186.00	151.28	22.32	0.69	0.20	0.00	0.00		
0.90	0.24	0.03	0.05	0.33	2.44	0.01	0.24	949.16	122.00	39.04	36.60	7.32	0.63	0.15	0.00	0.00		
0.25	1.24	0.07	0.26	0.92	7.44	0.07	0.55	1046.56	272.80	181.04	151.28	17.36	0.67	0.67	0.00	0.00		

Food Name	Amount	Measure	Weight (g)	Calories	Protein (g)	Total Carb (g)	Dietary Fiber (g)	Total Fat (g)	Sat Fat (g)	Mono Fat (g)	Poly Fat (g)	Chol (mg)	Vit A (mcg RAE)	Vit D (mcg)
SOUPS, STEWS AND CHILIS (*continued*)														
Soup, cream of mushroom, prep f/cnd w/water, cmrcl	1	Cup	244.00	129.32	2.32	9.30	0.49	8.98	2.44	1.71	4.22	2.44	14.64	
Soup, cream of onion, cond, cnd, cmrcl	0.5	Cup	125.50	110.44	2.76	13.05	0.50	5.27	1.47	2.10	1.46	15.06	35.14	
Soup, cream of potato, prep w/milk	1	Cup	248.00	148.80	5.78	17.16	0.50	6.45	3.77	1.74	0.57	22.32	52.08	
Soup, cream of shrimp, prep f/cnd w/milk, cmrcl	1	Cup	248.00	163.68	6.82	13.91	0.25	9.30	5.78	2.68	0.35	34.72	62.00	
Soup, lentil, rts, cnd Progresso Healthy Classics	1	Cup	242.00	125.84	7.79	20.30	5.57	1.50	0.27	0.82	0.24	0.00		
Soup, lentil vegetable, cnd Amy's	1	Cup	205.50	150.00	8.00	23.00	9.00	4.00	0.50			0.00		0.00
Soup, minestrone, chunky, rts, can	1	Cup	240.00	127.20	5.11	20.74	5.76	2.81	1.49	0.91	0.26	4.80	213.60	
Soup, onion, cond, cnd, cmrcl	0.5	Cup	123.00	56.58	3.76	8.22	0.86	1.75	0.26	0.75	0.65	0.00	3.69	
Soup, red lentil, curried Pacific Foods of Oregon Pacific Natural Foods	1	Cup	242.00	140.00	5.00	19.00	5.00	4.50	4.00			0.00		
Soup, split pea, w/ham, chunky, rducd fat & sod, rts, cnd	8	Ounce-weight	226.80	172.37	11.80	25.63		2.49	0.68	0.91	0.45	13.61	297.11	
Soup, tomato rice, prep f/cnd w/water, cmrcl	1	Cup	247.00	118.56	2.10	21.93	1.48	2.72	0.52	0.59	1.36	2.47	34.58	
Soup, tomato, prep f/cnd w/milk, cmrcl	1	Cup	248.00	161.20	6.10	22.30	2.73	6.00	2.90	1.61	1.12	17.36	64.48	
Soup, tomato, prep f/cnd w/water, cmrcl	1	Cup	244.00	85.40	2.05	16.59	0.49	1.93	0.37	0.44	0.95	0.00	24.40	
Soup, turkey noodle, cond, cnd, cmrcl	0.5	Cup	125.50	69.02	3.90	8.63	0.75	2.00	0.55	0.80	0.49	5.02	16.31	
Soup, turkey vegetable, cond, cnd, cmrcl	0.5	Cup	123.00	73.80	3.10	8.67	0.62	3.04	0.90	1.33	0.68	1.23	130.38	
Soup, vegetable beef, prep f/cnd w/water, cmrcl	1	Cup	244.00	78.08	5.59	10.17	0.49	1.90	0.85	0.81	0.12	4.88	95.16	
Soup, vegetable, vegetarian, cond, cnd, cmrcl	0.5	Cup	123.00	72.57	2.12	12.03	0.62	1.94	0.30	0.84	0.73	0.00	174.66	
Soup, won ton	1	Cup	241.00	181.69	14.08	14.28	0.90	7.03	2.26	3.01	0.98	52.95	56.01	
Spring Roll, fried, shrimp, wild, Chinese, fzn Blue Horizon Seafood	3	Each	60.00	110.00	3.00	16.00	1.00	4.00	1.50			0.00		
Spring Roll, fried, shrimp, wild, Thai, fzn Blue Horizon Seafood	3	Each	60.00	130.00	3.00	16.00	1.00	4.00	1.50			0.00		
Stew, beef, cnd Chef-Mate	1	Cup	252.00	191.52	15.02	18.93	3.28	6.15	2.27	2.50	0.32	32.76	154.98	
Stew, beef, hearty, family size, ckd f/fzn Banquet	1	Cup	245.70	170.00	10.00	18.00	4.00	7.00	3.00			30.00		
Stir Fry, chicken, ginger garlic, w/veg & rice, fzn Nestle Stouffer's Lean Cuisine	1	Each	278.54	290.00	17.00	46.00	4.00	4.00	1.00	1.00	1.50	30.00		0.18
Stir Fry, chicken, sesame, w/veg & vermicelli, fzn Nestle Stouffer's Lean Cuisine	1	Each	278.54	300.00	20.00	41.00	5.00	6.00	1.00	2.00	2.00	40.00		0.13
Stir Fry, chicken, teriyaki, w/rice & vegetables, fzn Nestle Stouffer's Lean Cuisine	1	Each	255.15	250.00	12.00	46.00	3.00	2.00	0.50	0.50	0.00	20.00		0.10
Stir Fry, shrimp, Szechuan, w/pasta, fzn Nestle Stouffer's Lean Cuisine	1	Each	255.15	230.00	13.00	39.00	5.00	2.50	0.00	0.00	1.00	60.00		0.00
Dry and Prepared Soups and Chilis														
Dish, rice, chicken teriyaki, dry svg General Mills Betty Crocker Chicken Helper	1	Each	47.00	160.00	4.00	36.00	0.75	1.00	0.00			0.00		
Dish, couscous, all natural, low fat, dry mix Hain Celestial Group Casbah	0.4	Cup	45.00	160.00	6.00	34.00	2.00	1.00	0.00			0.00		
Dish, couscous, rstd garlic & olive oil, dry Fantastic World Foods	0.33	Cup	55.00	220.00	7.00	43.00	3.00	0.50	0.00			0.00	0.00	
Dish, noodles, sweet & sour, dry Unilever Lipton Asian Sides	0.75	Cup	70.00	260.00	9.00	50.00	2.00	2.00	0.50			50.00		
Dish, noodles, teriyaki, dry Unilever Lipton Asian Sides	0.75	Cup	66.00	250.00	8.00	46.00	2.00	3.00	0.50			50.00		
Dish, noodles, Thai sesame, dry Unilever Lipton Asian Sides	0.75	Cup	62.00	230.00	8.00	42.00	2.00	3.50	1.00			50.00		
Dish, rice, Cajun, dry Unilever Lipton Cajun Sides	0.5	Cup	68.00	250.00	8.00	50.00	2.00	1.50	0.00			5.00		
Dish, rice, teriyaki, dry Unilever Lipton Asian Sides	0.5	Cup	65.00	240.00	6.00	50.00	1.00	1.00	0.00			0.00		
Falafel, all natural, dry mix Hain Celestial Group Casbah	0.33	Cup	45.00	180.00	7.00	29.00	3.00	5.00	0.00			0.00		
Lo Mein, beef, dry Unilever Lipton Asian Sides	0.75	Cup	62.00	230.00	9.00	42.00	2.00	2.50	0.50			50.00		

Vit E (mg)	Vit C	Vit B₁ Thia (mg)	Vit B₂ Ribo (mg)	Vit B₃ Nia (mg)	Fol (mcg)	Vit B₆ (mg)	Vita B₁₂ (mcg)	Sodi (mg)	Pota (mg)	Cal (mg)	Phos (mg)	Magn (mg)	Iron (mg)	Zinc (mg)	Caff (mg)	Alco (g)	Sol Fiber (g)	Insol Fiber (g)
0.95	0.98	0.05	0.09	0.72	4.88	0.01	0.05	880.84	100.04	46.36	48.80	4.88	0.51	0.59	0.00	0.00		
0.54	1.25	0.05	0.08	0.50	7.53	0.03	0.05	953.80	122.99	33.88	37.65	6.27	0.63	0.15	0.00	0.00		
0.10	1.24	0.08	0.24	0.64	9.92	0.09	0.50	1061.44	322.40	166.16	161.20	17.36	0.55	0.67	0.00	0.00		
0.99	1.24	0.06	0.23	0.53	9.92	0.45	1.04	1036.64	248.00	163.68	146.32	22.32	0.60	0.79	0.00	0.00		
0.58	0.97	0.11	0.09	0.70	101.64	0.16	0.00	442.86	336.38	41.14	128.26	41.14	2.66	1.04	0.00	0.00		
1.08	12.00	0.18	0.09	1.19	149.11	0.26	0.00	680.00	472.54	60.00	160.88	39.58	2.70	1.13	0.00	0.00		
1.61	4.80	0.06	0.12	1.18	52.80	0.24	0.00	864.00	612.00	60.00	110.40	14.40	1.78	1.44	0.00	0.00		
0.27	1.23	0.03	0.02	0.60	14.76	0.05	0.00	1057.80	68.88	27.06	11.07	2.46	0.68	0.62	0.00	0.00		
	2.40							750.00		20.00			1.80		0.00	0.00		
	9.53							777.92					2.09		0.00	0.00		
2.45	14.82	0.06	0.05	1.05	14.82	0.08	0.00	815.10	330.98	22.23	34.58	4.94	0.79	0.52	0.00	0.00		
1.24	67.70	0.13	0.25	1.52	17.36	0.16	0.45	744.00	448.88	158.72	148.80	22.32	1.81	0.30	0.00	0.00		
2.32	66.37	0.09	0.05	1.42	14.64	0.11	0.00	695.40	263.52	12.20	34.16	7.32	1.76	0.24	0.00	0.00		
0.18	0.13	0.07	0.06	1.40	18.82	0.04	0.16	815.75	75.30	11.29	47.69	5.02	0.94	0.58	0.00	0.00		
0.42	0.00	0.03	0.04	1.01	4.92	0.05	0.17	908.97	175.89	17.22	40.59	3.69	0.76	0.62	0.00	0.00		
0.37	2.44	0.04	0.05	1.03	9.76	0.08	0.32	790.56	173.24	17.08	41.48	4.88	1.12	1.54	0.00	0.00		
1.44	1.48	0.05	0.05	0.92	11.07	0.06	0.00	826.56	210.33	20.91	34.44	7.38	1.08	0.47	0.00	0.00		
0.39	3.36	0.41	0.26	4.60	18.85	0.20	0.40	542.88	316.10	31.07	152.50	20.62	1.76	1.12	0.00	0.00		
	15.00							210.00		20.00			1.08		0.00	0.00		
	15.00							210.00		20.00			1.08		0.00	0.00		
0.56	2.52	0.18	0.25	3.10		0.30	0.55	1186.92	388.08	63.00	158.76	35.28	1.59	2.49	0.00	0.00		
	3.60							1120.00		20.00			1.44		0.00	0.00		
1.23	15.00	0.16	0.16	7.17	40.92	0.46	0.28	640.00	550.00	60.00	194.89	53.18	1.94	1.08	0.00	0.00		
1.31	18.00	0.16	0.23	6.89	58.78	0.46	0.24	680.00	450.00	60.00	241.40	69.62	3.33	1.47	0.00	0.00		
0.46	4.80	0.32	0.10	6.38	109.17	0.39	0.16	570.00	470.00	60.00	153.36	30.73	3.18	0.85	0.00	0.00		
1.27	6.00	0.15	0.10	2.12	20.24	0.31	0.48	680.00	220.00	80.00	150.39	48.82	2.75	1.35	0.00	0.00		
	0.00	0.15	0.03	0.80	40.00			850.00	115.00	40.00			1.08		0.00	0.00		
	1.20							400.00		20.00			1.08		0.00	0.00		
	0.00							540.00		20.00			0.72		0.00	0.00		
	6.00	0.60	0.25	4.00	120.00			850.00	0.00	20.00			2.70		0.00	0.00		
	1.20	0.52	0.25	4.00	120.00			900.00	0.00	20.00			2.70		0.00	0.00		
	6.00	0.60	0.25	4.00	120.00			820.00	0.00	40.00			2.70		0.00	0.00		
	6.00	0.45	0.10	4.00	100.00			830.00	0.00	40.00			2.70		0.00	0.00		
	0.00	0.45	0.10	3.00	120.00			800.00	0.00	0.00			2.70		0.00	0.00		
	2.40							680.00		40.00			2.70		0.00	0.00		
	0.00	0.52	0.25	4.00	120.00			900.00	0.00	20.00			2.70		0.00	0.00		

Food Name	Amount	Measure	Weight (g)	Calories	Protein (g)	Total Carb (g)	Dietary Fiber (g)	Total Fat (g)	Sat Fat (g)	Mono Fat (g)	Poly Fat (g)	Chol (mg)	Vit A (mcg RAE)	Vit D (mcg)
SOUPS, STEWS AND CHILIS *(continued)*														
Macaroni & Cheese, Easy Mac, dry mix, pkt Kraft	1	Each	61.00	240.00	7.00	40.00	1.00	6.00	2.50			5.00		
Macaroni & Cheese, original, w/cheddar, dry mix, svg Kraft Deluxe	1	Serving	98.00	320.00	12.00	46.00	2.00	9.00	3.00			20.00		
Soup, beefy mushroom, dry mix Lipton Recipe Secrets	1.5	Tablespoon	11.00	32.78	0.85	6.62	0.11	0.38	0.05			0.22		
Soup, beefy onion, dry mix Lipton Recipe Secrets	1	Tablespoon	8.00	25.12	0.52	4.68	0.35	0.63	0.14			0.00	0.00	
Soup, broccoli cheese & rice, dry mix Uncle Ben's Inc.	1	Ounce-weight	28.35	101.90	4.20	16.74	0.70	2.00	1.10			4.20		
Soup, chicken, supreme, hearty, in a cup, dry Lipton Cup-A-Soup	1	Each	100.00	429.00	5.02	64.87	3.10	17.86	6.62			3.00		
Soup, cream of vegetable, dehyd, svg, makes 1 cup prep	1	Each	23.60	105.26	1.89	12.30	0.71	5.69	1.42	2.53	1.48	0.47	141.60	
Soup, noodle, giggle, dry mix, svg Lipton Soup Secrets	1	Each	19.00	73.53	2.52	11.46	0.42	2.13	0.69			17.86		
Soup, noodle, ring shape, dry mix, svg Lipton Soup Secrets	1	Each	17.00	65.96	2.20	9.91	0.36	1.98	0.64			15.64		
Soup, noodle, Szechuan, in a cup, dry Spice Hunter	1	Individual Cup	42.53	190.00	7.00	39.00	3.00	0.50	0.00			0.00		
Soup, onion mushroom, dry mix Lipton Recipe Secrets	1	Ounce-weight	28.35	91.29	2.38	16.30	0.91	2.24	0.31			0.00	0.00	
Soup, ramen noodle, any flvr, dry USDA SR-23	1	Serving	43.00	187.48	4.51	27.27	0.99	6.72	3.25	2.81	0.63	0.00	0.26	0.00
Soup, ramen noodle, beef flvr, dry pkg USDA SR-23	1	Serving	43.00	187.48	4.42	27.21	0.95	6.76	3.31	2.82	0.63	0.00		
Soup, ramen noodle, chicken flvr, dry, Cup Of Noodles Nissin Foods	1	Each	64.00	296.32	5.57	36.80		14.08	6.25				19.84	
Soup, ramen noodle, rducd fat & sodium, asrtd flvrs, dry USDA SR-23	0.5	Package	40.00	140.00	4.36	28.38	1.08	1.00	0.00	0.27	0.58	0.00	0.04	0.00
Soup, ramen noodle, vegetable miso flvr, in a cup, dry Fantastic World Foods	1	Serving	38.00	130.00	5.00	25.00	2.00	1.00	0.00			0.00		
Soup, spicy Thai, in a cup, dry Spice Hunter	1	Individual Cup	45.36	170.00	6.00	36.00	2.00	1.00	0.00			0.00		
Soup, tomato vegetable, prep f/dry pkt w/water	1	Cup	253.00	55.66	2.00	10.22	0.51	0.86	0.38	0.30	0.08	0.00	10.12	
Homemade/Generic Soups and Chilis														
Soup, cheese, cond, cnd, cmrcl	0.5	Cup	218.50	264.38	9.22	17.90	1.75	17.81	11.34	5.05	0.50	50.25	159.50	
Soup, cheese, prep w/water, cmrcl, can	1	Cup	247.00	155.61	5.41	10.52	0.99	10.47	6.67	2.96	0.30	29.64	296.40	
Soup, egg drop USDA Survey Database	1	Cup	244.00	72.96	7.51	1.11	0.00	3.84	1.15	1.52	0.59	103.46	40.99	
Soup, wonton USDA SR-23 USDA SR-23: Chinese Restaurant	1	Cup	223.00	71.36	4.64	11.71	0.45	0.58	0.14	0.17	0.16	8.92	3.35	0.00
Stew, chicken, w/potatoes veg gravy	1	Cup	252.00	290.68	24.36	15.14	1.97	14.31	4.03	5.73	3.12	87.42	384.25	
SPICES, FLAVORS, AND SEASONINGS														
Basil, fresh, leaves	1	Each	0.50	0.14	0.01	0.02	0.02	0.00	0.00	0.00	0.00	0.00	1.32	0.00
Cilantro, leaves, fresh	0.25	Cup	4.00	0.92	0.09	0.15	0.11	0.02	0.00	0.01	0.00	0.00	13.48	
Cream of Tartar	1	Teaspoon	3.00	7.74	0.00	1.84	0.01	0.00	0.00	0.00	0.00	0.00	0.00	
Curry, pwd	1	Teaspoon	2.00	6.48	0.24	1.16	0.68	0.28	0.04	0.12	0.04	0.00	0.96	0.00
Flavor, vanilla extract	1	Teaspoon	4.33	12.47	0.00	0.52	0.00	0.00	0.00			0.00		
Garlic Salt McCormick & Co., Inc.	0.25	Teaspoon	0.90	0.00	0.00	0.00	0.00	0.00	0.00	0.00	0.00	0.00		
Ginger Root, fresh, slices, 2"	5	Piece	11.00	8.80	0.20	1.95	0.22	0.08	0.02	0.02	0.02	0.00		
Herb, parsley, dried USDA SR-23	1	Teaspoon	0.50	1.46	0.13	0.25	0.13	0.03	0.00	0.00	0.02	0.00	0.48	0.00
Herb, rosemary, dried USDA SR-23	1	Teaspoon	1.20	3.97	0.06	0.77	0.51	0.18	0.09	0.04	0.03	0.00	1.88	0.00
Marjoram, dried	1	Teaspoon	0.60	1.63	0.08	0.36	0.24	0.04	0.00	0.01	0.03	0.00	2.42	0.00
Salt Substitute Morton International Incorporated	0.25	Teaspoon	1.20	0.10	0.00	0.02		0.00	0.00	0.00	0.00			
Salt, table	0.25	Teaspoon	1.50	0.00	0.00	0.00	0.00	0.00	0.00	0.00	0.00	0.00	0.00	
Seasoning, lemon pepper Alberto-Culver Mrs. Dash	0.25	Teaspoon	0.70	0.00	0.00	0.00	0.00	0.00	0.00	0.00	0.00	0.00	0.00	
Seasoning, taco, dry mix Unilever Lawry's	2	Teaspoon	5.00	15.00	0.00	3.00		0.00	0.00	0.00	0.00			
Spice, garlic powder ASTA	1	Teaspoon	3.00	10.35	0.47	2.25	0.63	0.01					0.03	
Spice, pepper, black, ground USDA SR-23	1	Teaspoon	2.30	5.77	0.24	1.47	0.58	0.07	0.03	0.02	0.02	0.00	0.63	0.00

Vit E (mg)	Vit C	Vit B$_1$ Thia (mg)	Vit B$_2$ Ribo (mg)	Vit B$_3$ Nia (mg)	Fol (mcg)	Vit B$_6$ (mg)	Vita B$_{12}$ (mcg)	Sodi (mg)	Pota (mg)	Cal (mg)	Phos (mg)	Magn (mg)	Iron (mg)	Zinc (mg)	Caff (mg)	Alco (g)	Sol Fiber (g)	Insol Fiber (g)
	0.00							570.00		200.00			1.44		0.00	0.00		
	0.00							820.00		100.00			1.80		0.00	0.00		
	0.16	0.00	0.01	0.08	0.00			645.15		10.78			0.10		0.00	0.00		
	0.66	0.01	0.02	0.12	0.00			606.56		11.20			0.12		0.00	0.00		
	9.00							605.10		89.30			0.18		0.00	0.00		
	0.60	0.27	0.25	2.83	0.00			3023.00		109.00			0.89		0.00	0.00		
0.57	3.92	1.22	0.11	0.52	7.08	0.02	0.12	1169.85	96.29	31.62	53.81	11.33	0.61	0.38	0.00	0.00		
	0.06	0.26	0.10	1.29	25.27			736.06		3.61			0.65		0.00	0.00		
	0.07	0.23	0.09	1.12	21.76			724.03		3.40			0.56		0.00	0.00		
								820.00							0.00	0.00		
	1.47	0.60	0.06	0.85	0.00			1773.86		28.63			0.34		0.00	0.00		
0.65	0.13	0.44	0.11	1.76	48.59	0.04	0.11	875.48	76.97	12.47	51.17	9.89	1.72	0.37	0.00	0.00		
0.67	0.26	0.65	0.11	1.80	46.87	0.04	0.08	860.86	79.55	12.90	52.03	10.32	1.77	0.46	0.00	0.00		
								1433.60					2.18		0.00	0.00		
0.10	0.48	0.23	0.16	1.96	48.80	0.03	0.00	480.00	51.20	8.80	46.80	9.20	1.81	0.30	0.00	0.00		
	1.20							540.00		20.00			1.44		0.00	0.00		
								940.00							0.00	0.00		
0.35	6.07	0.06	0.05	0.79	10.12	0.05	0.00	1146.09	103.73	7.59	30.36	20.24	0.63	0.18	0.00	0.00		
1.22	0.00	0.03	0.23	0.68	6.55	0.04	0.00	1632.19	262.20	242.53	231.61	6.55	1.27	1.09	0.00	0.00		
	0.00	0.02	0.14	0.40	4.94	0.02	0.00	958.36	153.14	140.79	135.85	4.94	0.74	0.64	0.00	0.00		
0.29	0.00	0.02	0.19	3.03	15.13	0.05	0.49	728.58	219.60	20.98	107.85	4.64	0.75	0.48	0.00	0.00	0.00	0.00
0.13	1.56	0.05	0.04	1.29	28.99	0.17	0.20	905.38	71.36	11.15	40.14	6.69	0.47	0.27	0.00	0.00		
0.46	12.21	0.14	0.20	9.02	18.05	0.45	0.24	112.64	631.89	32.36	220.79	42.02	1.86	1.91	0.00	0.00		
0.00	0.09	0.00	0.00	0.00	0.32	0.00	0.00	0.02	2.31	0.77	0.35	0.41	0.02	0.00	0.00	0.00		
0.10	1.08	0.00	0.01	0.04	2.48	0.01	0.00	1.84	20.84	2.68	1.92	1.04	0.07	0.02	0.00	0.00		
0.00	0.00	0.00	0.00	0.00	0.00	0.00	0.00	1.56	495.00	0.24	0.15	0.06	0.11	0.01	0.00	0.00		
0.44	0.24	0.00	0.00	0.08	3.08	0.04	0.00	1.04	30.84	9.56	6.96	5.08	0.60	0.08	0.00	0.00		
0.00	0.00	0.00	0.00	0.00	0.00	0.00	0.00	0.35	6.41	0.43	0.26	0.52	0.00	0.00	0.00	1.47	0.00	0.00
								242.00							0.00	0.00	0.00	0.00
0.03	0.55	0.00	0.00	0.08	1.21	0.02	0.00	1.43	45.65	1.76	3.74	4.73	0.07	0.04	0.00	0.00		
0.04	0.62	0.00	0.01	0.05	0.90	0.00	0.00	2.26	13.41	5.70	2.18	2.00	0.11	0.03	0.00	0.00		
	0.73	0.01	0.01	0.01	3.68	0.02	0.00	0.60	11.46	15.36	0.84	2.64	0.35	0.04	0.00	0.00		
0.01	0.31	0.00	0.00	0.02	1.64	0.01	0.00	0.46	9.13	11.94	1.84	2.08	0.50	0.02	0.00	0.00		
							0.00	0.12	603.60	6.60	5.40	0.01			0.00	0.00		
0.00	0.00	0.00	0.00	0.00	0.00	0.00	0.00	581.37	0.12	0.36	0.00	0.02	0.00	0.00	0.00	0.00	0.00	0.00
	0.00						0.00	0.00	10.00	0.00			0.00		0.00	0.00	0.00	0.00
							0.00	300.00							0.00	0.00		
	0.06						0.00	1.83		4.80			0.16		0.00	0.00		
0.02	0.00	0.00	0.00	0.03	0.39	0.01	0.00	0.46	30.57	10.19	3.63	3.93	0.22	0.03	0.00	0.00		

Food Name	Amount	Measure	Weight (g)	Calories	Protein (g)	Total Carb (g)	Dietary Fiber (g)	Total Fat (g)	Sat Fat (g)	Mono Fat (g)	Poly Fat (g)	Chol (mg)	Vit A (mcg RAE)	Vit D (mcg)
SPICES, FLAVORS, AND SEASONINGS *(continued)*														
Tenderizer, unseasoned McCormick & Co., Inc.	0.25	Teaspoon	1.10	0.00	0.00	0.00	0.00	0.00	0.00	0.00	0.00	0.00		
SPORTS BARS AND DRINKS														
Bar, energy, apple cinnamon Power Bar	1	Each	65.00	230.00	10.00	45.00	3.00	2.50	0.50	1.50	0.50	0.00	0.00	
Bar, energy, apricot Clif Bar Inc	1	Each	68.00	221.78	8.55	43.15	5.35	2.29	0.35			0.04		
Bar, energy, caramel nut blast Balance Bar Co Gold	1	Each	50.00	200.00	15.00	23.00	1.00	7.00	4.00			0.00		2.00
Bar, energy, choc dipped strawberry Experimental & Applied Sciences Myoplex Carb Sense	1	Each	70.00	250.00	30.00	23.00	2.00	6.00	4.00			5.00		
Bar, energy, chocolate Balance Bar Co	1	Each	50.00	200.00	14.00	22.00	1.00	6.00	3.50			3.00		2.00
Bar, energy, chocolate Power Bar	1	Each	65.00	240.00	7.00	45.00	4.00	4.00	1.00			0.00	0.00	
Bar, energy, chocolate Power Bar	1	Each	65.00	230.00	10.00	45.00	3.00	2.00	0.50	0.50	1.00	0.00	0.00	
Bar, energy, chocolate almond fudge Clif Bar Inc	1	Each	68.00	230.80	10.43	38.43	5.23	4.80	0.93			0.07		
Bar, energy, chocolate celebration Balance Bar Co Oasis	1	Each	48.00	180.00	9.00	26.00	0.75	3.50	2.50			0.00	109.41	
Bar, energy, chocolate chip peanut crunch Clif Bar Inc	1	Each	68.00	241.40	11.82	38.64	5.36	5.43	1.06			0.05		
Bar, energy, chocolate crisp, uncoated Balance Bar Co Outdoor	1	Each	50.00	200.00	14.00	22.00	0.75	6.00	3.00			3.00		
Bar, energy, chocolate fudge Experimental & Applied Sciences Myoplex Lite	1	Each	56.00	190.00	15.00	27.00	1.00	4.00	3.00			10.00		5.00
Bar, energy, chocolate fudge brownie Power Bar	1	Each	78.00	290.00	24.00	38.00	4.00	5.00	4.00			5.00	0.00	
Bar, energy, chocolate peanut butter Balance Bar Co Gold	1	Each	50.00	210.00	15.00	22.00	0.75	7.00	4.00			0.00	131.26	
Bar, energy, chocolate peanut butter Power Bar	1	Each	78.00	290.00	24.00	38.00	3.00	5.00	3.50			5.00	0.00	
Bar, energy, chocolate peanut crisp Balance Bar Co Oasis	1	Each	48.00	190.00	9.00	25.00	0.75	5.00	2.50			0.00	109.41	
Bar, energy, chocolate raspberry fudge Balance Bar Co	1	Each	50.00	200.00	14.00	22.00	1.00	6.00	3.50			3.00		2.00
Bar, energy, chocolate raspberry truffle Power Bar	1	Each	53.00	180.00	10.00	28.00	3.00	4.00	3.00			0.00	0.00	
Bar, energy, cookies & cream Clif Bar Inc	1	Each	68.00	224.80	10.42	39.25	5.26	3.73	1.45			0.06		
Bar, energy, cranberry apple cherry Clif Bar Inc	1	Each	68.00	220.20	8.19	43.94	5.06	1.94	0.30			0.04		
Bar, energy, fresh wild berry Experimental & Applied Sciences Results for Women	1	Each	55.00	190.00	11.00	28.00	4.00	6.00	2.00			0.00		
Bar, energy, honey nut, plus ginseng Balance Bar Co	1	Each	50.00	200.00	14.00	22.00	0.75	6.00	3.50			3.00		2.00
Bar, energy, honey peanut Balance Bar Co	1	Each	50.00	200.00	14.00	22.00	1.00	6.00	3.50			3.00		2.00
Bar, energy, mocha Power Bar	1	Each	65.00	230.00	10.00	45.00	3.00	2.50	1.00	1.00	0.50	0.00	0.00	
Bar, energy, nutz over chocolate Clif Bar Inc Luna Bar	1	Each	48.00	173.48	9.63	25.25	1.69	4.38	2.74			0.03		
Bar, energy, oatmeal raisin Balance Bar Co Oasis	1	Each	48.00	180.00	8.00	29.00	0.75	3.00	2.00			0.00	109.41	
Bar, energy, oatmeal raisin Power Bar	1	Each	65.00	230.00	10.00	45.00	3.00	2.50	0.50	1.00	1.00	0.00	0.00	
Bar, energy, peanut butter Clif Bar Inc	1	Each	68.00	239.63	12.28	38.26	4.96	5.11	0.77			0.05		
Bar, energy, peanut butter honey, Tiger's Milk Weider Nutrition Company	1	Each	35.00	150.00	6.00	18.00	1.00	6.00	1.00			0.00		1.50
Bar, energy, peanut caramel crisp Experimental & Applied Sciences Myoplex Lite	1	Each	54.00	180.00	15.00	26.00	1.00	4.50	3.00			5.00		
Bar, energy, rocky road Balance Bar Co Gold	1	Each	50.00	210.00	15.00	22.00	1.00	7.00	4.00			0.00	131.26	

Vit E (mg)	Vit C	Vit B1 Thia (mg)	Vit B2 Ribo (mg)	Vit B3 Nia (mg)	Fol (mcg)	Vit B6 (mg)	Vita B12 (mcg)	Sodi (mg)	Pota (mg)	Cal (mg)	Phos (mg)	Magn (mg)	Iron (mg)	Zinc (mg)	Caff (mg)	Alco (g)	Sol Fiber (g)	Insol Fiber (g)
					400.00										0.00	0.00	0.00	0.00
18.35	60.00	1.50	1.70	20.00	400.00	2.00	6.00	90.00	110.00	300.00	350.00	140.00	6.30	5.25	0.00	0.00		
20.32	67.10	0.40	0.28	3.49	82.60	0.42	0.98	70.83	274.61	273.99	287.20	109.39	4.94	3.19	0.00	0.00		
13.64	60.00	0.60	0.51	9.00	80.00	6.00	1.20	90.00	160.00	100.00	100.00	40.00	3.60	3.00		0.00		
4.77	18.00	0.45	0.51	6.00	120.00	0.60	2.40	190.00	70.00	300.00	300.00	40.00	6.30	5.25		0.00		
13.64	60.00	0.60	0.51	9.00	80.00	0.60	1.20	230.00	180.00	100.00	100.00	40.00	3.60	3.00		0.00		
18.34	60.00	0.75	0.85	10.00	200.00	1.00	3.00	80.00		150.00	150.00	60.00	2.70	2.25		0.00		
18.35	60.00	1.50	1.70	20.00	400.00	2.00	6.00	90.00	145.00	300.00	350.00	140.00	6.30	5.25	15.00	0.00		
20.76	65.67	0.39	0.31	3.63	84.62	0.43	0.98	139.30	231.80	278.00	304.10	128.30	5.74	3.71	0.01	0.00		
4.77	6.00	0.53	0.60	7.00	140.00	0.70	2.10	230.00	300.00	350.00	250.00	140.00	6.30	5.25		0.00		
20.34	65.88	0.40	0.30	6.09	94.58	0.41	0.98	274.24	304.60	265.12	297.40	111.09	5.37	3.51		0.00		
	120.00							160.00	160.00	100.00			3.60			0.00		
6.82	30.00	0.75	0.85	10.00	200.00	1.00	3.00	150.00	150.00	300.00	250.00	160.00	7.20	5.25		0.00		
18.34	60.00	1.50	1.70	20.00	400.00	2.00	6.00	150.00		300.00	350.00	140.00	6.30	5.25		0.00		
13.64	60.00	0.38	0.43	5.00	100.00	0.50	1.50	125.00	125.00	100.00	150.00	40.00	4.50	3.75		0.00		
18.34	60.00	1.50	1.70	20.00	400.00	2.00	6.00	290.00		300.00	350.00	140.00	6.30	5.25		0.00		
4.77	6.00	0.53	0.60	7.00	140.00	0.70	2.10	270.00	290.00	350.00	250.00	140.00	6.30	5.25		0.00		
13.64	60.00	0.60	0.51	9.00	80.00	0.60	1.20	150.00	190.00	100.00	100.00	40.00	3.60	3.00		0.00		
18.34	60.00	0.75	0.85	10.00	200.00	1.00	6.00	100.00		500.00	150.00	100.00	4.50	3.75		0.00		
20.26	66.15	0.35	0.27	3.45	85.13	0.43	0.98	179.00	211.90	278.60	266.50	102.60	5.23	3.21	0.00	0.00		
20.32	66.77	0.36	0.27	3.46	82.02	0.40	0.98	132.10	234.70	267.40	272.20	99.11	4.71	3.06	0.00	0.00		
4.09	21.00	0.45	0.51	5.00	120.00	0.50	1.50	150.00	170.00	300.00	250.00	40.00	6.30	5.25	0.00	0.00		
13.64	60.00	0.60	0.51	9.00	80.00	0.60	1.20	220.00	125.00	100.00	100.00	40.00	3.60	3.00		0.00		
13.64	60.00	0.60	0.51	9.00	80.00	0.60	1.20	220.00	115.00	100.00	100.00	40.00	3.60	3.00		0.00		
18.35	60.00	1.50	1.70	20.00	400.00	2.00	6.00	90.00	145.00	300.00	350.00	140.00	6.30	5.25	20.00	0.00		
18.10	58.91	1.72	1.69	20.79	416.10	2.41	5.88	213.13	153.73	446.20	422.12	17.01	7.96	5.46		0.00		
4.77	60.00	0.53	0.60	7.00	140.00	0.70	2.10	220.00	250.00	350.00	250.00	140.00	6.30	5.25	0.00	0.00		
18.35	60.00	1.50	1.70	20.00	400.00	2.00	6.00	120.00	180.00	300.00	350.00	140.00	6.30	5.25	0.00	0.00		
20.36	65.83	0.40	0.30	6.25	96.24	0.42	0.98	289.03	300.58	268.34	305.03	113.70	5.31	3.57	0.00	0.00		
	6.00	1.28	0.60	3.00		0.60	1.50	70.00		300.00	100.00	100.00	2.70			0.00	0.00	
6.82	30.00	0.75	0.85	10.00	200.00	1.00	3.00	240.00	200.00	250.00	250.00	100.00	5.40	3.75	0.00	0.00		
13.64	60.00	0.38	0.43	5.00	100.00	0.50	1.50	80.00	140.00	100.00	150.00	40.00	4.50	3.75		0.00		

Food Name	Amount	Measure	Weight (g)	Calories	Protein (g)	Total Carb (g)	Dietary Fiber (g)	Total Fat (g)	Sat Fat (g)	Mono Fat (g)	Poly Fat (g)	Chol (mg)	Vit A (mcg RAE)	Vit D (mcg)
SPORTS BARS AND DRINKS *(continued)*														
Bar, energy, s'mores														
Clif Bar Inc Luna Bar	1	Each	48.00	178.03	9.86	26.32	2.08	4.33	3.01			0.03		
Bar, energy, tstd nuts & cranberries														
Clif Bar Inc Luna Bar	1	Each	48.00	167.23	9.86	25.53	1.35	3.33	0.50			0.03		
Bar, energy, yogurt honey peanut														
Balance Bar Co	1	Each	50.00	200.00	14.00	22.00	1.00	6.00	3.00			3.00		2.00
Carbohydrate Gel, chocolate, pkt														
Power Bar	1	Each	41.00	120.00	0.00	28.00	0.00	1.50	1.00			0.00	0.00	
Drink, Anabolic Activator III, chocolate, pwd, scoop Optimum Nutrition	2	Each	57.00	180.00	26.00	15.00	1.00	1.50	1.00			15.00		5.00
Drink, carbohydrate, Carbo Pump, pwd, scoop Optimum Nutrition	2.5	Each	85.05	320.00	0.00	80.00		0.00	0.00	0.00	0.00			
Drink, creatine, HP, lemon lime, pwd, scoop Experimental & Applied Sciences Phosphagen	1	Each	43.00	140.00	0.00	34.00	0.00	0.00	0.00	0.00	0.00		0.00	
Drink, energy, w/caff & vit B complex	1	Cup	240.00	103.20	0.94	26.33	0.00	0.00	0.00	0.00	0.00	0.00	0.00	
Drink, protein, muscle building mix, n atural, choc pwd scoop Optimum Nutrition Pro-Complex	2	Each	70.00	270.00	54.00	7.00		2.50	1.50			75.00		5.00
Drink, protein, Simply Protein, whey, chocolate, pwd, scoop Experimental & Applied Sciences Simply Protein	2	Each	28.35	115.00	20.00	4.00	1.00	2.00	1.00			45.00	0.00	0.00
Drink, protein, whey, 100%, natural, vanilla, pwd, scoop Optimum Nutrition	1	Each	31.40	120.00	22.00	5.00	0.75	1.50	0.50			15.00		
Drink, protein, whey, Precision Protein, choc, pwd, scoop Experimental & Applied Sciences	1	Each	25.50	100.00	20.00	2.50		1.00	0.50			15.00	0.00	0.00
Drink, thermogenic, straw kiwi, rtd Experimental & Applied Sciences Results for Women	1	Each	236.00	0.00	0.00	0.00	0.00	0.00	0.00	0.00	0.00	0.00	0.00	
Drink, weight gain, Mighty One 3000, chocolate, pwd, scoop Optimum Nutrition	1	Each	56.00	210.00	5.25	46.25		0.50	0.25			8.75		1.25
Sports Drink, fruit flvr, low cal	1	Cup	240.00	26.40	0.00	7.20	0.00	0.00	0.00	0.00	0.00	0.00	0.00	
Sports Drink, tropical punch, btld Thirst Quencher	1	Cup	240.90	60.22	0.00	15.18	0.00	0.00	0.00	0.00	0.00	0.00	0.00	0.00
Supplement Drink, chocolate, prep w/2% milk Balance Bar Co Total Balance	1	Cup	290.00	280.00	22.00	33.00	1.00	10.40	4.00			24.00		5.00
SUPPLEMENTAL FOODS AND FORMULAS														
Protein, whey, isolate, vanilla, pwd, svg Visical, LLC	1	Ounce-weight	28.35	101.25	24.30	0.00	0.00	0.00	0.00	0.00	0.00	5.06		
Medical Nutritionals														
Bar, supplement, chocolate crunch Mead Johnson	1	Each	44.00	190.00	4.00	29.00	1.00	7.00	3.50			5.00		1.50
Custard, supplement, vanilla, rts Hormel HealthLabs	1	Each	118.00	140.00	7.00	22.00	2.00	3.50	2.00			2.50		
Fiber, supplement, Opti-Fiber, pwd Optimum Nutrition	1	Teaspoon	5.60	15.00	0.00	4.00	4.00	0.00	0.00	0.00	0.00			
Formula, chocolate, rtu	1	Cup	259.79	366.30	13.41	51.65	0.00	11.74	1.56	2.97	7.21	5.20	387.09	2.58
Formula, light, chocolate supreme, rtu Ross Laboratories	1	Cup	253.87	200.00	10.00	33.00	0.00	3.00	0.31	1.90	0.57	5.00		2.50
Supplement Drink, Hi Protein, vanilla, rtu Mead Johnson	1	Cup	255.50	240.00	15.00	33.00	0.00	6.00	0.50			10.00		3.75
Supplement Drink, vanilla, rtu Mead Johnson	1	Cup	255.50	240.00	10.00	41.00	0.00	4.00	0.50			5.00		2.50
Soy Nutritionals														
Bar, soy milk, vegetarian Galaxy Nutritional Foods	1	Each	41.00	140.00	7.00	23.00		2.00	1.50			0.00		
Bar, soy, cafe mocha Genisoy Products	1	Each	61.50	220.00	14.00	34.00	1.00	3.50	2.50			0.00		2.50
Bar, soy, cookies n cream Genisoy Products	1	Each	61.50	220.00	14.00	33.00	2.00	4.00	3.00			0.00		2.50

Vit E (mg)	Vit C	Vit B₁ Thia (mg)	Vit B₂ Ribo (mg)	Vit B₃ Nia (mg)	Fol (mcg)	Vit B₆ (mg)	Vita B₁₂ (mcg)	Sodi (mg)	Pota (mg)	Cal (mg)	Phos (mg)	Magn (mg)	Iron (mg)	Zinc (mg)	Caff (mg)	Alco (g)	Sol Fiber (g)	Insol Fiber (g)
13.76	45.03	1.32	1.28	15.14	321.58	1.84	4.48	183.03	125.88	346.53	343.24	11.27	6.75	4.27	0.00	0.00		
18.35	58.72	1.70	1.68	19.67	412.78	2.39	5.82	189.06	142.95	447.89	436.10	23.63	7.54	5.61	0.00	0.00		
13.64	60.00	0.60	0.51	9.00	80.00	0.60	1.20	220.00	130.00	100.00	100.00	40.00	3.60	3.00	0.00	0.00		
2.77	9.00							50.00	40.00	0.00			0.00		25.00	0.00	0.00	0.00
9.24	30.00	0.75	0.85		200.00	1.00	3.00	240.00	490.00	250.00	250.00	100.00	4.50	3.75		0.00		
															0.00	0.00		
	0.00							95.00	80.00	0.00	200.00	60.00	0.00		0.00	0.00	0.00	0.00
0.00	0.00	0.00	0.01	18.81	0.00	4.70	4.70	187.20	273.60	196.80	24.00	26.40	0.36	0.05	74.40	0.00	0.00	0.00
10.07	30.00		0.85	10.00	200.00	1.00	7.50	420.00	200.00	243.00			0.64			0.00		
								60.00	200.00	160.00			0.40			0.00		
								75.00	200.00	138.00			0.80			0.00		
			0.00			1.00		50.00	80.00	50.00		100.00				0.00		
	0.00							10.00	33.00	0.00			0.00		206.00	0.00	0.00	0.00
1.69	7.50	0.19	0.21	2.50	50.00	0.25	0.75	205.00	417.50	125.00		25.50	1.38	0.92	0.00	0.00		
0.00	15.12	0.00	0.00	0.00	0.00	0.00	0.00	84.00	24.00	0.00	21.60	2.40	0.12	0.05	0.00	0.00	0.00	0.00
0.00	0.00	0.01	0.00	0.00	0.00	0.00	0.00	96.36	26.50	0.00	21.68	2.41	0.12	0.05	0.00	0.00	0.00	0.00
13.64	60.00	0.45	0.77	5.00	100.00	0.60	2.40	408.00	840.00	700.00	400.00	160.00	2.70	5.25		0.00		
								40.50	263.25	111.38	53.66				0.00	0.00	0.00	0.00
2.05	9.00	0.23	0.23	3.00	60.00	0.30	0.90	90.00	105.00	150.00	150.00	60.00	1.08	2.30		0.00		
	2.40							260.00		250.00			0.00		0.00	0.00		
	100.00														0.00	0.00		
3.48	30.92	0.39	0.44	5.15	103.92	0.51	1.56	246.80	454.63	205.23	205.23	103.92	4.65	3.92	0.00	0.00	0.00	0.00
3.41	30.00	0.38	0.43	5.00	100.00	0.50	1.50	200.00	370.00	250.00	250.00	100.00	4.50	3.80		0.00	0.00	0.00
13.64	60.00	0.38	0.43	5.00	140.00	0.70	2.10	170.00	380.00	330.00	310.00	105.00	4.50	4.50	0.00	0.00	0.00	0.00
13.64	60.00	0.38	0.43	5.00	140.00	0.70	2.10	130.00	400.00	300.00	250.00	100.00	3.60	4.50	0.00	0.00	0.00	0.00
								140.00	25.00	400.00	250.00				0.00	0.00		
13.64	15.00	0.38	0.43	5.00	100.00	0.50	1.50	150.00	250.00	250.00	250.00	100.00	4.50	3.75		0.00		
3.41	15.00	0.38	0.43	5.00	100.00	0.50	1.50	160.00	260.00	250.00	250.00	100.00	4.50	3.75		0.00		

Food Name	Amount	Measure	Weight (g)	Calories	Protein (g)	Total Carb (g)	Dietary Fiber (g)	Total Fat (g)	Sat Fat (g)	Mono Fat (g)	Poly Fat (g)	Chol (mg)	Vit A (mcg RAE)	Vit D (mcg)
SUPPLEMENTAL FOODS AND FORMULAS *(continued)*														
Bar, soy, hi prot, chocolate peanut butter Max Muscle	1	Each	56.70	234.00	19.00	20.20	0.00	8.00	3.00			3.00		
Drink, soy, Opti-Soy 50, natural, chocolate, pwd, scoop Optimum Nutrition	1	Each	35.00	130.00	14.00	16.00	1.00	1.00						
Vitamins, Food Additives, & Supplements—Retail														
Bar, nutrition, AdvantEDGE Carb Control, choc pnt btr Abbott EAS	1	Each	60.00	230.00	17.00	26.00	5.00	8.00	5.00			5.00		
Bar, nutrition, AdvantEDGE Carb Control, choc pnt btr crisp Abbott EAS	1	Each	60.00	240.00	17.00	27.00	6.00	8.00	4.50			5.00		
Bar, nutrition, AdvantEDGE Carb Control, cookies & cream Abbott EAS	1	Each	60.00	230.00	17.00	25.00	5.00	8.00	4.50			5.00		
Bar, nutrition, AdvantEDGE Carb Control, double choc crisp Abbott EAS	1	Each	60.00	240.00	17.00	27.00	6.00	8.00	6.00			5.00		
Drink, creatine, w/Ribose, punch, pwd, scoop Optimum Nutrition Pre-Load Plus	1	Scoop	46.00	140.00	0.00	34.00		0.00	0.00	0.00	0.00			
Drink, protein, Muscle Milk, light, pwd USDA SR-23 Cytosport	2	Scoop	50.00	198.00	25.00	11.00	1.00	6.00	0.54	4.24	0.62	5.00	525.00	3.50
Drink, supplement, Pedialyte, grape, pwd Abbott Abbott	1	Ind. Pkt.	8.50	23.00	0.00	5.70		0.00	0.00	0.00	0.00			
Fiber, flaxseed, pwd Hain Celestial Group Spectrum Essentials	1	Tablespoon	8.00	30.00	2.00	4.00	3.00	1.00				0.00	0.00	
Protein, soy, pwd Bob's Red Mill	1	Tablespoon	6.50	20.00	5.00	0.00	0.00	0.00	0.00	0.00	0.00	0.00	0.00	
Protein, whey, EAS, chocolate, pwd Abbott EAS	1	Scoop	30.00	120.00	23.00	3.00	1.00	2.00	1.00			65.00	0.00	
Pudding, nutrition, Ensure, homemade vanilla Abbott Abbott	1	Ind. Pkt.	113.00	170.00	4.00	30.00	3.00	5.00	1.00	1.00	2.00	5.00		1.00
Shake, nutrition, Ensure High Calcium, creamy milk choc, rtd Abbott Abbott	8	Fluid ounce	252.00	220.00	10.00	31.00	1.00	6.00	1.00	2.00	3.00	5.00		5.00
Shake, nutrition, Ensure High Protein, creamy milk choc, rtd Abbott Abbott	8	Fluid ounce	252.00	230.00	12.00	31.00	1.00	6.00	1.00	2.00	3.00	5.00		2.50
Shake, nutrition, Ensure Plus, homemade vanilla, rtd Abbott Abbott	8	Fluid ounce	252.00	350.00	13.00	50.00	3.00	11.00	1.00	5.00	4.50	10.00		2.50
Shake, nutrition, Ensure Plus, rich dark chocolate, rtd Abbott Abbott	8	Fluid ounce	252.00	350.00	13.00	51.00	3.00	11.00	1.50	5.00	4.50	10.00		2.50
Shake, nutrition, Myoplex Original, chocolate cream, pwd Abbott EAS	1	Ind. Pkt.	78.00	300.00	42.00	22.00	3.00	6.00	1.50			50.00		
Supplement, fish oil, capsules Hain Celestial Group Spectrum Essentials	2	Each	2.00	25.00	0.00	0.00	0.00	2.00	0.50			12.00		0.10
Supplement, flaxseed oil, softgel, capsules Hain Celestial Group Spectrum Essentials	6	Each	6.00	60.00	0.00	0.00	0.00	6.00	0.50			0.00	0.00	
Yeast, brewer's, debittered, pwd Now Foods	2	Tablespoon	16.21	50.00	8.00	5.00		0.00	0.00	0.00	0.00	0.00		
Zinc Lozenges Optimum Nutrition	1	Tablet	2.48	10.00	0.00	2.00	0.00	0.00	0.00	0.00	0.00	0.00		
SWEETENERS AND SWEET SUBSTITUTES														
Jams and Jellies														
Fruit Butter, apple	1	Tablespoon	18.00	31.14	0.07	7.70	0.27	0.00	0.00	0.00	0.00	0.00	0.18	
Fruit Spread, strawberry, All-Fruit, Polaner's B&G Foods, Inc.	1	Tablespoon	18.00	41.58	0.13	10.26		0.00	0.00	0.00	0.00			
Jam	1	Tablespoon	20.00	55.60	0.07	13.77	0.22	0.01	0.00	0.01	0.00	0.00	0.00	
Jam, concord grape The J.M. Smucker Co.	1	Tablespoon	20.00	50.00	0.00	13.00	0.00	0.00	0.00	0.00	0.00	0.00		
Jam, rducd sug	1	Tablespoon	20.00	36.30	0.21	8.89	0.50	0.14	0.01	0.01	0.05	0.00	0.21	
Jam, strawberry The J.M. Smucker Co.	1	Tablespoon	20.00	50.00	0.00	13.00	0.00	0.00	0.00	0.00	0.00	0.00		
Jam/Preserves, any flvr, w/sod sacc, dietetic	1	Tablespoon	14.00	18.48	0.04	7.50	0.35	0.04	0.00	0.01	0.02	0.00	0.00	
Jelly	1	Tablespoon	19.00	50.54	0.03	13.29	0.19	0.00	0.00	0.00	0.00	0.00	0.05	
Jelly, rducd sug, prep f/recipe	1	Tablespoon	19.00	34.01	0.06	8.76	0.15	0.01	0.00	0.00	0.00	0.00	0.03	
Marmalade, orange	1	Tablespoon	20.00	49.20	0.06	13.26	0.14	0.00	0.00	0.00	0.00	0.00	0.60	
Preserves, strawberry The J.M. Smucker Co.	1	Tablespoon	20.00	50.00	0.00	13.00	0.00	0.00	0.00	0.00	0.00	0.00		
Sugars, Sugar Substitutes, and Syrups														
Honey, amber light Pure Sweet Honey Farm Incorporated	1	Tablespoon	21.00	63.84	0.15	17.01	0.00	0.00	0.00	0.00	0.00	0.00	0.00	0.00

Vit E (mg)	Vit C	Vit B₁ Thia (mg)	Vit B₂ Ribo (mg)	Vit B₃ Nia (mg)	Fol (mcg)	Vit B₆ (mg)	Vita B₁₂ (mcg)	Sodi (mg)	Pota (mg)	Cal (mg)	Phos (mg)	Magn (mg)	Iron (mg)	Zinc (mg)	Caff (mg)	Alco (g)	Sol Fiber (g)	Insol Fiber (g)
								162.00								0.00	0.00	0.00
40.27	60.00				200.00					310.00			5.00			0.00		
	18.00	0.45	0.51	6.00	80.00	0.60	1.80	230.00	160.00	300.00	150.00	40.00	5.40	4.50		0.00		
	18.00	0.45	0.51	7.00	120.00	0.60	1.80	350.00	140.00	350.00	250.00	60.00	5.40	4.50		0.00		
	18.00	0.45	0.51	6.00	120.00	0.60	1.80	120.00	120.00	500.00	100.00	40.00	5.40	4.50		0.00		
	18.00	0.45	0.51	6.00	120.00	0.60	1.80	340.00	230.00	300.00	200.00	60.00	6.30	4.50		0.00		
								40.00	80.00		239.00				0.00	0.00		
4.72	21.00	0.50	0.60	7.00	140.00	0.70	2.10	125.00	420.00	600.00	350.00	140.00	6.00	5.00	0.00	0.00		
								243.80	183.30						0.00	0.00		
	0.00							0.00	0.00	0.00			0.00		0.00	0.00		
	0.00							60.00		0.00			0.72		0.00	0.00	0.00	0.00
	0.00							50.00	170.00	100.00			0.36			0.00		
	9.00	0.23	0.26	2.00	60.00	0.30	0.60	85.00	110.00	100.00	100.00	40.00	1.80	1.50	0.00	0.00		
	42.00	0.38	0.43	5.00	120.00	0.50	1.80	290.00	500.00	500.00	250.00	100.00	4.50	3.70		0.00		
	30.00	0.38	0.43	5.00	100.00	0.50	1.50	290.00	500.00	300.00	250.00	100.00	4.50	5.70		0.00		
	36.00	0.38	0.43	5.00	100.00	0.50	1.50	220.00	420.00	300.00	300.00	100.00	4.50	3.80		0.00		
	36.00	0.38	0.43	5.00	100.00	0.50	1.50	230.00	700.00	300.00	300.00	100.00	4.50	4.50		0.00		
	24.00	0.60	0.85	9.00	200.00	0.90	3.60	250.00	875.00	600.00	450.00	200.00	7.20	7.50		0.00		
	0.00							0.00	0.00	0.00			0.00		0.00	0.00	0.00	0.00
	0.00							0.00	0.00	0.00			0.00		0.00	0.00	0.00	0.00
		2.40	0.51	6.00	120.00	0.50	3.00	20.00	320.00	20.00		40.00	1.44	1.50	0.00	0.00		
	30.00													23.00	0.00	0.00	0.00	0.00
0.00	0.18	0.00	0.00	0.01	0.18	0.01	0.00	2.70	16.38	2.52	1.26	0.90	0.06	0.01	0.00	0.00		
								3.60							0.00	0.00		
0.02	1.76	0.00	0.02	0.01	2.20	0.00	0.00	6.40	15.40	4.00	3.80	0.80	0.10	0.01	0.00	0.00		
	0.00							0.00		0.00			0.00		0.00	0.00	0.00	0.00
0.03	7.62	0.00	0.02	0.06	1.73	0.03	0.00	4.81	102.33	5.98	8.15	5.00	0.24	0.05	0.00	0.00		
	0.00							0.00		0.00			0.00		0.00	0.00	0.00	0.00
0.01	0.00	0.00	0.00	0.00	1.26	0.00	0.00	0.00	9.66	1.26	1.26	0.70	0.06	0.01	0.00	0.00		
0.00	0.17	0.00	0.00	0.01	0.38	0.00	0.00	5.70	10.26	1.33	1.14	1.14	0.04	0.01	0.00	0.00		
0.00	0.00	0.00	0.00	0.03	0.19	0.01	0.00	0.38	13.49	0.95	1.14	1.14	0.03	0.01	0.00	0.00		
0.01	0.96	0.00	0.01	0.01	1.80	0.00	0.00	11.20	7.40	7.60	0.80	0.40	0.03	0.01	0.00	0.00		
	0.00							0.00		0.00			0.00		0.00	0.00	0.00	0.00
0.00	0.10	0.00	0.06	0.06	2.10	0.00	0.00	0.60	10.50	1.01	1.05	0.42	0.05	0.03	0.00	0.00	0.00	0.00

Food Name	Amount	Measure	Weight (g)	Calories	Protein (g)	Total Carb (g)	Dietary Fiber (g)	Total Fat (g)	Sat Fat (g)	Mono Fat (g)	Poly Fat (g)	Chol (mg)	Vit A (mcg RAE)	Vit D (mcg)
SWEETENERS AND SWEET SUBSTITUTES *(continued)*														
Honey, strained/extracted	1	Tablespoon	21.19	64.41	0.06	17.46	0.04	0.00	0.00	0.00	0.00	0.00	0.00	
Molasses	1	Tablespoon	20.50	59.45	0.00	15.32	0.00	0.02	0.00	0.01	0.01	0.00	0.00	
Molasses, blackstrap	1	Tablespoon	20.50	48.17	0.00	12.46	0.00	0.00	0.00	0.00	0.00	0.00	0.00	
Sugar Substitute, Sweet 'N Low, granular														
Brooklyn Premium Corp.	1	Teaspoon	4.00	0.00	0.00	4.00	0.00	0.00	0.00	0.00	0.00	0.00	0.00	
Sugar, brown, packed	1	Teaspoon	4.60	17.34	0.00	4.47	0.00	0.00	0.00	0.00	0.00	0.00	0.00	
Sugar, confectioners/powdered, unsftd	1	Teaspoon	2.50	9.72	0.00	2.49	0.00	0.00	0.00	0.00	0.00	0.00	0.00	
Sugar, white, granulated, cubed	1	Each	2.50	9.68	0.00	2.50	0.00	0.00	0.00	0.00	0.00	0.00	0.00	
Syrup, corn, dark	2	Tablespoon	41.00	117.26	0.00	31.82	0.00	0.00	0.00	0.00	0.00	0.00	0.00	0.00
Syrup, maple	2	Tablespoon	40.00	104.40	0.00	26.84	0.00	0.08	0.01	0.03	0.04	0.00	0.00	
Syrup, pancake, w/2% maple	2	Tablespoon	39.40	104.41	0.00	27.42	0.00	0.04	0.01	0.01	0.03	0.00	0.00	
VEGETABLES AND LEGUMES														
Vegetables														
Raw Vegetables														
Agave, Southwestern, fresh USDA SR-23	1	Serving	140.00	95.20	0.73	22.72	9.24	0.21				0.00	2.59	0.00
Alfalfa Sprouts, fresh	0.5	Cup	16.50	4.79	0.66	0.62	0.41	0.11	0.01	0.01	0.07	0.00	1.32	
Artichokes, Calif, fresh	1	Each	340.00	85.00	6.80	20.40	10.20	0.00	0.00	0.00	0.00	0.00	0.00	
Arugula, chpd, fresh, cup	1	Cup	20.00	5.00	0.52	0.73	0.32	0.13	0.02	0.01	0.06	0.00	23.80	0.00
Asparagus, fresh, cup	0.5	Cup	67.00	13.40	1.47	2.60	1.39	0.08	0.02	0.00	0.05	0.00	25.46	
Asparagus, spears, tips, fresh, 2" long or less	10	Each	35.00	7.00	0.80	1.40	0.70	0.00	0.00	0.00	0.00	0.00	13.30	
Beans, broad, immature USDA SR-23	0.5	Cup	54.50	39.24	3.05	6.38	2.29	0.33	0.08	0.01	0.17	0.00	9.54	0.00
Beans, fava, immature USDA SR-23	0.5	Cup	54.50	39.24	3.05	6.38	2.29	0.33	0.08	0.01	0.17	0.00	9.54	0.00
Bean Sprouts, navy, mature, fresh	0.5	Cup	52.00	34.84	3.20	6.78	1.99	0.37	0.04	0.02	0.21	0.00	0.10	
Broccoli, bunch, fresh, each	1	Each	608.00	206.72	17.15	40.37	15.81	2.25	0.24	0.07	0.23	0.00	200.64	
Broccoli, florets, fresh	0.5	Cup	35.50	9.94	1.06	1.86	1.03	0.13	0.02	0.01	0.06	0.00	53.25	
Broccoli, stalk, fresh USDA SR-23	1	Each	114.00	31.92	3.40	5.97	3.42	0.40	0.06	0.03	0.19	0.00	22.80	0.00
Brussels Sprouts, fresh USDA SR-23	0.5	Cup	44.00	18.92	1.49	3.94	1.67	0.13	0.03	0.01	0.07	0.00	16.59	0.00
Cabbage, fresh harvest, fresh, shredded	0.5	Cup	35.00	8.40	0.42	1.88	0.81	0.06	0.01	0.00	0.03	0.00	2.10	0.00
Cabbage, kale, curly, fresh, chpd USDA SR-23	1	Cup	67.00	33.50	2.21	6.71	1.34	0.47	0.06	0.03	0.23	0.00	515.10	0.00
Cabbage, kohlrabi, fresh USDA SR-23	1	Cup	135.00	36.45	2.30	8.37	4.86	0.14	0.02	0.01	0.06	0.00	2.43	0.00
Cabbage, pickled, Japanese, fresh	0.5	Cup	75.00	22.50	1.20	4.25	2.33	0.08	0.01	0.01	0.04	0.00	6.75	
Cabbage, red, fresh, shredded	0.5	Cup	35.00	10.85	0.50	2.58	0.74	0.06	0.01	0.00	0.04	0.00	19.60	
Cactus, nopales, slices, fresh	0.5	Cup	43.00	6.88	0.57	1.43	0.94	0.04	0.00	0.01	0.02	0.00	9.89	
Capers Mezzetta	1	Teaspoon	5.00	0.22	0.20	0.08		0.00				0.00	0.60	
Carrots, baby, fresh, med	1	Each	10.00	3.50	0.06	0.82	0.18	0.01	0.00	0.00	0.01	0.00	69.00	
Carrots, fresh, chpd	0.5	Cup	64.00	26.24	0.59	6.13	1.79	0.15	0.02	0.01	0.08	0.00	385.28	
Carrots, fresh, med	1	Each	61.00	25.01	0.57	5.84	1.71	0.15	0.02	0.01	0.07	0.00	367.22	
Cauliflower, green, fresh	0.5	Cup	32.00	9.92	0.94	1.95	1.01	0.10	0.02	0.01	0.04	0.00	2.56	
Celery, stalk, sml, 5" long, fresh	1	Each	17.00	2.38	0.12	0.50	0.25	0.03	0.01	0.01	0.01	0.00	3.74	
Chili Peppers, green, hot, fresh, whole	0.5	Cup	75.00	30.00	1.50	7.10	1.12	0.15	0.02	0.00	0.08	0.00	44.25	
Chili Peppers, jalapeno, fresh USDA SR-23	1	Each	14.00	4.06	0.13	0.91	0.37	0.05	0.01	0.00	0.02	0.00	7.55	0.00
Chili Peppers, jalapeno, fresh, sliced USDA SR-23	0.25	Cup	22.50	6.52	0.20	1.46	0.59	0.08	0.02	0.01	0.03	0.00	12.13	0.00
Chili Peppers, serrano, fresh USDA SR-23	1	Each	6.10	1.95	0.11	0.41	0.20	0.03	0.00	0.00	0.01	0.00	2.86	0.00
Corn, white, sweet, kernels f/sml ear, 5.5"–6.5" long, fresh USDA SR-23	1	Each	73.00	62.78	2.35	13.88	1.97	0.86	0.13	0.25	0.41	0.00	0.04	0.00
Corn, white, sweet, kernels, fresh USDA SR-23	0.5	Cup	77.00	66.22	2.48	14.65	2.08	0.91	0.14	0.27	0.43	0.00	0.04	0.00
Corn, yellow, sweet, ear, fresh, med, 6.75"–7.5" long USDA SR-23	1	Each	102.00	87.72	3.34	19.07	2.04	1.38	0.33	0.44	0.50	0.00	9.54	0.00
Cornsalad, fresh	0.5	Cup	28.00	5.88	0.56	1.01	0.42	0.11				0.00	99.40	
Cucumber, Japanese, fresh Frieda's	0.66	Cup	85.00	10.00	1.00	2.00	1.00	0.00	0.00	0.00	0.00	0.00	10.00	
Cucumber, w/skin, fresh, slices	0.5	Cup	52.00	7.80	0.34	1.89	0.26	0.06	0.02	0.00	0.03	0.00	2.60	
Dish, falafel, prep f/recipe, patty, 2 1/4"	1	Each	17.00	56.61	2.26	5.41		3.03	0.41	1.73	0.71	0.00	0.17	
Eggplant, fresh, cubes USDA SR-23	0.5	Cup	41.00	9.84	0.41	2.34	1.38	0.08	0.01	0.01	0.03	0.00	0.55	0.00
Endive, fresh, chpd	0.5	Cup	25.00	4.25	0.31	0.84	0.78	0.05	0.01	0.00	0.02	0.00	27.00	
Fennel, bulb, fresh, slices	0.5	Cup	43.50	13.48	0.54	3.17	1.35	0.08				0.00	3.04	
Garlic, cloves, fresh USDA SR-23	1	Each	3.00	4.47	0.19	0.99	0.06	0.01	0.00	0.00	0.01	0.00	0.01	0.00
Greens, mustard spinach, tendergreen, fresh USDA SR-23	1	Cup	150.00	33.00	3.30	5.85	4.20	0.45	0.02	0.21	0.09	0.00	742.50	0.00

Vit E (mg)	Vit C	Vit B₁ Thia (mg)	Vit B₂ Ribo (mg)	Vit B₃ Nia (mg)	Fol (mcg)	Vit B₆ (mg)	Vita B₁₂ (mcg)	Sodi (mg)	Pota (mg)	Cal (mg)	Phos (mg)	Magn (mg)	Iron (mg)	Zinc (mg)	Caff (mg)	Alco (g)	Sol Fiber (g)	Insol Fiber (g)
0.00	0.11	0.00	0.01	0.03	0.42	0.01	0.00	0.85	11.02	1.27	0.85	0.42	0.09	0.05	0.00	0.00		
0.00	0.00	0.01	0.00	0.19	0.00	0.14	0.00	7.58	300.12	42.02	6.35	49.61	0.97	0.06	0.00	0.00	0.00	0.00
0.00	0.00	0.01	0.01	0.22	0.20	0.14	0.00	11.27	510.86	176.30	8.20	44.07	3.59	0.20	0.00	0.00	0.00	0.00
	0.00							0.00		0.00			0.00		0.00	0.00	0.00	0.00
0.00	0.00	0.00	0.00	0.00	0.05	0.00	0.00	1.79	15.92	3.91	1.01	1.33	0.09	0.01	0.00	0.00	0.00	0.00
0.00	0.00	0.00	0.00	0.00	0.00	0.00	0.00	0.02	0.05	0.02	0.00	0.00	0.00	0.00	0.00	0.00	0.00	0.00
0.00	0.00	0.00	0.00	0.00	0.00	0.00	0.00	0.00	0.05	0.03	0.00	0.00	0.00	0.00	0.00	0.00	0.00	0.00
0.00	0.00	0.00	0.00	0.01	0.00	0.00	0.00	63.55	18.04	7.38	4.51	3.28	0.15	0.01	0.00	0.00	0.00	0.00
0.00	0.00	0.00	0.00	0.01	0.00	0.00	0.00	3.60	81.60	26.80	0.80	5.60	0.48	1.67	0.00	0.00	0.00	0.00
0.00	0.00	0.00	0.01	0.00	0.00	0.00	0.00	24.03	2.36	1.97	3.94	0.79	0.03	0.09	0.00	0.00	0.00	0.00
0.32	5.60	0.04	0.05	0.23	9.80	0.08	0.00	19.60	177.80	583.80	9.80	77.00	2.52	0.21	0.00	0.00		
0.00	1.35	0.01	0.02	0.08	5.94	0.01	0.00	0.99	13.04	5.28	11.55	4.46	0.16	0.15	0.00	0.00	0.08	0.33
1.36	20.40	0.12	0.12	2.72	136.00	0.12		255.00	578.00	68.00	204.00	136.00	2.44		0.00	0.00		
0.09	3.00	0.01	0.02	0.06	19.40	0.01	0.00	5.40	73.80	32.00	10.40	9.40	0.29	0.09	0.00	0.00		
0.76	3.75	0.09	0.09	0.65	34.84	0.06	0.00	1.34	135.34	16.08	34.84	9.38	1.43	0.36	0.00	0.00		
0.40	2.00	0.10	0.00	0.30	18.20	0.00	0.00	0.70	70.70	8.40	18.20	4.90	0.70	0.20	0.00	0.00		
	17.99	0.09	0.06	0.82	52.32	0.02	0.00	27.25	136.25	11.99	51.78	20.71	1.04	0.32	0.00	0.00		
	17.99	0.09	0.06	0.82	52.32	0.02	0.00	27.25	136.25	11.99	51.78	20.71	1.04	0.32	0.00	0.00		
0.02	9.78	0.20	0.11	0.64	68.64	0.10	0.00	6.76	159.64	78.00	52.00	52.52	1.00	0.46	0.00	0.00		
4.74	542.34	0.43	0.71	3.89	383.04	1.06	0.00	200.64	1921.28	285.76	401.28	127.68	4.44	2.49	0.00	0.00	1.46	14.35
0.16	33.09	0.03	0.04	0.23	25.21	0.06	0.00	9.59	115.38	17.04	23.43	8.88	0.31	0.14	0.00	0.00	0.11	0.91
	106.25	0.07	0.14	0.73	80.94	0.18	0.00	30.78	370.50	54.72	75.24	28.50	1.00	0.46	0.00	0.00	0.38	3.04
0.39	37.40	0.06	0.04	0.33	26.84	0.10	0.00	11.00	171.16	18.48	30.36	10.12	0.62	0.18	0.00	0.00	0.88	0.79
0.04	17.85	0.02	0.01	0.11	19.95	0.03	0.00	6.30	86.10	16.45	8.05	5.25	0.20	0.06	0.00	0.00	0.27	0.53
	80.40	0.07	0.09	0.67	19.43	0.18	0.00	28.81	299.49	90.45	37.52	22.78	1.14	0.29	0.00	0.00	0.54	0.80
0.65	83.70	0.07	0.03	0.54	21.60	0.20	0.00	27.00	472.50	32.40	62.10	25.65	0.54	0.04	0.00	0.00	3.38	1.49
0.09	0.53	0.00	0.03	0.13	31.50	0.08	0.00	207.75	639.75	36.00	32.25	9.00	0.37	0.15	0.00	0.00		
0.04	19.95	0.02	0.02	0.15	6.30	0.07	0.00	9:45	85.05	15.75	10.50	5.60	0.28	0.08	0.00	0.00	0.04	0.70
0.00	4.00	0.00	0.02	0.18	1.29	0.03	0.00	9.03	110.51	70.52	6.88	22.36	0.26	0.11	0.00	0.00		
	0.00						0.00	105.40		1.81			0.05		0.00	0.00		
0.04	0.84	0.00	0.00	0.06	3.30	0.01	0.00	7.80	23.70	3.20	2.80	1.00	0.09	0.02	0.00	0.00	0.05	0.13
0.42	3.78	0.05	0.04	0.63	12.16	0.09	0.00	44.16	204.80	21.12	22.40	7.68	0.20	0.15	0.00	0.00	0.75	1.04
0.40	3.60	0.04	0.04	0.60	11.59	0.08	0.00	42.09	195.20	20.13	21.35	7.32	0.18	0.15	0.00	0.00	0.72	0.99
0.01	28.19	0.03	0.03	0.23	18.24	0.07	0.00	7.36	96.00	10.56	19.84	6.40	0.23	0.20	0.00	0.00		
0.05	0.53	0.00	0.01	0.05	6.12	0.01	0.00	13.60	44.20	6.80	4.08	1.87	0.03	0.02	0.00	0.00		
0.52	181.88	0.08	0.08	0.72	17.25	0.20	0.00	5.25	255.00	13.50	34.50	18.75	0.90	0.22	0.00	0.00	0.35	0.80
0.50	16.60	0.01	0.01	0.18	3.78	0.06	0.00	0.42	34.72	1.68	3.64	2.10	0.04	0.02	0.00	0.00		
0.81	26.68	0.01	0.02	0.29	6.07	0.09	0.00	0.67	55.80	2.70	5.85	3.37	0.06	0.03	0.00	0.00		
0.04	2.74	0.00	0.00	0.09	1.40	0.03	0.00	0.61	18.61	0.67	2.44	1.34	0.05	0.02	0.00	0.00		
0.05	4.96	0.15	0.04	1.24	33.58	0.04	0.00	10.95	197.10	1.46	64.97	27.01	0.38	0.33	0.00	0.00		
0.05	5.24	0.15	0.05	1.31	35.42	0.04	0.00	11.55	207.90	1.54	68.53	28.49	0.40	0.35	0.00	0.00		
0.07	6.94	0.16	0.06	1.81	42.84	0.09	0.00	15.30	275.40	2.04	90.78	37.74	0.53	0.47	0.00	0.00	0.08	1.96
0.03	10.70	0.02	0.02	0.12	3.92	0.08	0.00	1.12	128.52	10.64	14.84	3.64	0.61	0.17	0.00	0.00		
	4.80						0.00	0.00					0.00		0.00	0.00		
0.02	1.46	0.01	0.02	0.05	3.64	0.02	0.00	1.04	76.44	8.32	12.48	6.76	0.15	0.10	0.00	0.00	0.03	0.23
0.19	0.27	0.02	0.03	0.18	15.81	0.02	0.00	49.98	99.45	9.18	32.64	13.94	0.58	0.26	0.00	0.00		
0.12	0.90	0.02	0.02	0.27	9.02	0.03	0.00	0.82	94.30	3.69	10.25	5.74	0.10	0.07	0.00	0.00		
0.11	1.62	0.02	0.02	0.10	35.50	0.00	0.00	5.50	78.50	13.00	7.00	3.75	0.21	0.20	0.00	0.00	0.33	0.44
	5.22	0.00	0.02	0.28	11.74	0.02	0.00	22.62	180.09	21.32	21.75	7.40	0.32	0.08	0.00	0.00		
0.00	0.94	0.01	0.00	0.02	0.09	0.04	0.00	0.51	12.03	5.43	4.59	0.75	0.05	0.03	0.00	0.00		
	195.00	0.10	0.14	1.02	238.50	0.23	0.00	31.50	673.50	315.00	42.00	16.50	2.25	0.26	0.00	0.00		

Food Name	Amount	Measure	Weight (g)	Calories	Protein (g)	Total Carb (g)	Dietary Fiber (g)	Total Fat (g)	Sat Fat (g)	Mono Fat (g)	Poly Fat (g)	Chol (mg)	Vit A (mcg RAE)	Vit D (mcg)
VEGETABLES AND LEGUMES *(continued)*														
Greens, radicchio, fresh, shredded USDA SR-23	1	Cup	40.00	9.20	0.57	1.79	0.36	0.10	0.02	0.00	0.04	0.00	0.54	0.00
Greens, Swiss chard, fresh USDA SR-23	1	Cup	36.00	6.84	0.65	1.35	0.58	0.07	0.01	0.01	0.03	0.00	110.09	0.00
Greens, vine spinach, fresh USDA SR-23	1	Serving	85.00	16.15	1.53	2.89		0.26				0.00	340.00	0.00
Leeks, bulb & lower leaf, fresh, chpd	0.5	Cup	44.50	27.14	0.67	6.30	0.80	0.14	0.02	0.00	0.07	0.00	36.93	
Lemon Grass, fresh	0.5	Cup	33.50	33.17	0.60	8.49		0.16	0.04	0.02	0.07	0.00	0.11	
Lettuce, butterhead, fresh, leaf, med	2	Piece	15.00	1.95	0.20	0.34	0.17	0.03	0.00	0.00	0.02	0.00	24.90	
Lettuce, iceberg, fresh, leaf, med	2	Piece	16.00	2.24	0.14	0.47	0.19	0.02	0.00	0.00	0.01	0.00	4.00	
Lettuce, looseleaf, fresh, leaf	2	Piece	20.00	3.00	0.27	0.56	0.26	0.03	0.00	0.00	0.02	0.00	74.00	
Lettuce, romaine, fresh, inner leaf	2	Piece	20.00	3.40	0.25	0.66	0.42	0.06	0.01	0.00	0.03	0.00	58.00	
Lettuce, romaine, fresh, leaf Dole Food Company, Inc.	2	Piece	28.33	6.67	0.33	1.00	0.33	0.17	0.00			0.00	16.66	
Lotus Root, fresh, slices, 2 1/2" USDA SR-23	10	Piece	81.00	59.94	2.11	13.96	3.97	0.08	0.02	0.02	0.02	0.00	0.00	0.00
Mushrooms, brown, fresh Mushroom Council	6	Each	84.00	23.00	2.13	3.39	0.49	0.12				0.00	0.00	
Mushrooms, crimini, fresh	2	Each	28.00	6.16	0.70	1.15	0.17	0.03	0.00	0.00	0.01	0.00	0.00	
Mushrooms, enoki, lrg, fresh	6	Each	30.00	10.20	0.71	2.11	0.78	0.12	0.01	0.00	0.05	0.00	0.11	0.57
Mushrooms, fresh, pces/slices	0.5	Cup	35.00	7.70	1.09	1.13	0.42	0.12	0.02	0.00	0.05	0.00	0.00	0.67
Mushrooms, oyster, fresh, lrg	1	Each	148.00	54.76	6.13	9.21	3.55	0.75				0.00	2.96	
Mushrooms, portabella, fresh Mushroom Council	1	Each	84.00	27.00	2.07	4.33	1.28	0.13				0.00	0.00	
Mushrooms, portobello, fresh, chpd USDA SR-23	0.5	Cup	43.00	9.46	0.91	1.66	0.56	0.15	0.03	0.01	0.05	0.00	0.00	0.13
Mustard Greens, fresh, chpd	1	Cup	56.00	14.56	1.52	2.75	1.85	0.11	0.01	0.05	0.02	0.00	294.00	
Okra, fresh, pods, 3" long USDA SR-23	8	Each	95.00	29.45	1.90	6.68	3.04	0.09	0.02	0.02	0.03	0.00	17.81	0.00
Onion, pearl, fresh, chpd	0.5	Cup	80.00	33.60	0.73	8.08	1.12	0.07	0.02	0.01	0.04	0.00	0.08	
Onion, scallions, tops & bulb, fresh, chpd	0.5	Cup	50.00	16.00	0.92	3.67	1.30	0.09	0.02	0.01	0.04	0.00	25.00	
Onion, white, fresh, chpd	0.5	Cup	80.00	33.60	0.73	8.08	1.12	0.07	0.02	0.01	0.04	0.00	0.08	
Onion, yellow, fresh, chpd	0.5	Cup	80.00	33.60	0.73	8.08	1.12	0.07	0.02	0.01	0.04	0.00	0.08	
Parsnips, fresh, slices	0.5	Cup	66.50	49.88	0.80	11.96	3.26	0.20	0.04	0.08	0.03	0.00	0.00	
Pea Pods, sugar snap, fresh, whole USDA SR-23	10	Each	34.00	14.28	0.95	2.57	0.88	0.07	0.01	0.01	0.03	0.00	18.48	0.00
Peppers, bell, green, sweet, fresh, chpd	0.5	Cup	74.50	14.90	0.64	3.46	1.27	0.13	0.04	0.01	0.05	0.00	13.41	
Peppers, bell, red, sweet, fresh, chpd	0.5	Cup	74.50	19.37	0.74	4.49	1.47	0.22	0.04	0.01	0.12	0.00	116.97	
Peppers, bell, yellow, sweet, fresh, lrg, 3 3/4" long	1	Each	186.00	50.22	1.86	11.76	1.67	0.39	0.06	0.05	0.21	0.00	18.60	0.00
Potatoes, russet, w/skin, fresh, med 2 1/4"–3 1/4" USDA SR-23	1	Each	213.00	168.27	4.56	38.49	2.77	0.17	0.06	0.00	0.09	0.00	0.11	0.00
Potatoes, w/skin, fresh, med 2 1/4"–3 1/4", USDA USDA SR-23	1	Each	213.00	146.97	3.58	33.46	5.11	0.21	0.06	0.00	0.09	0.00	0.85	0.00
Prickly Pears, fresh, Northern Plains USDA SR-23	1	Serving	140.00	58.80	0.17	14.24	7.42	0.15				0.00		
Pumpkin, fresh, 1" cubes USDA SR-23	0.5	Cup	58.00	15.08	0.58	3.77	0.29	0.06	0.03	0.01	0.00	0.00	214.14	0.00
Radicchio, fresh, leaf	2	Each	16.00	3.68	0.23	0.72	0.14	0.04	0.01	0.00	0.02	0.00	0.16	
Radish Sprouts, fresh	0.5	Cup	19.00	8.17	0.72	0.68	0.50	0.48	0.14	0.08	0.22	0.00	3.80	
Radishes, fresh, med, 3/4" to 1"	10	Each	45.00	7.20	0.31	1.53	0.69	0.04	0.01	0.01	0.02	0.00	0.16	
Seaweed, nori, fresh, sheets, Porphyra tenera, for sushi	1	Each	2.60	0.91	0.15	0.13	0.01	0.01	0.00	0.00	0.00	0.00	6.76	
Shallots, chpd, fresh	1	Tablespoon	10.00	7.20	0.25	1.68	0.07	0.01	0.00	0.00	0.00	0.00	6.00	
Soybean Sprouts, mature, fresh	1	Cup	70.00	85.40	9.16	6.70	0.77	4.69	0.65	1.06	2.65	0.00	0.70	
Spinach, fresh, chpd	1	Cup	30.00	6.90	0.86	1.09	0.66	0.12	0.02	0.00	0.05	0.00	140.70	
Squash, bitter melon, fresh USDA SR-23	1	Each	124.00	21.08	1.24	4.59	3.47	0.21				0.00	29.20	0.00
Squash, butternut, fresh, cubes USDA SR-23	0.5	Cup	70.00	31.50	0.70	8.18	1.40	0.07	0.01	0.00	0.03	0.00	372.05	0.00
Squash, summer, all types, fresh, sml	1	Each	118.00	18.88	1.43	3.95	1.30	0.21	0.05	0.02	0.11	0.00	11.80	
Tomatillo, fresh, chpd/diced	0.5	Cup	66.00	21.12	0.63	3.85	1.25	0.67	0.09	0.10	0.28	0.00	3.96	
Tomatoes, Italian/plum, fresh, year round avg USDA SR-23	1	Each	62.00	11.16	0.55	2.41	0.74	0.12	0.02	0.02	0.05	0.00	25.82	0.00
Tomatoes, red, cherry, fresh, year round avg USDA SR-23	1	Each	17.00	3.06	0.15	0.66	0.20	0.03	0.00	0.01	0.01	0.00	7.08	0.00
Tomatoes, red, June-Oct, fresh, chpd	0.5	Cup	90.00	18.90	0.76	4.18	0.99	0.30	0.04	0.04	0.12	0.00	27.90	
Tomatoes, red, stwd f/fresh	0.5	Cup	50.50	39.89	0.99	6.59	0.86	1.35	0.26	0.53	0.44	0.00	16.66	
Tomatoes, roma, fresh, year round avg, fresh	1	Each	62.00	11.16	0.55	2.43	0.74	0.12	0.02	0.03	0.07	0.00	26.04	

Vit E (mg)	Vit C	Vit B₁ Thia (mg)	Vit B₂ Ribo (mg)	Vit B₃ Nia (mg)	Fol (mcg)	Vit B₆ (mg)	Vita B₁₂ (mcg)	Sodi (mg)	Pota (mg)	Cal (mg)	Phos (mg)	Magn (mg)	Iron (mg)	Zinc (mg)	Caff (mg)	Alco (g)	Sol Fiber (g)	Insol Fiber (g)
0.90	3.20	0.01	0.01	0.10	24.00	0.02	0.00	8.80	120.80	7.60	16.00	5.20	0.23	0.25	0.00	0.00		
0.68	10.80	0.01	0.03	0.14	5.04	0.04	0.00	76.68	136.44	18.36	16.56	29.16	0.65	0.13	0.00	0.00		
	86.70	0.04	0.13	0.43	119.00	0.20	0.00	20.40	433.50	92.65	44.20	55.25	1.02	0.37	0.00	0.00		
0.41	5.34	0.03	0.02	0.18	28.48	0.10	0.00	8.90	80.10	26.25	15.57	12.46	0.94	0.05	0.00	0.00	0.37	0.43
	0.87	0.02	0.04	0.38	25.13	0.02	0.00	2.01	242.21	21.78	33.84	20.10	2.75	0.74	0.00	0.00		
0.03	0.56	0.01	0.01	0.05	10.95	0.01	0.00	0.75	35.70	5.25	4.95	1.95	0.19	0.03	0.00	0.00		
0.03	0.45	0.01	0.00	0.02	4.64	0.01	0.00	1.60	22.56	2.88	3.20	1.12	0.07	0.02	0.00	0.00		
0.06	3.60	0.01	0.02	0.08	7.60	0.02	0.00	5.60	38.80	7.20	5.80	2.60	0.17	0.04	0.00	0.00		
0.03	4.80	0.01	0.01	0.06	27.20	0.01	0.00	1.60	49.40	6.60	6.00	2.80	0.19	0.05	0.00	0.00		
	0.80				13.33			0.00		6.67			0.12		0.00	0.00		
	35.64	0.13	0.18	0.32	10.53	0.21	0.00	32.40	450.36	36.45	81.00	18.63	0.94	0.32	0.00	0.00	1.46	2.51
	0.84	0.08	0.41	0.28	11.76	0.09	0.08	5.00	376.00	14.70	0.10		0.34	0.92	0.00	0.00		
0.03	0.00	0.03	0.14	1.06	3.92	0.03	0.03	1.68	125.44	5.04	33.60	2.52	0.11	0.31	0.00	0.00		
0.02	3.57	0.02	0.03	1.09	9.00	0.01	0.00	0.90	114.30	0.30	33.90	4.80	0.27	0.17	0.00	0.00		
0.00	0.84	0.03	0.14	1.35	5.60	0.04	0.01	1.40	109.90	1.05	29.75	3.15	0.18	0.18	0.00	0.00	0.07	0.35
	0.00	0.08	0.53	5.30	69.56	0.18	0.00	45.88	763.68	8.88	208.68	29.60	2.58	1.15	0.00	0.00		
	0.84	0.06	0.40	3.18	18.48	0.08	0.04	5.50	407.00	6.80	0.11		0.50	0.50	0.00	0.00		
0.01	0.00	0.03	0.06	1.93	12.04	0.06	0.02	3.87	156.52	1.29	46.44		0.13	0.23	0.00	0.00		
1.13	39.20	0.05	0.06	0.45	104.72	0.10	0.00	14.00	198.24	57.68	24.08	17.92	0.82	0.11	0.00	0.00	0.88	0.96
0.34	20.04	0.19	0.06	0.95	83.60	0.20	0.00	7.60	287.85	76.95	59.85	54.15	0.76	0.57	0.00	0.00		
0.02	5.12	0.04	0.02	0.07	15.20	0.11	0.00	2.40	115.20	17.60	21.60	8.00	0.15	0.13	0.00	0.00	0.07	1.05
0.28	9.40	0.03	0.04	0.26	32.00	0.03	0.00	8.00	138.00	36.00	18.50	10.00	0.74	0.19	0.00	0.00	0.40	0.90
0.02	5.12	0.04	0.02	0.07	15.20	0.11	0.00	2.40	115.20	17.60	21.60	8.00	0.15	0.13	0.00	0.00	0.07	1.05
0.02	5.12	0.04	0.02	0.07	15.20	0.11	0.00	2.40	115.20	17.60	21.60	8.00	0.15	0.13	0.00	0.00	0.07	1.05
0.99	11.30	0.06	0.04	0.46	44.56	0.06	0.00	6.65	249.38	23.94	47.22	19.28	0.39	0.39	0.00	0.00	1.00	2.26
0.13	20.40	0.05	0.03	0.20	14.28	0.05	0.00	1.36	68.00	14.62	18.02	8.16	0.71	0.09	0.00	0.00	0.24	0.65
0.28	59.90	0.04	0.02	0.36	8.20	0.17	0.00	2.24	130.38	7.45	14.90	7.45	0.25	0.10	0.00	0.00	0.15	1.12
1.18	141.55	0.04	0.06	0.73	13.41	0.22	0.00	1.49	157.20	5.22	19.37	8.94	0.32	0.19	0.00	0.00		
1.28	341.31	0.05	0.05	1.66	48.36	0.31	0.00	3.72	394.32	20.46	44.64	22.32	0.86	0.32	0.00	0.00	0.50	1.17
0.02	12.14	0.17	0.07	2.20	29.82	0.73	0.00	10.65	888.21	27.69	117.15	48.99	1.83	0.62	0.00	0.00		
0.02	41.96	0.15	0.07	2.27	38.34	0.43	0.00	34.08	866.91	19.17	132.06	44.73	1.11	0.62	0.00	0.00		
	15.40	0.01	0.04	0.41		0.11		5.60	182.00	252.00	15.40	96.60	0.28	0.20	0.00	0.00		
0.61	5.22	0.03	0.06	0.35	9.28	0.04	0.00	0.58	197.20	12.18	25.52	6.96	0.46	0.19	0.00	0.00		
0.36	1.28	0.00	0.00	0.04	9.60	0.01	0.00	3.52	48.32	3.04	6.40	2.08	0.09	0.10	0.00	0.00		
	5.49	0.02	0.02	0.54	18.05	0.06	0.00	1.14	16.34	9.69	21.47	8.36	0.16	0.10	0.00	0.00		
0.00	6.66	0.01	0.02	0.11	11.25	0.03	0.00	17.55	104.85	11.25	9.00	4.50	0.15	0.13	0.00	0.00		
0.03	1.01	0.00	0.01	0.04	3.80	0.00	0.00	1.25	9.26	1.82	1.51	0.05	0.05	0.03	0.00	0.00		
0.01	0.80	0.01	0.00	0.02	3.40	0.03	0.00	1.20	33.40	3.70	6.00	2.10	0.12	0.04	0.00	0.00	0.03	0.04
0.01	10.71	0.24	0.08	0.80	120.40	0.12	0.00	9.80	338.80	46.90	114.80	50.40	1.47	0.82	0.00	0.00		
0.61	8.43	0.02	0.06	0.22	58.20	0.06	0.00	23.70	167.40	29.70	14.70	23.70	0.81	0.16	0.00	0.00		
	104.16	0.05	0.05	0.50	89.28	0.05	0.00	6.20	367.04	23.56	38.44	21.08	0.53	0.99	0.00	0.00		
1.01	14.70	0.07	0.01	0.84	18.90	0.11	0.00	2.80	246.40	33.60	23.10	23.80	0.49	0.10	0.00	0.00		
0.14	20.06	0.06	0.17	0.57	34.22	0.26	0.00	2.36	309.16	17.70	44.84	20.06	0.41	0.34	0.00	0.00		
0.25	7.72	0.03	0.02	1.22	4.62	0.04	0.00	0.66	176.88	4.62	25.74	13.20	0.41	0.15	0.00	0.00		
0.33	8.49	0.02	0.01	0.37	9.30	0.05	0.00	3.10	146.94	6.20	14.88	6.82	0.17	0.11	0.00	0.00		
0.09	2.33	0.01	0.00	0.10	2.55	0.01	0.00	0.85	40.29	1.70	4.08	1.87	0.05	0.03	0.00	0.00		
0.31	23.40	0.05	0.04	0.57	13.50	0.07	0.00	8.10	199.80	4.50	21.60	9.90	0.40	0.08	0.00	0.00	0.23	0.76
0.64	9.19	0.05	0.04	0.56	5.55	0.04	0.00	229.77	124.73	13.13	19.19	7.57	0.54	0.09	0.00	0.00	0.20	0.66
0.33	7.87	0.02	0.01	0.37	9.30	0.05	0.00	3.10	146.94	6.20	14.88	6.82	0.17	0.11	0.00	0.00		

Food Name	Amount	Measure	Weight (g)	Calories	Protein (g)	Total Carb (g)	Dietary Fiber (g)	Total Fat (g)	Sat Fat (g)	Mono Fat (g)	Poly Fat (g)	Chol (mg)	Vit A (mcg RAE)	Vit D (mcg)
VEGETABLES AND LEGUMES *(continued)*														
Tomatoes, yellow, fresh USDA SR-23	1	Each	212.00	31.80	2.08	6.32	1.48	0.55	0.08	0.08	0.23	0.00	0.00	0.00
Turnips, ckd, drained, cubes	0.5	Cup	78.00	17.16	0.55	3.95	1.56	0.06	0.01	0.00	0.04	0.00	0.00	
Vegetables, stir fry, Oriental, fresh, rtu Frieda's Specialty Produce	3	Ounce-weight	85.05	15.01	1.00	3.00	1.00	0.00	0.00	0.00	0.00	0.00	75.04	
Waterchestnuts, Chinese, fresh, slices USDA SR-23	0.5	Cup	62.00	60.14	0.87	14.84	1.86	0.06	0.02	0.00	0.03	0.00	0.00	0.00
Yams, domestic, fresh, 5" USDA SR-23	1	Each	130.00	111.80	2.04	26.16	3.90	0.06	0.02	0.00	0.02	0.00	922.15	0.00
Cooked Vegetables														
Asparagus, ckd, drained	0.5	Cup	90.00	19.80	2.16	3.70	1.80	0.20	0.06	0.01	0.13	0.00	45.00	
Asparagus, spears, ckd f/fzn, drained	4	Each	60.00	10.80	1.77	1.15	0.96	0.25	0.06	0.01	0.11	0.00	24.00	
Bean Sprouts, mung, mature, stir fried	0.5	Cup	62.00	31.00	2.67	6.56	1.18	0.13	0.02	0.04	0.04	0.00	1.24	
Beets, ckd, drained, sliced	0.5	Cup	85.00	37.40	1.43	8.47	1.70	0.15	0.03	0.03	0.05	0.00	1.70	
Broccoli, Chinese, ckd USDA SR-23	0.5	Cup	44.00	9.68	0.50	1.68	1.10	0.32	0.05	0.02	0.15	0.00	36.04	0.00
Broccoli, chpd, ckd f/fzn w/o salt, drained	0.5	Cup	92.00	25.76	2.86	4.92	2.76	0.11	0.02	0.01	0.05	0.00	51.52	
Broccoli, spears, ckd f/fzn, drained	0.5	Cup	92.00	25.76	2.86	4.92	2.76	0.10	0.02	0.01	0.05	0.00	51.52	
Brussels Sprouts, ckd, drained	0.5	Cup	78.00	28.08	1.99	5.54	2.03	0.39	0.08	0.03	0.20	0.00	30.42	
Cabbage, napa/nappa	0.5	Cup	54.50	6.54	0.60	1.22		0.09				0.00	7.08	
Carrots, ckd f/fzn w/o salt, drained, slices	0.5	Cup	73.00	27.01	0.42	5.64	2.41	0.50	0.09	0.03	0.24	0.00	606.63	
Cauliflower, ckd f/fzn w/o salt, drained, 1" pces	0.5	Cup	90.00	17.10	1.45	3.38	2.44	0.20	0.03	0.01	0.10	0.00	0.46	
Cauliflower, ckd, drained, 1" pces	0.5	Cup	62.00	14.26	1.14	2.55	1.68	0.28	0.04	0.02	0.13	0.00	0.62	
Cauliflower, green, ckd, head	0.2	Each	90.00	28.80	2.73	5.65	2.98	0.28	0.04	0.02	0.13	0.00	6.30	
Celeriac, ckd, drained, pces	0.5	Cup	77.50	20.92	0.75	4.58	0.93	0.15	0.04	0.03	0.08	0.00	0.00	
Collards, chpd, ckd, drained	0.5	Cup	80.00	20.80	1.68	3.92	2.24	0.29	0.04	0.02	0.14	0.00	324.80	
Corn, white, sweet, cob, kernels, ckd f/fzn, drained	0.5	Cup	82.00	77.08	2.55	18.31	1.72	0.61	0.09	0.18	0.29	0.00	0.16	
Corn, yellow, sweet kernels ckd f/fzn w/salt drained, pkg	3	Ounce-weight	85.05	68.89	2.17	16.42	2.04	0.57	0.06	0.11	0.17	0.00	8.51	0.00
Corn, yellow, sweet, kernels, ckd f/fzn, drained	0.5	Cup	82.00	66.42	2.09	15.83	1.97	0.55	0.08	0.16	0.26	0.00	8.20	
Dasheen, ckd, slices, cup, Tahitian, Colocassia	0.5	Cup	68.50	30.14	2.85	4.69	0.69	0.47	0.10	0.04	0.19	0.00	60.28	
Dish, succotash, ckd f/fzn w/salt, drained	0.5	Cup	85.00	79.05	3.66	16.96	3.48	0.76	0.14	0.14	0.36	0.00	8.50	
Eggplant, ckd, drained, 1" cubes	0.5	Cup	49.50	17.32	0.41	4.32	1.24	0.12	0.02	0.01	0.04	0.00	0.99	
Eggplant, stir fried w/o oil	0.5	Cup	48.00	12.48	0.49	2.92	1.20	0.08	0.02	0.01	0.04	0.00	1.82	0.00
Gobo Root, ckd, drained, 1" pces	0.5	Cup	62.50	55.00	1.31	13.22	1.12	0.09	0.01	0.02	0.04	0.00	0.00	
Gourd, wax, ckd, drained	0.5	Cup	87.50	12.25	0.35	2.66	0.88	0.18	0.01	0.03	0.07	0.00	0.00	
Greens, Swiss chard, bld, drnd, chpd USDA SR-23	0.5	Cup	87.50	17.50	1.64	3.61	1.84	0.07	0.01	0.01	0.02	0.00	267.92	0.00
Kale, Chinese, ckd USDA SR-23	0.5	Cup	44.00	9.68	0.50	1.68	1.10	0.32	0.05	0.02	0.15	0.00	36.04	0.00
Kale, ckd, drained	0.5	Cup	65.00	18.20	1.24	3.66	1.30	0.26	0.04	0.02	0.12	0.00	442.65	0.00
Kohlrabi, ckd, drained, slices	0.5	Cup	82.50	23.92	1.48	5.52	0.91	0.09	0.01	0.01	0.05	0.00	1.65	
Lambsquarters, ckd, drained	0.5	Cup	90.00	28.80	2.88	4.50	1.90	0.64	0.04	0.12	0.28	0.00	436.50	
Leeks, bulb & lower leaf, ckd, drnd USDA SR-23	1	Each	124.00	38.44	1.00	9.45	1.24	0.25	0.03	0.00	0.14	0.00	50.34	0.00
Lotus Root, ckd w/salt, drained, slices	0.5	Cup	60.00	39.60	0.95	9.62	1.86	0.04	0.01	0.01	0.01	0.00	0.00	
Mushrooms, batter dipped, fried	5	Each	70.00	155.52	1.91	11.18	0.84	11.80	1.55	3.63	5.99	1.95	5.99	
Mushrooms, shiitake, ckd, pces	0.5	Cup	72.50	39.87	1.13	10.35	1.53	0.16	0.04	0.05	0.03	0.00	0.00	
Mushrooms, stuffed	2	Each	48.00	137.67	5.21	13.08	0.89	7.33	2.18	3.09	1.57	6.11	44.67	0.62
Onion, ckd w/salt, drained	0.5	Cup	105.00	46.20	1.43	10.66	1.47	0.20	0.04	0.02	0.07	0.00	0.11	
Peppers, bell, red, sweet, ckd, drnd, chpd USDA SR-23	0.5	Cup	68.00	19.04	0.63	4.56	0.82	0.14	0.02	0.01	0.07	0.00	99.99	0.00
Soybeans, green, ckd, drnd USDA SR-23	0.5	Cup	90.00	126.90	11.11	9.94	3.78	5.76	0.67	1.09	2.71	0.00	7.02	0.00
Spinach, ckd, drnd USDA SR-23	0.5	Cup	90.00	20.70	2.67	3.37	2.16	0.23	0.04	0.01	0.10	0.00	471.64	0.00
Sprouts, lentil bean, stir fried USDA SR-23	0.5	Cup	62.00	62.62	5.46	13.18	2.48	0.28	0.03	0.06	0.12	0.00	1.27	0.00
Sprouts, pea, immature, ckd, drnd USDA SR-23	1	Serving	85.00	83.30	5.99	14.52	3.40	0.43	0.08	0.04	0.20	0.00	4.55	0.00
Squash, acorn, bkd, cubes USDA SR-23	0.5	Cup	102.50	57.40	1.15	14.94	4.51	0.14	0.03	0.01	0.06	0.00	21.93	0.00
Squash, acorn, ckd, mashed	0.5	Cup	122.50	41.65	0.82	10.77	3.18	0.10	0.01	0.01	0.04	0.00	50.22	
Squash, butternut, bkd, cubes	0.5	Cup	102.50	41.00	0.93	10.76	2.87	0.10	0.02	0.01	0.04	0.00	571.95	
Squash, crookneck, ckd f/fzn, drnd, slices USDA SR-23	0.5	Cup	96.00	24.00	1.23	5.32	1.34	0.19	0.04	0.01	0.08	0.00	9.65	0.00

Vit E (mg)	Vit C	Vit B₁ Thia (mg)	Vit B₂ Ribo (mg)	Vit B₃ Nia (mg)	Fol (mcg)	Vit B₆ (mg)	Vita B₁₂ (mcg)	Sodi (mg)	Pota (mg)	Cal (mg)	Phos (mg)	Magn (mg)	Iron (mg)	Zinc (mg)	Caff (mg)	Alco (g)	Sol Fiber (g)	Insol Fiber (g)
	19.08	0.09	0.10	2.50	63.60	0.12	0.00	48.76	546.96	23.32	76.32	25.44	1.04	0.59	0.00	0.00		
0.02	9.05	0.02	0.02	0.23	7.02	0.06	0.00	12.48	138.06	25.74	20.28	7.02	0.14	0.09	0.00	0.00	0.71	0.85
	21.01							35.02		60.04			0.00		0.00	0.00		
0.74	2.48	0.09	0.12	0.62	9.92	0.20	0.00	8.68	362.08	6.82	39.06	13.64	0.04	0.31	0.00	0.00		
0.34	3.12	0.10	0.08	0.72	14.30	0.27	0.00	71.50	438.10	39.00	61.10	32.50	0.79	0.39	0.00	0.00		
1.36	6.94	0.15	0.13	0.97	134.10	0.07	0.00	12.60	201.60	20.70	48.60	12.60	0.82	0.54	0.00	0.00	0.29	1.51
0.72	14.64	0.04	0.06	0.62	81.00	0.01	0.00	1.80	103.20	10.80	29.40	6.00	0.34	0.25	0.00	0.00	0.16	0.80
0.01	9.92	0.09	0.11	0.74	43.40	0.08	0.00	5.58	135.78	8.06	48.98	20.46	1.18	0.56	0.00	0.00	0.23	0.94
0.03	3.06	0.03	0.03	0.28	68.00	0.06	0.00	65.45	259.25	13.60	32.30	19.55	0.67	0.29	0.00	0.00	0.56	1.14
1.21	36.90	0.05	0.08	0.42	51.52	0.12	0.00	10.12	130.64	30.36	45.08	11.96	0.56	0.26	0.00	0.00	1.46	1.30
0.21	12.41	0.04	0.06	0.19	43.56	0.03	0.00	3.08	114.84	44.00	18.04	7.92	0.25	0.17	0.00	0.00		
1.21	36.90	0.05	0.08	0.42	27.60	0.12	0.00	22.08	165.60	46.92	50.60	18.40	0.56	0.28	0.00	0.00	1.35	1.41
0.34	48.36	0.08	0.06	0.48	46.80	0.14	0.00	16.38	247.26	28.08	43.68	15.60	0.94	0.26	0.00	0.00	0.94	1.09
	1.74	0.00	0.01	0.26	23.43	0.02	0.00	5.99	47.41	15.80	10.35	4.36	0.40	2.05	0.00	0.00		
0.74	1.68	0.03	0.03	0.30	8.03	0.06	0.00	43.07	140.16	25.55	22.63	8.03	0.39	0.26	0.00	0.00		
0.05	28.18	0.03	0.05	0.28	36.90	0.07	0.00	16.20	125.10	15.30	21.60	8.10	0.37	0.12	0.00	0.00	0.94	1.48
0.04	27.47	0.03	0.03	0.26	27.28	0.11	0.00	9.30	88.04	9.92	19.84	5.58	0.20	0.11	0.00	0.00	0.53	1.14
0.03	65.34	0.06	0.10	0.61	36.90	0.19	0.00	20.70	250.20	28.80	51.30	17.10	0.65	0.57	0.00	0.00		
0.15	2.79	0.02	0.03	0.33	2.32	0.08	0.00	47.27	134.07	20.15	51.15	9.30	0.34	0.15	0.00	0.00	0.13	0.80
0.71	14.56	0.03	0.08	0.46	74.40	0.10	0.00	12.80	92.80	112.00	24.00	16.00	0.93	0.19	0.00	0.00	1.01	1.23
0.04	3.94	0.14	0.06	1.24	25.42	0.18	0.00	3.28	205.82	2.46	61.50	23.78	0.50	0.52	0.00	0.00	0.08	1.64
0.06	2.98	0.03	0.05	1.11	29.77	0.08	0.00	208.37	198.17	2.55	67.19	23.81	0.40	0.54	0.00	0.00	0.09	1.96
0.06	2.87	0.02	0.05	1.08	28.70	0.08	0.00	0.82	191.06	2.46	64.78	22.96	0.39	0.52	0.00	0.00		
1.85	26.03	0.03	0.14	0.33	4.79	0.08	0.00	36.99	426.75	102.06	45.89	34.93	1.07	0.07	0.00	0.00		
0.16	5.01	0.06	0.06	1.11	28.05	0.08	0.00	238.85	225.25	12.75	59.50	19.55	0.76	0.38	0.00	0.00	0.24	3.24
0.20	0.64	0.04	0.01	0.30	6.93	0.04	0.00	0.50	60.88	2.97	7.42	5.44	0.12	0.06	0.00	0.00	0.20	1.04
0.02	0.70	0.02	0.02	0.28	7.30	0.04	0.00	1.44	104.16	3.36	10.56	6.72	0.13	0.06	0.00	0.00	0.48	0.72
0.29	1.62	0.02	0.04	0.20	12.50	0.18	0.00	2.50	225.00	30.62	58.12	24.37	0.48	0.24	0.00	0.00		
0.34	9.19	0.03	0.00	0.34	3.50	0.03	0.00	93.63	4.38	15.75	14.88	8.75	0.33	0.51	0.00	0.00		
1.65	15.75	0.03	0.08	0.32	7.88	0.07	0.00	156.62	480.38	50.75	28.88	75.25	1.98	0.29	0.00	0.00		
0.21	12.41	0.04	0.06	0.19	43.56	0.03	0.00	3.08	114.84	44.00	18.04	7.92	0.25	0.17	0.00	0.00		
0.55	26.65	0.04	0.04	0.32	8.45	0.09	0.00	14.95	148.20	46.80	18.20	11.70	0.58	0.16	0.00	0.00	0.58	0.72
0.43	44.55	0.03	0.02	0.32	9.90	0.13	0.00	17.32	280.50	20.62	37.12	15.67	0.33	0.25	0.00	0.00	0.27	0.63
1.66	33.30	0.10	0.23	0.82	12.60	0.16	0.00	26.10	259.20	232.20	40.50	20.70	0.64	0.28	0.00	0.00		
0.62	5.21	0.03	0.02	0.25	29.76	0.14	0.00	12.40	107.88	37.20	21.08	17.36	1.36	0.07	0.00	0.00	0.56	0.68
0.01	16.44	0.08	0.01	0.18	4.80	0.13	0.00	168.60	217.80	15.60	46.80	13.20	0.54	0.20	0.00	0.00	0.72	1.14
2.34	1.20	0.11	0.26	2.25	8.26	0.04	0.03	111.70	154.27	15.30	119.48	6.78	1.22	0.42	0.00	0.00		
0.02	0.22	0.03	0.12	1.09	15.22	0.12	0.00	2.90	84.82	2.17	21.02	10.15	0.32	0.96	0.00	0.00		
0.83	2.81	0.15	0.26	2.64	11.00	0.07	0.10	297.57	208.61	99.82	107.44	14.29	1.49	0.70	0.00	0.08	0.08	0.81
0.02	5.46	0.05	0.02	0.17	15.75	0.14	0.00	250.95	174.30	23.10	36.75	11.55	0.25	0.22	0.00	0.00	0.53	0.95
1.12	116.28	0.04	0.02	0.32	10.88	0.16	0.00	1.36	112.88	6.12	12.24	6.80	0.31	0.08	0.00	0.00	0.27	0.54
	15.30	0.23	0.14	1.12	99.90	0.05	0.00	12.60	485.10	130.50	142.20	54.00	2.25	0.82	0.00	0.00		
1.87	8.82	0.09	0.21	0.44	131.40	0.22	0.00	63.00	419.40	122.40	50.40	78.30	3.21	0.68	0.00	0.00	0.65	1.51
	7.81	0.14	0.06	0.74	41.54	0.10	0.00	6.20	176.08	8.68	94.86	21.70	1.92	0.99	0.00	0.00	0.77	1.71
	5.61	0.18	0.24	0.91	30.60	0.11	0.00	2.55	227.80	22.10	20.40	34.85	1.42	0.66	0.00	0.00	0.81	2.59
	11.07	0.17	0.01	0.90	19.47	0.20	0.00	4.10	447.92	45.10	46.12	44.07	0.95	0.17	0.00	0.00	0.45	4.06
0.14	7.97	0.13	0.01	0.65	13.47	0.14	0.00	3.67	322.17	31.85	33.07	31.85	0.69	0.13	0.00	0.00	0.32	2.87
1.33	15.48	0.07	0.01	0.99	19.47	0.13	0.00	4.10	291.10	42.02	27.67	29.72	0.61	0.13	0.00	0.00	0.30	2.57
0.14	6.53	0.03	0.05	0.42	12.48	0.10	0.00	5.76	242.88	19.20	39.36	25.92	0.50	0.33	0.00	0.00		

Food Name	Amount	Measure	Weight (g)	Calories	Protein (g)	Total Carb (g)	Dietary Fiber (g)	Total Fat (g)	Sat Fat (g)	Mono Fat (g)	Poly Fat (g)	Chol (mg)	Vit A (mcg RAE)	Vit D (mcg)
VEGETABLES AND LEGUMES *(continued)*														
Squash, spaghetti, bkd/ckd, drained	0.5	Cup	77.50	20.92	0.51	5.01	1.08	0.20	0.05	0.02	0.10	0.00	4.65	
Squash, summer, all types, ckd, drained, slices	0.5	Cup	90.00	18.00	0.82	3.88	1.26	0.28	0.05	0.02	0.12	0.00	9.90	
Squash, winter, all types, bkd, cubes	0.5	Cup	102.50	37.92	0.92	9.07	2.87	0.36	0.11	0.04	0.22	0.00	267.52	
Squash, zucchini, w/skin, ckd, drnd, slices USDA SR-23	0.5	Cup	90.00	13.50	1.03	2.42	0.89	0.32	0.06	0.03	0.14	0.00	50.26	0.00
Sweet Potatoes, dark orange, bkd in skin w/salt USDA SR-23	0.5	Cup	100.00	92.00	2.01	20.71	3.30	0.15	0.05	0.00	0.09	0.00	960.90	0.00
Swiss Chard, ckd, drained, chpd	0.5	Cup	87.50	17.50	1.64	3.61	1.84	0.07	0.01	0.01	0.02	0.00	267.75	
Taro, poi USDA SR-23	0.5	Cup	120.00	134.40	0.46	32.68	0.48	0.17	0.03	0.01	0.07	0.00	3.96	0.00
Vegetables, mixed, broccoli cauliflower carrots, fzn Birds Eye Foods	0.5	Cup	92.00	25.26	1.69	5.37	2.48	0.23	0.05			0.00	250.10	
Frozen, Dehydrated, and Dried Vegetables														
Artichokes, globe/French, fzn, pkg	3	Ounce-weight	85.05	32.32	2.24	6.60	3.32	0.37	0.08	0.01	0.15	0.00	6.80	
Asparagus, fzn, 10oz pkg USDA SR-23	4	Ounce-weight	113.40	27.22	3.66	4.65	2.15	0.26	0.06	0.01	0.11	0.00	53.75	0.00
Beans, lima, baby, immature, fzn, 10 oz pkg USDA SR-23	0.5	Cup	82.00	108.24	6.22	20.61	4.92	0.36	0.08	0.02	0.18	0.00	7.75	0.00
Broccoli, florets, fzn Birds Eye Foods	0.5	Cup	42.50	15.00	0.50	2.00	1.00	0.00	0.00	0.00	0.00	0.00	0.00	
Chile Peppers, anaheim, dried Frieda's	2	Tablespoon	4.00	14.11	1.13	1.98	0.56	0.00	0.00	0.00	0.00	0.00	148.15	
Chile Peppers, California, dried Frieda's	2	Tablespoon	4.00	14.11	1.13	1.98	0.56	0.00	0.00	0.00	0.00	0.00	148.15	
Chili Peppers, hot, sun dried USDA SR-23	1	Each	0.50	1.62	0.05	0.35	0.14	0.03	0.00	0.00	0.02	0.00	6.62	0.00
Chips, yucca, salted USDA SR-23	1	Ounce-weight	28.35	146.00	0.38	19.63	1.05	7.35	2.46	2.11	1.96			
Corn, yellow, sweet, kernels, fzn, 10oz pkg USDA SR-23	0.5	Cup	68.00	59.84	2.05	14.08	1.43	0.53	0.08	0.15	0.25	0.00	6.63	0.00
Dish, broccoli, w/cheese flvd sauce, fzn Green Giant	0.5	Cup	84.00	56.28	1.93	7.48		2.10	0.40	0.85	0.22			
Grass, barley, dehyd, pwd	1	Teaspoon	3.50	10.00	0.80	1.30	1.30	0.11					87.50	0.00
Greens, collard, fzn, chpd, 10oz pkg USDA SR-23	4	Ounce-weight	113.40	37.42	3.05	7.33	4.08	0.42	0.05	0.03	0.20	0.00	520.68	0.00
Okra, fzn, 10oz pkg USDA SR-23	4	Ounce-weight	113.40	34.02	1.92	7.52	2.49	0.28	0.07	0.05	0.07	0.00	19.85	0.00
Peas, green, fzn, 10oz pkg USDA SR-23	0.5	Cup	67.00	51.59	3.50	9.13	3.02	0.27	0.04	0.02	0.12	0.00	68.94	0.00
Spinach, chpd/leaf, fzn, unprep, pkg	0.5	Cup	78.00	24.18	3.07	3.38	2.42	0.58	0.23	0.00	0.13	0.00	457.08	
Tomatoes, sun dried	0.5	Cup	27.00	69.66	3.81	15.06	3.32	0.80	0.12	0.13	0.30	0.00	11.88	
Tomatoes, sun dried, oil pack, drained	0.5	Cup	55.00	117.15	2.78	12.83	3.19	7.74	1.04	4.76	1.13	0.00	35.20	
Vegetables, Asian blend, fzn Birds Eye Foods C & W	0.75	Cup	85.00	60.00	3.00	9.00	2.00	1.00	0.00			0.00	0.00	
Vegetables, broccoli & cauliflower, fzn Birds Eye Foods Birds Eye Steamfresh	0.5	Cup	47.50	15.00	0.50	2.00	1.00	0.00	0.00	0.00	0.00	0.00	0.00	
Vegetables, Chinese stirfry, fzn General Mills Cascadian Farm	1	Cup	85.00	25.00	2.00	6.00	2.00	0.00	0.00	0.00	0.00	0.00	175.00	
Vegetables, corn broccoli & red peppers, fzn Birds Eye Foods C & W	0.67	Cup	85.00	50.00	2.00	8.00	2.00	0.50	0.00			0.00		
Vegetables, corn carrots peas & green beans, fzn Birds Eye Foods Birds Eye Steamfresh	0.67	Cup	90.00	60.00	2.00	12.00	2.00	0.00	0.00	0.00	0.00	0.00		
Canned Vegetables														
Artichokes, hearts, marinated, appetizers, cnd Progresso	2	Each	32.00	50.00	0.00	2.00	0.00	5.00	1.00			0.00	0.00	
Asparagus, drained, can	0.5	Cup	121.00	22.99	2.59	2.98	1.82	0.78	0.18	0.03	0.34	0.00	49.61	
Bamboo Shoots, slices, drained, can	0.5	Cup	65.50	12.44	1.12	2.11	0.90	0.26	0.06	0.00	0.12	0.00	0.66	
Beets, julienne, cnd S & W	0.5	Cup	123.00	30.00	1.00	7.00	1.00	0.00	0.00			0.00	0.00	
Carrots, cnd, drained, mashed	0.5	Cup	114.00	28.50	0.72	6.32	1.72	0.21	0.04	0.01	0.11	0.00	636.12	
Chili Peppers, green, cnd	0.5	Cup	69.50	14.59	0.51	3.20	1.18	0.19	0.02	0.02	0.12	0.00	4.17	
Chili Peppers, jalapeno, cnd, not drained, chpd	0.5	Cup	68.00	18.36	0.63	3.22	1.77	0.63	0.07	0.05	0.34	0.00	57.80	
Chili Peppers, jalapeno, dices, cnd, drained La Victoria Foods	1	Ounce-weight	28.35	6.75	0.00	1.35	1.35	0.00	0.00	0.00	0.00	0.00	0.00	
Corn, cream style, w/starch, cnd S & W	0.5	Cup	128.00	100.00	2.00	24.00	1.00	1.00	0.00			0.00	0.00	
Corn, yellow, sweet, cream style, can	0.5	Cup	128.00	92.16	2.23	23.21	1.54	0.54	0.08	0.16	0.26	0.00	5.12	
Corn, yellow, sweet, kernels, drained, can	0.5	Cup	82.00	66.42	2.15	15.25	1.64	0.82	0.13	0.24	0.38	0.00	3.28	
Corn, yellow, sweet, kernels, unsalted, cnd, not drained	0.5	Cup	128.00	81.92	2.49	19.72	2.18	0.64	0.10	0.19	0.30	0.00	3.84	

Vit E (mg)	Vit C	Vit B₁ Thia (mg)	Vit B₂ Ribo (mg)	Vit B₃ Nia (mg)	Fol (mcg)	Vit B₆ (mg)	Vita B₁₂ (mcg)	Sodi (mg)	Pota (mg)	Cal (mg)	Phos (mg)	Magn (mg)	Iron (mg)	Zinc (mg)	Caff (mg)	Alco (g)	Sol Fiber (g)	Insol Fiber (g)
0.09	2.72	0.03	0.02	0.63	6.20	0.07	0.00	13.95	90.67	16.27	10.85	8.52	0.26	0.15	0.00	0.00	0.11	0.98
0.13	4.96	0.04	0.03	0.47	18.00	0.06	0.00	0.90	172.80	24.30	35.10	21.60	0.33	0.35	0.00	0.00	0.48	0.78
0.12	9.84	0.01	0.07	0.51	20.50	0.17	0.00	1.02	447.92	22.55	19.47	13.32	0.45	0.23	0.00	0.00	0.31	2.57
0.11	11.61	0.03	0.02	0.46	25.20	0.07	0.00	2.70	237.60	16.20	33.30	17.10	0.33	0.30	0.00	0.00		
0.71	19.60	0.11	0.11	1.49	6.00	0.29	0.00	246.00	475.00	38.00	54.00	27.00	0.69	0.32	0.00	0.00		
1.65	15.75	0.03	0.08	0.32	7.88	0.07	0.00	156.62	480.38	50.75	28.88	75.25	1.98	0.29	0.00	0.00		
2.76	4.80	0.16	0.05	1.32	25.20	0.33	0.00	14.40	219.60	19.20	46.80	28.80	1.06	0.26	0.00	0.00		
	43.69	0.05	0.07	0.46	49.96	0.15	0.00	27.59	192.28	30.65	38.64	12.88	0.52		0.00	0.00		
0.14	4.51	0.05	0.12	0.73	107.16	0.07	0.00	39.97	210.92	16.16	49.33	22.96	0.43	0.27	0.00	0.00		
	36.06	0.14	0.15	1.36	216.59	0.13	0.00	9.07	286.90	28.35	72.58	15.88	0.83	0.67	0.00	0.00	0.31	1.85
	6.81	0.09	0.06	0.84	22.96	0.13	0.00	42.64	370.64	28.70	85.28	41.00	1.81	0.52	0.00	0.00	1.28	3.64
	15.00							10.00		10.00			0.00		0.00	0.00		
	1.02							1.98		5.64			0.00		0.00	0.00		
	1.02							1.98		5.64			0.00		0.00	0.00		
0.02	0.16	0.00	0.01	0.04	0.25	0.00	0.00	0.45	9.35	0.22	0.79	0.44	0.03	0.01	0.00	0.00		
0.79		0.01	0.01	0.34		0.04		83.92	246.08	14.74	28.07	13.04	0.20	0.24	0.00	0.00		
0.05	4.35	0.06	0.05	1.18	24.48	0.11	0.00	2.04	144.84	2.72	47.60	12.24	0.29	0.26	0.00	0.00	0.43	1.00
	29.74							403.20		45.36			0.54		0.00	0.00		
0.00	11.00	0.01	0.07	0.26	38.00	0.05	1.00	1.00	112.00	18.00	18.00	3.60	2.00	0.02	0.00	0.00		
	45.36	0.06	0.12	0.73	82.78	0.13	0.00	54.43	286.90	227.93	30.62	32.89	1.21	0.29	0.00	0.00	1.63	2.45
0.37	14.06	0.10	0.12	0.80	167.83	0.05	0.00	3.40	239.27	91.85	47.63	48.76	0.65	0.60	0.00	0.00		
0.01	12.06	0.17	0.07	1.15	35.51	0.06	0.00	72.36	102.51	14.74	54.94	17.42	1.03	0.55	0.00	0.00	0.29	2.73
2.26	18.95	0.08	0.18	0.45	101.40	0.12	0.00	57.72	290.16	120.90	40.56	56.94	1.58	0.35	0.00	0.00		
0.00	10.58	0.14	0.13	2.44	18.36	0.09	0.00	565.65	925.29	29.70	96.12	52.38	2.45	0.54	0.00	0.00	0.84	2.48
0.29	55.99	0.11	0.21	2.00	12.65	0.18	0.00	146.30	860.75	25.85	76.45	44.55	1.47	0.43	0.00	0.00	0.80	2.39
	9.00							180.00		40.00			0.72		0.00	0.00		
	15.00							12.50		10.00			0.18		0.00	0.00		
	18.00							15.00	160.00	20.00			0.36		0.00	0.00		
	18.00							10.00		20.00			0.36		0.00	0.00		
	3.60							20.00		20.00			0.36		0.00	0.00		
	3.60							110.00		0.00			0.00		0.00	0.00	0.00	0.00
0.37	22.26	0.07	0.12	1.15	116.16	0.13	0.00	347.27	208.12	19.36	52.03	12.10	2.22	0.48	0.00	0.00		
0.42	0.72	0.02	0.02	0.09	1.96	0.09	0.00	4.58	52.40	5.24	16.38	2.62	0.21	0.42	0.00	0.00		
	0.00						0.00	230.00	0.00	0.00			0.72		0.00	0.00		
0.84	3.08	0.03	0.04	0.63	10.26	0.13	0.00	275.88	204.06	28.50	27.36	9.12	0.72	0.30	0.00	0.00	0.87	0.83
	23.77	0.00	0.02	0.44	37.53	0.09	0.00	275.91	78.53	25.02	7.64	2.78	0.93	0.07	0.00	0.00		
0.48	6.80	0.02	0.02	0.27	9.52	0.14	0.00	1136.28	131.24	15.64	12.24	10.20	1.27	0.23	0.00	0.00	0.54	1.22
	1.62							168.75	33.75	0.00			0.00		0.00	0.00		
	1.20						0.00	340.00	0.00	0.00			3.60		0.00	0.00		
0.09	5.89	0.03	0.07	1.23	57.60	0.08	0.00	364.80	171.52	3.84	65.28	21.76	0.48	0.68	0.00	0.00	0.08	1.46
0.03	6.97	0.03	0.06	0.98	40.18	0.04	0.00	175.48	159.90	4.10	53.30	16.40	0.71	0.32	0.00	0.00	0.08	1.56
0.04	7.04	0.03	0.08	1.20	48.64	0.05	0.00	15.36	209.92	5.12	65.28	20.48	0.52	0.46	0.00	0.00	0.10	2.08

Food Name	Amount	Measure	Weight (g)	Calories	Protein (g)	Total Carb (g)	Dietary Fiber (g)	Total Fat (g)	Sat Fat (g)	Mono Fat (g)	Poly Fat (g)	Chol (mg)	Vit A (mcg RAE)	Vit D (mcg)
VEGETABLES AND LEGUMES *(continued)*														
Garlic, crushed, wet McCormick & Co., Inc.	1	Teaspoon	5.00	15.00	0.00	0.00	0.00	0.50				0.00		
Giant Butterbur, cnd, chpd USDA SR-23	0.5	Cup	62.00	1.86	0.07	0.24		0.08				0.00	0.00	0.00
Hominy, white, cnd	0.5	Cup	82.50	59.40	1.22	11.77	2.06	0.72	0.10	0.19	0.33	0.00	0.04	
Hominy, yellow, cnd	0.5	Cup	80.00	57.60	1.18	11.41	2.00	0.70	0.10	0.18	0.32	0.00	4.80	
Mushrooms, cnd, drained, slices	10	Each	40.00	10.00	0.75	2.04	0.96	0.12	0.02	0.00	0.05	0.00	0.00	
Olives, black, sml, w/o pits, cnd	1	Each	3.20	3.68	0.03	0.20	0.10	0.34	0.05	0.25	0.03	0.00	0.64	
Olives, green, queen, cnd S & W	1	Each	6.50	10.00	0.00	0.50	0.00	1.00		0.75	0.25	0.00	0.00	
Palm Hearts, cnd	0.5	Cup	73.00	20.44	1.84	3.37	1.75	0.45	0.10	0.07	0.15	0.00	0.00	
Peas, black eyed, unsalted, cnd Eden	0.5	Cup	130.00	90.00	6.00	16.00	4.00	1.00	0.00			0.00	0.00	
Pickles, dill, kosher, halves Kraft Claussen	0.5	Each	28.00	5.00	0.00	1.00		0.00	0.00	0.00	0.00	0.00	0.00	
Pumpkin, cnd, unsalted	0.5	Cup	122.50	41.65	1.35	9.91	3.55	0.34	0.18	0.05	0.02	0.00	953.05	
Sauerkraut, cnd, drained	0.5	Cup	71.00	13.49	0.65	3.04	1.77	0.10	0.02	0.01	0.04	0.00	0.71	
Spinach, cnd, unsalted, drained	0.5	Cup	107.00	24.61	3.01	3.64	2.57	0.54	0.09	0.01	0.22	0.00	524.30	
Tomatoes, crushed, cnd	0.5	Cup	50.50	16.16	0.83	3.68	0.96	0.14	0.02	0.02	0.06	0.00	17.67	
Tomatoes, puree, cnd	0.5	Cup	125.00	47.50	2.06	11.23	2.37	0.27	0.02	0.02	0.08	0.00	32.50	
Tomatoes, red, cnd, whole, lrg	1	Each	164.00	27.88	1.31	6.41	1.48	0.21	0.03	0.03	0.09	0.00	9.84	
Tomatoes, red, stwd, cnd, not drained	0.5	Cup	127.50	33.15	1.16	7.89	1.27	0.24	0.03	0.04	0.10	0.00	11.47	
Tomatoes, red, w/green chilis, cnd	0.5	Cup	120.50	18.08	0.83	4.36	1.21	0.10	0.01	0.01	0.04	0.00	24.10	
Tomatoes, red, whole, unsalted, can	1	Each	190.00	36.10	1.75	8.30	1.90	0.25	0.04	0.04	0.10	0.00	13.30	
Vegetables, garden medley, cnd Green Giant	0.5	Cup	121.00	40.00	1.00	9.00	2.00	0.00	0.00	0.00	0.00	0.00	100.00	
Vegetables, mixed, cnd, drained	0.5	Cup	81.50	39.94	2.11	7.55	2.45	0.20	0.04	0.01	0.09	0.00	474.33	
Waterchestnuts, Chinese, cnd, not drained, each	4	Each	28.00	14.00	0.25	3.44	0.70	0.02	0.00	0.00	0.01	0.00	0.00	
Legumes														
Bean Cakes, Japanese style	1	Each	32.00	130.46	1.72	15.83	0.91	6.85	1.02	2.90	2.58	0.00	0.00	0.00
Beans, adzuki, mature, ckd w/salt	0.5	Cup	115.00	147.20	8.65	28.48	8.40	0.12	0.04			0.00	0.35	0.00
Beans, black turtle soup, mature, cnd	0.5	Cup	120.00	109.20	7.24	19.87	8.28	0.35	0.09	0.03	0.15	0.00	0.24	
Beans, black, cnd Bush's Best	0.5	Cup	130.00	100.00	7.00	20.00	7.00	0.50	0.00			0.00	0.00	
Beans, black, fermented, Szechuan	0.5	Cup	86.00	164.26	16.60	10.66		6.11						
Beans, blackeyed, immature, ckd, drained	0.5	Cup	82.50	80.03	2.61	16.77	4.13	0.31	0.08	0.03	0.13	0.00	33.00	
Beans, cannellini, cnd Progresso	0.5	Cup	130.00	100.00	5.00	18.00	5.00	0.50	0.00	0.00	0.50	0.00	0.00	
Beans, chickpea, mature, ckd	0.5	Cup	82.00	134.48	7.26	22.49	6.23	2.12	0.22	0.47	0.95	0.00	0.82	
Beans, chickpea/garbanzo, unsalted, cnd	0.5	Cup	130.00	120.00	7.00	19.00	5.00	1.50				0.00		
Beans, cowpeas, mature, ckd	0.5	Cup	86.00	99.76	6.65	17.85	5.59	0.46	0.11	0.04	0.19	0.00	0.86	
Beans, fava/broad, cnd Progresso	0.5	Cup	130.00	110.00	6.00	20.00	5.00	0.50				0.00	0.00	
Beans, fava/broad, mature, cnd, not drained	0.5	Cup	128.00	90.88	7.00	15.89	4.74	0.28	0.04	0.06	0.11	0.00	1.28	
Beans, frijoles, w/cheese, fast food	0.5	Cup	83.50	112.73	5.68	14.36		3.89	2.04	1.31	0.35	18.37	17.54	
Beans, garbanzo, cnd Old El Paso	0.5	Cup	130.00	100.00	6.00	16.00	4.00	1.50	0.00	0.60	0.90	0.00	0.00	
Beans, garbanzo, mature, cnd	0.5	Cup	120.00	142.80	5.94	27.15	5.28	1.37	0.14	0.30	0.61	0.00	1.20	
Beans, great northern, cnd Bush's Best	0.5	Cup	130.00	110.00	7.00	18.00	7.00	0.50	0.00			0.00		
Beans, great northern, mature, cnd	0.5	Cup	131.00	149.34	9.65	27.55	6.42	0.51	0.16	0.02	0.21	0.00	0.06	
Beans, green, French cut, cnd Green Giant	0.5	Cup	118.00	20.00	1.00	4.00	1.00	0.00	0.00	0.00	0.00	0.00	15.00	
Beans, green, French cut, fzn Birds Eye Foods	0.5	Cup	83.00	25.00	1.33	5.75	1.91	0.15	0.03			0.00	19.04	
Beans, green, snap, fresh	0.5	Cup	55.00	17.05	1.00	3.93	1.87	0.06	0.01	0.00	0.03	0.00	19.25	
Beans, green, whole, deluxe, fzn Birds Eye Foods	10	Each	40.00	10.68	0.60	2.38	0.92	0.09	0.02			0.00	13.73	
Beans, Italian, cut, cnd Del Monte Foods	0.5	Cup	121.00	30.00	1.00	6.00	3.00	0.00	0.00	0.00	0.00	0.00	10.00	
Beans, kidney, dark red, cnd Bush's Best	0.5	Cup	130.00	130.00	8.00	21.00	7.00	1.00	0.00			0.00		
Beans, lentils, ckd f/dry w/o salt	0.5	Cup	99.00	114.84	8.93	19.93	7.82	0.37	0.06	0.07	0.18	0.00	0.40	
Beans, lentils, cnd Westbrae Natural	0.5	Cup	130.00	100.00	8.00	17.00	9.00	0.00	0.00	0.00	0.00	0.00	0.00	
Beans, lima, baby, immature, ckd f/fzn, drained, cup	0.5	Cup	90.00	94.50	5.98	17.50	5.40	0.27	0.06	0.02	0.13	0.00	7.20	
Beans, lima, green, cnd Del Monte Foods	0.5	Cup	126.00	80.00	4.00	15.00	4.00	0.00	0.00	0.00	0.00	0.00	5.00	
Beans, navy, mature, cnd	0.5	Cup	131.00	148.03	9.87	26.78	6.68	0.56	0.15	0.05	0.24	0.00	0.00	
Beans, pinto, cnd Bush's Best	0.5	Cup	130.00	110.00	6.00	19.00	6.00	0.00	0.00	0.00	0.00	0.00		
Beans, refried, fat free, cnd Bush's Best	0.5	Cup	125.00	130.00	9.00	24.00	7.00	0.00	0.00	0.00	0.00	0.00		
Beans, refried, spicy, cnd Rosarita	0.5	Cup	128.00	100.00	6.00	18.00	6.00	2.00	1.00			0.00	0.00	
Beans, refried, vegetarian, cnd Old El Paso	0.5	Cup	118.00	100.00	6.00	17.00	6.00	1.00	0.00	0.00	1.00	0.00	0.00	

Vit E (mg)	Vit C	Vit B$_1$ Thia (mg)	Vit B$_2$ Ribo (mg)	Vit B$_3$ Nia (mg)	Fol (mcg)	Vit B$_6$ (mg)	Vita B$_{12}$ (mcg)	Sodi (mg)	Pota (mg)	Cal (mg)	Phos (mg)	Magn (mg)	Iron (mg)	Zinc (mg)	Caff (mg)	Alco (g)	Sol Fiber (g)	Insol Fiber (g)
										0.00					0.00	0.00	0.00	0.00
	7.38	0.00	0.00	0.09	1.86	0.02	0.00	2.48	7.44	21.08	2.48	1.24	0.39	0.04	0.00	0.00		
0.04	0.00	0.00	0.01	0.03	0.82	0.01	0.00	173.25	7.42	8.25	28.87	13.20	0.51	0.86	0.00	0.00	0.08	1.98
0.08	0.00	0.00	0.01	0.02	0.80	0.01	0.00	168.00	7.20	8.00	28.00	12.80	0.50	0.84	0.00	0.00	0.10	1.90
0.00	0.00	0.03	0.01	0.64	4.80	0.02	0.00	170.00	51.60	4.40	26.40	6.00	0.32	0.29	0.00	0.00	0.08	0.88
0.05	0.03	0.00	0.00	0.00	0.00	0.00	0.00	27.90	0.26	2.82	0.10	0.13	0.11	0.01	0.00	0.00	0.01	0.10
	0.00						0.00	110.00	0.00	0.00			0.00		0.00	0.00	0.00	0.00
	5.77	0.01	0.04	0.32	28.47	0.02	0.00	310.98	129.21	42.34	47.45	27.74	2.29	0.84	0.00	0.00		
	0.00	0.52	0.13	0.13	24.00			25.00	210.00	30.00	104.00	58.20	1.65	1.60	0.00	0.00	0.00	4.00
	0.00							330.00		0.00			0.00		0.00	0.00		
1.30	5.15	0.03	0.07	0.45	14.70	0.07	0.00	6.13	252.35	31.85	42.88	28.18	1.70	0.21	0.00	0.00	0.60	2.95
0.07	10.44	0.01	0.02	0.10	17.04	0.09	0.00	469.31	120.70	21.30	14.20	9.23	1.04	0.13	0.00	0.00	0.80	0.97
2.08	15.30	0.02	0.15	0.42	104.86	0.11	0.00	28.89	370.22	135.89	47.08	81.32	2.46	0.49	0.00	0.00	0.64	1.93
0.27	4.65	0.04	0.03	0.62	6.56	0.08	0.00	66.66	147.96	17.17	16.16	10.10	0.66	0.14	0.00	0.00		
2.46	13.25	0.04	0.10	1.83	13.75	0.17	0.00	498.75	548.75	22.50	50.00	28.75	2.23	0.46	0.00	0.00		
1.16	14.76	0.07	0.08	1.21	13.12	0.15	0.00	209.92	308.32	50.84	31.16	18.04	1.59	0.23	0.00	0.00	0.21	1.26
1.06	10.07	0.06	0.04	0.91	6.37	0.02	0.00	281.77	263.92	43.35	25.50	15.30	1.70	0.22	0.00	0.00	0.32	0.96
0.46	7.47	0.04	0.02	0.77	10.85	0.12	0.00	483.21	128.94	24.10	16.87	13.26	0.31	0.16	0.00	0.00	0.30	0.90
1.52	26.98	0.09	0.06	1.40	15.20	0.17	0.00	19.00	431.30	57.00	36.10	22.80	1.04	0.30	0.00	0.00	0.42	1.48
	0.00							360.00		0.00			0.72		0.00	0.00		
0.28	4.08	0.04	0.04	0.47	19.56	0.06	0.00	121.44	237.17	22.01	34.23	13.04	0.85	0.33	0.00	0.00	0.93	1.52
0.14	0.36	0.00	0.01	0.10	1.68	0.04	0.00	2.24	33.04	1.12	5.32	1.40	0.24	0.11	0.00	0.00		
1.24	0.00	0.08	0.05	0.55	9.10	0.02	0.00	0.53	57.70	3.15	20.86	6.15	0.67	0.16	0.00	0.00		
0.12	0.00	0.13	0.08	0.83	139.15	0.12	0.00	280.60	611.80	32.20	193.20	59.80	2.30	2.03	0.00	0.00		
0.31	3.24	0.17	0.15	0.75	73.20	0.06	0.00	460.80	369.60	42.00	129.60	42.00	2.28	0.65	0.00	0.00	1.16	7.12
	0.00							460.00		40.00			1.80		0.00	0.00		
		0.11	0.21	2.75			0.00				156.52	170.28	4.73		0.00	0.00		
0.18	1.82	0.08	0.12	1.16	104.78	0.06	0.00	3.30	344.85	105.60	42.08	42.90	0.93	0.85	0.00	0.00	0.50	3.63
	0.00							270.00		40.00			1.80		0.00	0.00		
0.28	1.07	0.09	0.05	0.43	141.04	0.12	0.00	5.74	238.62	40.18	137.76	39.36	2.37	1.26	0.00	0.00	1.93	4.30
		0.09	0.07	0.40					250.00	60.00	100.00	60.00	1.44	1.50				
0.24	0.34	0.17	0.05	0.43	178.88	0.09	0.00	3.44	239.08	20.64	134.16	45.58	2.16	1.11	0.00	0.00	0.70	4.89
	0.00							250.00		20.00			1.44		0.00	0.00		
0.10	2.30	0.03	0.06	1.22	42.24	0.06	0.00	579.84	309.76	33.28	101.12	40.96	1.28	0.80	0.00	0.00	1.14	3.60
	0.75	0.07	0.17	0.75	55.95	0.10	0.34	440.88	302.27	94.36	87.68	42.59	1.12	0.87	0.00	0.00		
	0.00							340.00		40.00			1.44		0.00	0.00		
0.18	4.56	0.04	0.04	0.17	80.40	0.56	0.00	358.80	206.40	38.40	108.00	34.80	1.62	1.27	0.00	0.00	1.27	4.01
	1.20							400.00		40.00			1.44		0.00	0.00		
0.34	1.70	0.19	0.08	0.60	106.11	0.14	0.00	5.24	459.81	69.43	178.16	66.81	2.06	0.85	0.00	0.00	1.09	5.33
	2.40							390.00		20.00			0.36		0.00	0.00		
	7.59	0.05	0.07	0.25	11.12	0.04	0.00	3.25	141.10	37.61	20.75	18.26	0.79		0.00	0.00		
0.23	8.97	0.05	0.06	0.41	20.35	0.04	0.00	3.30	114.95	20.35	20.90	13.75	0.57	0.13	0.00	0.00	0.77	1.10
	4.34	0.02	0.04	0.12	4.68	0.02	0.00	0.86	70.80	15.43	10.00	8.00	0.31		0.00	0.00		
	2.40							390.00		20.00			0.72		0.00	0.00		
	1.20							260.00		80.00			1.80		0.00	0.00		
0.11	1.49	0.17	0.08	1.05	179.19	0.18	0.00	1.98	365.31	18.81	178.20	35.64	3.30	1.25	0.00	0.00	1.29	6.53
								150.00							0.00	0.00		
0.58	5.22	0.06	0.05	0.69	14.40	0.10	0.00	26.10	369.90	25.20	100.80	50.40	1.76	0.49	0.00	0.00	1.46	3.94
	4.80							390.00		20.00			1.44		0.00	0.00		
1.02	0.92	0.18	0.07	0.63	81.22	0.13	0.00	586.88	377.28	61.57	175.54	61.57	2.42	1.01	0.00	0.00	4.01	2.67
	1.20							390.00		40.00			1.80		0.00	0.00		
	0.00							490.00		60.00			2.70		0.00	0.00		
	0.00							630.00		40.00			1.98		0.00	0.00		
	0.00							490.00		40.00			1.80		0.00	0.00		

Food Name	Amount	Measure	Weight (g)	Calories	Protein (g)	Total Carb (g)	Dietary Fiber (g)	Total Fat (g)	Sat Fat (g)	Mono Fat (g)	Poly Fat (g)	Chol (mg)	Vit A (mcg RAE)	Vit D (mcg)
VEGETABLES AND LEGUMES *(continued)*														
Beans, refried/frijoles, cnd	0.5	Cup	126.40	118.82	6.94	19.63	6.70	1.59	0.60	0.70	0.20	10.11	0.00	
Beans, white, sml, cnd S & W	0.5	Cup	122.00	80.00	7.00	19.00	6.00	0.50	0.00			0.00	0.00	
Beans, yardlong, ckd, drained	0.5	Cup	52.00	24.44	1.32	4.77	2.60	0.05	0.01	0.01	0.02	0.00	11.96	
Beans, yellow, snap, fresh	0.5	Cup	55.00	17.05	1.00	3.93	1.87	0.07	0.01	0.00	0.03	0.00	2.75	
Jicama, fresh, chpd	0.5	Cup	65.00	24.70	0.47	5.74	3.19	0.06	0.02	0.00	0.03	0.00	0.65	
Peas, edible pod, ckd, drained	0.5	Cup	80.00	33.60	2.62	5.64	2.24	0.19	0.04	0.02	0.08	0.00	41.60	
Peas, green, ckd, drained	0.5	Cup	80.00	67.20	4.29	12.51	4.40	0.18	0.03	0.02	0.08	0.00	32.00	
Peas, green, drained, can	0.5	Cup	85.00	58.65	3.76	10.69	3.48	0.29	0.05	0.03	0.14	0.00	22.95	
Peas, pigeon, mature, ckd w/salt	0.5	Cup	84.00	101.64	5.68	19.53	5.63	0.32	0.07	0.00	0.17	0.00	0.13	0.00
Peas, split, mature, ckd w/salt	0.5	Cup	98.00	115.64	8.17	20.68	8.14	0.38	0.06	0.08	0.16	0.00	0.35	
Soybeans, edamame, in pods, edible parts only Seapoint Farms	0.5	Cup	75.00	100.00	8.00	9.00	4.00	3.00	0.00			0.00	22.50	
Soybeans, edamame, shelled Seapoint Farms	0.5	Cup	75.00	100.00	8.00	9.00	4.00	3.00	0.00			0.00	22.50	
Soybeans, green, ckd w/salt, drained	0.5	Cup	90.00	126.90	11.11	9.94	3.78	5.76	0.67	1.09	2.71	0.00	7.20	
Soybeans, mature, dry rstd	0.5	Cup	86.00	387.86	34.04	28.14	6.97	18.60	2.69	4.11	10.50	0.00	0.00	
Vegetables, peas & carrots, ckd f/fzn, drnd, pkg	3	Ounce-weight	85.05	40.82	2.63	8.61	2.64	0.36	0.07	0.03	0.17	0.00	398.03	
Vegetables, peas & carrots, cnd, not drained	0.5	Cup	127.50	48.45	2.77	10.81	2.55	0.34	0.06	0.03	0.17	0.00	368.47	
Potatoes														
Dish, baked potato & bacon, w/cheese sauce	1	Each	299.00	451.49	18.42	44.43		25.89	10.13	9.71	4.75	29.90	188.37	
Dish, baked potato & broccoli, w/cheese sauce	1	Each	339.00	403.41	13.66	46.58		21.42	8.51	7.68	4.18	20.34	267.81	
Dish, baked potato, w/cheese sauce	1	Each	296.00	473.60	14.62	46.50		28.74	10.56	10.70	6.04	17.76	251.60	
Dish, baked potato, w/cheese sauce & chili	1	Each	395.00	481.90	23.23	55.85		21.84	13.04	6.84	0.90	31.60	185.65	
Dish, baked potato, w/sour cream & chives	1	Each	302.00	392.60	6.67	50.01		22.32	10.01	7.87	3.32	24.16	265.76	
Dish, mashed potatoes, granules prep w/milk water margarine	0.5	Cup	105.00	121.80	2.30	16.88	1.36	5.03	1.27	2.05	1.41	2.10	49.35	0.23
Dish, mashed potatoes, w/whole milk & margarine	0.5	Cup	105.00	118.65	2.10	17.76	1.57	4.40	1.05	1.83	1.27	1.05	43.05	0.15
Dish, potatoes au gratin, prep f/dry w/water milk&butter svg	1	Each	137.00	127.41	3.15	17.59	1.23	5.64	3.54	1.61	0.18	20.55	71.24	
Dish, potatoes o'brien, fzn	0.5	Cup	97.09	73.79	1.78	16.96	1.84	0.14	0.03	0.01	0.06		6.80	
Dish, scalloped potatoes, prep f/dry w/whl milk & butter svg	1	Each	137.00	127.41	2.90	17.49	1.51	5.89	3.61	1.66	0.27	15.07	47.95	
Potatoes, baked, peeled, unsalted, 2 1/3" × 4 3/4"	1	Each	156.00	145.08	3.06	33.62	2.34	0.16	0.04	0.00	0.07	0.00	0.00	
Potatoes, baked, unsalted, lrg, 3" to 4 1/4"	1	Each	298.90	277.98	7.47	63.22	6.58	0.39	0.10	0.01	0.17	0.00	2.99	
Potatoes, ckd in skin, peeled, unsalted, 2 1/2", each	1	Each	136.00	118.32	2.54	27.38	2.45	0.14	0.04	0.00	0.06	0.00	0.20	
Potatoes, french fries, heated f/fzn w/o salt	10	Each	50.00	100.00	1.58	15.60	1.60	3.78	0.63	2.38	0.39	0.00	0.12	0.00
Potatoes, hash browns, plain, fzn, pkg	0.5	Cup	105.00	86.10	2.16	18.61	1.47	0.65	0.17	0.01	0.28	0.00	0.00	
Potatoes, peeled, ckd, lrg, 3" to 4 1/4"	1	Each	299.60	257.66	5.12	59.95	5.39	0.30	0.08	0.01	0.13	0.00	0.45	
Potatoes, red, w/skin, baked, med, 2 1/4" to 3 1/4"	1	Each	173.00	153.97	3.98	33.89	3.11	0.26	0.04	0.00	0.07	0.00	1.73	
Potatoes, skin, bkd	1	Each	58.00	114.84	2.49	26.71	4.58	0.06	0.02	0.00	0.02	0.00	0.58	
Potatoes, w/skin, baked, lrg, 3" to 4 1/4"	1	Each	299.00	281.06	6.28	63.03	6.28	0.45	0.07	0.01	0.11	0.00	2.99	
Potatoes, wedges, USDA, fzn	3	Ounce-weight	85.05	104.61	2.30	21.69	1.70	1.87	0.47	1.23	0.09	0.00	0.00	
Sweetpotatoes, bkd in skin, unsalted, peeled	0.5	Cup	100.00	90.00	2.01	20.71	3.31	0.15	0.05	0.00	0.09	0.00	961.00	
Sweetpotatoes, candied, prep f/recipe, 2 1/2" × 2" pce	1	Piece	105.00	151.20	0.92	29.25	2.52	3.41	1.42	0.66	0.16	8.40	0.00	
Yams, orange, bkd in skin, unsalted, peeled	0.5	Cup	100.00	90.00	2.01	20.71	3.31	0.15	0.05	0.00	0.09	0.00	961.00	
WEIGHT LOSS BARS AND DRINKS														
Weight Loss Bars														
Bar, diet, banana nut, low carb, snack Slim Fast Low Carb	1	Each	32.00	120.00	6.00	18.00	1.00	3.00	2.00			5.00		1.50

Vit E (mg)	Vit C	Vit B$_1$ Thia (mg)	Vit B$_2$ Ribo (mg)	Vit B$_3$ Nia (mg)	Fol (mcg)	Vit B$_6$ (mg)	Vita B$_{12}$ (mcg)	Sodi (mg)	Pota (mg)	Cal (mg)	Phos (mg)	Magn (mg)	Iron (mg)	Zinc (mg)	Caff (mg)	Alco (g)	Sol Fiber (g)	Insol Fiber (g)
0.00	7.58	0.03	0.01	0.39	13.90	0.18	0.00	377.94	337.49	44.24	108.70	41.71	2.09	1.47	0.00	0.00	2.54	4.16
	0.00							440.00	350.00	60.00			1.44		0.00	0.00		
0.12	8.42	0.05	0.05	0.33	23.40	0.01	0.00	2.08	150.80	22.88	29.64	21.84	0.51	0.18	0.00	0.00		
0.05	8.96	0.05	0.05	0.42	20.35	0.04	0.00	3.30	114.95	20.35	20.90	13.75	0.57	0.13	0.00	0.00	0.41	1.45
0.30	13.13	0.02	0.02	0.13	7.80	0.03	0.00	2.60	97.50	7.80	11.70	7.80	0.39	0.11	0.00	0.00		
0.31	38.32	0.10	0.06	0.43	23.20	0.11	0.00	3.20	192.00	33.60	44.00	20.80	1.57	0.29	0.00	0.00	0.96	1.28
0.11	11.36	0.21	0.12	1.62	50.40	0.17	0.00	2.40	216.80	21.60	93.60	31.20	1.23	0.95	0.00	0.00	1.20	3.20
0.03	8.16	0.10	0.07	0.62	37.40	0.05	0.00	214.20	147.05	17.00	56.95	14.45	0.80	0.60	0.00	0.00	0.34	3.14
0.09	0.00	0.12	0.05	0.65	93.24	0.04	0.00	202.44	322.56	36.12	99.96	38.64	0.93	0.76	0.00	0.00	2.53	3.10
0.03	0.39	0.18	0.06	0.88	63.70	0.05	0.00	233.24	354.76	13.72	97.02	35.28	1.27	0.98	0.00	0.00	2.77	5.37
	5.40							30.00		50.00			1.62		0.00	0.00		
	5.40							30.00		50.00			1.62		0.00	0.00		
0.01	15.30	0.23	0.14	1.12	99.90	0.05	0.00	225.00	485.10	130.50	142.20	54.00	2.25	0.82	0.00	0.00		
3.96	3.96	0.37	0.65	0.91	176.30	0.19	0.00	1.72	1173.04	120.40	558.14	196.08	3.39	4.10	0.00	0.00	2.99	3.98
0.44	6.89	0.19	0.05	0.98	22.11	0.07	0.00	57.83	134.38	19.56	41.67	13.61	0.80	0.38	0.00	0.00	0.21	2.42
0.24	8.41	0.10	0.07	0.75	22.95	0.11	0.00	331.50	127.50	29.32	58.65	17.85	0.95	0.74	0.00	0.00	0.23	2.32
	28.70	0.27	0.24	3.98	29.90	0.75	0.33	971.75	1178.06	307.97	346.84	68.77	3.14	2.15	0.00	0.00		
	48.48	0.27	0.27	3.59	61.02	0.78	0.34	484.77	1440.75	335.61	345.78	77.97	3.32	2.03	0.00	0.00		
	26.05	0.24	0.21	3.34	26.64	0.71	0.18	381.84	1166.24	310.80	319.68	65.12	3.02	1.89	0.00	0.00		
	31.60	0.28	0.36	4.19	47.40	0.95	0.24	699.15	1572.10	410.80	497.70	110.60	6.12	3.79	0.00	0.00		
	33.82	0.27	0.18	3.71	33.22	0.79	0.21	181.20	1383.16	105.70	184.22	69.46	3.11	0.91	0.00	0.00		
0.54	6.82	0.09	0.09	0.91	8.40	0.17	0.10	180.60	162.75	33.60	65.10	21.00	0.22	0.25	0.00	0.00		
0.44	11.02	0.10	0.05	1.23	9.45	0.26	0.07	349.65	342.30	21.00	50.40	19.95	0.27	0.31	0.00	0.00		
1.64	4.25	0.03	0.11	1.29	9.59	0.05	0.00	601.43	300.03	113.71	130.15	20.55	0.44	0.33	0.00	0.00	0.25	0.99
0.17	10.97	0.05	0.04	1.10	7.77	0.20	0.00	32.04	241.75	12.62	47.57	17.48	1.00	0.28	0.00	0.00		
0.21	4.52	0.03	0.08	1.41	13.70	0.06	0.00	467.17	278.11	49.32	76.72	19.18	0.52	0.34	0.00	0.00	0.30	1.21
0.06	19.97	0.16	0.03	2.18	14.04	0.47	0.00	7.80	609.96	7.80	78.00	39.00	0.55	0.45	0.00	0.00	0.56	1.78
0.12	28.69	0.19	0.14	4.21	83.69	0.93	0.00	29.89	1599.11	44.83	209.23	83.69	3.23	1.08	0.00	0.00	1.64	4.93
0.01	17.68	0.14	0.03	1.96	13.60	0.41	0.00	5.44	515.44	6.80	59.84	29.92	0.42	0.41	0.00	0.00	0.54	1.90
0.10	5.05	0.06	0.01	1.04	6.00	0.15	0.00	15.00	209.00	4.00	41.00	11.00	0.62	0.20	0.00	0.00	0.27	1.33
0.18	8.61	0.10	0.01	1.75	4.20	0.09	0.00	23.10	299.25	10.50	49.35	11.55	1.03	0.22	0.00	0.00		
0.03	22.17	0.29	0.06	3.93	26.96	0.81	0.00	14.98	982.69	23.97	119.84	59.92	0.93	0.81	0.00	0.00	2.04	3.36
0.07	21.80	0.12	0.09	2.76	46.71	0.37	0.00	13.84	942.85	15.57	124.56	48.44	1.21	0.69	0.00	0.00		
0.02	7.83	0.07	0.06	1.78	12.76	0.36	0.00	12.18	332.34	19.72	58.58	24.94	4.08	0.28	0.00	0.00		
0.12	37.67	0.14	0.13	4.57	113.62	0.63	0.00	20.93	1626.56	29.90	224.25	80.73	1.91	1.05	0.00	0.00		
	9.53	0.09	0.03	1.31		0.30	0.00	41.67	335.10	12.76	73.99	16.16	0.60	0.31	0.00	0.00		
0.71	19.60	0.11	0.11	1.48	6.00	0.28	0.00	36.00	475.00	38.00	54.00	27.00	0.69	0.32	0.00	0.00		
3.99	7.04	0.02	0.04	0.41	11.55	0.04	0.00	73.50	198.45	27.30	27.30	11.55	1.18	0.16	0.00	0.00	1.03	1.49
0.71	19.60	0.11	0.11	1.48	6.00	0.28	0.00	36.00	475.00	38.00	54.00	27.00	0.69	0.32	0.00	0.00		
2.05	9.00	0.23	0.26	3.00	60.00	0.30	0.90	80.00	20.00	250.00	100.00		2.70			0.00		

Food Name	Amount	Measure	Weight (g)	Calories	Protein (g)	Total Carb (g)	Dietary Fiber (g)	Total Fat (g)	Sat Fat (g)	Mono Fat (g)	Poly Fat (g)	Chol (mg)	Vit A (mcg RAE)	Vit D (mcg)
WEIGHT LOSS BARS AND DRINKS (*continued*)														
Bar, diet, chewy trail mix, granola Slim Fast	1	Each	56.00	220.00	8.00	33.00	2.00	5.00	1.00			5.00		3.50
Bar, diet, chocolate chip Carb Options	1	Each	50.00	200.00	16.00	17.00	0.50	8.00	4.00			3.00		3.50
Bar, diet, chocolate chip, granola Slim Fast	1	Each	56.00	220.00	8.00	35.00	1.00	6.00	3.50			5.00		3.50
Bar, diet, hi prot & low carbohydrate, chocolate banana Optimum Nutrition Complete Protein Diet	1	Each	50.00	180.00	21.00	3.00	0.50	4.50	3.00			0.00		
Bar, diet, hi prot, chocolate raspberry Optimum Nutrition Pro-Complex	1	Each	70.00	260.00	31.00	11.00	1.00	5.00	3.50			0.00		
Bar, diet, honey peanut	1	Each	56.00	220.00	8.00	34.00	2.00	5.00	3.50			3.00		3.50
Bar, diet, Metabolift, chocolate coconut Twin Laboratories	1	Each	35.00	120.00	12.00	7.00	5.00	4.00	2.00					
Bar, diet, milk chocolate peanut Slim Fast Meal on the Go	1	Each	56.00	220.00	8.00	36.00	2.00	5.00	3.00			3.00		3.50
Bar, diet, toasted oats & spice Slim Fast Meal on the Go	1	Each	56.00	220.00	8.00	37.00	2.00	5.00	3.50			3.00		3.50
Bar, nutrition, AdvantEDGE Carb Control, choc pnt btr Abbott EAS	1	Each	60.00	230.00	17.00	26.00	5.00	8.00	5.00			5.00		
Bar, nutrition, AdvantEDGE Carb Control, choc pnt btr crisp Abbott EAS	1	Each	60.00	240.00	17.00	27.00	6.00	8.00	4.50			5.00		
Bar, nutrition, AdvantEDGE Carb Control, cookies & cream Abbott EAS	1	Each	60.00	230.00	17.00	25.00	5.00	8.00	4.50			5.00		
Bar, nutrition, AdvantEDGE Carb Control, double choc crisp Abbott EAS	1	Each	60.00	240.00	17.00	27.00	6.00	8.00	6.00			5.00		
Weight Loss Drinks														
Drink, diet, café mocha, soy prot, pwd scp Slim Fast Ultra	2	Each	48.00	170.00	15.00	26.00	5.00	1.50	0.50	0.50	0.50	0.00		3.50
Drink, diet, choc fudge, milk base, rtd can Slim Fast	1	Each	345.00	220.00	10.00	42.00	5.00	3.00	1.00	1.50	0.50	5.00		3.50
Drink, diet, hi prot & low carbohydrate, choc, dry pkt Optimum Nutrition Complete Protein Diet	1	Each	49.00	200.00	35.00	3.00	0.00	5.00	1.00			20.00		4.00
Drink, diet, straw cream, milk base, rtd can Slim Fast	1	Each	345.00	220.00	10.00	40.00	5.00	2.50	0.50	1.50	0.50	5.00		3.50
Drink, diet, vanilla cream, low carb, rtd can Slim Fast Low Carb	1	Each	350.00	190.00	20.00	7.00	5.00	9.00	1.50	6.00	1.50	15.00		3.50
MISCELLANEOUS														
Baking Chips, Chocolates, Coatings, and Cocoas														
Baking Bar, chocolate, semi sweet Hershey Foods	0.5	Ounce-weight	14.18	70.88	1.01	9.11		4.05	2.53				0.00	
Baking Chips, chocolate morsels, semi sweet Toll House	1	Tablespoon	14.18	70.00	1.00	9.00	1.00	4.00	2.50			0.00	0.00	
Baking Chips, M & M's, milk chocolate, mini bits	1	Tablespoon	14.20	70.72	0.68	9.56	0.38	3.31	2.05	1.08	0.10	2.13		
Baking Chips, M & M's, semi sweet chocolate, mini bits	1	Tablespoon	14.00	72.52	0.62	9.23	0.94	3.68	2.19	1.23	0.12	0.42	0.56	
Baking Chips, Reese's peanut butter Hershey Foods	1	Tablespoon	15.00	80.00	3.00	7.00		4.00	4.00			0.00	0.00	
Baking Chips, white morsels, premier Toll House	1	Tablespoon	14.18	80.00	1.00	9.00	0.00	4.00	3.50			0.00	0.00	
Baking Chocolate, Mexican, square	1	Each	20.00	85.20	0.73	15.48	0.80	3.12	1.72	1.01	0.23	0.00	0.00	
Baking Chocolate, unswntd, liquid	1	Tablespoon	15.00	70.80	1.82	5.09	2.72	7.16	3.79	1.38	1.61	0.00	0.15	
Cocoa Powder, unswntd, w/alkali, dry	0.25	Cup	21.50	47.73	3.89	11.78	6.41	2.82	1.67	0.95	0.09	0.00	0.00	
Baking Ingredients														
Baking Powder, double acting, sodium aluminum sulfate	1	Teaspoon	4.60	2.44	0.00	1.27	0.01	0.00	0.00	0.00	0.00	0.00	0.00	
Baking Soda	1	Teaspoon	4.60	0.00	0.00	0.00	0.00	0.00	0.00	0.00	0.00	0.00	0.00	
Yeast, baker's, dry active, pkg	1	Each	7.00	20.65	2.66	2.66	1.47	0.35	0.07	0.21	0.00	0.00	0.00	

Vit E (mg)	Vit C	Vit B₁ Thia (mg)	Vit B₂ Ribo (mg)	Vit B₃ Nia (mg)	Fol (mcg)	Vit B₆ (mg)	Vita B₁₂ (mcg)	Sodi (mg)	Pota (mg)	Cal (mg)	Phos (mg)	Magn (mg)	Iron (mg)	Zinc (mg)	Caff (mg)	Alco (g)	Sol Fiber (g)	Insol Fiber (g)
4.77	21.00	0.23	0.60	7.00	60.00	0.70	2.10	150.00	400.00	300.00		140.00	2.70	2.25	0.00	0.00		
4.77	21.00	0.23	0.60	7.00	60.00	0.70	2.10	200.00	400.00	300.00	400.00	140.00	2.70	2.25		0.00		
4.77	21.00	0.23	0.60	7.00	60.00	0.70	2.10	270.00	400.00	300.00	400.00	140.00	2.70	2.25		0.00		
								95.00		60.00	100.00		0.72			0.00		
							0.60	130.00		200.00	200.00		1.08			0.00		
4.77	21.00	0.53	0.60	7.00	120.00	0.70	2.10	160.00	170.00	300.00	250.00	140.00	2.70	2.25	0.00	0.00		
								80.00		256.00			0.50		5.00	0.00		
4.77	21.00	0.53	0.60	7.00	120.00	0.70	2.10	125.00	160.00	300.00	250.00	140.00	2.70	2.25		0.00		
4.77	21.00	0.53	0.60	7.00	60.00	0.70	2.10	160.00	65.00	300.00	250.00	140.00	2.70	2.25	0.00	0.00		
	18.00	0.45	0.51	6.00	80.00	0.60	1.80	230.00	160.00	300.00	150.00	40.00	5.40	4.50		0.00		
	18.00	0.45	0.51	7.00	120.00	0.60	1.80	350.00	140.00	350.00	250.00	60.00	5.40	4.50		0.00		
	18.00	0.45	0.51	6.00	120.00	0.60	1.80	120.00	120.00	500.00	100.00	40.00	5.40	4.50		0.00		
	18.00	0.45	0.51	6.00	120.00	0.60	1.80	340.00	230.00	300.00	200.00	60.00	6.30	4.50		0.00		
13.64	60.00	0.53	0.60	7.00	200.00	2.00	6.00	270.00	400.00	600.00	400.00	120.00	6.30	5.25		0.00		
13.64	60.00	0.53	0.60	7.00	120.00	0.70	2.10	220.00	600.00	400.00	400.00	140.00	2.70	2.25		0.00		
8.18	60.00	0.90	0.85	20.00	200.00	1.20	3.00	70.00	380.00	490.00	290.00	148.00	0.20	6.00		0.00	0.00	0.00
13.64	60.00	0.53	0.60	7.00	120.00	0.70	2.10	220.00	600.00	400.00	400.00	140.00	2.70	2.25	0.00	0.00		
13.64	60.00	0.53	0.60	2.00	120.00	0.20	0.60	200.00	400.00	400.00	400.00	140.00	2.70	2.25	0.00	0.00		
	0.00							0.00		0.00			0.36			0.00		
	0.00	0.01		0.06				0.00	45.23	0.00	22.40		0.00		7.66	0.00		
0.13	0.09	0.01	0.03	0.03	0.71	0.00	0.04	9.66	41.61	16.47	23.57	6.53	0.17	0.15	2.51	0.00		
0.15	0.00	0.01	0.01	0.06	3.92	0.01	0.00	0.42	47.04	4.76	17.08	14.84	0.41	0.21	9.10	0.00		
	0.00							35.00		0.00			0.00			0.00	0.00	
	0.00							20.00		20.00			0.00		0.00	0.00	0.00	0.00
0.07	0.02	0.01	0.02	0.37	1.00	0.01	0.00	0.60	79.40	6.80	28.40	19.00	0.44	0.25	2.80	0.00		
0.91	0.00	0.01	0.04	0.32	2.85	0.01	0.00	1.80	174.90	8.10	51.00	39.75	0.62	0.55	7.05	0.00		
0.02	0.00	0.02	0.10	0.52	6.88	0.03	0.00	4.08	539.43	23.86	156.52	102.34	3.34	1.37	16.77	0.00		
0.00	0.00	0.00	0.00	0.00	0.00	0.00	0.00	487.60	0.92	270.30	100.79	1.24	0.51	0.00	0.00	0.00		
0.00	0.00	0.00	0.00	0.00	0.00	0.00	0.00	1258.56	0.00	0.00	0.00	0.00	0.00	0.00	0.00	0.00	0.00	0.00
0.00	0.00	0.14	0.35	2.80	163.80	0.14	0.00	3.50	140.00	4.48	90.30	6.86	1.19	0.42	0.00	0.00		

Food Name	Amount	Measure	Weight (g)	Calories	Protein (g)	Total Carb (g)	Dietary Fiber (g)	Total Fat (g)	Sat Fat (g)	Mono Fat (g)	Poly Fat (g)	Chol (mg)	Vit A (mcg RAE)	Vit D (mcg)
MISCELLANEOUS (continued)														
Condiments														
Bacon Bits, Bac O Bits General Mills, Inc.	1	Tablespoon	6.00	24.96	2.46	1.62		0.96				0.00		
Catsup	1	Tablespoon	15.00	15.00	0.26	3.87	0.14	0.07	0.01	0.01	0.03	0.00	7.05	
Catsup, low sod	1	Tablespoon	15.00	15.60	0.23	4.09	0.20	0.05	0.01	0.01	0.02	0.00	7.80	
Horseradish, prep, tsp	1	Teaspoon	5.00	2.40	0.06	0.56	0.17	0.03	0.00	0.01	0.02	0.00	0.01	
Ketchup, pkt	1	Each	6.00	6.00	0.10	1.55	0.05	0.03	0.00	0.00	0.01	0.00	2.82	
Mustard, deli Hebrew National	1	Teaspoon	5.00	4.00	0.00	0.00	0.00	0.00	0.00	0.00	0.00	0.00		
Mustard, yellow Westbrae Natural	1	Teaspoon	5.00	0.00	0.00	0.00	0.00	0.00	0.00	0.00	0.00			
Pepperoncini, Greek GL Mezzetta	1	Ounce-weight	28.35	7.65	0.21	1.42	0.38	0.13	0.04	0.02	0.08	0.00		
Pickles, bread & butter	1	Each	8.00	6.16	0.07	1.43	0.12	0.02	0.00	0.00	0.01	0.00	0.56	
Pickles, dill, slices	5	Piece	35.00	6.30	0.22	1.45	0.40	0.07	0.01	0.00	0.02	0.00	3.15	
Pickles, sour, slices	5	Piece	35.00	3.85	0.12	0.79	0.42	0.07	0.02	0.00	0.02	0.00	2.45	
Pickles, sour, spears	1	Piece	30.00	3.30	0.10	0.68	0.36	0.06	0.02	0.00	0.02	0.00	2.10	
Pickles, sweet, lrg, 3" long	1	Each	35.00	40.95	0.13	11.13	0.38	0.09	0.02	0.00	0.03	0.00	3.15	
Relish, cranberry orange, cnd, cup	0.25	Cup	68.75	122.38	0.21	31.76	0.00	0.07	0.01	0.01	0.04	0.00	2.75	
Sauce, hot dog chili, rts, pkg Chef-Mate	0.25	Cup	63.00	69.30	2.69	9.23	1.70	2.38	0.97	0.97	0.22	4.41		
Sauce, hot, jalapeno, svg	1	Each	14.00	4.94	0.00	0.99	0.00	0.00	0.00	0.00	0.00	0.00	0.00	
Sauce, soy, f/soy & wheat	2	Tablespoon	32.00	16.96	2.01	2.44	0.26	0.01	0.00	0.00	0.01	0.00	0.00	
Sauce, steak Carb Options	1	Tablespoon	16.00	5.00	0.00	1.00	0.00	0.00	0.00	0.00	0.00	0.00	0.00	
Sauce, tabasco, rts	1	Teaspoon	4.70	0.56	0.06	0.04	0.03	0.04	0.00	0.00	0.02	0.00	3.85	
Sauce, taco, green, mild														
La Victoria Foods	2	Tablespoon	30.18	9.05	0.24	1.76	0.18	0.11				0.00	1.21	
Sauce, taco, hot Old El Paso	2	Tablespoon	30.00	10.00	0.00	2.00	0.00	0.00	0.00	0.00	0.00	0.00	0.00	
Sauce, worcestershire	1	Tablespoon	17.00	11.39	0.00	3.31	0.00	0.00	0.00	0.00	0.00	0.00	0.85	
Vinegar, balsamic, 60 grain														
Fleischmann's Vinegars&Wines	1	Tablespoon	15.00	21.00	0.00	5.33	0.00	0.00	0.00	0.00	0.00	0.00		
Salsas														
Salsa La Victoria Foods	2	Tablespoon	30.00	10.00	0.00	2.00	0.00	0.00	0.00	0.00	0.00	0.00	0.00	
Salsa, chili, chunky, cnd														
La Victoria Foods	2	Tablespoon	30.00	9.30	0.24	1.96	0.15	0.05					3.30	
Salsa, green, Jalapena La Victoria Foods	2	Tablespoon	30.16	9.65	0.28	1.42	0.27	0.33				0.00	4.22	
Sauce, picante Pace	2	Tablespoon	32.40	10.00	0.00	2.00	0.83	0.00	0.00	0.00	0.00	0.00		
Sauce, picante, rts, pkg Ortega	2	Tablespoon	30.00	10.20	0.37	2.00	0.00	0.07	0.01	0.01	0.03	0.00		

Vit E (mg)	Vit C	Vit B$_1$ Thia (mg)	Vit B$_2$ Ribo (mg)	Vit B$_3$ Nia (mg)	Fol (mcg)	Vit B$_6$ (mg)	Vita B$_{12}$ (mcg)	Sodi (mg)	Pota (mg)	Cal (mg)	Phos (mg)	Magn (mg)	Iron (mg)	Zinc (mg)	Caff (mg)	Alco (g)	Sol Fiber (g)	Insol Fiber (g)
		0.52	0.02	0.11				102.60	163.80	13.20			0.40		0.00	0.00		
0.22	2.27	0.00	0.07	0.23	1.50	0.02	0.00	166.50	56.55	2.70	4.80	2.85	0.08	0.04	0.00	0.00	0.03	0.10
0.24	2.27	0.01	0.01	0.21	2.25	0.03	0.00	3.00	72.15	2.85	5.85	3.30	0.11	0.03	0.00	0.00	0.05	0.15
0.00	1.25	0.00	0.00	0.02	2.85	0.00	0.00	15.70	12.30	2.80	1.55	1.35	0.02	0.04	0.00	0.00		
0.09	0.91	0.00	0.03	0.09	0.60	0.01	0.00	66.60	22.62	1.08	1.92	1.14	0.03	0.01	0.00	0.00	0.01	0.04
								65.00							0.00	0.00	0.00	0.00
								75.00							0.00	0.00	0.00	0.00
	1.83							368.55		10.75			0.17		0.00	0.00		
0.01	0.72	0.00	0.00	0.00	0.32	0.00	0.00	53.84	16.00	2.56	2.16	0.16	0.03	0.00	0.00	0.00		
0.03	0.66	0.00	0.01	0.02	0.35	0.00	0.00	448.70	40.60	3.15	7.35	3.85	0.19	0.05	0.00	0.00		
0.02	0.35	0.00	0.00	0.00	0.35	0.00	0.00	422.80	8.05	0.00	4.90	1.40	0.14	0.01	0.00	0.00	0.00	0.42
0.02	0.30	0.00	0.00	0.00	0.30	0.00	0.00	362.40	6.90	0.00	4.20	1.20	0.12	0.01	0.00	0.00	0.00	0.36
0.03	0.42	0.00	0.01	0.06	0.35	0.00	0.00	328.65	11.20	1.40	4.20	1.40	0.21	0.02	0.00	0.00	0.00	0.38
0.03	12.38	0.02	0.01	0.07	2.06	0.02	0.00	22.00	26.13	7.56	5.50	2.75	0.14	0.06	0.00	0.00	0.00	0.00
0.29	0.06	0.05	0.05	0.66	22.05	0.07	0.13	398.79	149.31	19.53	39.69	12.60	0.98	0.55	0.00	0.00		
	0.00							108.64		0.00			0.00		0.00	0.00	0.00	0.00
0.00	0.00	0.01	0.05	0.70	4.48	0.05	0.00	1803.84	69.44	6.08	40.00	13.76	0.62	0.17	0.00	0.00		
	0.00							200.00		0.00			0.00		0.00	0.00	0.00	0.00
	0.21	0.00	0.00	0.01	0.05	0.01	0.00	29.75	6.02	0.56	1.08	0.56	0.05	0.01	0.00	0.00		
	1.45							191.34		2.41			0.02		0.00	0.00		
	0.00							180.00		0.00			0.00		0.00	0.00	0.00	0.00
0.01	2.21	0.01	0.02	0.12	1.36	0.00	0.00	166.60	136.00	18.19	10.20	2.21	0.90	0.03	0.00	0.00	0.00	0.00
	0.15	0.15	0.15	0.15				3.00	10.50	1.80	3.00		0.15		0.00	0.00	0.00	0.00
	2.40							115.00	55.00	0.00			0.00		0.00	0.00	0.00	0.00
	3.15							147.90		4.20			0.01		0.00	0.00		
	3.62							180.96		4.83			0.12		0.00	0.00		
	0.00							230.00		0.00			0.00		0.00	0.00		
0.37	0.57	0.02	0.01	0.29	3.00	0.04	0.00	252.00	80.40	12.60	8.40	4.50	0.15	0.05	0.00	0.00	0.00	0.00

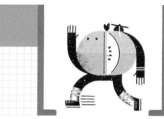

BY LIZ APPLEGATE, PH.D.

[PersonalBest]

Fridge Wisdom
NUTRITION ADVICE FOR HEALTHY, HUNGRY RUNNERS

Get Milk
Why runners need more of this nutrient-rich beverage

FEW DRINKS ARE as high in health-boosting nutrients as milk. This staple contains protein, carbs, and key vitamins and minerals that make it a smart choice—especially for runners. (But choose fat-free or one-percent varieties to reduce your intake of saturated fat.) Now, thanks to new processing techniques that help suspend tiny micro particles of fat in milk, even fat-free varieties (which actually have about half a gram per cup) have a creamier taste. Here's how milk can do the runner's body good.

BUILD STRENGTH → As a kid, you learned milk is a standout source of calcium (vital for bone health and muscle contraction), supplying about 30 percent of your Daily Value (DV). Milk also contains more than 10 percent of your DV for potassium, which supports both fluid balance and healthy blood pressure.

BEAT SORENESS → Eight ounces of milk provides 18 percent of the DV for protein. Studies show that milk protein (made of whey and casein) may stave off muscle soreness. And a new study concludes that milk does a better job of lowering markers of muscle damage postworkout than sports drinks do.

REFUEL MUSCLES → Milk has about 12 grams of carbs per serving in the form of lac-tose, a sugar that helps refuel muscles. Lactose intolerant runners have trouble digesting this sugar, and drinking milk can cause GI issues. Fortunately, lactose-free versions make it possible for sensitive runners to enjoy milk.

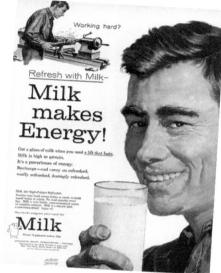

Working hard?

Refresh with Milk—
Milk makes Energy!

Milk

STILL A GOOD CHOICE
Besides calcium, milk provides protein, potassium, and healthy fats.

IMPROVE PERFORMANCE → Milk is fortified with about 25 percent of your DV for vitamin D, which many runners fall short on and may be important for endurance and speeding recovery. Milk has a quarter of your needs for vitamin B_3, which runners—especially women—need to help maintain high mileage.

LOSE WEIGHT → Organic milk may be more expensive, but it also contains higher levels of the essential fat alpha-linolenic acid (or ALA). Some studies suggest this fatty acid may help with long-term weight control. Brands such as Organic Horizon are now fortifying some of their milk products with omega-3 fatty acids, which fight inflammatory disorders and may help runners recover faster.

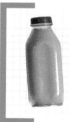

ADD TO YOUR CART
Chocolate Milk

Yet another happy study (this one from the U.K.) finds drinking chocolate milk between exhaustive bouts of exercise improves endurance more than a carb recovery drink. Researchers think chocolate milk has a superior ratio of fat, carbs, and protein, making it ideal for recovery.

Don't Have A Cow
Choose the healthiest nondairy "milks"

SOY MILK
Made from ground soybeans and water, it has nearly as much protein as cow's milk and some fiber, and it's fortified with calcium and vitamins A, D, and B_{12}. It also has nutrients that may help lower cancer risk, cholesterol, and heart-disease risk.

ALMOND MILK
This rich, cream-colored beverage is made of ground almonds and water. A cup has only one gram of protein, but supplies 50 percent of your DV for vitamin E, which may stave off muscle soreness. Look for varieties fortified with calcium and vitamin D.

RICE MILK
Produced by combining water and ground rice, it's very low in protein, so it's not a good milk substitute for postrun recovery. Choose brands with added calcium and vitamin D to make up for its nutritional shortfalls.

HEMP MILK
This "milk" is made of ground hemp seeds and water. It has more fat than whole milk, but some of it is essential omega-3 fatty acids. While hemp milk is tasty, not all brands are fortified with vitamins A, D, and B_{12}, and it is also lower in protein.

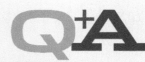

[PersonalBest]

Fridge Wisdom
NUTRITION ADVICE FOR HEALTHY, HUNGRY RUNNERS

BY LIZ APPLEGATE, PH.D.

Don't Kick the Can

A new generation of preserved foods are healthy—and tasty

CANNED FOODS ARE often dismissed as lacking both taste and nutrients. But neither criticism is necessarily true anymore. Thanks to technological advances, these foods can retain much of their flavor and nutrition—and in some cases they're actually healthier than fresh. One thing that hasn't changed: They're still cheap and convenient. Here's how to make the most of this overlooked pantry staple.

FRUITS FOR ANTIOXIDANTS
→ Buy fruit packed in juice (not syrup) to avoid added sugar; choose ones with vitamin C for an immune boost. Mix canned peaches and pears with yogurt. Or try canned pumpkin. It's great in smoothies, and a half-cup has 300 percent of your vitamin A needs—that's 10 times more than fresh.

VEGETABLES FOR FAST FIBER
→ Peas, green beans, okra, and other canned veggies are high in fiber—but with the washing and chopping done, they're ready fast. Use reduced-sodium versions if you have high blood pressure. Canned tomatoes are easier to cook than fresh, provide rich flavor, and are higher in the cancer-fighting antioxidant lycopene.

SEAFOOD FOR PROTEIN
→ Canned tuna supplies muscle-building protein but can contain mercury, so limit your consumption to two six-ounce cans per week. Canned salmon is rich in both omega-3s and protein, and canned clams (great in spaghetti sauce) are loaded with zinc and selenium—important for immune health and preventing muscle damage.

BEANS FOR VERSATILITY
→ Canned beans are loaded with 35 percent of your daily fiber needs, along with protein and iron. Use them in salads and soups. Stuff them into wraps, or blend into a dip. Beans that are different colors contain different antioxidants, so eat a variety for a wide range of nutrients.

SOUPS FOR LUNCH
→ Choose those with fewer than 600 milligrams of sodium, five grams of fat or less, and at least eight grams of protein per serving. Add tofu, canned chicken, or clams for a protein boost. Minestrone is often low in calories but high in fiber; chicken with vegetables and black bean soups are both rich in protein and carbs.

CHILI FOR RECOVERY
→ Canned turkey, beef, or vegetarian chili provides postrun recovery nutrients; make sure it has fewer than six grams of fat and at least 10 grams of protein per cup. Even canned pasta (yes, Spaghetti-Os) makes a healthy fallback meal supplying a dose of protein with five grams of fat or less—just round out the meal with a salad and fruit.

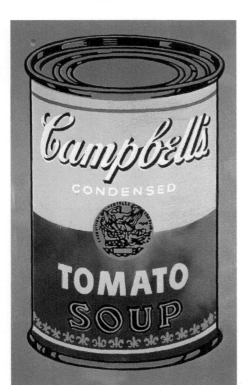

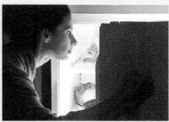

Q Is it healthy to "starve a cold"?
A Never starve yourself, especially when it comes to immune health. Instead, eat ample calories so your body is fueled to produce virus-fighting cells. Have vegetables and protein at every meal to maintain immune strength. Consider taking a multivitamin with zinc during cold season. And eat yogurt. A new study found that eating a cup of yogurt daily can cut upper-respiratory-tract infections by 25 percent.

Can-Do's (And Don'ts)
Keep preserved foods healthy

 DO KEEP 'EM COOL Store cans in a cool, dry pantry—not over the stove or near the oven.

 DO CLEAN BEFORE OPENING Wipe the top of the can before opening it to avoid getting any dirt or debris in your food.

DON'T BUY DAMAGED GOODS Pass by cans with dents, signs of leakage, or bulges (which indicate spoilage).

DO THINK ABOUT BPA Most cans contain bisphenol A (BPA), which some studies link to cancer in lab animals. If you're concerned about exposure, consider buying cans labeled "BPA-free."

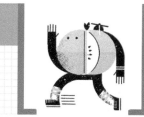

[PersonalBest]

Fridge Wisdom

NUTRITION ADVICE FOR HEALTHY, HUNGRY RUNNERS

BY LIZ APPLEGATE, PH.D.

The Runner's Pie

Feel good creating (and eating!) tasty, low-fat pizza

RUNNERS LOVE PIZZA so much that most eat about one medium pie every month. Trouble is, many are high-fat disasters with few nutritionally redeeming qualities. One solution? Make your own at home and load it with good-for-you ingredients. Choose your crust, sauce, cheese, and toppings, then assemble the pizza on a baking sheet lined with parchment paper. Bake at 450°F for 10 to 15 minutes.

CHOOSE YOUR CRUST

→ Look for uncooked whole-wheat dough in your grocer's refrigerated or freezer case. Or use prebaked options, like focaccia, naan, whole-wheat pita, or French bread. Sprinkle crust with flaxseed meal or wheat germ for an extra boost of nutrients.

SPREAD ON THE SAUCE

→ Marinara sauce is rich in lycopene, a cancer-fighting antioxidant. One study found eating a red-sauce pizza every week can lower your risk for certain cancers. Jarred varieties are convenient, but you can also make your own in less than 20 minutes. Or spread on a thin layer of pesto or stir-fry sauce.

BE CHEESE SAVVY

→ Shredded, part-skim mozzarella has just 72 calories, four grams of fat, and 20 percent of your daily calcium needs per ounce. A tablespoon of Parmesan adds big flavor with only 21 calories. Or give your pizza Greek or Mexican flare with feta cheese or queso fresco.

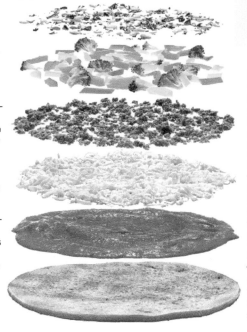

Marinara Sauce

5	seeded Roma tomatoes
½	small white onion
¼	cup fresh basil, or 1 teaspoon dried
	Garlic powder to taste
	Oregano to taste
	Salt and pepper to taste

Place all ingredients in food processor; blend until smooth. In a skillet, simmer sauce 10 to 15 minutes, or until thick. Spread ½ to ¾ cup on 12-inch crust.

SELECT YOUR PROTEIN

→ Choose lean options, such as grilled chicken, baby shrimp, ground beef, smoked salmon, pork tenderloin, or Canadian bacon—all provide about 40 percent of your daily protein needs. Or go meatless and add tofu or beans.

PILE ON VEGETABLES

→ Vegetables are low-calorie and nutrient-rich, so add as many as you like. Chop raw veggies into small pieces so they cook faster, or lightly sauté them to shorten cooking time and prevent the pizza from getting soggy.

ADD FINISHING TOUCHES

→ Give your pizza extra pizzazz: Add chopped nuts and spices; sprinkle with fresh herbs in the last few minutes of baking. Finish with a drizzle of olive or sesame oil for heart-healthy flavor. **RW**

Heat and Eat
Healthy frozen pies have fiber and fewer than 11 fat grams per serving

AMERICAN FLATBREAD
The thin-crust Ionian Awakening is topped with olives and rosemary.
300 CAL, **10** G FAT, **2** G FIBER

AMY'S PIZZA
Lactose-intolerant runners will enjoy the soy cheese option.
290 CAL, **11** G FAT, **2** G FIBER

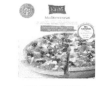

KASHI PIZZA
The crust on the Mediterranean pie includes whole grains and flaxseeds.
290 CAL, **9** G FAT, **5** G FIBER

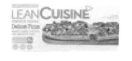

LEAN CUISINE PIZZA
The French Bread Pizza has a hearty crust; a small amount of pepperoni and sausage add big flavor.
340 CAL, **8** G FAT, **4** G FIBER

PHOTOGRAPHS BY **MITCH MANDEL**

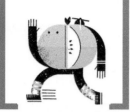

[PersonalBest]

Fridge Wisdom
NUTRITION ADVICE FOR HEALTHY, HUNGRY RUNNERS

BY LIZ APPLEGATE, PH.D.

Fill 'r Up

Alternative carb sources keep you fueled on runs

SPRING'S HERE, and chances are you're logging longer runs. So it's important to have a smart midrun fueling strategy to keep your energy high. Start by eating a prerun meal that consists of a couple hundred calories (up to 500) two to three hours before your run. If you run for one to two hours, consume 30 to 60 grams of carbs per hour of exercise. Run longer than that and you'll need 60 to 90 grams per hour. Luckily, runners have plenty of options for fueling up on the road, including sports drinks, energy gels, and energy bars. But when you don't have your go-to product handy, these alternatives will keep you just as energized so you can finish your run feeling strong.

SPORTS DRINKS

Products like Gatorade supply 14 to 18 grams of carbs per eight ounces and often contain several carb types, such as glucose and fructose, which speed energy absorption. Most also have electrolytes to help maintain fluid balance.

DIY → Mix 8 teaspoons sugar, 2 teaspoons honey, 1/3 teaspoon salt, and 1 teaspoon lime juice in 24 ounces of water.

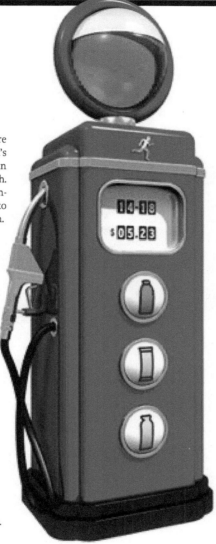

ENERGY GELS

One gel has 22 to 29 grams of carbs—usually from multiple sources—along with electrolytes. Take these with water to speed delivery of energy into your system.

DIY → Mild-tasting and easy to swallow, jelly packs (those mini jams found at diners) contain 13 grams of carbs and provide two types of sugar.

ENERGY CHEWS

These bite-sized, candylike products contain about five grams of carbs per chew. You can eat chews a few at a time, making it easy to customize your energy intake.

DIY → Old-fashioned gumdrops contain about four grams of carbs per candy. Take 10 with you for a hit of midrun energy.

CAFFEINATED CARBS

Caffeine-boosted gels and chews contain 50 to 100 milligrams of caffeine per packet. The caffeine jolt helps boost your energy and may prolong endurance.

DIY → A can of Starbucks Doubleshot (made from espresso, milk, and sugar) supplies 130 milligrams of caffeine. Unlike gels and chews, it's not overly sweet.

ENERGY BARS

Products like PowerBar and Clif Bar supply 22 to 45 grams of carbohydrate, plus a good dose of protein, which will keep your stomach from growling on runs.

DIY → Two hearty fig bars supply 90 calories and 22 grams of carbohydrate from flour, figs, and sugar. **RW**

BOTTOM: MITCH MANDEL (3)

Road Food New, tasty, midrun fuel will energize your workouts

CLIF C BARS
→ Small and soft, these tasty bars (flavors include cherry pomegranate, blueberry, and raspberry) are made from dried fruit, juice, and nuts. Each contains 130 calories, 25 g carbs, and 4.5 g fat. clifbar.com

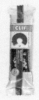

HONEY STINGER WAFFLES
→ These honey-filled "waffles" are thin and slightly crisp. One contains 160 calories, 21 g carbs, and 7 g fat. honeystinger.com

GREATER THAN
→ This sports drink is made with coconut water and sugar. It supplies 30 calories and 7 g carbs per eight ounces (half of regular sports drinks) but contains extra electrolytes. drinkgt.com

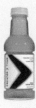

ILLUSTRATION BY **FAIYAZ JAFRI**

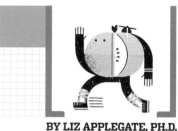

BY LIZ APPLEGATE, PH.D.

[**Personal**Best]

Fridge Wisdom

NUTRITION ADVICE FOR HEALTHY, HUNGRY RUNNERS

One-Dish Wonders

Best ways to cook tasty, healthy, low-mess meals

IN THE OVEN

GOOD FOR → Tenderizing meat and bringing out sweetness in veggies.

COOK IT → Pork Tenderloin with Winter Vegetables (pictured, right)
Mix two tablespoons mustard with crushed garlic and pepper. Spread on a one-pound pork tenderloin. Roast in casserole with Brussels sprouts, sweet potato, fennel, and carrots, and seven ounces of chicken stock at 375°F for 45 minutes.

ON THE STOVETOP

GOOD FOR → Adding ingredients at different stages of cooking.

COOK IT → Chicken, Rice, and Veggies
In a Dutch oven, brown four chicken thighs in olive oil; set aside. Sauté diced onion and minced garlic, then sauté sliced mushrooms. Add a cup of brown rice, salt, pepper, and seasoning. Lightly toast. Add two cups of stock, then chicken. Cover and simmer 30 minutes. Add a cup and a half of asparagus tips; simmer 15 minutes.

IN THE MICROWAVE

GOOD FOR → Quick meals that preserve nutrients lost in longer, hotter cooking.

COOK IT → Vegetarian Chili
In a casserole, combine eight ounces crumbled faux meat or extra-firm tofu,
two cans of beans, one can of Mexican-style tomatoes, one and a half cups of corn, and chili powder. Cover; cook eight minutes. Stir, then sprinkle with grated cheddar cheese. Cook four more minutes.

IN A SLOW COOKER

GOOD FOR → Tossing in ingredients before you leave for work.

COOK IT → Meat and Potatoes
Cover a pound of cut-up top sirloin with steak rub and garlic powder. Line a slow cooker with red potatoes, carrots, and red onion wedges. Place beef on top. Add a can of stock. Cook on low for eight hours.

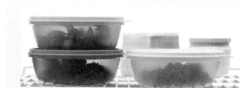

Cold Storage

Put away leftovers properly for delicious (and safe) meals

CHILL OUT Cool slightly, then refrigerate or freeze in an airtight container. Don't leave out longer than two hours.

REMEMBER TO EAT Finish leftovers within three to four days, or freeze and use within one to two months.

DEFROST SAFELY Thaw frozen leftovers in the fridge, making sure the container stays at 40°F or cooler.

BE CONTAINER SMART Stick to microwave-safe containers. Plastic tubs or bags may transfer chemicals.

FOOD STYLIST: JOAN PARKIN; DUTCH OVEN COURTESY LA CREUSET
RIGHT: HAMMOND/PHOTOCUISINE/CORBIS

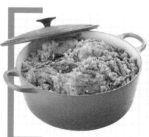

KITCHEN ESSENTIALS
Dutch Oven

Ideal for one-dish meals on the stovetop or in the oven, cast-iron Dutch ovens provide even heating. Enameled versions are easy to clean and don't require seasoning as do exposed-iron models. A tight-fitting lid keeps food moist.

PHOTOGRAPHS BY **MITCH MANDEL**

2015-2020 Dietary Guidelines

Executive Summary

In this section:

1. **The Guidelines**

2. **Key Recommendations**

Over the past century, deficiencies of essential nutrients have dramatically decreased, many infectious diseases have been conquered, and the majority of the U.S. population can now anticipate a long and productive life. At the same time, rates of chronic diseases—many of which are related to poor quality diet and physical inactivity—have increased. About half of all American adults have one or more preventable, diet-related chronic diseases, including cardiovascular disease, type 2 diabetes, and overweight and obesity.

However, a large body of evidence now shows that healthy eating patterns and regular physical activity can help people achieve and maintain good health and reduce the risk of chronic disease throughout all stages of the lifespan. The *2015-2020 Dietary Guidelines for Americans* reflects this evidence through its recommendations.

The *Dietary Guidelines* is required under the 1990 National Nutrition Monitoring and Related Research Act, which states that every 5 years, the U.S. Departments of Health and Human Services (HHS) and of Agriculture (USDA) must jointly publish a report containing nutritional and dietary information and guidelines for the general public. The statute (Public Law 101-445, 7 U.S.C. 5341 et seq.) requires that the *Dietary Guidelines* be based on the preponderance of current scientific and medical knowledge. The 2015-2020 edition of the *Dietary Guidelines* builds from the 2010 edition with revisions based on the *Scientific Report of the 2015 Dietary Guidelines Advisory Committee* and consideration of Federal agency and public comments.

The *Dietary Guidelines* is designed for professionals to help all individuals ages 2 years and older and their families consume a healthy, nutritionally adequate diet. The information in the *Dietary Guidelines* is used in developing Federal food, nutrition, and health policies and programs. It also is the basis for Federal nutrition education materials designed for the public and for the nutrition education components of HHS and USDA food programs. It is developed for use by policymakers and nutrition and health professionals. Additional audiences who may use *Dietary Guidelines* information to develop programs, policies, and communication for the general public include businesses, schools, community groups, media, the food industry, and State and local governments.

Previous editions of the *Dietary Guidelines* focused primarily on individual dietary components such as food groups and nutrients. However, people do not eat food groups and nutrients in isolation but rather in combination, and the totality of the diet forms an overall eating pattern. The components of the eating pattern can have interactive and potentially cumulative effects on health. These patterns can be tailored to an individual's personal preferences, enabling Americans to choose the diet that is right for them. A growing body of research has examined the relationship between overall eating patterns, health, and risk of chronic disease, and findings on these relationships are sufficiently well established to support dietary guidance. As a result, eating patterns and their food and nutrient characteristics are a focus of the recommendations in the *2015-2020 Dietary Guidelines*.

The *2015-2020 Dietary Guidelines* provides five overarching Guidelines that encourage healthy eating patterns, recognize that individuals will need to make shifts in their food and beverage choices to achieve a healthy pattern, and acknowledge that all segments of our society have a role to play in supporting healthy choices. These Guidelines also embody the idea that a healthy eating pattern is not a rigid prescription, but rather, an adaptable framework in which individuals can enjoy foods that meet their personal, cultural, and traditional preferences and fit within their budget. Several examples of healthy eating patterns that translate and integrate the recommendations in overall healthy ways to eat are provided.

The Guidelines

1. **Follow a healthy eating pattern across the lifespan.** All food and beverage choices matter. Choose a healthy eating pattern at an appropriate calorie level to help achieve and maintain a healthy body weight, support nutrient adequacy, and reduce the risk of chronic disease.

2. **Focus on variety, nutrient density, and amount.** To meet nutrient needs within calorie limits, choose a variety of nutrient-dense foods across and within all food groups in recommended amounts.

3. **Limit calories from added sugars and saturated fats and reduce sodium intake.** Consume an eating pattern low in added sugars, saturated fats, and sodium. Cut back on foods and beverages higher in these components to amounts that fit within healthy eating patterns.

4. **Shift to healthier food and beverage choices.** Choose nutrient-dense foods and beverages across and within all food groups in place of less healthy choices.

Consider cultural and personal preferences to make these shifts easier to accomplish and maintain.

5. **Support healthy eating patterns for all.** Everyone has a role in helping to create and support healthy eating patterns in multiple settings nationwide, from home to school to work to communities.

Key Recommendations provide further guidance on how individuals can follow the five Guidelines:

Key Recommendations

The *Dietary Guidelines'* Key Recommendations for healthy eating patterns should be applied in their entirety, given the interconnected relationship that each dietary component can have with others.

Consume a healthy eating pattern that accounts for all foods and beverages within an appropriate calorie level.

A healthy eating pattern includes:[1]

- A variety of vegetables from all of the subgroups—dark green, red and orange, legumes (beans and peas), starchy, and other

- Fruits, especially whole fruits

- Grains, at least half of which are whole grains

- Fat-free or low-fat dairy, including milk, yogurt, cheese, and/or fortified soy beverages

- A variety of protein foods, including seafood, lean meats and poultry, eggs, legumes (beans and peas), and nuts, seeds, and soy products

- Oils

A healthy eating pattern limits:

- Saturated fats and *trans* fats, added sugars, and sodium

Key Recommendations that are quantitative are provided for several components of the diet that should be limited. These components are of particular public health concern in the United States, and the specified limits can help individuals achieve healthy eating patterns within calorie limits:

- Consume less than 10 percent of calories per day from added sugars[2]

- Consume less than 10 percent of calories per day from saturated fats[3]

- Consume less than 2,300 milligrams (mg) per day of sodium[4]

- If alcohol is consumed, it should be consumed in moderation—up to one drink per day for women and up to two drinks per day for men—and only by adults of legal drinking age.[5]

In tandem with the recommendations above, Americans of all ages—children, adolescents, adults, and older adults—should meet the *Physical Activity Guidelines for Americans* to help promote health and reduce the risk of chronic disease. Americans should aim to achieve and maintain a healthy body weight. The relationship between diet and physical activity contributes to calorie balance and managing body weight. As such, the *Dietary Guidelines* includes a Key Recommendation to

- Meet the *Physical Activity Guidelines for Americans*.[6]

Terms To Know

Several terms are used to operationalize the principles and recommendations of the *2015-2020 Dietary Guidelines*. These terms are essential to understanding the concepts discussed herein:

Eating pattern—The combination of foods and beverages that constitute an individual's complete dietary intake over time. Often referred to as a "dietary pattern," an eating pattern may describe a customary way of eating or a combination of foods recommended for consumption. Specific examples include USDA Food Patterns and the Dietary Approaches to Stop Hypertension (DASH) Eating Plan.

Nutrient dense—A characteristic of foods and beverages that provide vitamins, minerals, and other substances that contribute to adequate nutrient intakes or may have positive health effects, with little or no solid fats and added sugars, refined starches, and sodium. Ideally, these foods and beverages also are in forms that retain naturally occurring components, such as dietary fiber. All vegetables, fruits, whole grains, seafood, eggs, beans and peas, unsalted nuts and seeds, fat-free and low-fat dairy products, and lean meats and poultry—when prepared with little or no added solid fats, sugars, refined starches, and sodium—are nutrient-dense foods. These foods contribute to meeting food group recommendations within calorie and sodium limits. The term "nutrient dense" indicates the nutrients and other beneficial substances in a food have not been "diluted" by the addition of calories from added solid fats, sugars, or refined starches, or by the solid fats naturally present in the food.

Variety—A diverse assortment of foods and beverages across and within all food groups and subgroups selected to fulfill the recommended amounts without exceeding the limits for calories and other dietary components. For example, in the vegetables food group, selecting a variety of foods could be accomplished over the course of a week by choosing from all subgroups, including dark green, red and orange, legumes (beans and peas), starchy, and other vegetables.

An underlying premise of the *Dietary Guidelines* is that nutritional needs should be met primarily from foods. All forms of foods, including fresh, canned, dried, and frozen, can be included in healthy eating patterns. Foods in nutrient-dense forms contain essential vitamins and minerals and also dietary fiber and other naturally occurring substances that may have positive health effects. In some cases, fortified foods and dietary supplements may be useful in providing one or more nutrients that otherwise may be consumed in less-than-recommended amounts.

For most individuals, achieving a healthy eating pattern will require changes in food and beverage choices. This edition of the *Dietary Guidelines* focuses on **shifts** to emphasize the need to make substitutions—that is, choosing nutrient-dense foods and beverages in place of less healthy choices—rather than increasing intake overall. Most individuals would benefit from shifting food choices both within and across food groups. Some needed shifts are minor and can be accomplished by making simple substitutions, while others will require greater effort to accomplish.

Although individuals ultimately decide what and how much to consume, their personal relationships; the settings in which they live, work, and shop; and other contextual factors strongly influence their choices. Concerted efforts among health professionals, communities, businesses and industries, organizations, governments, and other segments of society are needed to support individuals and families in making dietary and physical activity choices that align with the *Dietary Guidelines*. Everyone has a role, and these efforts, in combination and over time, have the potential to meaningfully improve the health of current and future generations.

Figure ES-1.
2015-2020 Dietary Guidelines for Americans at a Glance

The *2015-2020 Dietary Guidelines* focuses on the big picture with recommendations to help Americans make choices that add up to an overall healthy eating pattern. To build a healthy eating pattern, combine healthy choices from across all food groups—while paying attention to calorie limits, too.

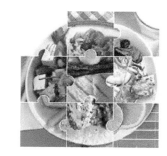

Check out the 5 Guidelines that encourage healthy eating patterns:

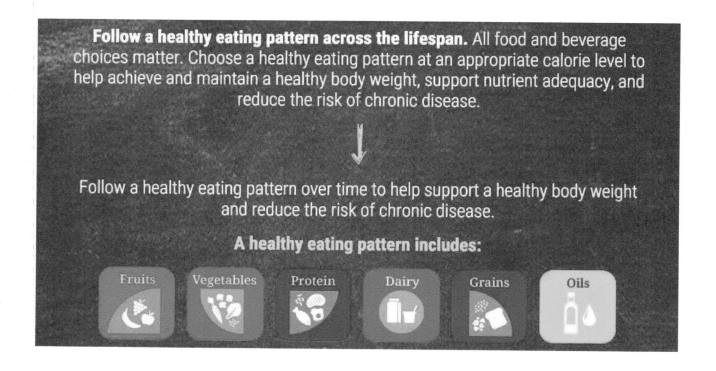

Follow a healthy eating pattern across the lifespan. All food and beverage choices matter. Choose a healthy eating pattern at an appropriate calorie level to help achieve and maintain a healthy body weight, support nutrient adequacy, and reduce the risk of chronic disease.

Follow a healthy eating pattern over time to help support a healthy body weight and reduce the risk of chronic disease.

A healthy eating pattern includes:

Fruits   Vegetables   Protein   Dairy   Grains   Oils

Notes

[1] Definitions for each food group and subgroup are provided throughout Chapter 1. Key Elements of Healthy Eating Patterns (/dietaryguidelines/2015/guidelines/chapter-1/) and are compiled in Appendix 3. USDA Food Patterns: Healthy U.S.-Style Eating Pattern (/dietaryguidelines/2015/guidelines/appendix-3/).

[2] The recommendation to limit intake of calories from added sugars to less than 10 percent per day is a target based on food pattern modeling and national data on intakes of calories from added sugars that demonstrate the public health need to limit calories from added sugars to meet food group and nutrient needs within calorie limits. The limit on calories from added sugars is not a Tolerable Upper Intake Level (UL) set by the Institute of Medicine (IOM). For most calorie levels, there are not enough calories available after meeting food group needs to consume 10 percent of calories from added sugars and 10 percent of calories from saturated fats and still stay within calorie limits.

[3] The recommendation to limit intake of calories from saturated fats to less than 10 percent per day is a target based on evidence that replacing saturated fats with unsaturated fats is associated with reduced risk of cardiovascular disease. The limit on calories from saturated fats is not a UL set by the IOM. For most calorie levels, there are not enough calories available after meeting food group needs to consume 10 percent of calories from added sugars and 10 percent of calories from saturated fats and still stay within calorie limits.

[4] The recommendation to limit intake of sodium to less than 2,300 mg per day is the UL for individuals ages 14 years and older set by the IOM. The recommendations for children younger than 14 years of age are the IOM age- and sex-appropriate ULs (See Appendix 7. Nutritional Goals for Age-Sex Groups Based on Dietary Reference Intakes and Dietary Guidelines Recommendations (/dietaryguidelines/2015/guidelines/appendix-7/)).

[5] It is not recommended that individuals begin drinking or drink more for any reason. The amount of alcohol and calories in beverages varies and should be accounted for within the limits of healthy eating patterns. Alcohol should be consumed only by adults of legal drinking age. There are many circumstances in which individuals should not drink, such as during pregnancy. See Appendix 9. Alcohol (/dietaryguidelines/2015/guidelines/appendix-9/) for additional information.

[6] U.S. Department of Health and Human Services. *2008 Physical Activity Guidelines for Americans*. Washington (DC): U.S. Department of Health and Human Services; 2008. ODPHP Publication No. U0036. Available at: http://www.health.gov/paguidelines (http://www.health.gov/paguidelines). Accessed August 6, 2015.

2015-2020 Dietary Guidelines

Introduction

Nutrition and Health Are Closely Related

Over the past century, essential nutrient deficiencies have dramatically decreased, many infectious diseases have been conquered, and the majority of the U.S. population can now anticipate a long and productive life. However, as infectious disease rates have dropped, the rates of noncommunicable diseases—specifically, chronic diet-related diseases—have risen, due in part to changes in lifestyle behaviors. A history of poor eating and physical activity patterns have a cumulative effect and have contributed to significant nutrition- and physical activity-related health challenges that now face the U.S. population. About half of all American adults—117 million individuals—have one or more preventable chronic diseases, many of which are related to poor quality eating patterns and physical inactivity. These include cardiovascular disease, high blood pressure, type 2 diabetes, some cancers, and poor bone health. More than two-thirds of adults and nearly one-third of children and youth are overweight or obese. These high rates of overweight and obesity and chronic disease have persisted for more than two decades and come not only with increased health risks, but also at high cost. In 2008, the medical costs associated with obesity were estimated to be $147 billion. In 2012, the total estimated cost of diagnosed diabetes was $245 billion, including $176 billion in direct medical costs and $69 billion in decreased productivity.[1]

Table I-1 describes the high rates of nutrition- and physical activity-related chronic diseases and their related risk factors. These diseases affect all ages—children, adolescents, adults, and older adults—though rates vary by several factors, including race/ethnicity, income status, and body weight status.

Table I-1.

Facts About Nutrition- and Physical Activity-Related Health Conditions in the United States

Health Condition	Facts
Overweight and Obesity	• For more than 25 years, more than half of the adult population has been overweight or obese. • Obesity is most prevalent in those ages 40 years and older and in African American adults, and is least prevalent in adults with highest incomes. • Since the early 2000s, abdominal obesity[a] has been present in about half of U.S. adults of all ages. Prevalence is higher with increasing age and varies by sex and race/ethnicity. • In 2009-2012, 65% of adult females and 73% of adult males were overweight or obese. • In 2009-2012, nearly one in three youth ages 2 to 19 years were overweight or obese.

Cardiovascular Disease (CVD) and Risk Factors:

- Coronary heart disease

- Stroke

- Hypertension

- High total blood cholesterol

- In 2010, CVD affected about 84 million men and women ages 20 years and older (35% of the population).

- In 2007-2010, about 50% of adults who were normal weight, and nearly three-fourths of those who were overweight or obese, had at least one cardiometabolic risk factor (i.e., high blood pressure, abnormal blood lipids, smoking, or diabetes).

- Rates of hypertension, abnormal blood lipid profiles, and diabetes are higher in adults with abdominal obesity.

- In 2009-2012, almost 56% of adults ages 18 years and older had either prehypertension (27%) or hypertension (29%).[b]

- In 2009-2012, rates of hypertension among adults were highest in African Americans (41%) and in adults ages 65 years and older (69%).

- In 2009-2012, 10% of children ages 8 to 17 years had either borderline hypertension (8%) or hypertension (2%).[c]

- In 2009-2012, 100 million adults ages 20 years or older (53%) had total cholesterol levels ≥200 mg/dL; almost 31 million had levels ≥240 mg/dL.

- In 2011-2012, 8% of children ages 8 to 17 years had total cholesterol levels ≥200 mg/dL.

Diabetes

- In 2012, the prevalence of diabetes (type 1 plus type 2) was 14% for men and 11% for women ages 20 years and older (more than 90% of total diabetes in adults is type 2).

- Among children with type 2 diabetes, about 80% were obese.

| **Cancer[d]**

• Breast cancer

• Colorectal cancer | • Breast cancer is the third leading cause of cancer death in the United States.

• In 2012, an estimated 3 million women had a history of breast cancer.

• Colorectal cancer is the second leading cause of cancer death in the United States.

• In 2012, an estimated 1.2 million adult men and women had a history of colorectal cancer. |
| **Bone Health** | • A higher percent of women are affected by osteoporosis (15%) and low bone mass (51%) than men (about 4% and 35%, respectively).

• In 2005-2010, approximately 10 million (10%) adults ages 50 years and older had osteoporosis and 43 million (44%) had low bone mass. |

[a] Abdominal obesity, as measured by waist circumference, is defined as a waist circumference of >102 centimeters in men and >88 centimeters in women.

[b] For adults, prehypertension was defined as a systolic blood pressure of 120-139 mm mercury (Hg) or diastolic blood pressure of 80-89 mm Hg among those who were not currently being treated for hypertension. Hypertension was defined as systolic blood pressure (SBP) >140 mm Hg, diastolic blood pressure (DBP) >90 mm Hg, or taking antihypertensive medication.

[c] For children, borderline hypertension was defined as systolic or diastolic blood pressure at the 90th percentile or higher but lower than the 95th percentile or as blood pressure levels of 120/80 mm Hg or higher (but less than the 95th percentile). Hypertension was defined as a systolic or diastolic blood pressure at the 95th percentile or higher.

[d] The types of cancer included here are not a complete list of all diet- and physical activity-related cancers.

Concurrent with these diet-related health problems persisting at high levels, trends in food intake over time show that, at the population level, Americans are not consuming healthy eating patterns. For example, the prevalence of overweight and obesity has risen and remained high for the past 25 years, while Healthy Eating Index (HEI) scores, a measure of how food choices align with the *Dietary Guidelines*, have remained low (Figure I-1). Similarly, physical activity levels have remained low over time (Figure I-2). The continued high rates of overweight and obesity and low levels of progress toward meeting *Dietary Guidelines* recommendations highlight the need to improve dietary and physical activity education and behaviors across the U.S. population. Progress in reversing these trends will require comprehensive and coordinated strategies, built on the *Dietary Guidelines* as the scientific foundation, that can be maintained over time. The *Dietary Guidelines* is an important part of a complex and multifaceted solution to promoting health and helping to reduce the risk of chronic disease.

Figure I-1.

Adherence of the U.S. Population Ages 2 Years and Older to the *2010 Dietary Guidelines*, as Measured by Average Total Healthy Eating Index-2010 (HEI-2010) Scores

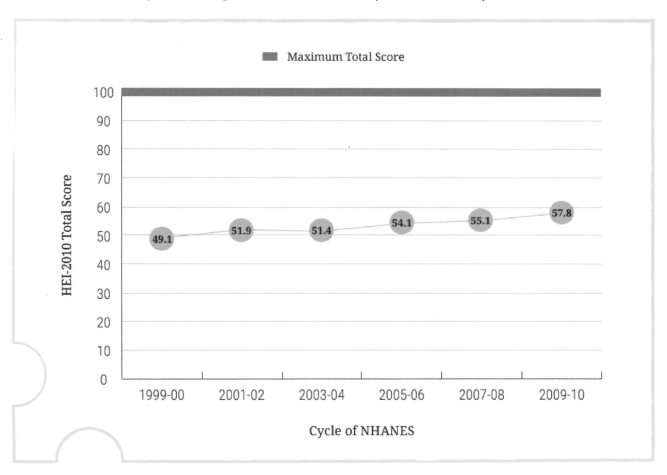

Read text description of Figure I-1

DATA SOURCE:
Analyses of What We Eat in America, National Health and Nutrition Examination Survey (NHANES) data from 1999-2000 through 2009-2010.

NOTE:
HEI-2010 total scores are out of 100 possible points. A score of 100 indicates that recommendations on average were met or exceeded. A higher total score indicates a higher quality diet.

Figure I-2.

Percentage of Adults Meeting the *Physical Activity Guidelines* (Aerobic and Muscle-Strengthening Recommendations)

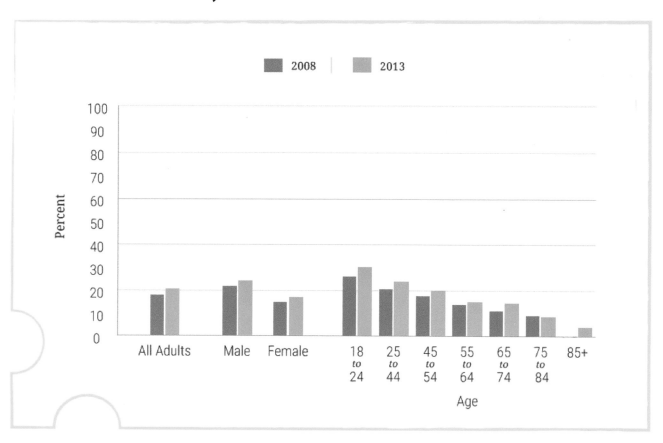

Read text description of Figure I-2

DATA SOURCE:

Analyses of the National Health Interview Survey, 2008 and 2013.

Healthy People 2020 PA-2.4. Increase the proportion of adults who meet the objectives for aerobic physical activity and for muscle-strengthening activity. Washington, DC: U.S. Department of Health and Human Services, Office of Disease Prevention and Health Promotion, June 3, 2015. Available at: http://www.healthypeople.gov/2020/data-search/Search-the-Data?nid=5072 (http://www.healthypeople.gov/2020/data-search/Search-the-Data?nid=5072).

The Importance of Physical Activity in a Healthy Lifestyle

Although the primary focus of the *Dietary Guidelines* is on nutrition recommendations, physical activity is mentioned throughout this edition because of its critical and complementary role in promoting good health and preventing disease, including many diet-related chronic diseases. The following chapters note the role of physical activity in improving health and reducing chronic disease risk; describe the gap between current physical activity recommendations and reported levels of activity; and discuss how the settings in which people live, learn, work, and play can be enhanced to encourage increased physical activity. For more information, see the *Physical Activity Guidelines for Americans* at www.health.gov/paguidelines (http://www.health.gov/paguidelines).

Notes

[1] For more information, see: Centers for Disease Control and Prevention (CDC). Chronic Disease Overview. August 26, 2015. Available at http://www.cdc.gov/chronicdisease/overview/ (http://www.cdc.gov/chronicdisease/overview/). Accessed November 3, 2015.

2015-2020 Dietary Guidelines

CHAPTER 1
Key Elements of Healthy Eating Patterns

A Closer Look Inside Healthy Eating Patterns

In this section:

1. **Food Groups**

2. **Other Dietary Components**

The following sections describe a healthy eating pattern and how following such a pattern can help people meet the Guidelines and its Key Recommendations. Throughout, it uses the Healthy U.S.-Style Eating Pattern as an example to illustrate the specific amounts and limits for food groups and other dietary components that make up healthy eating patterns. The Healthy U.S.-Style Eating Pattern is one of three USDA Food Patterns and is based on the types and proportions of foods Americans typically consume, but in nutrient-dense forms and appropriate amounts. Because calorie needs vary based on age, sex, height, weight, and level of physical activity (see Appendix 2. Estimated Calorie Needs per Day, by Age, Sex, and Physical Activity Level (/dietaryguidelines/2015/guidelines/appendix-2/)), the pattern has been provided at 12 different calorie levels (see Appendix 3. USDA Food Patterns: Healthy U.S.-Style Eating Pattern (/dietaryguidelines/2015/guidelines/appendix-3/)). The 2,000-calorie level of the Pattern is shown in Table 1-1.

The Healthy U.S.-Style Eating Pattern is the same as the primary USDA Food Patterns of the *2010 Dietary Guidelines*. Two additional USDA Food Patterns—the Healthy Mediterranean-Style Eating Pattern and the Healthy Vegetarian Eating Pattern—are found at the end of this chapter and reflect other styles of eating (see Appendix 4. USDA Food Patterns: Healthy Mediterranean-Style Eating Pattern (/dietaryguidelines/2015/guidelines/appendix-4/) and Appendix 5. USDA Food Patterns: Healthy Vegetarian Eating Pattern (/dietaryguidelines/2015/guidelines/appendix-5/)). These three patterns are examples of healthy eating patterns that can be adapted based on cultural and personal preferences. The

USDA Food Patterns also can be used as guides to plan and serve meals not only for the individual and household but in a variety of other settings, including schools, worksites, and other community settings.

Table 1-1.

Healthy U.S.-Style Eating Pattern at the 2,000-Calorie Level, With Daily or Weekly Amounts From Food Groups, Subgroups, and Components

Food Group[a]	Amount[b] in the 2,000-Calorie-Level Pattern
Vegetables	2½ c-eq/day
Dark green	1½ c-eq/wk
Red and orange	5½ c-eq/wk
Legumes (beans and peas)	1½ c-eq/wk
Starchy	5 c-eq/wk
Other	4 c-eq/wk
Fruits	2 c-eq/day
Grains	6 oz-eq/day
Whole grains	≥ 3 oz-eq/day
Refined grains	≤ 3 oz-eq/day
Dairy	3 c-eq/day
Protein Foods	5½ oz-eq/day
Seafood	8 oz-eq/wk

Meats, poultry, eggs	26 oz-eq/wk
Nuts, seeds, soy products	5 oz-eq/wk
Oils	27 g/day
Limit on Calories for Other Uses (% of calories)[c]	270 kcal/day (14%)

[a] Definitions for each food group and subgroup are provided throughout the chapter and are compiled in Appendix 3. (/dietaryguidelines/2015/guidelines/appendix-3/)

[b] Food group amounts shown in cup-(c) or ounce-(oz) equivalents (eq). Oils are shown in grams (g). Quantity equivalents for each food group are defined in Appendix 3. (/dietaryguidelines/2015/guidelines/appendix-3/) Amounts will vary for those who need less than 2,000 or more than 2,000 calories per day. See Appendix 3 (/dietaryguidelines/2015/guidelines/appendix-3/) for all 12 calorie levels of the pattern.

[c] Assumes food choices to meet food group recommendations are in nutrient-dense forms. Calories from added sugars, added refined starches, solid fats, alcohol, and/or to eat more than the recommended amount of nutrient-dense foods are accounted for under this category.

Note: The total eating pattern should not exceed *Dietary Guidelines* limits for intake of calories from added sugars and saturated fats and alcohol and should be within the Acceptable Macronutrient Distribution Ranges for calories from protein, carbohydrate, and total fats. Most calorie patterns do not have enough calories available after meeting food group needs to consume 10 percent of calories from added sugars *and* 10 percent of calories from saturated fats and still stay within calorie limits. Values are rounded.

The Healthy U.S.-Style Eating Pattern is designed to meet the Recommended Dietary Allowances (RDA) and Adequate Intakes for essential nutrients, as well as Acceptable Macronutrient Distribution Ranges (AMDR) set by the Food and Nutrition Board of the IOM. This eating pattern also conforms to limits set by the IOM or *Dietary Guidelines* for other nutrients or food components (see Appendix 6. Glossary of Terms (/dietaryguidelines/2015/guidelines/appendix-6/) and Appendix 7. Nutritional Goals for Age-Sex Groups Based on Dietary Reference Intakes and Dietary Guidelines Recommendations (/dietaryguidelines/2015/guidelines/appendix-7/)). Nutritional goals for almost all nutrients are met (see Appendix 3 (/dietaryguidelines/2015/guidelines/appendix-3/) for additional information).

Figure 1-1.

Cup- and Ounce-Equivalents

Within a food group, foods can come in many forms and are not created equal in terms of what counts as a cup or an ounce. Some foods are more concentrated, and some are more airy or contain more water. Cup- and ounce-equivalents identify the amounts of foods from each food group with similar nutritional content. In addition, portion sizes do not always align with one cup-equivalent or one ounce-equivalent. See examples below for variability.

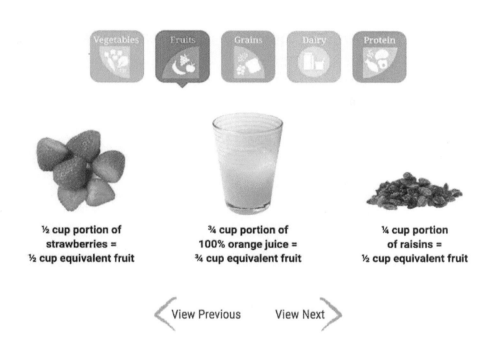

½ cup portion of
strawberries =
½ cup equivalent fruit

¾ cup portion of
100% orange juice =
¾ cup equivalent fruit

¼ cup portion
of raisins =
½ cup equivalent fruit

⟨ View Previous   View Next ⟩

Importance of Calorie Balance Within Healthy Eating Patterns

Managing calorie intake is fundamental to achieving and maintaining calorie balance—the balance between the calories taken in from foods and the calories expended from metabolic processes and physical activity. The best way to determine whether an eating pattern is at an appropriate number of calories is to monitor body weight and adjust calorie intake and expenditure in physical activity based on changes in weight over time.

All foods and many beverages contain calories, and the total number of calories varies depending on the macronutrients in a food. On average, carbohydrates and protein contain 4 calories per gram, fats contain 9 calories per gram, and alcohol has 7 calories per gram. The total number of calories a person needs each day varies depending on a number of factors, including the person's age, sex, height, weight, and level of physical activity (see Appendix 2 (/dietaryguidelines/2015/guidelines/appendix-2/)). In addition, a need to lose, maintain, or gain weight and other factors affect how many calories should be consumed.

All Americans—children, adolescents, adults, and older adults—are encouraged to achieve and/or maintain a healthy body weight. General guidance for achieving and maintaining a healthy body weight is provided below, and Appendix 8. Federal Resources for Information on Nutrition and Physical Activity (/dietaryguidelines/2015/guidelines/appendix-8/) provides additional resources, including an evolving array of tools to facilitate Americans' adoption of healthy choices.

- Children and adolescents are encouraged to maintain calorie balance to support normal growth and development without promoting excess weight gain. Children and adolescents who are overweight or obese should change their eating and physical activity behaviors to maintain or reduce their rate of weight gain while linear growth occurs, so that they can reduce body mass index (BMI) percentile toward a healthy range.

- Before becoming pregnant, women are encouraged to achieve and maintain a healthy weight, and women who are pregnant are encouraged to gain weight within gestational weight gain guidelines.[8]

- Adults who are obese should change their eating and physical activity behaviors to prevent additional weight gain and/or promote weight loss. Adults who are overweight should not gain additional weight, and those with one or more CVD risk factors (e.g., hypertension and hyperlipidemia) should change their eating and physical activity behaviors to lose weight. To lose weight, most people need to reduce the number of calories they get from foods and beverages and increase their physical activity. For a weight loss of 1 to 1½ pounds per week, daily intake should be reduced by 500 to 750 calories. Eating patterns that contain 1,200 to 1,500 calories each day can help most women lose weight safely, and eating patterns that contain 1,500 to 1,800 calories each day are suitable for most men for weight loss. In adults who are overweight or obese, if reduction in total calorie intake is achieved, a variety of eating patterns can produce weight loss, particularly in the first 6 months to 2 years;[9] however, more research is needed on the health implications of consuming these eating patterns long-term.

- Older adults, ages 65 years and older, who are overweight or obese are encouraged to prevent additional weight gain. Among older adults who are obese, particularly those with CVD risk factors, intentional weight loss can be beneficial and result in improved quality of life and reduced risk of chronic diseases and associated disabilities.

Food Groups

Eating an appropriate mix of foods from the food groups and subgroups—within an appropriate calorie level—is important to promote health. Each of the food groups and their subgroups provides an array of nutrients, and the amounts recommended reflect eating patterns that have been associated with positive health outcomes. Foods from all of the food groups should be eaten in nutrient-dense forms. The following sections describe the recommendations for each of the food groups, highlight nutrients for which the food group is a key contributor, and describe special considerations related to the food group.

Vegetables

Healthy intake: Healthy eating patterns include a variety of vegetables from all of the five vegetable subgroups—dark green, red and orange, legumes (beans and peas), starchy, and other.[10] These include all fresh, frozen, canned, and dried options in cooked or raw forms, including vegetable juices. The recommended amount of vegetables in the Healthy U.S.-Style Eating Pattern at the 2,000-calorie level is 2½ cup-equivalents of vegetables per day. In addition, weekly amounts from each vegetable subgroup are recommended to ensure variety and meet nutrient needs.

Key nutrient contributions: Vegetables are important sources of many nutrients, including dietary fiber, potassium, vitamin A,[11] vitamin C, vitamin K, copper, magnesium, vitamin E, vitamin B_6, folate, iron, manganese, thiamin, niacin, and choline. Each of the vegetable subgroups contributes different combinations of nutrients, making it important for individuals to consume vegetables from all the subgroups. For example, dark-green vegetables provide the most vitamin K, red and orange vegetables the most vitamin A, legumes the most dietary fiber, and starchy vegetables the most potassium. Vegetables in the "other" vegetable subgroup provide a wide range of nutrients in varying amounts.

Considerations: To provide all of the nutrients and potential health benefits that vary across different types of vegetables, the Healthy U.S.-Style Eating Pattern includes weekly recommendations for each subgroup. Vegetable choices over time should vary and include many different vegetables. Vegetables should be consumed in a nutrient-dense form, with limited additions such as salt, butter, or creamy sauces. When selecting frozen or canned vegetables, choose those lower in sodium.

About Legumes (Beans and Peas)

Legumes include kidney beans, pinto beans, white beans, black beans, garbanzo beans (chickpeas), lima beans (mature, dried), split peas, lentils, and edamame (green soybeans).

Legumes are excellent sources of protein. In addition, they provide other nutrients that also are found in seafood, meats, and poultry, such as iron and zinc. They are excellent sources of dietary fiber and of nutrients, such as potassium and folate that also are found in other vegetables.

Because legumes have a similar nutrient profile to foods in both the protein foods group and the vegetable group, they may be thought of as either a vegetable or a protein food and thus, can be counted as a vegetable or a protein food to meet recommended intakes.

Green peas and green (string) beans are not counted in the legume subgroup, because their nutrient compositions are not similar to legumes. Green peas are similar to starchy vegetables and are grouped with them. Green beans are grouped with the other vegetables subgroup, which includes onions, iceberg lettuce, celery, and cabbage, because their nutrient content is not similar to legumes.

Fruits

Healthy intake: Healthy eating patterns include fruits, especially whole fruits. The fruits food group includes whole fruits and 100% fruit juice. Whole fruits include fresh, canned, frozen, and dried forms. The recommended amount of fruits in the Healthy U.S.-Style Eating Pattern at the 2,000-calorie level is 2 cup-equivalents per day. One cup of 100% fruit juice counts as 1 cup of fruit. Although fruit juice can be part of healthy eating patterns, it is lower than whole fruit in dietary fiber and when consumed in excess can contribute extra calories. Therefore, at least half of the recommended amount of fruits should come from whole fruits. When juices are consumed, they should be 100% juice, without added sugars. Also, when selecting canned fruit, choose options that are lowest in added sugars. One-half cup of dried fruit counts as one cup-equivalent of fruit. Similar to juice, when consumed in excess, dried fruits can contribute extra calories.

Key nutrient contributions: Among the many nutrients fruits provide are dietary fiber, potassium, and vitamin C.

Considerations: Juices may be partially fruit juice, and only the proportion that is 100% fruit juice counts (e.g., 1 cup of juice that is 50% juice counts as ½ cup of fruit juice). The remainder of the product may contain added sugars. Sweetened juice products with minimal juice content, such as juice drinks, are considered to be sugar-sweetened beverages rather than fruit juice because they are primarily composed of water with added sugars (see the Added Sugars section below). The percent of juice in a beverage may be found on the package label, such as "contains 25% juice" or "100% fruit juice." The amounts of fruit juice allowed in the USDA Food Patterns for young children align with the recommendation from the American Academy of Pediatrics that young children consume no more than 4 to 6 fluid ounces of 100% fruit juice per day.[12] Fruits with small amounts of added sugars can be accommodated in the diet as long as calories from added sugars do not exceed 10 percent per day and total calorie intake remains within limits.

Grains

Healthy Intake: Healthy eating patterns include whole grains and limit the intake of refined grains and products made with refined grains, especially those high in saturated fats, added sugars, and/or sodium, such as cookies, cakes, and some snack foods. The grains food group includes grains as single foods (e.g., rice, oatmeal, and popcorn), as well as products that include grains as an ingredient (e.g., breads, cereals, crackers, and pasta). Grains are either whole or refined. Whole grains (e.g., brown rice, quinoa, and oats) contain the entire kernel, including the endosperm, bran, and germ. Refined grains differ from whole grains in that the grains have been processed to remove the bran and germ, which removes dietary fiber, iron, and other nutrients. The recommended amount of grains in the Healthy U.S.-Style Eating Pattern at the 2,000-calorie level is 6 ounce-equivalents per day. At least half of this amount should be whole grains (see the How To Make at Least Half of Grains Whole Grains call-out box).

Key nutrient contributions: Whole grains are a source of nutrients, such as dietary fiber, iron, zinc, manganese, folate, magnesium, copper, thiamin, niacin, vitamin B_6, phosphorus, selenium, riboflavin, and vitamin A.[13] Whole grains vary in their dietary fiber content. Most refined grains are enriched, a process that adds back iron and four B vitamins (thiamin, riboflavin, niacin, and folic acid). Because of this process, the term "enriched grains" is often used to describe these refined grains.

Considerations: Individuals who eat refined grains should choose enriched grains. Those who consume all of their grains as whole grains should include some grains, such as some whole-grain ready-to-eat breakfast cereals, that have been fortified with folic acid. This is particularly important for women who are or are capable of becoming pregnant, as folic acid fortification in the United States has been successful in reducing the incidence of neural tube defects during fetal development. Although grain products that are high in added sugars and saturated fats, such as cookies, cakes, and some snack foods, should be limited, as discussed in the Added Sugars and Saturated Fats sections below, grains with some added sugars and saturated fats can fit within healthy eating patterns.

How To Make at Least Half of Grains Whole Grains

A food is a 100-percent whole-grain food if the only grains it contains are whole grains. One ounce-equivalent of whole grains has 16 g of whole grains. The recommendation to consume at least half of total grains as whole grains can be met in a number of ways.

The most direct way to meet the whole grain recommendation is to choose 100 percent whole-grain foods for at least half of all grains consumed. The relative amount of whole grain in the food can be inferred by the placement of the grain in the ingredients list. The whole grain should be the first ingredient—or the second ingredient, after water. For foods with multiple whole-grain ingredients, they should appear near the beginning of the ingredients list.

Many grain foods contain both whole grains and refined grains. These foods also can help people meet the whole grain recommendation, especially if a considerable proportion of the grain ingredients is whole grains. Another way to meet the recommendation to make at least half of grains whole grains is to choose products with at least 50 percent of the total weight as whole-grain ingredients.[14][15] If a food has at least 8 g of whole grains per ounce-equivalent, it is at least half whole grains.[16] Some product labels show the whole grains health claim or the grams of whole grain in the product. This information may help people identify food choices that have a substantial amount of whole grains.

Dairy

Healthy intake: Healthy eating patterns include fat-free and low-fat (1%) dairy, including milk, yogurt, cheese, or fortified soy beverages (commonly known as "soymilk"). Soy beverages fortified with calcium, vitamin A, and vitamin D, are included as part of the dairy group because they are similar to milk based on nutrient composition and in their use in meals. Other products sold as "milks" but made from plants (e.g., almond, rice, coconut, and hemp "milks") may contain calcium and be consumed as a source of calcium, but they are not included as part of the dairy group because their overall nutritional content is not similar to dairy milk and fortified soy beverages (soymilk). The recommended amounts of dairy in the Healthy U.S.-Style Pattern are based on age rather than calorie level and are 2 cup-equivalents per day for children ages 2 to 3 years, 2½ cup-equivalents per day for children ages 4 to 8 years, and 3 cup-equivalents per day for adolescents ages 9 to 18 years and for adults.

Key nutrient contributions: The dairy group contributes many nutrients, including calcium, phosphorus, vitamin A, vitamin D (in products fortified with vitamin D), riboflavin, vitamin B_{12}, protein, potassium, zinc, choline, magnesium, and selenium.

Considerations: Fat-free and low-fat (1%) dairy products provide the same nutrients but less fat (and thus, fewer calories) than higher fat options, such as 2% and whole milk and regular cheese. Fat-free or low-fat milk and yogurt, in comparison to cheese, contain less saturated fats and sodium and more potassium, vitamin A, and vitamin D. Thus, increasing the proportion of dairy intake that is fat-free or low-fat milk or yogurt and decreasing the proportion that is cheese would decrease saturated fats and sodium and increase potassium, vitamin A, and vitamin D provided from the dairy group. Individuals who are lactose intolerant can choose low-lactose and lactose-free dairy products. Those who are unable or choose not to consume dairy products should consume foods that provide the range of nutrients generally obtained from dairy, including protein, calcium, potassium, magnesium, vitamin D, and vitamin A (e.g., fortified soy beverages [soymilk]). Additional sources of potassium, calcium, and vitamin D are found in Appendix 10 (/dietaryguidelines/2015/guidelines/appendix-10/), Appendix 11 (/dietaryguidelines/2015/guidelines/appendix-11/), and Appendix 12 (/dietaryguidelines/2015/guidelines/appendix-12/), respectively.

Protein Foods

Healthy intake: Healthy eating patterns include a variety of protein foods in nutrient-dense forms. The protein foods group comprises a broad group of foods from both animal and plant sources and includes several subgroups: seafood; meats, poultry, and eggs; and nuts, seeds, and soy products. Legumes (beans and peas) may also be considered part of the protein foods group as well as the vegetables group (see the About Legumes (Beans and Peas) call-out box). Protein also is found in some foods from other food groups (e.g., dairy). The recommendation for protein foods in the Healthy U.S.-Style Eating Pattern at the 2,000-calorie level is 5½ ounce-equivalents of protein foods per day.

Key nutrient contributions: Protein foods are important sources of nutrients in addition to protein, including B vitamins (e.g., niacin, vitamin B_{12}, vitamin B_6, and riboflavin), selenium, choline, phosphorus, zinc, copper, vitamin D, and vitamin E). Nutrients provided by various types of protein foods differ. For example, meats provide the most zinc, while poultry provides the most niacin. Meats, poultry, and seafood provide heme iron, which is more bioavailable than the non-heme iron found in plant sources. Heme iron is especially important for young children and women who are capable of becoming pregnant or who are pregnant. Seafood provides the most vitamin B_{12} and vitamin D, in addition to almost all of the polyunsaturated omega-3 fatty acids, eicosapentaenoic acid (EPA), and docosahexaenoic acid (DHA), in the Patterns (see the About Seafood call-out box). Eggs provide the most choline, and nuts and seeds provide the most vitamin E. Soy products are a source of copper, manganese, and iron, as are legumes.

Considerations: For balance and flexibility within the food group, the Healthy U.S.-Style Eating Pattern includes weekly recommendations for the subgroups: seafood; meats, poultry, and eggs; and nuts, seeds, and soy products. A specific recommendation for at least 8 ounce-equivalents of seafood per week also is included for the 2,000-calorie level (see the About Seafood call-out box). One-half ounce of nuts or seeds counts as 1 ounce-equivalent of protein foods, and because they are high in calories, they should be eaten in small portions and used to replace other protein foods rather than being added to the diet. When selecting protein foods, nuts and seeds should be unsalted, and meats and poultry should be consumed in lean forms. Processed meats and processed poultry are sources of sodium and saturated fats, and intake of these products can be accommodated as long as sodium, saturated fats, added sugars, and total calories are within limits in the resulting eating pattern (see the About Meats and Poultry call-out box). The inclusion of protein foods from plants allows vegetarian options to be accommodated.

About Seafood

Seafood, which includes fish and shellfish, received particular attention in the *2010 Dietary Guidelines* because of evidence of health benefits for the general populations as well as for women who are pregnant or breastfeeding. For the general population, consumption of about 8 ounces per week of a variety of seafood, which provide an average consumption of 250 mg per day of EPA and DHA, is associated with reduced cardiac deaths among individuals with and without preexisting CVD. Similarly, consumption by women who are pregnant or breastfeeding of at least 8 ounces per week from seafood choices that are sources of DHA is associated with improved infant health outcomes.

The recommendation to consume 8 or more ounces per week (less for young children) of seafood is for the total package of nutrients that seafood provides, including its EPA and DHA content. Some seafood choices with higher amounts of EPA and DHA should be included.

Strong evidence from mostly prospective cohort studies but also randomized controlled trials has shown that eating patterns that include seafood are associated with reduced risk of CVD, and moderate evidence indicates that these eating patterns are associated with reduced risk of obesity. As described earlier, eating patterns consist of multiple, interacting food components and the relationships to health exist for the overall eating pattern, not necessarily to an isolated aspect of the diet.

Mercury is a heavy metal found in the form of methyl mercury in seafood in varying levels. Seafood choices higher in EPA and DHA but lower in methyl mercury are encouraged.[17] Seafood varieties commonly consumed in the United States that are higher in EPA and DHA and lower in methyl mercury include salmon, anchovies, herring, shad, sardines, Pacific oysters, trout, and Atlantic and Pacific mackerel (*not* king mackerel, which is high in methyl mercury). Individuals who regularly consume more than the recommended amounts of seafood that are in the Healthy U.S-Style Pattern should choose a mix of seafood that emphasizes choices relatively low in methyl mercury.

Some canned seafood, such as anchovies, may be high in sodium. To keep sodium intake below recommended limits, individuals can use the Nutrition Facts label to compare sodium amounts.

Women who are pregnant or breastfeeding should consume at least 8 and up to 12 ounces[18] of a variety of seafood per week, from choices that are lower in methyl mercury. Obstetricians and pediatricians should provide guidance on how to make healthy food choices that include seafood. Women who are pregnant or breastfeeding and young children should not eat certain types of fish that are high in methyl mercury.[19]

About Meats and Poultry

Meat, also known as red meat, includes all forms of beef, pork, lamb, veal, goat, and non-bird game (e.g., venison, bison, and elk). Poultry includes all forms of chicken, turkey, duck, geese, guineas, and game birds (e.g., quail and pheasant). Meats and poultry vary in fat content and include both fresh and processed forms. Lean meats and poultry contain less than 10 g of fat, 4.5 g or less of saturated fats, and less than 95 mg of cholesterol per 100 g and per labeled serving size (e.g., 95% lean ground beef, pork tenderloin, and skinless chicken or turkey breast). Processed meats and processed poultry (e.g., sausages, luncheon meats, bacon, and beef jerky) are products preserved by smoking, curing, salting, and/or the addition of chemical preservatives.

Strong evidence from mostly prospective cohort studies but also randomized controlled trials has shown that *eating patterns* that include lower intake of meats as well as processed meats and processed poultry are associated with reduced risk of CVD in adults. Moderate evidence indicates that these *eating patterns* are associated with reduced risk of obesity, type 2 diabetes, and some types of cancer in adults. As described earlier, eating patterns consist of multiple, interacting food components, and the relationships to health exist for the overall eating pattern, not necessarily to an isolated aspect of the diet. Much of this research on eating patterns has grouped together all meats and poultry, regardless of fat content or processing, though some evidence has identified lean meats and lean poultry in healthy eating patterns. In separate analyses, food pattern modeling has demonstrated that lean meats and lean poultry can contribute important nutrients within limits for sodium, calories from saturated fats and added sugars, and total calories when consumed in recommended amounts in healthy eating patterns, such as the Healthy U.S.-Style and Mediterranean-Style Eating Patterns.

The recommendation for the meats, poultry, and eggs subgroup in the Healthy U.S.-Style Eating Pattern at the 2,000-calorie level is 26 ounce-equivalents per week. This is the same as the amount that was in the primary USDA Food Patterns of the *2010 Dietary Guidelines*. As discussed in Chapter 2 (/dietaryguidelines/2015/guidelines/chapter-2/), average intakes of meats, poultry, and eggs for teen boys and adult men are above recommendations in the Healthy U.S.-Style Eating Pattern. For those who eat animal products, the recommendation for the protein foods subgroup of meats, poultry, and eggs can be met by consuming a variety of lean meats, lean poultry, and eggs. Choices within these eating patterns may include processed meats and processed poultry as long as the resulting eating pattern is within limits for sodium, calories from saturated fats and added sugars, and total calories.

Oils

Healthy intake: Oils are fats that contain a high percentage of monounsaturated and polyunsaturated fats and are liquid at room temperature. Although they are not a food group, oils are emphasized as part of healthy eating patterns because they are the major source of essential fatty acids and vitamin E. Commonly consumed oils extracted from plants include canola, corn, olive, peanut, safflower, soybean, and sunflower oils. Oils also are naturally present in nuts, seeds, seafood, olives, and avocados. The fat in some tropical plants, such as coconut oil, palm kernel oil, and palm oil, are not included in the oils category because they do not resemble other oils in their composition. Specifically, they contain a higher percentage of saturated fats than other oils (see Dietary Fats: The Basics call-out box). The recommendation for oils in the Healthy U.S.-Style Eating Pattern at the 2,000-calorie level is 27 g (about 5 teaspoons) per day.

Key nutrient contributions: Oils provide essential fatty acids and vitamin E.

Considerations: Oils are part of healthy eating patterns, but because they are a concentrated source of calories, the amount consumed should be within the AMDR for total fats without exceeding calorie limits. Oils should replace solid fats rather than being added to the diet. More information on types of fats is provided in the Dietary Fats: The Basics call-out box, and information on the relationship between dietary fats and health is discussed in the **Saturated Fats, *Trans* Fats, and Cholesterol** section, below.

Dietary Fats: The Basics

Dietary fats are found in both plant and animal foods. They supply calories and help with the absorption of the fat-soluble vitamins A, D, E, and K. Some also are good sources of two essential fatty acids—linoleic acid and α-linolenic acid.

All dietary fats are composed of a mix of polyunsaturated, monounsaturated, and saturated fatty acids, in varied proportions (Figure 1-2). For example, most of the fatty acids in butter are saturated, but it also contains some monounsaturated and polyunsaturated fatty acids. Oils are mostly unsaturated fatty acids, though they have small amounts of saturated fatty acids.

Figure 1-2.
Fatty Acid Profiles of Common Fats and Oils

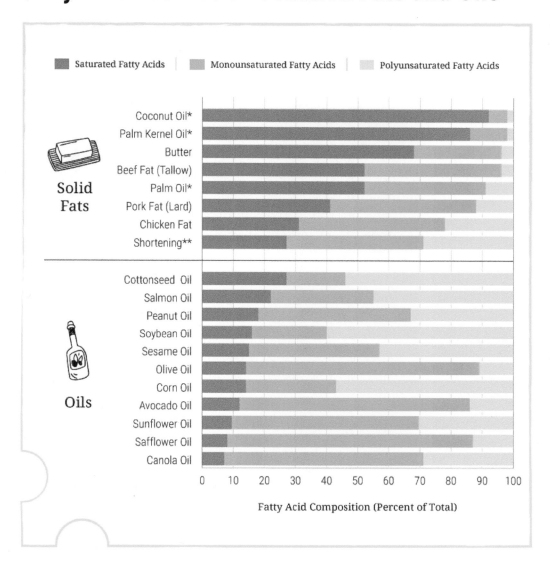

Read text description of Figure 1-2

* Coconut, palm kernel, and palm oil are called oils because they come from plants. However, they are solid or semi-solid at room temperature due to their high content of short-chain saturated fatty acids. They are considered solid fats for nutritional purposes.

** Shortening may be made from partially hydrogenated vegetable oil, which contains *trans* fatty acids.

DATA SOURCE:

U.S. Department of Agriculture, Agricultural Research Service, Nutrition Data Laboratory. USDA National Nutrient Database for Standard Reference. Release 27, 2015. Available at http://ndb.nal.usda.gov/ (http://ndb.nal.usda.gov/). Accessed August 31, 2015.

- **Polyunsaturated fatty acids (polyunsaturated fats[20])** are found in greatest amounts in corn, soybean, and cottonseed oils; walnuts; pine nuts; and sesame, pumpkin, and flax seeds. Only small amounts of polyunsaturated fats are found in most animal fats. Omega-3 (n-3) fatty acids are a type of polyunsaturated fats found in seafood, such as salmon, trout, herring, tuna, and mackerel, and in flax seeds and walnuts. EPA and DHA are long chain n-3 fatty acids found in seafood.

- **Monounsaturated fatty acids (monounsaturated fats)** are found in greatest amounts in olive, canola, peanut, sunflower, and safflower oils, and in avocados, peanut butter, and most nuts. Monounsaturated fats also are part of most animal fats such as fats from chicken, pork, beef, and wild game.

- **Saturated fatty acids (saturated fats)** are found in the greatest amounts in coconut and palm kernel oils, in butter and beef fats, and in palm oil. They also are found in other animal fats, such as pork and chicken fats and in other plant fats, such as nuts.

- ***Trans* fatty acids (*trans* fats)** are unsaturated fats found primarily in partially hydrogenated vegetable oils and foods containing these oils and in ruminant (animal) fats. They are structurally different from the unsaturated fatty acids that occur naturally in plant foods and differ in their health effects.

The proportions of fatty acids in a particular fat determine the physical form of the fat:

- Fats with a higher amount of polyunsaturated and monounsaturated fatty acids are usually liquid at room temperature and are referred to as "oils."

- Fats with a higher amount of saturated fatty acids are usually solid at room temperature and are referred to as "solid fats." Fats containing *trans* fatty acids are also classified as solid fats, although they may or may not be solid at room temperature.

A relevant detail in the complexity of making food-based recommendations that consider nutrients is the difference between the terms "saturated fats" and "solid fats." Although they are closely related terms, saturated fats and solid fats are not synonymous. The term "saturated fats" refers to saturated fatty acids, a nutrient found in foods, while the term "solid fats" describes the physical manifestation of the fats in a food. Some solid fats, such as the strip of fat around a piece of meat, can easily be seen. Other solid fats are not so visible. For example, the solid fats in whole milk are suspended in the fluid milk by the process of homogenization.

Margarines and margarine-like vegetable oil spreads are food products composed of one or more oils or solid fats designed to replace butter, which is high in saturated fats. These products may be sold in sticks, tubs, bottles, or sprays. Margarine and vegetable oil spreads generally contain less saturated fats than butter. However, they vary in their total fat and calorie content and in the fat and oil blends used to make them and, thus, in the proportions of saturated, unsaturated, and *trans* fats they contain. It is important to read the Nutrition Facts label to identify the calorie and saturated and *trans* fats content of the spread and choose foods with no *trans* fats and lower amounts of saturated fats.

The *Dietary Guidelines* provides recommendations on saturated fats as well as on solid fats because its aim is to improve the health of the U.S. population through food-based guidance. It includes recommendations on saturated fats because of the strong relationship of this nutrient to a health outcome (CVD risk). It includes recommendations on solid fats because, as discussed in Chapter 2 (/dietaryguidelines/2015/guidelines/chapter-2/), they are abundant in the diets of the U.S. population, and reducing solid fats when making food choices is an important way to reduce saturated fats and excess calories.

Limits on Calories That Remain After Food Group Needs Are Met in Nutrient-Dense Forms

The USDA Food Patterns are designed to meet food group and nutrient recommendations while staying within calorie needs. To achieve this goal, the Patterns are based on consuming foods in their nutrient-dense forms (i.e., without added sugars and in the leanest and lowest fat forms, see Appendix 6 (/dietaryguidelines/2015/guidelines/appendix-6/)). For nearly all calorie levels, most of the calories in the USDA Food Patterns are needed for nutrient-dense food choices, and only a limited number remain for other uses. These calories are indicated in the USDA Food Patterns as "limits on calories for other uses." For example, after food group needs are met in the Healthy U.S.-Style Eating Pattern from 1,000 to 1,600 calories, only 100 to 170 calories per day remain within the limit for other uses. In the 2,000-calorie pattern, the limit for other uses is 270 calories and in the 2,800-calorie pattern, 400 calories (see Appendix 3 (/dietaryguidelines/2015/guidelines/appendix-3/), Appendix 4 (/dietaryguidelines/2015/guidelines/appendix-4/), and Appendix 5 (/dietaryguidelines/2015/guidelines/appendix-5/)). Calories up to the limit for the specific pattern can be used to eat foods that are not in nutrient-dense forms (e.g., to accommodate calories from added sugars, added refined starches, or solid fats) or to eat more than the recommended amount of nutrient-dense foods. If alcohol is consumed, calories from alcoholic beverages should also be accounted for within this limit to keep total calorie intake at an appropriate level.

As discussed in Chapter 2 (/dietaryguidelines/2015/guidelines/chapter-2/), in contrast to the healthy choices that make up the Patterns, foods from most food groups as they are typically consumed in the United States are not in nutrient-dense forms. In addition, foods and beverages are consumed that are primarily composed of added sugars and/or solid fats, and provide excess calories without contributing to meeting food group recommendations. The excess calories consumed from these sources far exceed the limited number of calories available for choices other than nutrient-dense foods in each food group.

From a public health perspective, it is important to identify the calories that are needed to meet food group needs to help inform guidance on limits from calories from added sugars, solid fats, alcohol[21], or other sources, in order to help individuals move toward healthy eating patterns within calorie limits. The USDA Food Patterns can be used to plan and serve meals for individuals, households, and in a variety of organizational settings (e.g., schools, worksites, and other community settings). The limit on calories for other uses can assist in determining how to plan and select foods that can fit within healthy eating patterns, such as how many calories are available to select foods from a food group that are not in nutrient-dense forms. As discussed in the next portion of the chapter, additional constraints apply related to other dietary components when building healthy eating patterns.

Figure 1-3.

Hidden Components in Eating Patterns

Many of the foods and beverages we eat contain sodium, saturated fats, and added sugars. Making careful choices, as in this example, keeps amounts of these components within their limits while meeting nutrient needs to achieve a healthy eating pattern.

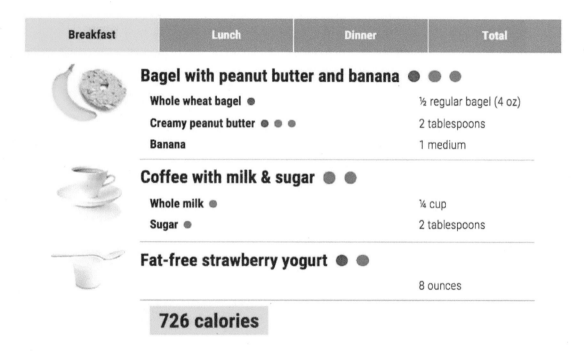

Breakfast	Lunch	Dinner	Total
Bagel with peanut butter and banana ● ● ●			
Whole wheat bagel ●			½ regular bagel (4 oz)
Creamy peanut butter ● ● ●			2 tablespoons
Banana			1 medium
Coffee with milk & sugar ● ●			
Whole milk ●			¼ cup
Sugar ●			2 tablespoons
Fat-free strawberry yogurt ● ●			
			8 ounces

726 calories

Other Dietary Components

In addition to the food groups, it is important to consider other food components when making food and beverage choices. The components discussed below include added sugars, saturated fats, *trans* fats, cholesterol, sodium, alcohol, and caffeine. For each component, information is provided on how the component relates to eating patterns and outlines considerations related to the component. See Chapter 2 (/dietaryguidelines/2015/guidelines/chapter-2/) for a further discussion of each of these components, current intakes, and shifts that are needed to help individuals align with a healthy eating pattern.

Added Sugars

Healthy intake: Added sugars include syrups and other caloric sweeteners. When sugars are added to foods and beverages to sweeten them, they add calories without contributing essential nutrients. Consumption of added sugars can make it difficult for individuals to meet their nutrient needs while staying within calorie limits. Naturally occurring sugars, such as those in fruit or milk, are not added sugars. Specific examples of added sugars that can be listed as an ingredient include brown sugar, corn sweetener, corn syrup, dextrose, fructose, glucose, high-fructose corn syrup, honey, invert sugar, lactose, malt syrup, maltose, molasses, raw sugar, sucrose, trehalose, and turbinado sugar.

Healthy eating patterns limit added sugars to less than 10 percent of calories per day. This recommendation is a target to help the public achieve a healthy eating pattern, which means meeting nutrient and food group needs through nutrient-dense food and beverage choices and staying within calorie limits. When added sugars in foods and beverages exceed 10 percent of calories, a healthy eating pattern may be difficult to achieve. This target also is informed by national data on intakes of calories from added sugars, which as discussed in Chapter 2, (/dietaryguidelines/2015/guidelines/chapter-2/) account on average for almost 270 calories, or more than 13 percent of calories per day in the U.S. population.

The USDA Food Patterns show that an eating pattern with enough foods from all food groups to meet nutrient needs without eating too many calories has only limited room for calories from added sugars. At most lower calorie levels (i.e., 1,200 to 1,800 calories), the calories that remain after meeting food group recommendations in nutrient-dense forms ("limits on calories for other uses") are less than 10 percent per day of calories; however, at higher calorie levels, the limits on calories for other uses are more than 10 percent per day. The recommendation to limit added sugars to no more than 10 percent of calories is a target that applies to all calorie levels to help individuals move toward healthy eating patterns within calorie limits.

Although the evidence for added sugars and health outcomes is still developing, the recommendation to limit calories from added sugars is consistent with research examining *eating patterns* and health. Strong evidence from mostly prospective cohort studies but also randomized controlled trials has shown that *eating patterns* that include lower intake of sources of added sugars are associated with reduced risk of CVD in adults, and moderate evidence indicates that these *eating patterns* are associated with reduced risk of obesity, type 2 diabetes, and some types of cancer in adults. As described earlier, eating patterns consist of multiple, interacting food components, and the relationships to health exist for the overall eating pattern, not necessarily to an isolated aspect of the diet. Moderate evidence indicates a relationship between added sugars and dental caries in children and adults.

Considerations: Added sugars provide sweetness that can help improve the palatability of foods, help with preservation, and/or contribute to functional attributes such as viscosity, texture, body, color, and browning capability. As discussed in Chapter 2 (/dietaryguidelines/2015/guidelines/chapter-2/), the two main sources of added sugars in U.S. diets are sugar-sweetened beverages and snacks and sweets. Many foods high in calories from added sugars provide few or no essential nutrients or dietary fiber and, therefore, may contribute to excess calorie intake without contributing to diet quality; intake of these foods should be limited to help achieve healthy eating patterns within calorie limits. There is room for Americans to include limited amounts of added sugars in their eating patterns, including to improve the palatability of some nutrient-dense foods, such as fruits and vegetables that are naturally tart (e.g., cranberries and rhubarb). Healthy eating patterns can accommodate other nutrient-dense foods with small amounts of added sugars, such as whole-grain breakfast cereals or fat-free yogurt, as long as calories from added sugars do not exceed 10 percent per day, total carbohydrate intake remains within the AMDR, and total calorie intake remains within limits.

It should be noted that replacing added sugars with high-intensity sweeteners may reduce calorie intake in the short-term, yet questions remain about their effectiveness as a long-term weight management strategy. High-intensity sweeteners that have been approved by the U.S. Food and Drug Administration (FDA) include saccharin, aspartame, acesulfame potassium (Ace-K), and sucralose.[22] Based on the available scientific evidence, these high-intensity sweeteners have been determined to be safe for the general population. This means that there is reasonable certainty of no harm under the intended conditions of use because the estimated daily intake is not expected to exceed the acceptable daily intake for each sweetener. The FDA has determined that the estimated daily intake of these high-intensity sweeteners would not exceed the acceptable daily intake, even for high consumers of each substance.

Saturated Fats, *Trans* Fats, and Cholesterol

Saturated Fats

Healthy intake: Intake of saturated fats should be limited to less than 10 percent of calories per day by replacing them with unsaturated fats and while keeping total dietary fats within the age-appropriate AMDR. The human body uses some saturated fats for physiological and structural functions, but it makes more than enough to meet those needs. Individuals 2 years and older therefore have no dietary requirement for saturated fats.

Strong and consistent evidence shows that replacing saturated fats with unsaturated fats, especially polyunsaturated fats, is associated with reduced blood levels of total cholesterol and of low-density lipoprotein-cholesterol (LDL-cholesterol). Additionally, strong and consistent evidence shows that replacing saturated fats with polyunsaturated fats is associated with a reduced risk of CVD events (heart attacks) and CVD-related deaths.

Some evidence has shown that replacing saturated fats with plant sources of monounsaturated fats, such as olive oil and nuts, may be associated with a reduced risk of CVD. However, the evidence base for monounsaturated fats is not as strong as the evidence base for replacement with polyunsaturated fats. Evidence has also shown that replacing saturated fats with carbohydrates reduces blood levels of total and LDL-cholesterol, but increases blood levels of triglycerides and reduces high-density lipoprotein-cholesterol (HDL-cholesterol). Replacing total fat or saturated fats with carbohydrates is not associated with reduced risk of CVD. Additional research is needed to determine whether this relationship is consistent across categories of carbohydrates (e.g., whole versus refined grains; intrinsic versus added sugars), as they may have different associations with various health outcomes. Therefore, saturated fats in the diet should be replaced with polyunsaturated and monounsaturated fats.

Considerations: As discussed in Chapter 2 (/dietaryguidelines/2015/guidelines/chapter-2/), the main sources of saturated fats in the U.S. diet include mixed dishes containing cheese, meat, or both, such as burgers, sandwiches, and tacos; pizza; rice, pasta, and grain dishes; and meat, poultry, and seafood dishes. Although some saturated fats are inherent in foods, others are added. Healthy eating patterns can accommodate nutrient-dense foods with small amounts of saturated fats, as long as calories from saturated fats do not exceed 10 percent per day, intake of total fats remains within the AMDR, and total calorie intake remains within limits. When possible, foods high in saturated fats should be replaced with foods high in unsaturated fats, and other choices to reduce solid fats should be made (see Chapter 2 (/dietaryguidelines/2015/guidelines/chapter-2/)).

Trans Fats

Individuals should limit intake of *trans* fats to as low as possible by limiting foods that contain synthetic sources of *trans* fats, such as partially hydrogenated oils in margarines, and by limiting other solid fats. A number of studies have observed an association between increased intake of *trans* fats and increased risk of CVD. This increased risk is due, in part, to its LDL-cholesterol-raising effect.

Trans fats occur naturally in some foods and also are produced in a process called hydrogenation. Hydrogenation is used by food manufacturers to make products containing unsaturated fatty acids solid at room temperature (i.e., more saturated) and therefore more resistant to becoming spoiled or rancid. Partial hydrogenation means that some, but not all, unsaturated fatty acids are converted to saturated fatty acids; some of the unsaturated fatty acids are changed from a *cis* to *trans* configuration. *Trans* fatty acids produced this way are referred to as "artificial" or "industrially produced" *trans* fatty acids. Artificial *trans* fatty acids are found in the partially hydrogenated oils[23] used in some margarines, snack foods, and prepared desserts as a replacement for saturated fatty acids. Although food manufacturers and restaurants have reduced the amounts of artificial *trans* fats in many foods in recent years, these fats can still be found in some processed foods, such as some desserts, microwave popcorn, frozen pizza, margarines, and coffee creamers.

Naturally occurring *trans* fats, known as "natural" or "ruminant" *trans* fats, are produced by ruminant animals. Natural *trans* fats are present in small quantities in dairy products and meats, and consuming fat-free or low-fat dairy products and lean meats and poultry will reduce the intake of natural *trans* fats from these foods. Because natural *trans* fats are present in dairy products and meats in only small quantities and these foods can be important sources of nutrients, these foods do not need to be eliminated from the diet.

Dietary Cholesterol

The body uses cholesterol for physiological and structural functions but makes more than enough for these purposes. Therefore, people do not need to obtain cholesterol through foods.

The Key Recommendation from the *2010 Dietary Guidelines* to limit consumption of dietary cholesterol to 300 mg per day is not included in the 2015 edition, but this change does not suggest that dietary cholesterol is no longer important to consider when building healthy eating patterns. As recommended by the IOM,[24] individuals should eat as little dietary cholesterol as possible while consuming a healthy eating pattern. In general, foods that are higher in dietary cholesterol, such as fatty meats and high-fat dairy products, are also higher in saturated fats. The USDA Food Patterns are limited in saturated fats, and because of the commonality of food sources of saturated fats and dietary cholesterol, the Patterns are also low in dietary cholesterol. For example, the Healthy U.S.-Style Eating Pattern contains approximately 100 to 300 mg of cholesterol across the 12 calorie levels. Current average intake of dietary cholesterol among those 1 year and older in the United States is approximately 270 mg per day.

Strong evidence from mostly prospective cohort studies but also randomized controlled trials has shown that *eating patterns* that include lower intake of dietary cholesterol are associated with reduced risk of CVD, and moderate evidence indicates that these eating patterns are associated with reduced risk of obesity. As described earlier, *eating patterns* consist of multiple, interacting food components and the relationships to health exist for the overall eating pattern, not necessarily to an isolated aspect of the diet. More research is needed regarding the dose-response relationship between dietary cholesterol and blood cholesterol levels. Adequate evidence is not available for a quantitative limit for dietary cholesterol specific to the *Dietary Guidelines*.

Dietary cholesterol is found only in animal foods such as egg yolk, dairy products, shellfish, meats, and poultry. A few foods, notably egg yolks and some shellfish, are higher in dietary cholesterol but not saturated fats. Eggs and shellfish can be consumed along with a variety of other choices within and across the subgroup recommendations of the protein foods group.

Sodium

Healthy intake: The scientific consensus from expert bodies, such as the IOM, the American Heart Association, and Dietary Guidelines Advisory Committees, is that average sodium intake, which is currently 3,440 mg per day (see Chapter 2 (/dietaryguidelines/2015/guidelines/chapter-2/)), is too high and should be reduced. Healthy eating patterns limit sodium to less than 2,300 mg per day for adults and children ages 14 years and older and to the age- and sex-appropriate Tolerable Upper Intake Levels (UL) of sodium for children younger than 14 years (see Appendix 7 (/dietaryguidelines/2015/guidelines/appendix-7/)). Sodium is an essential nutrient and is needed by the body in relatively small quantities, provided that substantial sweating does not occur.[25] Sodium is primarily consumed as salt (sodium chloride).

The limits for sodium are the age- and sex-appropriate ULs. The UL is the highest daily nutrient intake level that is likely to pose no risk of adverse health effects to almost all individuals in the general population. The recommendation for adults and children ages 14 years and older to limit sodium intake to less than 2,300 mg per day is based on evidence showing a linear dose-response relationship between increased sodium intake and increased blood pressure in adults. In addition, moderate evidence suggests an association between increased sodium intake and increased risk of CVD in adults. However, this evidence is not as consistent as the evidence on blood pressure, a surrogate indicator of CVD risk.

Calorie intake is highly associated with sodium intake (i.e., the more foods and beverages people consume, the more sodium they tend to consume). Because children have lower calorie needs than adults, the IOM established lower ULs for children younger than 14 years of age based on median intake of calories. Similar to adults, moderate evidence also indicates that the linear dose-response relationship between sodium intake and blood pressure is found in children as well.

Adults with prehypertension and hypertension would particularly benefit from blood pressure lowering. For these individuals, further reduction to 1,500 mg per day can result in even greater blood pressure reduction. Because of the linear dose-response relationship between sodium intake and blood pressure, every incremental decrease in sodium intake that moves toward recommended limits is encouraged. Even without reaching the limits for sodium intake, strong evidence indicates that reductions in sodium intake can lower blood pressure among people with prehypertension and hypertension. Further, strong evidence has demonstrated that adults who would benefit from blood pressure lowering should combine the Dietary Approaches to Stop Hypertension (DASH) dietary pattern with lower sodium intake (see Dietary Approaches to Stop Hypertension call-out box).

Considerations: As a food ingredient, sodium has multiple uses, such as in curing meat, baking, thickening, enhancing flavor (including the flavor of other ingredients), as a preservative, and in retaining moisture. For example, some fresh meats have sodium solutions added to help retain moisture in cooking. As discussed in Chapter 2 (/dietaryguidelines/2015/guidelines/chapter-2/), sodium is found in foods across the food supply, including mixed dishes such as burgers, sandwiches, and tacos; rice, pasta, and grain dishes; pizza; meat, poultry, and seafood dishes; and soups. Multiple strategies should be implemented to reduce sodium intake to the recommended limits (see Chapter 3. Everyone Has a Role in Supporting Healthy Eating Patterns (/dietaryguidelines/2015/guidelines/chapter-3/)).

Dietary Approaches to Stop Hypertension (DASH)

The DASH dietary pattern is an example of a healthy eating pattern and has many of the same characteristics as the Healthy U.S.-Style Eating Pattern. The DASH dietary pattern and several variations have been tested in randomized controlled clinical trials to study the effect of the DASH dietary pattern on CVD risk factors. The original DASH trial demonstrated that the DASH dietary pattern lowered blood pressure and LDL-cholesterol levels, resulting in reduced CVD risk, compared to diets that resembled a typical American diet. The DASH-Sodium trial confirmed the beneficial blood pressure and LDL-cholesterol effects of the DASH eating pattern at three levels of dietary sodium intake and also demonstrated a step-wise lowering of blood pressure as sodium intake was reduced. The OmniHeart Trial found that replacing some of the carbohydrates in DASH with the same amount of either protein or unsaturated fats lowered blood pressure and LDL-cholesterol levels more than the original DASH dietary pattern.

The DASH Eating Plan is high in vegetables, fruits, low-fat dairy products, whole grains, poultry, fish, beans, and nuts and is low in sweets, sugar-sweetened beverages, and red meats. It is low in saturated fats and rich in potassium, calcium, and magnesium, as well as dietary fiber and protein. It also is lower in sodium than the typical American diet, and includes menus with two levels of sodium, 2,300 and 1,500 mg per day. Additional details on DASH are available at http://www.nhlbi.nih.gov/health/health-topics/topics/dash (http://www.nhlbi.nih.gov/health/health-topics/topics/dash).

Alcohol

Alcohol is not a component of the USDA Food Patterns. The *Dietary Guidelines* does not recommend that individuals who do not drink alcohol start drinking for any reason. If alcohol is consumed, it should be in moderation—up to one drink per day for women and up to two drinks per day for men—and only by adults of legal drinking age.[6] There are also many circumstances in which individuals should not drink, such as during pregnancy. For the purposes of evaluating amounts of alcohol that may be consumed, the *Dietary Guidelines* includes drink-equivalents. One alcoholic drink-equivalent is described as containing 14 g (0.6 fl oz) of pure alcohol.[26] The following are reference beverages that are one alcoholic drink-equivalent: 12 fluid ounces of regular beer (5% alcohol), 5 fluid ounces of wine (12% alcohol), or 1.5 fluid ounces of 80 proof distilled spirits (40% alcohol).[27] The amount of alcohol and calories in beverages varies and should be accounted for within the limits of healthy eating patterns so that calorie limits are not exceeded. See Appendix 9. Alcohol (/dietaryguidelines/2015/guidelines/appendix-9/) for additional information.

Caffeine

Caffeine is not a nutrient; it is a dietary component that functions in the body as a stimulant. Caffeine occurs naturally in plants (e.g., coffee beans, tea leaves, cocoa beans, kola nuts). It also is added to foods and beverages (e.g., caffeinated soda, energy drinks). If caffeine is added to a food, it must be included in the listing of ingredients on the food label.[28] Most intake of caffeine in the United States comes from coffee, tea, and soda. Caffeinated beverages vary widely in their caffeine content. Caffeinated coffee beverages include drip/brewed coffee (12 mg/fl oz), instant coffee (8 mg/fl oz), espresso (64 mg/fl oz), and specialty beverages made from coffee or espresso, such as cappuccinos and lattes. Amounts of caffeine in other beverages such as brewed black tea (6 mg/fl oz), brewed green tea (2-5 mg/fl oz), and caffeinated soda[29] (1-4 mg/fl.oz) also vary. Beverages within the energy drinks category have the greatest variability (3-35 mg/fl oz).

Much of the available evidence on caffeine focuses on coffee intake. Moderate coffee consumption (three to five 8-oz cups/day or providing up to 400 mg/day of caffeine) can be incorporated into healthy eating patterns. This guidance on coffee is informed by strong and consistent evidence showing that, in healthy adults, moderate coffee consumption is not associated with an increased risk of major chronic diseases (e.g., cancer) or premature death, especially from CVD. However, individuals who do not consume caffeinated coffee or other caffeinated beverages are not encouraged to incorporate them into their eating pattern. Limited and mixed evidence is available from randomized controlled trials examining the relationship between those energy drinks which have high caffeine content and cardiovascular risk factors and other health outcomes. In addition, caffeinated beverages, such as some sodas or energy drinks, may include calories from added sugars, and although coffee itself has minimal calories, coffee beverages often contain added calories from cream, whole or 2% milk, creamer, and added sugars, which should be limited. The same considerations apply to calories added to tea or other similar beverages.

Those who choose to drink alcohol should be cautious about mixing caffeine and alcohol together or consuming them at the same time; see Appendix 9. Alcohol (/dietaryguidelines/2015/guidelines/appendix-9/) for additional discussion. In addition, women who are capable of becoming pregnant or who are trying to, or who are pregnant, and those who are breastfeeding should consult their health care providers for advice concerning caffeine consumption.

Notes

[6] It is not recommended that individuals begin drinking or drink more for any reason. The amount of alcohol and calories in beverages varies and should be accounted for within the limits of healthy eating patterns. Alcohol should be consumed only by adults of legal drinking age. There are many circumstances in which individuals should not drink, such as during pregnancy. See Appendix 6. Alcohol (/dietaryguidelines/2015/guidelines/appendix-9/) for additional information.

[8] Institute of Medicine (IOM) and National Research Council (NRC). Weight gain during pregnancy: Reexamining the guidelines. Washington (DC): The National Academies Press; 2009.

[9] Jensen MD, Ryan DH, Apovian CM, Ard JD, Comuzzie AG, Donato KA, et al. 2013 AHA/ACC/TOS guideline for the management of overweight and obesity in adults: a report of the American College of Cardiology/American Heart Association Task Force on Practice Guidelines and The Obesity Society. J Am Coll Cardiol. 2014;63(25 Pt B):2985-3023. PMID: 24239920. Available at: http://www.ncbi.nlm.nih.gov/pubmed/24239920 (http://www.ncbi.nlm.nih.gov/pubmed/24239920).

[10] Definitions for each food group and subgroup are provided throughout the chapter and are compiled in Appendix 3 (/dietaryguidelines/2015/guidelines/appendix-3/).

[11] In the form of provitamin A carotenoids

[12] American Academy of Pediatrics. Healthy Children, Fit Children: Answers to Common Questions From Parents About Nutrition and Fitness. 2011.

[13] In the form of provitamin A carotenoids

[14] Products that bear the U.S. Food and Drug Administration (FDA) health claim for whole grains have at least 51 percent of the total ingredients by weight as whole-grain ingredients; they also meet other criteria.

[15] Foods that meet the whole grain-rich criteria for the school meal programs contain 100 percent whole grain or a blend of whole-grain meal and/or flour and enriched meal and/or flour of which at least 50 percent is whole grain. The remaining 50 percent or less of grains, if any, must be enriched. http://www.fns.usda.gov/sites/default/files/WholeGrainResource.pdf [PDF - 1.3 MB] (http://www.fns.usda.gov/sites/default/files/WholeGrainResource.pdf). Accessed October 22, 2015.

[16] Adapted from the Food Safety and Inspection Service (FSIS) guidance on whole-grain claims. Available at http://www.fsis.usda.gov/wps/portal/fsis/home (http://www.fsis.usda.gov/wps/portal/fsis/home). Accessed November 25, 2015.

[17] State and local advisories provide information to guide consumers who eat fish caught from local waters. See the EPA website, "Fish Consumption Advisories, General Information." Available at http://water.epa.gov/scitech/swguidance/fishshellfish/fishadvisories/general.cfm (http://water.epa.gov/scitech/swguidance/fishshellfish/fishadvisories/general.cfm). Accessed September 26, 2015.

[18] Cooked, edible portion

[19] The U.S. Food and Drug Administration (FDA) and the U.S. Environmental Protection Agency (EPA) provide joint guidance regarding seafood consumption for women who are pregnant or breastfeeding and young children. For more information, see the FDA and EPA websites www.FDA.gov/fishadvice (http://www.FDA.gov/fishadvice); www.EPA.gov/fishadvice (http://www.EPA.gov/fishadvice).

[20] The term "fats" rather than "fatty acids" is generally used in this document when discussing categories of fatty acids (e.g., unsaturated, saturated, *trans*) for consistency with the Nutrition Facts label and other Federal materials.

[21] It is not recommended that individuals begin drinking or drink more for any reason. The amount of alcohol and calories in beverages varies and should be accounted for within the limits of healthy eating patterns. Alcohol should be consumed only by adults of legal drinking age. There are many circumstances in which individuals should not drink, such as during pregnancy. See Appendix 9. Alcohol (/dietaryguidelines/2015/guidelines/appendix-9/) for additional information.

[22] For more information, see: FDA. High-Intensity Sweeteners. May 19, 2014. [Updated November 5, 2014.] Available at: http://www.fda.gov/food/ingredientspackaginglabeling/foodadditivesingredients/ucm397716.htr (http://www.fda.gov/food/ingredientspackaginglabeling/foodadditivesingredients/ucm397716.ht Accessed October 19, 2015. This page provides a link to "Additional Information about High-Intensity Sweeteners Permitted for use in Food in the United States" which includes more information on types and uses of high-intensity sweeteners and the scientific evidence evaluated by the FDA for safety for the general population.

[23] The FDA has determined that partially hydrogenated oils, which are the primary dietary source of industrially produced *trans* fats, are no longer generally recognized as safe (GRAS), with compliance expected by June 18, 2018. FDA. Final Determination Regarding Partionally Hydrogenated Oils. Federal Register. June 17, 2015;80(116):34650-34670. Available at: https://www.federalregister.gov/articles/2015/06/17/2015-14883/final-determination-regarding-partially-hydrogenated-oils (https://www.federalregister.gov/articles/2015/06/17/2015-14883/final-determination-regarding-partially-hydrogenated-oils). Accessed October 20, 2015.

[24] Institute of Medicine. Dietary Reference Intakes for Energy, Carbohydrate, Fiber, Fat, Fatty Acids, Cholesterol, Protein, and Amino Acids. Washington (DC): The National Academies Press; 2002.

[25] The IOM set an Adequate Intake (AI) level for sodium to meet the sodium needs of healthy and moderately active individuals. Because of increased loss of sodium from sweat, the AI does not apply to highly active individuals and workers exposed to extreme heat stress, estimated to be less than 1 percent of the U.S. population. Institute of Medicine. Dietary Reference Intakes for Water, Potassium, Sodium, Chloride, and Sulfate. Washington (DC): The National Academies Press; 2005.

[26] Bowman SA, Clemens JC, Friday JE, Thoerig RC, and Moshfegh AJ. 2014. Food Patterns Equivalents Database 2011-12: Methodology and User Guide [Online]. Food Surveys Research Group, Beltsville Human Nutrition Research Center, Agricultural Research Service, U.S. Department of Agriculture, Beltsville, Maryland. Available at: http://www.ars.usda.gov/nea/bhnrc/fsrg (http://www.ars.usda.gov/nea/bhnrc/fsrg). Accessed November 3, 2015. For additional information, see the National Institute on Alcohol Abuse and Alcoholism (NIAAA) webpage available at: http://rethinkingdrinking.niaaa.nih.gov/ (http://rethinkingdrinking.niaaa.nih.gov/).

[27] Drink-equivalents are not intended to serve as a standard drink definition for regulatory purposes.

[28] Some dietary supplements such as energy shots also contain caffeine, but the amount of caffeine in these products is not required to be disclosed.

[29] Caffeine is a substance that is generally recognized as safe (GRAS) in cola-type beverages by the U.S. Food and Drug Administration for use by adults and children. Code of Federal Regulation Title 21, Subchapter B, Part 182, Subpart B. Caffeine. U.S. Government Printing Office. November 23, 2015. Available at: http://www.ecfr.gov/cgi-bin/retrieveECFR? gp=1&SID=f8c3068e9ec0062a3b4078cfa6361cf6&ty=HTML&h=L&mc=true&r=SECTION&n=se21 (http://www.ecfr.gov/cgi-bin/retrieveECFR? gp=1&SID=f8c3068e9ec0062a3b4078cfa6361cf6&ty=HTML&h=L&mc=true&r=SECTION&n=se21

Documents in PDF format require Adobe Acrobat Reader (http://get.adobe.com/reader/). If you have problems with PDF documents, please download the latest version of the Reader (http://get.adobe.com/reader/).

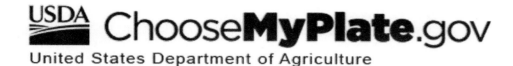

United States Department of Agriculture

Home / Popular Topics   Dietary Guidelines

Today, about half of all American adults have one or more chronic diseases, often related to poor diet. The *2015-2020 Dietary Guidelines for Americans* emphasizes the importance of creating a healthy eating pattern to maintain health and reduce the risk of disease. Everything we eat and drink — the food and beverage choices we make day to day and over our lifetime — matters.

MyPlate offers messages, resources, and tools to help you make the choices that are right for you.

2015-2020 Dietary Guidelines: Answers to Your Questions

Find answers to questions about caffeine, cholesterol, fat, and more.

MyPlate Messages

Find MyPlate tips and solutions that reflect your personal preferences, values, traditions, culture, and budget. The MyPlate consumer messages to help communicate the *2015-2020 Dietary Guidelines for Americans* are:

Everything you eat and drink over time matters. The right mix can help you be healthier now and in the future. Start with small changes to make healthier choices you can enjoy.

Find your healthy eating style and maintain it for a lifetime. This means:

- Make half your plate fruits and vegetables.

  - Focus on whole fruits.

  - Vary your veggies.

- Make half your grains whole grains.

- Move to low-fat and fat-free milk or yogurt.

- Vary your protein routine.

- Drink and eat less sodium, saturated fat, and added sugars.

New MyPlate Resources and Tools for Professionals

Find personalized information and ideas to use with individuals and communities.

MyPlate, MyWins	Use this tip sheet with your audience to help them find their healthy eating solutions for everyday life and create personal MyPlate, MyWins.
SuperTracker	Get a personalized nutrition and physical activity plan for better health! Track food intake and physical activity and see how individuals and groups stack up to their goals!
MyPlate Daily Checklist	The MyPlate Daily Checklist (formerly Daily Food Plan) shows food group targets and components to limit – what and how much to eat within your calorie allowance.
MyPlate Style Guide	Updated images and graphics to support MyPlate promotions and communications.

Stay Up-to-Date with MyPlate

Visit ChooseMyPlate.gov frequently to find updates, new resources, and other tools to help you bring MyPlate to life. Follow us on Facebook and Twitter or sign up for email updates to stay informed about the latest MyPlate activities. Become a National Strategic Partner, Community Partner, or Campus Ambassador.

Dietary Guidelines Resources for Professionals

Provides guidance on key elements of healthy eating patterns and focuses on preventing the diet-related chronic diseases that continue to affect Americans.

2015-2020 Dietary Guidelines for Americans	Find the *2015-2020 Dietary Guidelines* and related resources, including the Executive Summary, press release, Q&As, and previous Dietary Guidelines.
Communicator's Guide	Resource designed to help others create consumer nutrition education materials and messages based on the *2015-2020 Dietary Guidelines for Americans*.
Top 10 Things You Need to Know about the New DGAs	Lists the top things Americans should know when it comes to the *Dietary Guidelines*.
Dietary Guidelines Answers	Find answers to questions about caffeine, cholesterol, fat, and more.

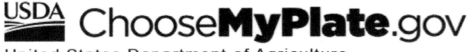

United States Department of Agriculture

2015-2020 Dietary Guidelines: Answers to Your Questions

What are "eating patterns" and why does the *2015-2020 Dietary Guidelines* focus on them?

An eating pattern refers to the combination of *all* of the foods and beverages a person eats and drinks regularly over time. A large body of science now shows that healthy eating *patterns* and regular physical activity can help people achieve and maintain good health and reduce the risk of chronic disease throughout life.

While the core parts of healthy eating patterns in the *2015-2020 Dietary Guidelines* are the same as those from previous *Dietary Guidelines* (vegetables, fruits, whole grains, low-fat and fat-free dairy, and protein foods — all with little to no added sugars, saturated fats, and sodium), the emphasis of the *2015-2020 Dietary Guidelines* is on the importance of the *totality* of what you eat and drink as a whole package. Food groups and nutrients are not eaten as individual components — they're eaten in combination with each other over time. And together those individual parts of an eating pattern can act synergistically and have potentially cumulative effects on health. In other words, an eating pattern is more than the sum of its parts.

The *2015-2020 Dietary Guidelines* embodies the idea that a healthy eating pattern is not a rigid plan. Rather, it can be adapted to include foods people enjoy that meet their personal preferences and fit within their budget. In essence, a personalized healthy eating pattern could be considered the way or style in which a person makes healthy choices they can maintain over time. For that reason, MyPlate uses "healthy eating style" to speak to consumers when referring to "healthy eating patterns" that are highlighted in the *Dietary Guidelines*. All of the food and beverage choices you make matter. Start with small changes to make healthier choices you can enjoy and create your own *healthy eating style*! Find your healthy eating style with MyPlate, MyWins.

What is the recommendation for added sugars?

According to the *2015-2020 Dietary Guidelines*, we should limit our total daily consumption of added sugars to less than 10% of calories per day. This recommendation is to help achieve a healthy eating style. After eating foods from all food groups to meet nutrient needs, there is limited room for calories from added sugars. When added sugars in foods and beverages exceed 10% of calories, it may be difficult to achieve a healthy eating style that meets personal calorie limits.

A large body of science shows that eating styles with less added sugars are associated with reduced risk of cardiovascular disease in adults, and some evidence indicates that these styles are also associated with reduced risk of obesity, type 2 diabetes, and some types of cancer in adults.

Added sugars, such as syrups and other caloric sweeteners, are used as a sweetener in many food products. Learn more about different types and common sources of added sugars and ways to limit your intake.

Does the *Dietary Guidelines* promote a low-fat diet?

The *2015-2020 Dietary Guidelines* does not encourage a low-fat diet (meaning low in total fats) — in fact its healthy eating style examples can contain up to 35% of total calories per day from fat.

Consistent with the previous edition of the *Dietary Guidelines, the 2015-2020* edition encourages eating styles that emphasize unsaturated fats and are low in *saturated* fat. Specifically, the *Dietary Guidelines* recommends keeping saturated fat consumption to less than 10% of calories per day. This recommendation is based on scientific evidence that replacing saturated fat with unsaturated fats is associated with reduced risk of cardiovascular disease. However, it is important to note that replacing saturated fat with carbohydrates *does not* reduce the risk of cardiovascular disease.

Learn more about the difference between saturated and unsaturated fats and common sources of each.

What is the sodium recommendation?

For most people ages 14 years and older, sodium intake should not exceed 2,300 mg/day. Intake below this level is recommended for children younger than 14 years old and people who have prehypertension or hypertension (i.e., high blood pressure).

The relationship between sodium intake and blood pressure is well-documented. As one goes up, so does the other. Since most people typically consume too much sodium, most of us need to reduce our intake. Sodium is found in many of the foods we commonly eat. Learn more about sources of sodium and ways to limit your intake.

Is caffeine okay to include in my day?

Much of the available scientific studies on caffeine focuses on coffee intake, thus the *2015-2020 Dietary Guidelines* provides guidance that centers around coffee. According to the *2015-2020 Dietary Guidelines*, moderate coffee consumption — up to three to five 8-oz cups/day or providing up to 400 mg/day of caffeine — can be incorporated into healthy eating styles since it is not associated with an increased risk of major chronic diseases (e.g., cancer) or premature death, especially from cardiovascular disease.

However, the *Dietary Guidelines* notes that people who currently do not consume caffeinated coffee or other caffeinated beverages are not encouraged to start. The *Dietary Guidelines* also includes an important note that some coffee or other caffeinated beverages may include calories from added sugars and/or saturated fat (such as cream, whole or 2% milk, and creamer), both of which should be limited.

Do I still need to watch my cholesterol intake?

While adequate evidence is not available for a *quantitative* limit for dietary cholesterol in the *2015-2020 Dietary Guidelines*, cholesterol is still important to consider when building a healthy eating style. In fact, the *Dietary Guidelines* states that people should eat as little dietary cholesterol as possible.

In general, foods that are higher in dietary cholesterol, such as fatty meats and high-fat dairy products, are also higher in saturated fats (which should be limited to 10% of total calories per day). The primary healthy eating style described in the *Dietary Guidelines* is limited in saturated fats, and thus, dietary cholesterol (about 100-300 mg across the various calorie levels).

MyPlate Daily Checklist

Write down the foods you ate today and track your daily MyPlate, MyWins!

Food group targets for a 1,600 calorie* pattern are:

	Write your food choices for each food group	Did you reach your target?

Fruits

1 1/2 cups
1 cup of fruits counts as
- 1 cup raw or cooked fruit; or
- 1/2 cup dried fruit; or
- 1 cup 100% fruit juice.

Did you reach your target? ☐ Y ☐ N

Vegetables

2 cups
1 cup vegetables counts as
- 1 cup raw or cooked vegetables; or
- 2 cups leafy salad greens; or
- 1 cup 100% vegetable juice.

Did you reach your target? ☐ Y ☐ N

Grains

5 ounce equivalents
1 ounce of grains counts as
- 1 slice bread; or
- 1 ounce ready-to-eat cereal; or
- 1/2 cup cooked rice, pasta, or cereal.

Did you reach your target? ☐ Y ☐ N

Protein

5 ounce equivalents
1 ounce of protein counts as
- 1 ounce lean meat, poultry, or seafood; or
- 1 egg; or
- 1 Tbsp peanut butter; or
- 1/4 cup cooked beans or peas; or
- 1/2 ounce nuts or seeds.

Did you reach your target? ☐ Y ☐ N

Dairy

3 cups
1 cup of dairy counts as
- 1 cup milk; or
- 1 cup yogurt; or
- 1 cup fortified soy beverage; or
- 1 1/2 ounces natural cheese or 2 ounces processed cheese.

Did you reach your target? ☐ Y ☐ N

Limit:
- Sodium to **2,300 milligrams** a day.
- Saturated fat to **18 grams** a day.
- Added sugars to **40 grams** a day.

☐ Y ☐ N

Be active your way:

Adults:
- Be physically active at least **2 1/2 hours** per week.

Children 6 to 17 years old:
- Move at least **60 minutes** every day.

☐ Y ☐ N

* This 1,600 calorie pattern is only an estimate of your needs. Monitor your body weight and adjust your calories if needed.

Track your MyPlate, MyWins

MyWins

_____

_____

Center for Nutrition Policy and Promotion
January 2016
USDA is an equal opportunity provider and employer.

MyPlate Daily Checklist

Write down the foods you ate today and track your daily MyPlate, MyWins!

Food group targets for a 1,800 calorie* pattern are:

		Write your food choices for each food group	Did you reach your target?
Fruits	**1 1/2 cups** 1 cup of fruits counts as • 1 cup raw or cooked fruit; or • 1/2 cup dried fruit; or • 1 cup 100% fruit juice.	_____ _____ _____	Y N
Vegetables	**2 1/2 cups** 1 cup vegetables counts as • 1 cup raw or cooked vegetables; or • 2 cups leafy salad greens; or • 1 cup 100% vegetable juice.	_____ _____ _____	Y N
Grains	**6 ounce equivalents** 1 ounce of grains counts as • 1 slice bread; or • 1 ounce ready-to-eat cereal; or • 1/2 cup cooked rice, pasta, or cereal.	_____ _____ _____	Y N
Protein	**5 ounce equivalents** 1 ounce of protein counts as • 1 ounce lean meat, poultry, or seafood; or • 1 egg; or • 1 Tbsp peanut butter; or • 1/4 cup cooked beans or peas; or • 1/2 ounce nuts or seeds.	_____ _____ _____	Y N
Dairy	**3 cups** 1 cup of dairy counts as • 1 cup milk; or • 1 cup yogurt; or • 1 cup fortified soy beverage; or • 1 1/2 ounces natural cheese or 2 ounces processed cheese.	_____ _____ _____	Y N

Limit:
• Sodium to **2,300 milligrams** a day.
• Saturated fat to **20 grams** a day.
• Added sugars to **45 grams** a day.

Y   N

Be active your way:

Adults:
• Be physically active at least **2 1/2 hours** per week.

Children 6 to 17 years old:
• Move at least **60 minutes** every day.

Y   N

* This 1,800 calorie pattern is only an estimate of your needs. Monitor your body weight and adjust your calories if needed.

Center for Nutrition Policy and Promotion
January 2016
USDA is an equal opportunity provider and employer.

Track your MyPlate, MyWins

MyWins _____

ChooseMyPlate.gov

MyPlate Daily Checklist

Write down the foods you ate today and track your daily MyPlate, MyWins!

Food group targets for a 2,000 calorie* pattern are:

	Write your food choices for each food group	Did you reach your target?

Fruits

2 cups

1 cup of fruits counts as
- 1 cup raw or cooked fruit; or
- 1/2 cup dried fruit; or
- 1 cup 100% fruit juice.

Did you reach your target? Y / N

Vegetables

2 1/2 cups

1 cup vegetables counts as
- 1 cup raw or cooked vegetables; or
- 2 cups leafy salad greens; or
- 1 cup 100% vegetable juice.

Did you reach your target? Y / N

Grains

6 ounce equivalents

1 ounce of grains counts as
- 1 slice bread; or
- 1 ounce ready-to-eat cereal; or
- 1/2 cup cooked rice, pasta, or cereal.

Did you reach your target? Y / N

Protein

5 1/2 ounce equivalents

1 ounce of protein counts as
- 1 ounce lean meat, poultry, or seafood; or
- 1 egg; or
- 1 Tbsp peanut butter; or
- 1/4 cup cooked beans or peas; or
- 1/2 ounce nuts or seeds.

Did you reach your target? Y / N

Dairy

3 cups

1 cup of dairy counts as
- 1 cup milk; or
- 1 cup yogurt; or
- 1 cup fortified soy beverage; or
- 1 1/2 ounces natural cheese or 2 ounces processed cheese.

Did you reach your target? Y / N

Limit:
- Sodium to **2,300 milligrams** a day.
- Saturated fat to **22 grams** a day.
- Added sugars to **50 grams** a day.

Y / N

Be active your way:

Adults:
- Be physically active at least **2 1/2 hours** per week.

Children 6 to 17 years old:
- Move at least **60 minutes** every day.

Y / N

Track your MyPlate, MyWins

MyWins

ChooseMyPlate.gov

* This 2,000 calorie pattern is only an estimate of your needs. Monitor your body weight and adjust your calories if needed.

Center for Nutrition Policy and Promotion
January 2016
USDA is an equal opportunity provider and employer.

MyPlate Daily Checklist

Write down the foods you ate today and track your daily MyPlate, MyWins!

Food group targets for a 2,400 calorie* pattern are:

	Write your food choices for each food group	Did you reach your target?
Fruits — **2 cups** 1 cup of fruits counts as • 1 cup raw or cooked fruit; or • 1/2 cup dried fruit; or • 1 cup 100% fruit juice.		Y / N
Vegetables — **3 cups** 1 cup vegetables counts as • 1 cup raw or cooked vegetables; or • 2 cups leafy salad greens; or • 1 cup 100% vegetable juice.		Y / N
Grains — **8 ounce equivalents** 1 ounce of grains counts as • 1 slice bread; or • 1 ounce ready-to-eat cereal; or • 1/2 cup cooked rice, pasta, or cereal.		Y / N
Protein — **6 1/2 ounce equivalents** 1 ounce of protein counts as • 1 ounce lean meat, poultry, or seafood; or • 1 egg; or • 1 Tbsp peanut butter; or • 1/4 cup cooked beans or peas; or • 1/2 ounce nuts or seeds.		Y / N
Dairy — **3 cups** 1 cup of dairy counts as • 1 cup milk; or • 1 cup yogurt; or • 1 cup fortified soy beverage; or • 1 1/2 ounces natural cheese or 2 ounces processed cheese.		Y / N

Limit:
• Sodium to **2,300 milligrams** a day.
• Saturated fat to **27 grams** a day.
• Added sugars to **60 grams** a day.

Y / N

Be active your way:

Adults:
• Be physically active at least **2 1/2 hours** per week.

Children 6 to 17 years old:
• Move at least **60 minutes** every day.

Y / N

Track your MyPlate, MyWins

* This 2,400 calorie pattern is only an estimate of your needs. Monitor your body weight and adjust your calories if needed.

Center for Nutrition Policy and Promotion
January 2016
USDA is an equal opportunity provider and employer.

MyPlate Daily Checklist

Write down the foods you ate today and track your daily MyPlate, MyWins!

Food group targets for a 2,800 calorie* pattern are:

Food group	Write your food choices for each food group	Did you reach your target?
Fruits — **2 1/2 cups** — 1 cup of fruits counts as • 1 cup raw or cooked fruit; or • 1/2 cup dried fruit; or • 1 cup 100% fruit juice.	_____ _____ _____	Y N
Vegetables — **3 1/2 cups** — 1 cup vegetables counts as • 1 cup raw or cooked vegetables; or • 2 cups leafy salad greens; or • 1 cup 100% vegetable juice.	_____ _____ _____	Y N
Grains — **10 ounce equivalents** — 1 ounce of grains counts as • 1 slice bread; or • 1 ounce ready-to-eat cereal; or • 1/2 cup cooked rice, pasta, or cereal.	_____ _____ _____	Y N
Protein — **7 ounce equivalents** — 1 ounce of protein counts as • 1 ounce lean meat, poultry, or seafood; or • 1 egg; or • 1 Tbsp peanut butter; or • 1/4 cup cooked beans or peas; or • 1/2 ounce nuts or seeds.	_____ _____ _____	Y N
Dairy — **3 cups** — 1 cup of dairy counts as • 1 cup milk; or • 1 cup yogurt; or • 1 cup fortified soy beverage; or • 1 1/2 ounces natural cheese or 2 ounces processed cheese.	_____ _____ _____	Y N

Limit:
- Sodium to **2,300 milligrams** a day.
- Saturated fat to **31 grams** a day.
- Added sugars to **70 grams** a day.

Y   N

Be active your way:

Adults:
- Be physically active at least **2 1/2 hours** per week.

Children 6 to 17 years old:
- Move at least **60 minutes** every day.

Y   N

* This 2,800 calorie pattern is only an estimate of your needs. Monitor your body weight and adjust your calories if needed.

Track your MyPlate, MyWins

_____
_____

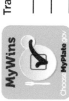

MyWins

Center for Nutrition Policy and Promotion
January 2016
USDA is an equal opportunity provider and employer.

ChooseMyPlate.gov

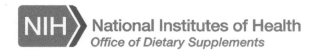

National Institutes of Health
Office of Dietary Supplements

Dietary Supplements: What You Need to Know

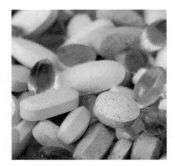

The majority of adults in the United States take one or more dietary supplements either every day or occasionally. Today's dietary supplements include vitamins, minerals, herbals and botanicals, amino acids, enzymes, and many other products. Dietary supplements come in a variety of forms: traditional tablets, capsules, and powders, as well as drinks and energy bars. Popular supplements include vitamins D and E; minerals like calcium and iron; herbs such as echinacea and garlic; and specialty products like glucosamine, probiotics, and fish oils.

The Dietary Supplement Label

All products labeled as a dietary supplement carry a Supplement Facts panel that lists the contents, amount of active ingredients per serving, and other added ingredients (like fillers, binders, and flavorings). The manufacturer suggests the serving size, but you or your health care provider might decide that a different amount is more appropriate for you.

Effectiveness

If you don't eat a nutritious variety of foods, some supplements might help you get adequate amounts of essential nutrients. However, supplements can't take the place of the variety of foods that are important to a healthy diet. Good sources of information on eating well include the Dietary Guidelines for Americans (http://health.gov/dietaryguidelines) and My Plate (http://www.choosemyplate.gov).

Scientific evidence shows that some dietary supplements are beneficial for overall health and for managing some health conditions. For example, calcium and vitamin D are important for keeping bones strong and reducing bone loss; folic acid decreases the risk of certain birth defects; and omega-3 fatty acids from fish oils might help some people with heart disease. Other supplements need more study to determine their value. The U.S. Food and Drug Administration (FDA) does not determine whether dietary supplements are effective before they are marketed.

Safety and Risk

Many supplements contain active ingredients that can have strong effects in the body. Always be alert to the possibility of unexpected side effects, especially when taking a new product.

Supplements are most likely to cause side effects or harm when people take them instead of prescribed medicines or when people take many supplements in combination. Some supplements can increase the risk of bleeding or, if a person takes them before or after surgery, they can affect the person's response to anesthesia. Dietary supplements can also interact with certain prescription drugs in ways that might cause problems. Here are just a few examples:

- Vitamin K can reduce the ability of the blood thinner Coumadin® to prevent blood from clotting.
- St. John's wort can speed the breakdown of many drugs (including antidepressants and birth control pills) and thereby reduce these drugs' effectiveness.
- Antioxidant supplements, like vitamins

C and E, might reduce the effectiveness of some types of cancer chemotherapy.

Keep in mind that some ingredients found in dietary supplements are added to a growing number of foods, including breakfast cereals and beverages. As a result, you may be getting more of these ingredients than you think, and more might not be better. Taking more than you need is always more expensive and can also raise your risk of experiencing side effects. For example, getting too much vitamin A can cause headaches and liver damage, reduce bone strength, and cause birth defects. Excess iron causes nausea and vomiting and may damage the liver and other organs.

Be cautious about taking dietary supplements if you are pregnant or nursing. Also, be careful about giving them (beyond a basic multivitamin/mineral product) to a child. Most dietary supplements have not been well tested for safety in pregnant women, nursing mothers, or children.

If you suspect that you have had a serious reaction from a dietary supplement, let your health care provider know. He or she may report your experience to the FDA. You may also submit a report to the FDA by calling 800-FDA-1088 or completing a form at http://www.fda.gov/Safety/MedWatch/HowToReport. In addition, report your reaction to the dietary supplement company by using the contact information on the product label.

Quality

Dietary supplements are complex products. The FDA has established quality standards for dietary supplements to help ensure their identity, purity, strength, and composition. These standards are designed to prevent the inclusion of the wrong ingredient, the addition of too much or too little of an ingredient, the possibility of contamination, and the improper packaging and labeling of a product. The FDA periodically inspects facilities that manufacture dietary supplements.

In addition, several independent organizations offer quality testing and allow products that pass these tests to display their seals of approval. These seals of approval provide assurance that the product was properly manufactured, contains the ingredients listed on the label, and does not contain harmful levels of contaminants. These seals of approval do not guarantee that a product is safe or effective. Organizations that offer this quality testing include:

- U.S. Pharmacopeia
- ConsumerLab.com
- NSF International

Keep in Mind

Don't decide to take dietary supplements to treat a health condition that you have diagnosed yourself, without consulting a health care provider.

- Don't take supplements in place of, or in combination with, prescribed medications without your health care provider's approval.
- Check with your health care provider about the supplements you take if you are scheduled to have any type of surgical procedure.
- The term "natural" doesn't always mean safe. A supplement's safety depends on many things, such as its chemical makeup, how it works in the body, how it is prepared, and the dose used. Certain herbs (for example, comfrey and kava) can harm the liver.
- Before taking a dietary supplement, ask yourself these questions:
  - What are the potential health benefits of this dietary supplement product?
  - What are its potential benefits for me?
  - Does this product have any safety risks?
  - What is the proper dose to take?
  - How, when, and for how long should I take it?

If you don't know the answers to these questions, use the information sources listed in this brochure and talk to your health care providers.

Talk with Your Health Care Provider

Let your health care providers (including doctors, pharmacists, and dietitians) know which dietary supplements you're taking so that you can discuss what's best for your overall health. Your health care provider can help you determine which supplements, if any, might be valuable for you.

Keep a record of the supplements you take in one place, just as you should be doing for all of your medicines. Note the specific product name, the dose you take, how often you take it, and the reason why you use each one. You can also bring the products you use with you when you see your health care provider.

Federal Regulation of Dietary Supplements

Dietary supplements are products intended to supplement the diet. They are not drugs and, therefore, are not intended to treat, diagnose, mitigate, prevent, or cure diseases. The FDA is the federal agency that oversees both dietary supplements and medicines.

In general, the FDA regulations for dietary supplements are different from those for prescription or over-the-counter drugs.

3 • Dietary Supplements: What You Need to Know

Unlike drugs, which must be approved by the FDA before they can be marketed, dietary supplements do not require premarket review or approval by the FDA. While the supplement company is responsible for having evidence that their products are safe and the label claims are truthful and not misleading, they do not have to provide that evidence to the FDA before the product is marketed.

Dietary supplement labels may carry certain types of health-related claims. Manufacturers are permitted to say, for example, that a dietary supplement addresses a nutrient deficiency, supports health, or is linked to a particular body function (like immunity or heart health). Such a claim must be followed by the words, "This statement has not been evaluated by the Food and Drug Administration. This product is not intended to diagnose, treat, cure, or prevent any disease."

Manufacturers must follow certain good manufacturing practices to ensure the identity, purity, strength, and composition of their products. If the FDA finds a product to be unsafe or otherwise unfit for human consumption, it may take enforcement action to remove the product from the marketplace or work with the manufacturer to voluntarily recall the product.

Also, once a dietary supplement is on the market, the FDA monitors information on the product's label and package insert to make sure that information about the supplement's content is accurate and that any claims made for the product are truthful and not misleading. The Federal Trade Commission, which polices product advertising, also requires all information about a dietary supplement product to be truthful and not misleading.

The federal government can take legal action against companies and Web sites that sell dietary supplements when the companies make false or deceptive statements about their products, if they promote them as treatments or cures for diseases, or if their products are unsafe.

Federal Government Information Sources on Dietary Supplements

NATIONAL INSTITUTES OF HEALTH
The National Institutes of Health supports research on dietary supplements.

- **Office of Dietary Supplements**
  http://ods.od.nih.gov

  The Office of Dietary Supplements provides accurate and up-to-date scientific information about dietary supplements.

- **National Center for Complementary and Alternative Medicine**
  http://nccam.nih.gov

  National Center for Complementary and Alternative Medicine Clearinghouse:
  1-888-644-6226

- **National Library of Medicine**
  http://www.nlm.nih.gov

  Medline Plus http://medlineplus.gov
  PubMed http://www.pubmed.gov

- **NIH Health Information**
  http://health.nih.gov

U.S. FOOD AND DRUG ADMINISTRATION
http://www.fda.gov/Food/DietarySupplements

The Food and Drug Administration issues rules and regulations and provides oversight of dietary supplement labeling, marketing, and safety.

FEDERAL TRADE COMMISSION
http://www.ftc.gov

The Federal Trade Commission polices health and safety claims made in advertising for dietary supplements.

U.S. DEPARTMENT OF AGRICULTURE
http://www.nutrition.gov
http://fnic.nal.usda.gov

The U.S. Department of Agriculture provides information on a variety of food and nutrition topics.

U.S. DEPARTMENT OF HEALTH AND HUMAN SERVICES
http://www.healthfinder.gov

The U.S. Department of Health and Human Services provides an encyclopedia of health topics, personal health tools, and health news.

National Institutes of Health

Office of Dietary Supplements | 6100 Executive Boulevard | Room 3B01, MSC 7517
Bethesda, MD 20892-7517 | E-mail: ods@nih.gov
Visit our Web site for more information about ODS: http://ods.od.nih.gov
Reviewed: June 17, 2011

American College of Sports Medicine (ACSM)
www.acsm.org

Academy of Nutrition and Dietetics
www.eatright.org

American Heart Association
http://www.heart.org/HEARTORG/

American Institute for Cancer Research
www.aicr.org

National Association of Anorexia Nervosa and Associated Disorders
http://www.anad.org/

Center for Nutrition Policy and Promotion, USDA
www.usda.gov/cnpp

Centers for Disease Control and Prevention
www.cdc.gov

Food and Drug Administration
www.fda.gov

Food and Nutrition Information Center
www.fns.usda.gov/fns

Healthfinder®—Gateway to Reliable Consumer Health Information
www.healthfinder.gov

National Heart, Lung, and Blood Institute Information Center
www.nhlbi.nih.gov

National Institute on Alcohol Abuse and Alcoholism
www.niaaa.nih.gov

National Institute of Diabetes and Digestive and Kidney Diseases
www.niddk.nih.gov

Office of Dietary Supplements, NIH
http://ods.od.nih.gov/

The World's Healthiest Foods
www.whfoods.com

WebMD
www.webmd.com

Dr. Liz Applegate, a nationally renowned expert on nutrition and fitness, is a faculty member in the nutrition department and the director of sports nutrition at the University of California at Davis.

Her enthusiasm for teaching and informal lecture style make her undergraduate nutrition classes the nation's largest with enrollments exceeding 3,000 students annually (over 60,000 students taught). Her Nutrition 10 course was voted "Best GE Course" in 2008, 2009, and 2010 by the *California Aggie*, the UC Davis student newspaper. In 2010, Dr. Applegate received the *Distinguished Undergraduate Teaching Award*. She has also received the *Excellence in Teaching Award* from the University of California, the *ASUCD Excellence in Education Award*, and *Distinguished Scholarly Public Service Award*. And most recently, Dr. Applegate received the prestigious 2016 regional *USDA Food and Agriculture Excellence in Teaching Award*.

Dr. Applegate is the author of several books including *Bounce Your Body Beautiful, Encyclopedia of Sports and Fitness Nutrition, Eat Smart, Play Hard,* and *101 Miracle Foods That Heal Your Heart.*

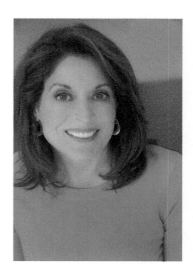

Dr. Applegate is also on the editorial board of the *International Journal of Sport Nutrition and Exercise Metabolism.* She is a fellow and past board of trustees member for the American College of Sports Medicine and a member of the Sports and Cardiovascular Nutritionists, a practice group of the American Dietetics Association. She frequently serves as a keynote speaker at industry, athletic, and scientific meetings.

In addition to her university duties, Dr. Applegate writes the popular "Fridge Wisdom" nutrition column for *Runner's World* magazine for over 30 years and has written more than 450 magazine articles on nutrition and fitness. She is frequently interviewed by national media outlets, including CNN, ESPN, Myth Busters, *The LA Times, Shape, Self,* KCBS Radio, *Redbook, Harper's Bazar,* ABC News, *Men's Health,* and *Men's Journal.*